SPORTS MEDICINE

Prevention, Evaluation, Management, and Rehabilitation

STEVEN ROY, M.D.

Center for Sports Medicine and Running Injuries, Eugene, Oregon

RICHARD IRVIN, A.T., C., Ed.D.

Oregon State University, Corvallis, Oregon

PRENTICE-HALL, INC., Englewood Cliffs, New Jersey 07632

Library of Congress Cataloging in Publication Data

ROY, STEVEN.
   Sports medicine for the athletic trainer.

   Bibliography: p.
   Includes index.   1. Sports medicine.   2. Physical education and
   training.   I. Irvin, Richard.   II. Title.   [DNLM:
   1. Athletic injuries.   2. Sports medicine.   QT 260 R888s]
   RC1210.R68   1983   617'.1027   82-18146
   ISBN 0-13-837807-X

Editorial/production supervision and interior design: Virginia Rubens
Cover design: Judith Matz and Donald Person
Manufacturing buyer: Harry Baisley

Printed in the United States of America

10   9   8   7   6   5   4

0-13-837807-X

PRENTICE-HALL INTERNATIONAL, INC., *London*
PRENTICE-HALL OF AUSTRALIA PTY. LIMITED, *Sydney*
EDITORA PRENTICE-HALL DO BRASIL, LTDA., *Rio de Janeiro*
PRENTICE-HALL CANADA INC., *Toronto*
PRENTICE-HALL OF INDIA PRIVATE LIMITED, *New Delhi*
PRENTICE-HALL OF JAPAN, INC., *Tokyo*
PRENTICE-HALL OF SOUTHEAST ASIA, PTE. LTD., *Singapore*
WHITEHALL BOOKS LIMITED, *Wellington, New Zealand*

CONTENTS

FOREWORD I

Every so often a textbook in a particular science field comes along which fills a unique need and mirrors the growth of knowledge in that profession where few people recognized that such a need existed. This new publication on sports medicine by Steven Roy, M.D., and Dick Irvin, A.T.,C., Ed. D. is such a book.

At the present time, interest in the proper prevention, diagnosis, and care of athletic-related injuries is at an all-time high, whether it be the painful leg problems of the recreational jogger or the rehabilitation of a prominent professional athlete. Medical clinics and rehabilitation centers devoted exclusively to the problems of the athlete are continuing to open and prosper around the country. Subspecialties in such related fields as podiatry and physical therapy are being developed. This book, being the first all-new publication for athletic trainers and related professionals in fifteen years, makes a timely and much-needed contribution to the sports medicine field.

Athletic training as a profession has changed markedly in the past decade and a half. No longer can one person be expected to "do it all" as an athletic trainer. Increasingly, specialization, and even subspecialization, has created the practitioner, the educator, and even the researcher within the athletic trainers' profession. Fifteen years ago there were only a few pioneering university curriculums designed specifically for the student wishing to become an athletic trainer. Each of these curriculums was unique and different from the others. Today, well over fifty college curriculums are approved by the National Athletic Trainers Association on both the graduate and the undergraduate levels. Very demanding and sophisticated educational guidelines are imposed, and many more curriculums have applied but failed to gain approval due to inadequate faculty, academic, or clinical standards.

The term "Certified Athletic Trainer" was given to only a few veteran male athletic trainers via the "grandfather" route fifteen years ago. Today, the initials A.T.,C. following one's name are highly sought by men and women alike. Certain players' associations on the professional sports level are demanding from management that certified athletic trainers be hired, and college positions advertising in placement publications invariably require it. This is equally true on the secondary school level, where most of the exciting new employment opportunities in sports medicine are opening up at the present time. It was my privilege to work with Dick Irvin during the formative years of the Board of Certification of the National Athletic Trainers Association. His energies and abilities have contributed immeasurably to the sophistication and reliability of the certification process, and NATA is fortunate that he continues to serve on the certification committee. It is fitting, therefore, that this new text, which so accurately reflects this new professionalism and sophistication in the athletic training profession, should appear at this time.

This text is unique in that it is co-authored by the "sports medicine team" at a university prominent in intercollegiate athletics, where an excellent NATA-approved athletic training curriculum is well established. Without the enthusiastic concern of a capable team physician to support and to exchange knowledge with the certified athletic trainer, the trainer cannot be effective. Conversely, I strongly feel that the team physician alone, no matter how capable and concerned, cannot be effective without his or her training-room partner on the sports medicine team. For six years Dick Irvin and Dr. Roy were a closely knit team at Oregon State University, and this association, reflected in the text, should immediately give the book greater acceptance in both the athletic trainer's and the team physician's office library.

This book is an accurate reflection of the advances made in the science of athletic training in recent years. It is a must for the serious, advanced student of athletic training, and it raises the level of expected competence in the treatment of sports-related injuries. It goes a full step beyond the basic textbook by incorporating the latest methods and theories into one publication, and it gives excellent reference sources for an even more complete study. The busy coach, physi-

cal therapist, and medical doctor will find it easy to use as a reference source for specific injury problems where essential information can be quickly found.

Dick Irvin's 23 years of experience as an athletic trainer, physical therapist, and clinical educator has combined with Dr. Steven Roy's equally outstanding background as a team physician and "sports doctor" to make this a must book for all individuals vitally interested in providing proper medical care to the athlete, young or old, at all levels of competition.

LINDSY MCLEAN
Head Athletic Trainer, San Francisco "Forty-Niners"
Former Chairman, Board of Certification, National Athletic Trainers Association

FOREWORD II

Sports medicine has received a considerable amount of attention in recent years. The publicity afforded a professional athlete and his or her injuries, the increased participation by individuals in physical fitness and recreational athletics and their associated injuries, and the government's role in encouraging physical fitness through the President's Council on Physical Fitness and Sports are some of the reasons for the increased awareness and interest.

Among the earliest purveyors of treatment to the injured athlete have been athletic trainers. Their role has become increasingly important in the overall care of the athlete. They have demonstrated a growing thirst for a more detailed and intimate knowledge not only of the treatment of injury, but also of the associated aspects such as prevention of injury, biomechanics, anatomy, and the physiology associated with sports activities. Athletic trainers have made great strides in recent years in upgrading their professional qualifications. This book serves as a very appropriate aid in their quest for a knowledgeable approach to the total field of sports medicine.

The authors have carefully reviewed much of the literature relating to sports medicine and have organized this material into a relevant and practical presentation for ready reference. Many of the tables, charts, and graphs provide a very concise visual aid for quick reference to a particular topic discussed in a chapter. The chapters on head and spinal injuries, for instance, have many helpful charts to which the reader can refer when confronted with this type of injury.

The breadth and detail of this book make it an appropriate reference for any of the medical and paramedical personnel that share in the care and well-being of the athlete.

Dr. Roy and Dr. Irvin have drawn on their close association with sports medicine and dedicated a considerable amount of effort and time to the development of this text. They are to be congratulated on the completion of this task and on the final results, which provide a much-needed reference for the athletic trainer.

ROBERT L. LARSON, M. D.
Director of Athletic Medicine, University of Oregon, Eugene, Oregon
Past President, American Orthopaedic Society for Sports Medicine

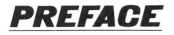

PREFACE

Sports medicine, and in particular athletic training, has come a long way since the days of the "bucket and sponge." Today the athlete is served by a team of professionals who are dedicated to the prevention, management, and rehabilitation of injuries. The athletic trainer is a key member of this team.

Sports medicine has developed at a considerable pace over the last decade. As with other areas of medicine where knowledge and understanding are rapidly expanding, it is necessary for the athletic trainer to first be given an adequate basic preparation, and then be reminded of the necessity to keep abreast of the latest developments and advances.

The goal of this book is to provide information relevant to the needs of those who serve the athlete, be they athletic trainers, coaches, emergency medical technicians, physical therapists, or non-orthopedic physicians. However, the major emphasis throughout the book has been directed at the needs of the athletic trainer's pre- and post-graduate education.

The athlete expects the trainer to be familiar with any athletically related injury— and this is not an unrealistic expectation. Therefore, injuries involving important anatomical areas are discussed in detail, but the rationale behind many of the statements made and the conclusions reached have frequently not been explored. Instead, references are included for those who wish a wider or a more profound understanding of a particular subject.

At the present time, the immediate care of many athletic injuries is administered by the coach, who may find guidance and information in the section on the prevention and immediate care of athletic injuries. There are also criteria to help in the evaluation of an injury, and guidelines for allowing the athlete to return to participation after an injury.

Though this text is directed mainly towards the athletic trainer, it includes information of major importance for physicians, physical therapists, podiatrists and coaches who are involved either directly or peripherally with athletic injuries and sports medicine. Non-orthopedic physicians involved with individual athletes or athletic teams may, we hope, find information applicable to their needs.

Many of our ideas are the result of an unselfish sharing of knowledge and experience that has been one of the hallmarks of practitioners of sports medicine in this country—a tradition that we hope will continue to flourish. To all those who have either knowingly or unknowingly helped us with the contents of this book we would like to express our sincere thanks.

However, we would be remiss not to acknowledge special help we received. To the illustrators, Kathy Sherwood and Lauretta Kaderlik, for their painstaking dedication to perfection, and to the typists, especially Janet McKelvey, for the countless hours of work on the manuscript, we extend a special thanks. We are also grateful to Dr. Caroline Houba for her expert help with the index; to Virginia Rubens, the production editor, for her patience and thoroughness; to Doris Michaels, the acquisitions editor; to William Winkler, Jr., M. S., who contributed much to the chapter on nutrition; and to Kenneth M. Singer, M. D., and Kenneth L. Knight, Ph.D., A.T.C., and others for reviewing the text and providing the behind-the-scenes assistance that transferred thought into action and reality.

DISCLAIMER STATEMENT
The procedures in this book are based on the most current research and recommendations of responsible medical sources. The authors and publisher, however, disclaim responsibility for any adverse effects or consequences resulting from the misapplication or injudicious use of the material contained herein.

Introduction to Sports Medicine

Sports medicine is a broad and very inclusive term that involves a variety of medical as well as paramedical personnel, including exercise physiologists, kinesiologists, athletic trainers, physical therapists, and physical educators, as they are involved with the various aspects of physical activity and athletics.

Ryan[1] has indicated that the concept of sports medicine consists of

1. medical supervision of the athlete
2. special (adapted) physical education
3. therapeutic exercise
4. exercise in the prevention of chronic degenerative disease

This text is mainly concerned with the physician's, the athletic trainer's, and the physical therapist's responsibilities to the athlete.

The Sports Medicine Physician

Physicians concerned with sports medicine may be divided into a number of categories:

1. The physician who only sees the occasional sports medicine patient, but who is interested in athletics and sports medicine.

2. The physician—especially the orthopedic surgeon, family practitioner or generalist, pediatrician, cardiologist, internist, or podiatrist—who spends a substantial portion of the professional day treating sports medicine patients. Many team physicians fall into this group.[2,3]

3. The full-time sports medicine physician. These professionals have come a long way from the days of the local team physician whose sports medicine practice was limited to attending games in his or her spare time. Today there are a number of sports medicine clinics staffed by physicians who have completely, or to a large extent, limited their practices to the prevention, diagnosis, and rehabilitation of athletically related injuries. This new breed is cutting through many of the traditional dividing lines that separated the specialties in the past. Sports medicine requires a special attitude, specific knowledge of many sports and their demands, and an empathy with the athlete. This group of physicians is attempting to meet the challenge. The direction of the professional growth of sports medicine physicians, as well as the granting of a specialty ranking, is under discussion at this time.[4,5,6]

Athletic Training

Athletic training is best defined by considering the major functions or responsibilities of the athletic trainer. These functions fall into the following categories:

1. Prevention of athletic trauma or conditions that adversely affect the health or the performance of the athlete
2. Management (first aid, evaluation, treatment, and rehabilitation) of athletic trauma or other medical problems that affect the athlete

3. Counseling of the athlete in various health-related areas such as
   a. nutrition
   b. relaxation and tension control
   c. personal health habits

Texas, in its state licensing bill,* has defined an athletic trainer as

"a person with specific qualifications . . . who upon the advice and consent of his team physician carries out the practice of prevention and/or physical rehabilitation of injuries incurred by athletes. To carry out these functions the athletic trainer is authorized to use physical modalities such as heat, light, sound, cold, electricity, or mechanical devices related to rehabilitation and treatment."

The two major organizations most closely associated with the athletic trainer and the therapist are: (1) the National Athletic Trainers Association (NATA) and (2) the American Physical Therapy Association (APTA), particularly the Sports Medicine Section.

The National Athletic Trainers Association was founded in 1949, mainly for the purpose of advancing, encouraging, and improving the athletic training profession in all its phases. It implements this goal by seeking to promote a better working relationship among those interested in the profession of athletic training, to further develop the ability of each member, and to better serve the common interest of its members by providing a means for a full exchange of ideas within the profession.[7]

The years since the formation of NATA have seen many advances. One area of achievement that needs to be mentioned is the establishment of the certification of athletic trainers. In August of 1970 the first NATA certification examination was held, and by the end of 1977 a total of 1,501 candidates had taken the examination.[8]

Another committee of NATA, the Professional Education Committee, has worked to improve and upgrade educational standards for athletic trainers. At present there are approximately fifty colleges and universities that offer approved NATA curriculums in undergraduate athletic training. In addition, five universities offer graduate-level programs.

There are two major sections under which an individual can qualify to apply to take the certification examination administered by NATA. These two sections are:

1. Students who have graduated from an approved undergraduate or graduate program
2. Internship program graduates

For complete details of specific certification requirements and procedures, the reader should consult the *Athletic Training Journal of the NATA* or write to:

National Athletic Trainers Association
Chairman, Board of Certification
Greenville, North Carolina 27834

The Sports Physical Therapy Section of the American Physical Therapy Association was established to provide those physical therapists interested in sports medicine with an opportunity to gain additional knowledge in sports medicine. The functions of the APTA Sports Medicine Section are to

1. provide information relative to evaluation, treatment, and rehabilitation of sports-related injuries
2. improve relationships among organizations associated with the treatment of athletic injuries
3. promote the development of sports medicine within physical therapy educational programs
4. provide a mechanism for therapists to become involved in research as well as in the practical aspects of sports medicine

*Texas Athletic Training Licensing Act

5. broaden the field of physical therapy in the areas of prevention, conditioning, treatment, and rehabilitation of athletic injuries, thereby providing employment opportunities

6. keep the membership informed, by dissemination of information, of current sports medicine trends and practices

Those involved in sports medicine should also be aware of organizations such as the American College of Sports Medicine (ACSM) which may be relevant to their needs. In addition, there are specialty sports medicine organizations such as the American Orthopaedic Society for Sports Medicine (AOSSM) and the American Academy of Podiatric Sports Medicine (AAPSM).

Ethical Problems and the Athletic Trainer

The trainer is frequently placed in situations which can only be regarded as less than enviable. It is necessary for those who are, or will be, involved with the athlete to be aware of potential ethical problems so that they will be somewhat prepared to deal with them.

The trainer is usually employed by the team management, and this may lead to an implicit expectation on the part of the management or coaching staff of loyalty to them. This arrangement may not always be in the best interests of the athlete, and in recent years there have been movements directed at organizing athletes so they may have their own athletic trainer and/or physician. This would theoretically limit management's power in potentially controlling the actions of medical personnel.

The player's welfare should be placed above all other considerations, including pressure from the coaches and management, fears of job security, or ego problems. This does not mean the coaches or the management do not have valid concerns, rather that the trainer must not allow a nonmedical con-

sideration to influence his or her judgment.

In order to serve both parties effectively, the trainer needs to be accepted by the athlete as well as by the coaches and management, but there should be no doubt in anyone's mind that decisions regarding the health and welfare of the athlete will be made on a sound medical basis and will not be subject to manipulation or influence by others. All too frequently, subtle or blatant pressure is exerted on the trainer "for the sake of the team," with little or no regard for the potential health hazards to which the athlete might be exposed. The athlete's best interests should always be given first priority. If pressure is exerted and a question of judgment arises, the trainer should call for a physician's opinion. The physician should be the person who makes the unpopular decision, not the trainer.

A trainer is often asked to defy the natural process of healing and frequently does an amazing job of helping an athlete to return to participation. There is the risk, however, of cutting corners or proclaiming athletes ready to return when they are not. This situation arises if the trainer feels that, in order to retain his or her status in the eyes of the coach or management, the player should be ready by a particular deadline. Sometimes, however, controlled activity ("rest") is the only answer, and the trainer needs to be able to decide, in spite of external pressures, when rest is indicated and to explain this in an acceptable manner to the athlete as well as to the coach and management without creating hostility on either side.

Sometimes an athlete may be medically able to return to participation, but due to the enforced layoff, his or her inadequate level of fitness may be a disadvantage to the team. Premature return to competition should first be discussed with the athlete, but the coaching staff should know of the trainer's opinion regarding the level of fitness of an athlete who has been injured.

Another potential source of conflict of which the trainer should be aware is the issue of confidentiality of the athlete's background of injuries. All too often, professional scouts or reporters may casually discuss a particular player. The trainer does not want to be caught in the trap of informally (or formally) disclosing private medical information without a player's written release. All information that is given out verbally or in writing should be cleared by the player as well as by the management and a notation made of the information, the date, and to whom it was released.

The trainer may on occasion find unsafe coaching practices or facilities. Should this occur, the trainer should first advise the appropriate person. If this advice is ignored, a report of the findings and recommendations should be sent to the highest authority. This does not mean the trainer should act like a "know-it-all." On the contrary, careful judgment is necessary to ensure that frivolous remarks are not made. If definite hazardous conditions exist, however, it is the trainer's professional duty to ensure that corrective action is taken. The same situation applies to the use of inappropriate, illegal, or banned drugs in an athletic setting.

As can be seen, the trainer will find strings pulling him or her in all directions and will often be confronted with extremely taxing situations. Mature judgment, a cool head, and frequent consultations with physicians, peers, and superiors can help lessen the load and allow wise decisions to be made.

Frequency of Injury in Athletes

The number of individuals participating in all types of athletic events at all ages is increasing yearly. To study the number of school and college students engaged in athletics, as well as the injury rate, a survey was conducted by the Department of Health, Education and Welfare (HEW) by authorization of the Congress of the United States (§826 of Public Law 93–380). This survey ran from July 1, 1975, to June 30, 1976, and was based upon a sample of 2,500 secondary schools and 1,300 colleges.[9] Some of the findings were as follows:

1. There were 5.4 million participants in varsity sports sponsored by secondary schools and colleges.

2. There were 1 million varsity (tackle) male football participants at the secondary level, and 70,000 in two- and four-year colleges.

3. In sports other than football, there were 2.8 million male and 1.7 million female participants.

4. Intramural sports accounted for 3.3 million male and 1.8 million female participants.

If there is value in participation in athletic activity, then the apparent trend towards increased participation in athletics would seem to be desirable. However, in evaluating the total worth of athletics, the possible negative as well as positive effects need to be considered, and the risk of injury is certainly a negative factor.

In this study the following statistics relate to the injury rate:

1. Over 1 million athletic injuries occurred in secondary schools and college programs (including intramural and physical education classes).

2. 776,893 injuries occurred in varsity sports.

3. 325,957 injuries occurred in tackle football.

4. 270,025 injuries occurred in other contact sports.

5. 150,911 injuries occurred in noncontact sports.

6. Females accounted for 28.7 percent of varsity athletic participants, and 15.9 percent of those injured.

The Garrick and Requa[10] study of injuries in high school sports for two academic years (1973–74 and 1974–75) revealed 1,197 injuries for 3,049 participants in 19 sports. These two authors also reported on the number of injuries for various specific sports (see Table 0.1).

In the area of high school football, the North Carolina study found an injury rate of 48.8 percent,[11,12] whereas the study of Garrick and Requa found an injury rate of 81 percent[10] (Table 0.2). This discrepancy in the findings may be accounted for by considering the definition of an injury as well as the method of data collection.

Graham and Bruce conducted a study investigating the injuries that occurred in women during intercollegiate competition in the 1974–75 school year in Virginia (Table 0.3), as well as the body part involved (Table 0.4).[13] The role of the trainer in minimizing

these injuries will be discussed throughout this book.

The Utilization of Athletic Trainers in Athletic Programs

The HEW study, as well as many other studies, points out that every sport has a potential for injury; however, some sports have greater risk factors than others. For instance, Garrick and Requa reported a 3 percent injury rate for tennis (males), but an 81 percent injury rate for football. There are critics of athletics and, in particular, contact sports who have suggested the elimination of athletic programs, principally because of the risk of injury. This risk factor could be decreased if greater utilization were made of qualified sports medicine physicians and certified athletic trainers. The HEW study found that the coach or assistant coach provided on-field care in 80% of injuries and decided on return to play in 60% of the cases because a NATA-certified or associated member athletic trainer was not available. Certified athletic trainers were employed in only 10.9 percent of the public secondary schools and 40.2 percent of the four-year colleges in 1976. While the need for the services of a certified athletic trainer working with a physician is important at all levels of athletics, there is a critical need for this service at the high-school level.

As is apparent, there are a great number of athletic programs that have not secured the services of a NATA-certified or associat-

TABLE 0.1 High School Injuries (per 100 participants)

Male	Injuries	Female	Injuries
Cross-country	29	Cross-country	35
Football	81	Volleyball	6
Volleyball	10	Basketball	25
Gymnastics	28	Gymnastics	40
Basketball	31	Swimming	9
Wrestling	75	Tennis	7
Swimming	1	Track and Field	35
Soccer	30	Softball	44
Baseball	18		
Tennis	3		
Track and Field	33		

Source: James G. Garrick and R. K. Requa, "Injuries in High School Sports," *Pediatrics* 61:465–469, 1978. Copyright American Academy of Pediatrics, 1978.

TABLE 0.2 Comparison of High School Football Injury Studies

Injury Study	Method of Data Collection or Source of Data	Year(s)	Injury Rate (in percentages)
1. Blyth and Mueller[11]	Direct interviews	1969–72	48.8
2. Irvin	Daily injury records	1974	47.5
3. Garrick and Requa[10]	Data collected by assigned athletic trainers	1973–74, 1974–75	81.0

TABLE 0.3 Injury Rate per Player and Percentage of Disabling Injuries by Sport

Sport	Number of Players	Number of Injuries	Percentage of Injuries	Number of Disabling Injuries[a]	Percentage of Disabling Injuries
Archery	44	1	2.3	0	0.0
Basketball	243	72	29.6	24	33.3
Fencing	64	0	0.0	0	0.0
Field Hockey	275	66	24.0	12	18.2
Golf	28	0	0.0	0	0.0
Lacrosse	237	21	8.9	6	28.5
Swimming	78	8	10.2	1	12.5
Tennis	157	1	0.6	0	0.0
Volleyball	84	16	19.0	7	43.8

[a]A disabling injury was defined as one that resulted in nonparticipation for seven or more days.

Source: G.P. Graham and P.J. Bruce, "Survey of Intercollegiate Athletic Injuries to Women," *Research Quarterly* 48: 217–220, 1977. Reprinted by permission of the publisher, AAHPER.

ed member athletic trainer. Once-proposed federal legislation might have required all educational institutions engaged in interscholastic athletics to employ a certified athletic trainer. At the present time, however, this goal is a long way from being achieved.

In response to this issue, many state medical associations have passed resolutions endorsing the concept of certified athletic trainers and their usefulness to the high school. However, even more needs to be done to ensure that all high school athletes are served by a sufficient number of adequately trained and certified athletic trainers.

TABLE 0.4 Body Parts Involved in Sports Injuries (in percentages)[a]

	Basketball	Field Hockey	Lacrosse	Swimming	Volleyball
Ankle	50.0	22.7	23.8		12.5
Arm		3.0		12.5	12.5
Foot	2.8	4.5	9.5		6.2
Hand	9.7	7.6	9.5		25.0
Hamstrings		3.0			
Head and Face	2.8	24.2	4.8		
Knee	13.9	10.6	19.0	25.0	25.0
Lower Leg	6.9	9.1	19.0		6.2
Pelvis			4.8		
Quadriceps	5.5	10.6		12.5	18.7
Ribs		4.5		12.5	
Shoulder			4.8	12.5	
Vertebrae		3.0		12.5	
Other	8.3	4.5	4.8	12.5	

[a]Numbers are percentages of the total injuries in that sport. Where totals are greater than 100%, multiple injuries were involved.

Source: G.P. Graham and P.J. Bruce, "Survey of Intercollegiate Athletic Injuries to Women," *Research Quarterly* 48: 217–220, 1977. Reprinted by permission of the publisher, AAHPER.

The Sports Medicine Center or Clinic

There is a need for the various medical and paramedical specialties of the sports medicine team to be efficiently organized in order to make them available to all participants. A centralized sports medicine center or clinic seems to be a logical and appropriate way to utilize and mobilize available services, and in many instances the college or the university community lends itself ideally to the development of such a clinic. The athlete and the medical and paramedical personnel are in residence, and it should be feasible to centralize the sports medicine services.

The college or university sports medicine center could provide the following services or functions:

1. preventive programs for various types of athletic endeavors
2. athletic first aid and emergency care
3. evaluation and diagnostic services
4. nonsurgical treatment
5. referral service when appropriate
6. rehabilitation
7. research
8. teaching modules for utilization by various curriculums in the sports medicine field

The sports medicine center could provide services to the following programs:

1. intercollegiate athletics
2. intramural athletics
3. clubs and recreational sports
4. physical education departments

Other types of sports medicine centers[14] designed to serve specific athletic needs have been developed for the pre- and post-college athlete and for the general public. They are usually organized as either a regional sports medicine center (usually associated with a medical school), or a private sports medicine center.

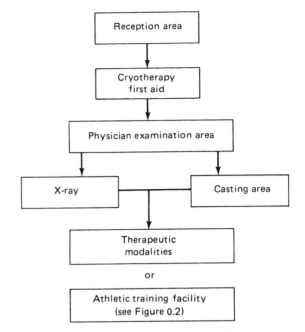

FIGURE 0.1 **Example of a sports medicine clinic flow pattern**

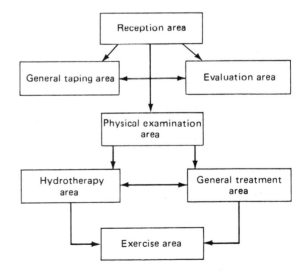

FIGURE 0.2 **Example of an athletic training facility flow pattern**

A sports medicine directory has been published which indicates the centers by location and provides information concerning the function, the services of the facility, and the staff of each center.[15]

Smodlaka[16] has proposed a national institute of sports medicine that would include the following departments:

Biology	Medical supervision
Epidemiology	and treatment
Pharmacology	Physical medicine
Physiology	and rehabilitation
Anatomy	Biomechanics
Pathophysiology	Psychology
Medicine	

All-inclusive sports complexes are being proposed to serve the ever-increasing interest in and need for a complete approach to health and fitness. This type of complex would use the services of a sports medicine team as part of the total organization.

REFERENCES

1. Ryan AJ, Allman FL, editors: *Sports Medicine*. New York, Academic Press, 1974.
2. Hirsch FJ: Generalist as team physician. *Phys Sportsmed* 7:88–90 and 92–95, August 1979.
3. Ryan AJ: Sports medicine history. *Phys Sportsmed* 6:77–82, October 1978.
4. Ryan AJ: Is sports medicine a "specialty"? *Phys Sportsmed* 6:3, January 1978.
5. Caldwell F: Physicians discuss sports medicine training. *Phys Sportsmed* 6:12, August 1978.
6. Prokop L: Sports medicine (Development and range of the field). *Olympian* 4:15–17, 1978.
7. Bell GW: Athletic training awareness. *Athletic Training* 13:200–205, 1978.
8. Westphalen SW, McLean L: Seven years of certification by the NATA. *Athletic Training* 13:86–88 and 91, 1978.
9. Calvert R: Athletic injuries and deaths in secondary schools and colleges, 1975–1976. National Center for Educational Statistics, Washington DC.
10. Garrick JG, Requa RK: Injuries in high school sports. *Pediatrics* 61:465–469, 1978.
11. Blyth CS, Mueller FO: An epidemiologic study of high school football injuries. Final report, distributed by US Consumer Product Safety Commission CPSC-C-74-18.
12. Mueller FO: Football injury update—1979 season. *Phys Sportsmed* 8:53–55, October 1980.
13. Graham GP, Bruce PJ: Survey of intercollegiate athletic injuries to women. *Res Q* 48:217–220, 1977.
14. Ferstle J: Olympic centers, money and muddle. *Phys Sportsmed* 6:22–23, June 1978.
15. Ryan AJ: Sports medicine directory. *Phys Sportsmed* 8:135–144, September 1980.
16. Smodlaka VN: A National Institute of Sports Medicine. *Phys Sportsmed* 6:115–118, April 1978.

RECOMMENDED READINGS

Adkinson JW, Requa RK, Garrick JG: Injury rates in high school football. *Clin Orthop* 99:131–136, 1974.

Garrick JG, Requa R: Medical care and injury surveillance in the high school setting. *Phys Sportsmed* 9:115–120, February 1981.

Goldberg B, Veres G, Nicholas JA: Sports medicine. *NY State J Med* 78:1406–1408, 1978.

Nicholas JA: What sports medicine is about. *Con Med* 42:4–8, 1979.

Ryan AJ: Do we need a federal institute? *Phys Sportsmed* 6:45, April 1978.

Ryan AJ: Sports medicine today. *Science* 200:919–924, 1978.

Shively RA, Grana WA, Ellis D: High school sports injuries. *Phys Sportsmed* 9:46–50, August 1981.

Vinger PF, Hoerner EF, editors: *Sports Injuries: The Unthwarted Epidemic*. Littleton, MA, PSG Publishing Company Inc., 1981.

Williams JG: International Federation of Sports Medicine. American Medical Association: *Proceedings of the Medical Aspects of Sports*. Chicago, 1974, pp 48–51.

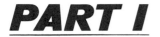

PART I

The Prevention of Athletic Injuries

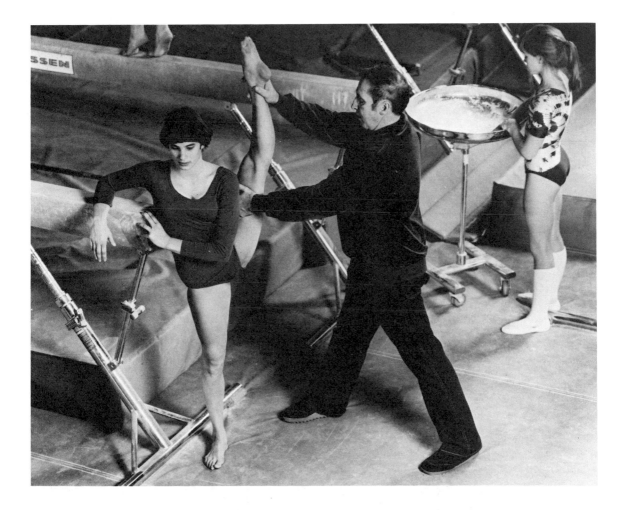

CHAPTER 1

The Preparticipation Physical Examination

A preparticipation physical examination should have a definite purpose according to the type of athlete being examined.[1] For instance, the examination of a young teen-ager entails a different orientation from that of a professional football player. To quote from Garrick[2]:

A child athlete offers the most potential for accomplishing something meaningful in the preparticipation examination. As athletes become more experienced one is less likely to discover significant medical problems during the course of an examination, as the first few participation examinations uncover conditions that will preclude specific athletic activities. Later in the athlete's career one usually looks for (and finds) only the residuals of previous injuries. For the experienced athlete the examination serves primarily as a quality control of treatment and rehabilitation of previous injuries.

The purpose of the examination is to

1. determine if any defects or conditions exist which might place that athlete at risk or increase the chances of injury in that particular sport
2. bring to the athlete's attention any weakness or imbalance, so that correction of these may be undertaken before beginning a particular athletic activity
3. determine whether an athlete may participate safely in spite of having a recognizable problem

The physical examination should ideally be conducted approximately one month before the beginning of the season in order to allow (1) further investigation of any questionable finding elicited during the examination, and (2) sufficient time to correct problems such as muscle weakness, infections, and other conditions.

The examination should ideally take place in a health care facility. At least one of the rooms should be in an area of complete quiet and privacy so that a cardiac and a medical examination can be satisfactorily undertaken. The trainer can assist with or perform many parts of the examination, and may be asked to be responsible for the organization and record keeping.

There are eight major areas involved in the physical examination:

1. *History.* In the case of the precollege athlete, the best medical history is usually obtained from the family physician in conjunction with the parents. However, the history form should be reviewed in detail with the athlete, either on an individual basis or in a group. The athlete should not just be given a form and told to fill it in. The questions should be phrased so that any *yes* answer can be further evaluated (see History Form, pages 12–14, and Sports Medicine Physical Examination Form, pages 14–15).

2. *Measurement.* This should include height, weight, and blood pressure.

3. *Medical examination.* This examination should be conducted in a quiet, private room and should include the cardiovascular,

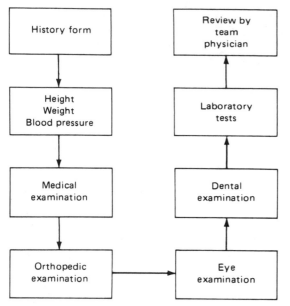

FIGURE 1.1 The physical examination—flow pattern (Adapted from Pediatric Clinics of North America, James G. Garrick, M.D., *Sports Medicine* 24:4, November 1977, p. 741.)

respiratory, abdominal, lymphatic, genital, dermatological, and ear, nose, and throat systems.

4. *Orthopedic examination.*

5. *Eye examination.*

6. *Dental screening examination.*

7. *Laboratory tests.* These should consist of a minimum of a hemoglobin or hematocrit estimation and a urinalysis.

8. *Review of the physical examination by the physician in charge.* This physician should decide on the status of each athlete, and each athlete should be assigned to one of four categories:

    a. no athletic participation

    b. limited participation, with specific sports mentioned

    c. clearance withheld until additional tests, examinations, or rehabilitation can be completed

    d. no reason found to restrict participation

History Form

I. *Past Injuries*

Do you have, or have you ever had, any of the following conditions? If so, please state when and who cared for you:

Injury	*Do you have this injury now?*
_____ Concussion(s) _____(number) _____	_____
_____ Skull fracture(s) _____(number) _____	_____
_____ Neck injuries	
_____ Shoulder injuries	
_____ Elbow injuries	
_____ Arm/wrist/hand injuries	
_____ Rib cage injuries	
_____ Back injuries	
_____ Hip injuries	
_____ Thigh injuries	
_____ Knee injuries	
_____ Lower leg injuries/"shin splints"	
_____ Ankle injuries	
_____ Foot injuries	
_____ Muscle strains (pulls)	
_____ Any injury to any part not mentioned?	
_____ Do you have false teeth or a bridge?	

History Form *(cont.)*

	Injury	*Do you have* *this injury now?*

_____ Have you been advised to restrict activity
during the past 5 years? _____

_____

_____

_____

_____

II. *Past Illnesses or Medical Problems*

Do you now have, or have you ever had, any of the following conditions? If so, please state when and who cared for you:

Surgical operations:

Confinement to hospital:

	Illness	*Do you have this* *illness/problem now?*

_____ Frequent headaches _____

_____ Fainting spells, dizziness or weakness _____

_____ Weakness or illness when exposed to high temperatures _____

_____ Epilepsy or convulsions _____

_____ Numbness or tingling _____

_____ Nosebleeds _____

_____ Difficulty hearing _____

_____ Frequent colds _____

_____ Pneumonia _____

_____ Tuberculosis _____

_____ Rheumatic fever _____

_____ Scarlet fever _____

_____ Heart murmur _____

_____ Have you ever had an electrocardiogram? yes __ no __
If so, when and by whom? _____

_____ High blood pressure _____

_____ Arthritis _____

_____ Diabetes _____

_____ Any abnormal bleeding tendencies _____

_____ Anemia _____

_____ Thyroid disorders _____

_____ Skin disorders _____

_____ Any allergies — food (that should not be taken) _____

_____   — drugs-medicines _____

_____   — skin _____

_____   — asthma _____

_____ Loss of, or serious impairment of, a paired organ
(e.g., kidney, eye, lung) _____

_____ Hepatitis or jaundice _____

_____ Infectious mononucleosis (mono) _____

_____ Bowel cramps or upsets _____

_____ Frequent indigestion or heartburn _____

_____ Stomach ulcer _____

_____ Kidney and bladder problems _____

_____ Menstrual problems _____

_____ Do you/should you wear glasses or contacts?   _____ yes   _____no

History Form *(cont.)*

Illness	Do you have this illness/problem now?
_____ Do you have prescription(s) available?	_____ yes _____ no
_____ Anything else not mentioned? _____	

_____

_____

_____

_____

_____

III. *Immunization Record and Disease History*
    Have you been immunized against: *Date*
    _____ Diptheria and/or tetanus   _____
    _____ Polio   _____

Sports Medicine Physical Examination Form

Name _____ Age _____ No. _____

Height _____   Weight _____   Blood Pressure _____ / _____

Vision: OK _____ Needs investigation _____

Medical Examination

	OK	Problem	Comment
Dental			
Eyes/Fundus			
Ears, Nose, Throat			
Head & Neck			
Skin & Scalp			
Lymphatics			
Thorax			
Lungs			
Heart			
Abdomen			
Hernia			
Genitalia			
Neurologic			
			Signature Date
Orthopedic Examination			
Neck & Shoulder			
Elbow, Hand & Wrist			
Back			
Knee			

Sports Medicine Physical Examination Form (*cont.*)

Ankle			
Feet			
Flexibility:			
Other:			
		Signature	Date

Laboratory Tests
    Hemoglobin/Hematocrit: _____ Gm. _____% Urinalysis: _____

    Other: _____
Review by Team Physician
    _____ No Athletic Participation
    _____ Limited Participation, e.g.: _____
    _____ Clearance Withheld Until: _____
    _____ Full Unlimited Participation. _____

Advice: _____

_____

Team Physician's Signature: _____ Date: _____

This physician may also review advice given to the athlete—for instance, "improve flexibility of the hamstrings, decrease body fat, increase strength of the quadriceps."

Some Characteristics to Note during the Physical Examination

Body build. The height and weight, when compared year by year, will help chart the physical development of the athlete. It is also useful to understand the concepts of the system of *somatotypes* which has been described by Sheldon[3,4] and subsequently further developed by Heath and Carter[5,6] and others. This theory states that people can be grouped according to the type of tissue that predominates in their body (Figure 1.2).

1. *Endomorphs.* Endodermal tissue in the embryo gives rise to abdominal viscera. People comprising this somatotype have large, efficient abdominal viscera and digest, ab-sorb, and store food efficiently, therefore tending to become obese. Extreme endomorphs are not very muscular or active physically and are seldom if ever seen in the more advanced classes of athletes. A less extreme endomorph may be able to participate in high-performance athletics by maintaining a strict diet and training regimen, but will tend to gain weight easily should the discipline become lax.

2. *Mesomorphs.* The mesomorph has much mesodermal tissue such as bone, muscle, and connective tissue and tends to be a muscular athlete with a large skeletal frame. Most athletes fall into the mesomorphic category. They are by nature very competitive and aggressive.

3. *Ectomorphs.* The ectomorph has a high proportion of skin and nervous tissue on a small skeletal frame, with very little subcutaneous fat. Ectomorphs tend to make good marathon runners and by their nature may avoid contact sports.

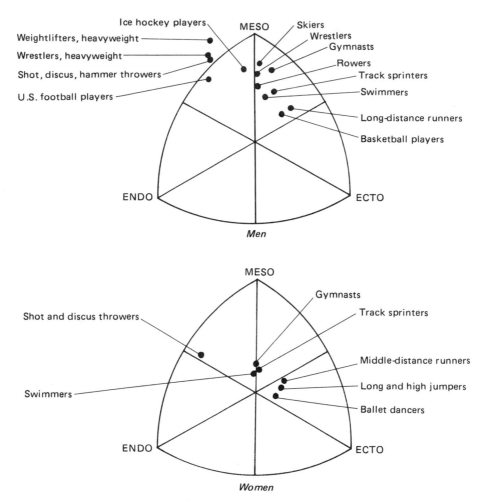

FIGURE 1.2 Somatotypes   An example of somatotypes of men and women athletes in different sports (Adapted from Carter, 1976.)

Posture.   Posture is not only a reflection of the state of muscle tone, but often reflects on some aspects of the athlete's psychology as well. During a screening examination it is necessary to become aware of each athlete's posture and what can be done to correct any abnormality. A useful guide for this examination is found in Figure 1.3.

Flexibility.   The subject of flexibility has produced a great deal of controversy in recent years. There is no doubt, however, that some athletes are "tight" while others are "loose." Assessment of an athlete's flexibility can be carried out by using the tests illustrated in Figure 1.4.

Some authorities[7,8] feel that a tight-jointed individual is more prone to muscle strains, whereas a loose-jointed individual is more subject to ligament sprains. However, others[9] disagree with this assessment and feel that one cannot predict the occurrence of injuries based on these criteria alone.

Irrespective of these arguments is the athlete's subjective feeling of improved performance and comfort if a slow, passive-

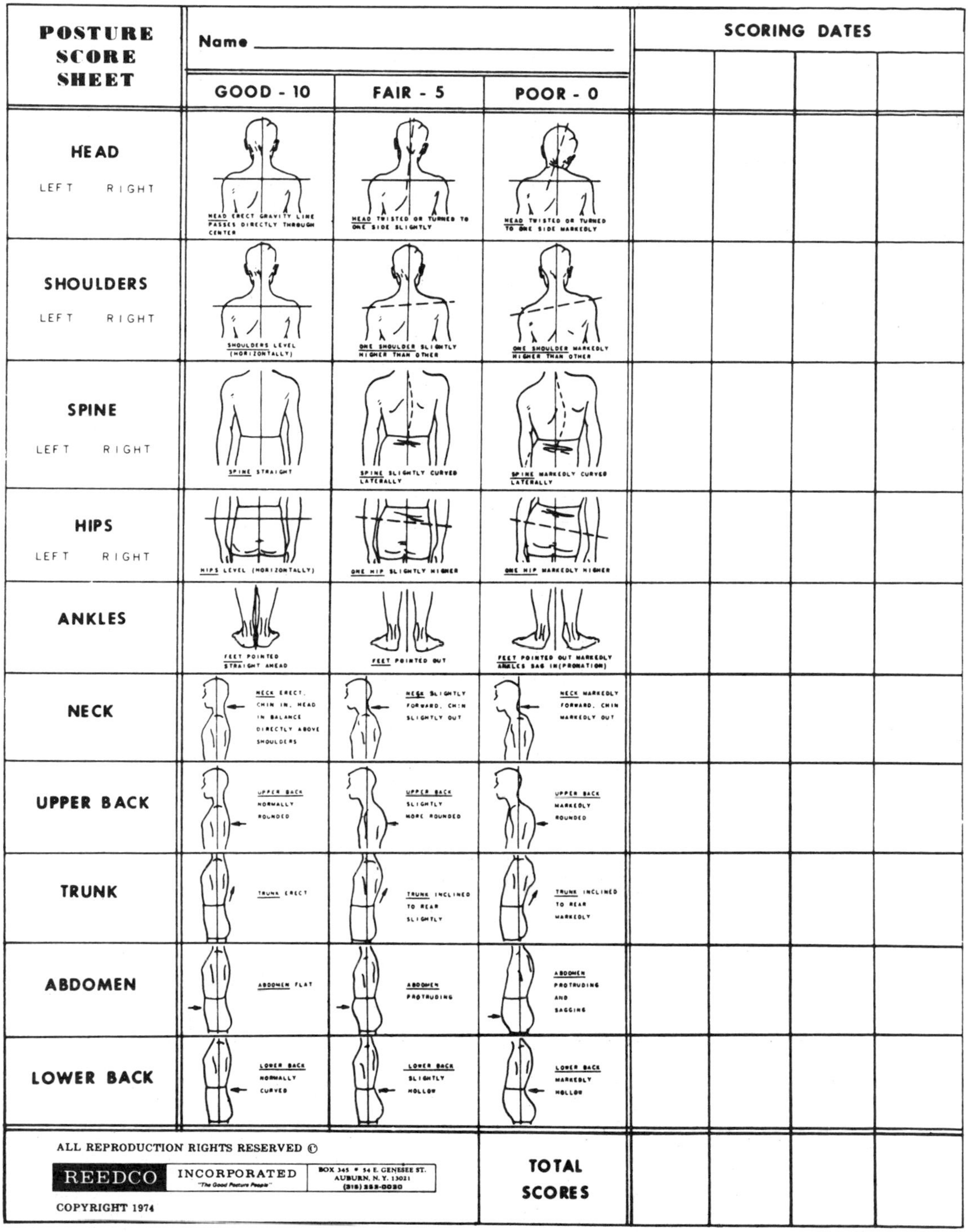

POSTURE SCORE SHEET	Name _____			SCORING DATES			
	GOOD - 10	FAIR - 5	POOR - 0				
HEAD LEFT RIGHT	HEAD ERECT GRAVITY LINE PASSES DIRECTLY THROUGH CENTER	HEAD TWISTED OR TURNED TO ONE SIDE SLIGHTLY	HEAD TWISTED OR TURNED TO ONE SIDE MARKEDLY				
SHOULDERS LEFT RIGHT	SHOULDERS LEVEL (HORIZONTALLY)	ONE SHOULDER SLIGHTLY HIGHER THAN OTHER	ONE SHOULDER MARKEDLY HIGHER THAN OTHER				
SPINE LEFT RIGHT	SPINE STRAIGHT	SPINE SLIGHTLY CURVED LATERALLY	SPINE MARKEDLY CURVED LATERALLY				
HIPS LEFT RIGHT	HIPS LEVEL (HORIZONTALLY)	ONE HIP SLIGHTLY HIGHER	ONE HIP MARKEDLY HIGHER				
ANKLES	FEET POINTED STRAIGHT AHEAD	FEET POINTED OUT	FEET POINTED OUT MARKEDLY ANKLES SAG IN(PRONATION)				
NECK	NECK ERECT, CHIN IN, HEAD IN BALANCE DIRECTLY ABOVE SHOULDERS	NECK SLIGHTLY FORWARD, CHIN SLIGHTLY OUT	NECK MARKEDLY FORWARD, CHIN MARKEDLY OUT				
UPPER BACK	UPPER BACK NORMALLY ROUNDED	UPPER BACK SLIGHTLY MORE ROUNDED	UPPER BACK MARKEDLY ROUNDED				
TRUNK	TRUNK ERECT	TRUNK INCLINED TO REAR SLIGHTLY	TRUNK INCLINED TO REAR MARKEDLY				
ABDOMEN	ABDOMEN FLAT	ABDOMEN PROTRUDING	ABDOMEN PROTRUDING AND SAGGING				
LOWER BACK	LOWER BACK NORMALLY CURVED	LOWER BACK SLIGHTLY HOLLOW	LOWER BACK MARKEDLY HOLLOW				
ALL REPRODUCTION RIGHTS RESERVED © REEDCO INCORPORATED BOX 345 • 54 E. GENESEE ST. AUBURN, N.Y. 13021 (319) 353-0030 "The Good Posture People" COPYRIGHT 1974		TOTAL SCORES					

FIGURE 1.3 **Posture score sheet** (Reproduced by permission of Reedco, Inc., Auburn, N.Y.)

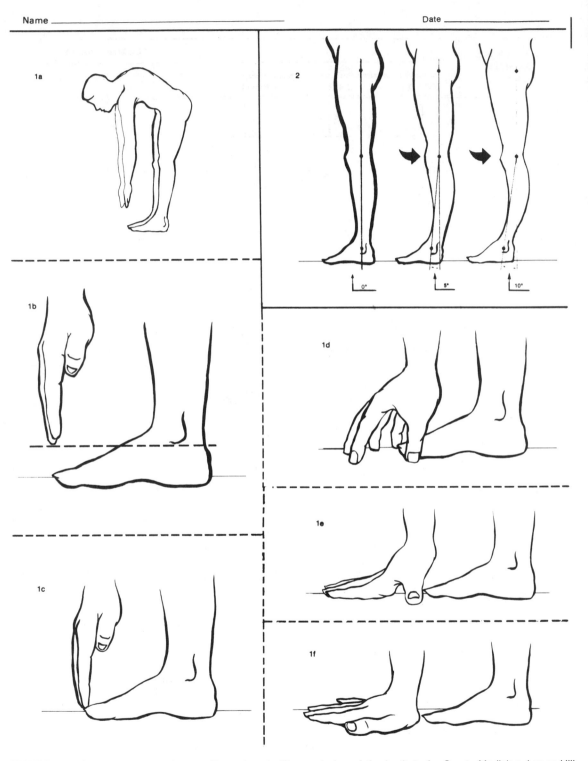

FIGURE 1.4   Flexibility score sheet   (Reproduced with permission of the Institute for Sports Medicine, Lenox Hill Hospital, New York, N.Y.)

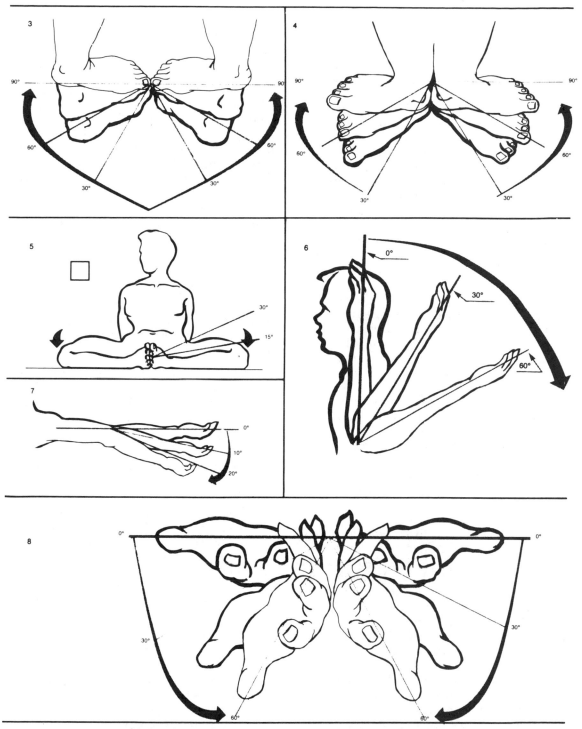

stretching program is performed routinely. It appears that this type of stretching program is useful in injury prevention, particularly with certain muscle groups that tend to become too tight with repeated use, for example, the hamstrings and the gastrocnemius-soleus-Achilles group. For these reasons it is considered desirable that athletes be encouraged to perform slow stretching exercises of specific muscle groups that might become tight in their particular sporting activity. On the other hand, however, there are certain high-performance athletes who are tight and do not wish to stretch, yet who do not appear to be prone to injury. Whether this is the exception that proves the rule is still a subject of debate.

Skinfold thickness. There are almost no sports (except perhaps long-distance swimming and sumu wrestling) in which a large amount of subcutaneous fat is an advantage. If an athlete needs to put on weight, it should be as muscle mass only and not as fat.

An estimation of percentage of body fat can be made by a number of methods, one of the most accurate being total body immersion in an underwater weighing tank. As this is not practical in many cases, skinfold thickness measurement by means of calipers is a useful technique, but one that needs to be continually practiced in order to achieve consistency and accuracy (Figure 1.5).

Women are normally considered to have a higher body fat content than men,[10] and most male athletes should fall below 12 percent to 15 percent body fat. Endurance athletes,[11] gymnasts of both sexes, and wrestlers are often below 7 percent but should not be below 5 percent. However, if an individual has a total body fat above the optimum for that sport, he or she is carrying excessive deadweight, which is detrimental to athletic performance as well as to health. Athletes should be educated in this area and advised accordingly (see Chapter 24).

A practical way to estimate the fluctuations in body fat is to measure a number of standard locations and add them together to obtain a total.[12,13,14] This procedure can be repeated on occasion throughout the season.

Strength. There are a number of different methods used to test muscle strength. One method is to place the extremity into the desired position and ask the athlete to maintain that position while a constant resistance is applied (Figure 1.6). Other methods include the use of a strain gauge for isometric contractions; a handgrip dynamometer (Figure 1.7); successive lifts on an isotonic machine (Universal Gym) until the maximum lift is achieved; or visual or printed readouts on one of the isokinetic machines (Cybex or Orthotron).

Maturation. The participation of a pre-adolescent or adolescent athlete should be determined not by age, but by size, weight, and degree of maturity. Two methods of evaluating physical maturity are:

1. *Skeletal development.* This is determined by comparing X-rays of the wrist with the norms found in a radiologic atlas (Figure 1.8).[15,16]

2. *Sexual development.* The presence and character of pubic or axillary hair is a satisfactory indication of the degree of maturity reached by that athlete. Such a classification might be:

Stage I	No pubic or axillary hair
Stage II	Slight amount of hair
Stage III	Hair darker and more curled and starting to spread
Stage IV	Adult in type but covering a smaller area than an adult's
Stage V	Adult in type and amount, extending over a larger area

According to Smith,[17] collision contact sports such as football, wrestling, lacrosse, and ice hockey should not be recommended for boys until they have reached Stage V development. On the other hand, the highly skilled junior-high school athlete with Stage IV or V pubic hair development may be a suitable participant in many high school pro-

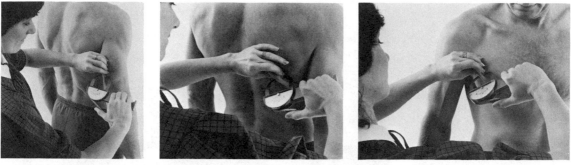

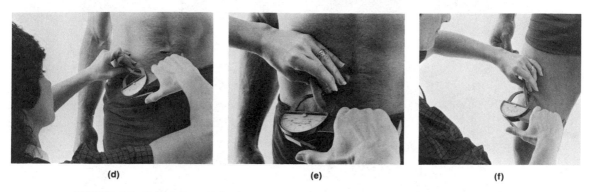

FIGURE 1.5 Estimation of body fat by the use of skinfold thickness calipers The skin should be lifted away from the underlying muscle. The most commonly used sites are illustrated: **(a)** mid triceps **(b)** scapula **(c)** anterior chest **(d)** iliac crest **(e)** just below and lateral to the umbilicus **(f)** the anterior thigh

TABLE 1.1 Simple Classification of Skinfold Measurements for Athletes

Classification	Triceps[a]	Scapula[b]	Abdomen[c]	Total
Lean (< 7% fat)	< 7 mm	< 8 mm	< 10 mm	< 25 mm
Acceptable (12–15% fat)	7–13 mm	8–15 mm	10–20 mm	25–48 mm
Over fat (> 15% fat)	> 13 mm	> 15 mm	> 20 mm	> 48 mm

[a]Back of upper arm, over triceps midway on upper arm—skinfold lifted to parellel to long axis of arm with the arm hanging.

[b]Below tip of right scapula, skinfold lifted along axis of body.

[c]Five centimeters lateral to umbilicus, avoid umbilical crease, skinfold lifted on axis with umbilicus.

Note: The scapular skinfold is the single best skinfold to measure; the triceps, the next best.

Source: E. S. Buskirk, *Sports Medicine* (A. J. Ryan, F. L. Allman, eds.). New York, Academic Press, 1974, p. 146.

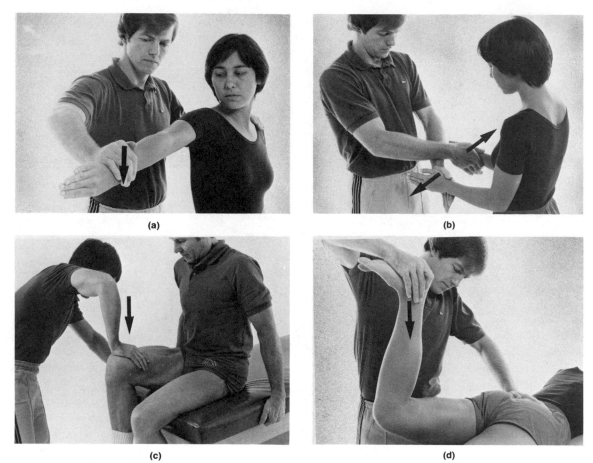

FIGURE 1.6 Manual resistive muscle testing Firm, constant pressure (not overpowering force) is applied by the examiner in order to detect muscle dysfunction or weakness. **(a)** deltoids **(b)** internal rotators **(c)** hip flexors **(d)** gluteals

grams. In adolescent females, the onset of menstruation may be a suitable index of their degree of maturation and development (see chart opposite, "Scale to Determine Physical Maturity of a Girl.")

Conditions That Might Disqualify an Athlete from Specific Athletic Participation

As mentioned in Table 1.2 (p. 24), some of the conditions listed as "disqualifying" apply only to particular sports. Other conditions are subject to the responsible physician's evaluating all the various factors involved.[18]

1. *Eye conditions.* An athlete with only one eye, severe myopia in one eye, or previous retinal detachment which has been repaired should be advised to refrain from contact sports.

The athlete should not wear hard contact lenses while boxing. Specially manufactured eyeglasses can be used for contact events if the athlete so chooses. However, soft contact lenses are usually readily accept-

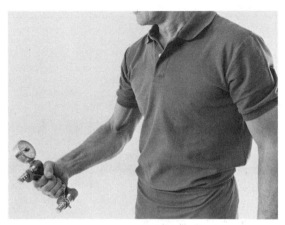

FIGURE 1.7   A handgrip dynamometer   An accurate way to determine handgrip strength

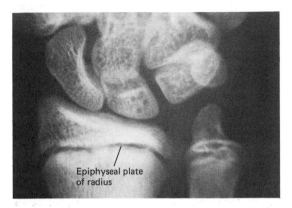

Epiphyseal plate of radius

FIGURE 1.8   Skeletal maturity   This wrist X-ray may be used to help determine the degree of bony maturity present. Note the epiphyseal plates which are still widely open. By using X-rays such as these, it may be possible to predict the potential height of the subject.

Scale to Determine Physical Maturity of a Girl

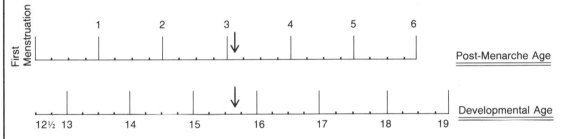

Mark a point on the line below to indicate months and years elapsed since her first menstruation. The point directly below on the second line shows the developmental age rating to use when considering programming this individual with girls of dissimilar chronological age.

Example: Trudy J.

First menstruation: August 1976
Date of current evaluation: September 1979
Time elapsed since the onset of menstruation and evaluation dates: 3 years, 1 month. (Mark this on top line.)

The point directly below on the second line indicates a developmental level of 15 years, 7 months, although Trudy's chronological age is 14 years, 4 months. (Date of birth May 6, 1965.)

Thus, Trudy may be considered for programming with girls 15–16 years of age if other factors indicate superior levels of fitness and skills.

Source: Institute of Sports Medicine and Athletic Trauma, Lenox Hill Hospital, 130 East 77th Street, New York, New York 10021.

TABLE 1.2 Disqualifying Conditions for Sports Participation

Condition	Collision[a]	Contact[b]	Noncontact[c]	Other[d]
General:				
Acute infections—respiratory, genito-urinary, infectious mononucleosis, hepatitis, active rheumatic fever, active tuberculosis	x	x	x	x
Obvious physical immaturity in comparison with other competitors	x	x		
Hemorrhagic disease—hemophilia, purpura, and other serious bleeding tendencies	x	x	x	
Diabetes, inadequately controlled . .	x	x	x	
Diabetes, controlled				x
Jaundice	x	x	x	x
Eyes:				
Absence or loss of function of one eye	x	x		
Respiratory:				
Tuberculosis (active or symptomatic)	x	x	x	x
Severe pulmonary insufficiency	x	x	x	x
Cardiovascular:				
Mitral stenosis, aortic stenosis, aortic insufficiency, coarctation of aorta, cyanotic heart disease, recent carditis of any etiology	x	x	x	x
Hypertension on organic basis	x	x	x	x
Previous heart surgery for congenital or acquired heart disease[e]				
Liver:				
Enlarged liver	x	x		
Skin:				
Boils, impetigo, and herpes simplex gladiatorum	x	x		
Spleen:				
Enlarged spleen	x	x		
Hernia:				
Inguinal or femoral hernia	x	x	x	
Musculoskeletal:				
Symptomatic abnormalities or inflammations	x	x	x	x
Functional inadequacy of the musculoskeletal system, congenital or acquired, incompatible with the contact or skill demands of the sport . .	x	x	x	
Neurological:				
History or symptoms of previous serious head trauma or repeated concussions	x			
Controlled convulsive disorder[f] . . .				

TABLE 1.2   Disqualifying Conditions for Sports Participation (*cont.*)

Condition	Collision[a]	Contact[b]	Noncontact[c]	Other[d]
Convulsive disorder not moderately well controlled by medication	x			
Previous head surgery	x	x		
Renal:				
Absence of one kidney	x	x		
Renal disease	x	x	x	x
Genitalia:[g]				
Absence of one testicle				
Undescended testicle				

[a]Football, rugby, hockey, lacrosse, etc.

[b]Baseball, soccer, basketball, wrestling, etc.

[c]Cross-country, track, tennis, crewing, swimming, etc.

[d]Bowling, golf, archery, field events, etc.

[e]Each patient should be judged on an individual basis in conjunction with his or her cardiologist and operating surgeon.

[f]Each patient should be judged on an individual basis. All things being equal, it is probably better to encourage a young boy or girl to participate in a noncontact sport rather than a contact sport. However, if a particular patient has a great desire to play a contact sport, and this is deemed a major ameliorating factor in his or her adjustment to school, associates, and the seizure disorder, serious consideration should be given to letting him or her participate if the seizures are moderately well controlled or the athlete is under good medical management.

[g]The Committee approves the concept of contact sports participation for youths with only one testicle or with an undescended testicle or testicles, except in specific cases such as an inguinal canal undescended testicle or testicles, following appropriate medical evaluation to rule out unusual injury risk. However, the athlete, parents, and school authorities should be fully informed that participation in contact sports for youths with only one testicle does carry a slight risk to the remaining healthy testicle. Following such an injury, fertility may be adversely affected. But the chances of an injury to a descended testicle are rare, and the injury risk can be further substantially minimized with an athletic supporter and protective device.

*Reprinted by permission of the American Medical Association, Committee on Medical Aspects of Sport.

ed by most athletes and are probably superior and safer to use than glasses.

2. *Cardiac conditions.* Heart murmurs are frequently heard in many athletes. In most cases these are functional in nature, but they usually need to be evaluated by a cardiologist in order to exclude more serious conditions which might result in sudden death during athletic participation (e.g., prolapsed mitral valve, idiopathic hypertrophic aortic stenosis, and congenital aortic stenosis).[19,20,21,22]

3. *Multiple concussions.* At present it is gen-

erally agreed that an athlete who has had three episodes of loss of consciousness with retrograde amnesia or other changes following the concussion should be disqualified from further contact sports. This figure should be used as a guide only and should not be an inflexible number. Some athletes should be advised to refrain from contact activities after only one severe head injury. Other athletes who have had multiple episodes of minor concussions ("bell rung") may be candidates for disqualificaton even though they have not actually lost consciousness. These cases should be examined in conjunction with a neurologist or neurosurgeon in order to reach the most satisfactory conclusion with regard to the athlete's ability to continue with contact participation.

4. *Convulsive disorders.* Participation in athletics, and even in contact sports, can be undertaken by children and teen-agers whose epilepsy is suitably controlled, if they are cooperative and emotionally stable. Those who suffer from epilepsy only while sleeping should be evaluated in the same manner as non-epileptics.[23,24,25]

There should, however, be restrictions on

1. mountain climbing
2. working at heights
3. swimming alone
4. scuba diving

There should be restrictions on participation among

1. those who experience daily or weekly seizures
2. those who display bizarre forms of psychomotor epilepsy
3. those whose postconvulsive state is prolonged or typically includes marked abnormal behavior.

REFERENCES

1. Tennant FS, Sorenson K, Day CM: Benefits of preparticipation sports examinations. *J Fam Pract* 13:287–288, 1981.
2. Garrick JG: Pre-participation sports assessment. *Pediatrics* 66:803–806, 1980.
3. Sheldon WH, Stevens SS: *The Varieties of Temperament.* New York, Harper and Brothers, third edition, 1942.
4. Sheldon WH, Stevens SS, Tucker WB: *Varieties of Human Physique.* New York, Harper and Brothers, 1954.
5. Carter JEL: The somatotypes of athletes. A review. *Hum Biol* 42:535–569, 1970.
6. Heath BH, Carter JEL: Modified somatotype method. *Am J Phys Anthrop* 27:57–74, 1967.
7. Nicholas JA: Risk factors: Sports medicine and the orthopedic system. An overview. *J Sports Med* 3:243–259, 1975.
8. Nicholas JA: Injuries to knee ligaments. Relationship to looseness and tightness in football players. *JAMA* 212:2236–2239, 1970.
9. Jackson DW, Jarrett H, Bailey D, et al: Injury prediction in the young athlete: A preliminary report. *Am J Sports Med* 6:6–14, 1978.
10. Durnin JV, Womersley J: Body fat assessed from total body density and its estimation from skinfold thickness: measurements on 481 men and women aged 16 to 72 years. *Br J Nutr* 32:77–97, 1974.
11. Costill DL, Bowers R, Kammer WF: Skinfold estimates of body fat among marathon runners. *Med Sci Sports* 2:93–95, 1970.
12. Wilmore JH, Behnke AR: An anthropometric estimation of body density and lean body weight in young men. *J Appl Physiol* 27:25–31, 1969.
13. Jackson AS, Pollock MC, Ward A: Generalized equations for predicting body density in women. *Med Sci Sports Exerci* 12:175–182, 1980.
14. Jackson AS, Pollock MC: Generalized equations for predicting body density of men. *Br J Nutr* 40:497–504, 1978.
15. Greulich WW, Pyle SI: *Radiographic Atlas of Skeletal Development of the Hand and Wrist.* Palo Alto, Stanford University Press, second edition, 1959.
16. Tanner JM, Whitehouse RH, Marshall WA, et al: *Assessment of Skeletal Maturity and Prediction of Adult Height.* London, Academic Press, 1975.
17. Smith NJ: *Sports Medicine and Physiology.* Strauss RH editor. Philadelphia, Saunders, 1979.
18. Shaffer TE: The health examination for participation in sports. *Pediatr Ann* 7:27–30, 1978.
19. Shaffer TE, Rose KD: Cardiac evaluation for participation in school sports. Questions and Answers in *JAMA* 228:398, 1974.
20. Rose KD: Which cardiovascular "problems" should disqualify athletes? *Phys Sportsmed* 3:62–68, June 1975.
21. Zeppilli P, Venerando A: Screening for mitral valve prolapse. Guest editorial. *Phys Sportsmed* 10–29, January 1982.
22. American Academy of Pediatrics Policy Statement: *Cardiac Evaluation for Participation in Sports.* April 1977.
23. Livingston S: *Comprehensive Management of Epilepsy in Infancy, Childhood and Adolescence.* Springfield, Ill., Charles C. Thomas, 1972.
24. Livingston S, Berman W: Participation of the epileptic child in contact sports. *J Sports Med* 2:170–174, 1974.
25. Livingston S: Should epileptics be athletes? *Phys Sportsmed* 3:67–72, April 1975.

RECOMMENDED READINGS

Allman Jr, FL: Moderator of Round Table on: The preparticipation physical examination. *Phys Sportsmed* 2:23–29, August 1974.

Behnke AR, Wilmore JH: *Evaluation and Regulation of Body Build and Composition.* Englewood Cliffs, New Jersey, Prentice-Hall, 1974.

Blackburn Jr, TA, editor: *Guidelines for Pre-Season Athletic Participation Evaluation.* Columbus, Georgia, Sports Medicine Section of the American Physical Therapists Association. 1979.

Gomolack C: Problems in matching young athletes: Baby fat, peach fuzz, muscle, and mustache. In Lockerroom, *Phys Sportsmed* 3:96–98, May 1975.

Kendall HO, Kendall FP, Wadsworth GE: *Muscles: Testing and Function.* Baltimore, Williams and Wilkins, second edition, 1971.

Nicholas JA, Strizak AM, Veras G: A study of thigh muscle weakness in different pathological states of the lower extremity. *Am J Sports Med* 4:241–248, 1976.

Salem DN, Isner JM: Cardiac screening for athletes. Symposium on sports injuries. *Othop Clin North Am* 11:687–695, 1980.

Sheldon WH, Dupertuis CW, McDermott E: *Atlas of Men.* New York, Harper Brothers, 1954.

Tanner JM: *The Physique of The Olympic Athlete.* London, George Allen and Unwin, 1964.

CHAPTER 2

The Athletic Conditioning Program

INTRODUCTION

The athlete who participates in a well-devised, scientifically based, and properly supervised athletic physical conditioning program should benefit in at least four areas:

a. enhanced athletic performance

b. decreased risk of injury

c. decreased severity should an injury occur

d. accelerated rehabilitation and return to activity after an injury

At the present time, it has not been definitely proven that improvement in the various components of conditioning or fitness offers the athlete a lessened risk of injury, though it has been suggested by many individuals that there are theoretical benefits for injury prevention from a preparticipation physical conditioning program. The following people have advanced a variety of thoughts on the effects of physical conditioning programs:

Reid and *Schiffbauer*—The importance of hypertrophy of muscle tissue as a protection against bodily injury should be stressed.[1]

Gallagher—To avoid injuries to the lower extremities and to the back area, athletes should supplement their normal activities with exercises to increase the size and the strength of the muscles, which will then protect the joints in these areas from injury.[2]

Rasch—The athlete who is in a fatigued state has less efficiency and slower reactions, and therefore may be unable to guard against situations that could result in an injury.[3]

Thorndike—Exercises to strengthen the ankle and the knee can reduce injuries to these areas.[4]

Adams—Habitual exercise can cause a significant increase in the strength of the ligaments surrounding the knee and therefore prevent injuries to the knee.[5]

Falls et al.—Improved movement skill is important in the avoidance of injury.[6]

Gallagher—Overdevelopment provides increased strength that helps to stabilize joints.[2]

Kraus—While general conditioning is an important factor in the prevention of athletic injury, it is also important in the prevention of re-injury.[7]

Cahill and *Griffith*—A pre-season general body conditioning program results in fewer and less severe knee injuries.[8]

Physical conditioning or athletic fitness can be classified in a variety of ways. Table 2.1 gives the specific physical conditioning components, a definition of each, and the application of the component to the prevention of injuries.

Injury, as well as injury prevention, is influenced by the position of the origin and insertion of a muscle, the relationship of this muscle to the joint, and the angle of pull of the muscles on the bone at a particular moment through the range of motion. For instance, if a muscle has its origin near the joint and its insertion at a distance from the joint, the major resultant action will be to keep the two articulating bones of the joint in close approximation. This type of muscle action contributes to the stability of the joint (a shunt muscle action).

An example of the stabilizing action of muscles on a joint is the glenohumeral joint, which consists of the head of the humerus articulating with the shallow glenoid fossa of the scapula. The joint capsule is loose and flexible, thus permitting a wide range of motion, and the supportive ligaments are relatively weak. The muscles around the shoulder need to be developed and conditioned in order to provide optimal stabilization of the shoulder.

Where a muscle primarily produces motion of the joint, proper conditioning can enable the muscle to prevent an unwanted or exaggerated movement. The knee joint is frequently at risk from a combination of internal forces (e.g., a pivoting or cutting action) and external forces (e.g., a tackle or block in football). Adequate conditioning of

TABLE 2.1 Athletic Conditioning Components

Conditioning Component	Definition	Application to Injury Prevention
Strength	A maximal voluntary force exerted in a single muscular effort.	To stabilize an anatomical area against applied forces.
Power	Force × distance × time; or, strength × speed.	To shorten the time required to perform and/or increase the applied force (explosive type of movement), such as may be required to rapidly respond to a threat of injury.
Muscular endurance	The ability to repeat a series of muscular contractions.	A low muscular endurance capacity increases the potential for injury.
Flexibility	The range of movement of a joint that is permitted by the surrounding tissues.	To respond to forced extensibility without injury to the involved tissue.
Agility	The involvement of coordination and speed to permit rapid control in the movement or change of direction of the body.	To change the direction or position of the body rapidly, efficiently, and with precision in response to avoiding collision and the resulting injury.
Balance	Equilibrium of the body over its supporting base.	To control and maintain effective static and/or dynamic body position to prevent any awkward position that might contribute to injury.
Proprioception	The awareness of body position in space.	To perceive the position of the various body segments or be aware of the segment-space relationship to prevent injury (*example:* position of the foot as it comes in contact with the floor or the ground after being airborne).
Cardiovascular-respiratory endurance	The adequate function or response of those physiological systems that deliver fuel and oxygen to the active muscles.	To enable continuous muscular effort to be exerted in order to avoid the onset of fatigue which might then contribute to the occurrence of injury.

the muscles could contribute to the prevention of some of these knee injuries. All the muscles around the knee (the quadriceps in front, the hamstrings behind, the pes anserinus group medially, and the popliteus and biceps tendons and the iliotibial tract laterally) help maintain the stability of the knee. In particular, the quadriceps (especially the vastus medialis) provides resistance to lateral subluxation of the patella.

Cahill and Griffith conducted an eight-year study of groups of high-school football players.[8] Those involved in an active preseason, general body-conditioning program (which included the thigh muscles) suffered fewer and less serious injuries than those who did not condition (see Table 2.2).

Well-conditioned and hypertrophied muscles or muscle groups can contribute to the protection of less stable underlying soft tissues. For example, adequate strength, hypertrophy, and reflexive action of the abdominal muscles can afford protection to the abdominal viscera.

These are just a few of the many possible examples where a degree of protection may be provided by adherence to a well-designed conditioning program. Other possible beneficial effects are discussed later in this chapter.

SKELETAL MUSCLE

Skeletal muscles are made up of motor units controlled by the central nervous system. In recent years, muscle biopsies have been used with increasing frequency to help define and clarify the different types of muscle fibers.[9,10] The trainer should be aware of the influence of conditioning and rehabilitation programs on these different muscle fibers.

Two basic types of motor units have been identified, and they may be classified according to their speed of contraction—*slow-twitch*, which are also called *Type I fibers*, and *fast-twitch*, also called *Type II fibers*. There are considerable individual variations in the percentage of these fibers in different athletes and in different muscles—as a generalization, endurance athletes usually have more Type I fibers in their muscles whereas successful sprinters have muscles containing a higher proportion of Type II fibers. The percentage of fiber types seems to be genetically determined and is probably minimally influenced by training.

Type I Fibers (Slow-twitch Fibers)

When Type I fibers are activated, they take nearly twice as long as Type II fibers to reach their peak tension. This speed of contraction is dependent upon the enzyme adenosine triphosphatase, which splits adenosine triphosphate (ATP) into adenosine diphosphate (ADP). Slow-twitch fibers are low in adenosine triphosphatase as well as in enzymes used for degrading glycogen to lactate, and take a prolonged period to generate a relatively low level of force.

As Type I fibers are concerned mainly with oxidative and aerobic metabolism (i.e.,

TABLE 2.2   Knee Injury Summary

	No Conditioning					Conditioning					Total
	1969	*1970*	*1971*	*1972*	*Total*	*1973*	*1974*	*1975*	*1976*	*Total*	*Total*
Number of players	318	312	307	317	1254	298	277	350	302	1227	2481
Number of injured	24	16	22	23	85	18	16	9	7	50	135
Number of operations	6	4	4	5	19	1	4	1	1	7	26

Source: B.R. Cahill and E.H. Griffith, "Effect of Preseason Conditioning on the Incidence and Severity of High School Football Knee Injuries," *American Journal of Sports Medicine* 6:180–183, 1978. Reprinted by permission of the American Orthopaedic Society for Sports Medicine.

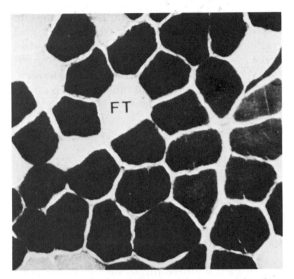

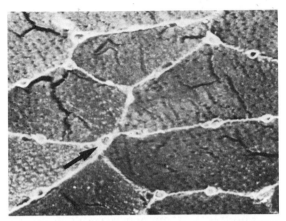

FIGURE 2.2 Muscle biopsy—low magnification showing a large number of capillaries which have developed as a result of intense aerobic training.

FIGURE 2.1 Muscle biopsy showing mainly slow-twitch fibers (dark staining) and a few fast-twitch fibers (FT, light stain). This biopsy was taken from the thigh of an Olympic marathon champion.

the ability to use oxygen for prolonged periods to synthesize and use ATP), they have many mitochondrial enzymes that can oxidize carbohydrates and fats, and are supplied with a greater number of capillaries per fiber than are the fast-twitch fibers. The slow-twitch fibers are more resistive to fatigue, and are the first to be recruited during submaximal exercise. However, when the exercise is continued until exhaustion, all fiber types are recruited.

If a limb is immobilized, Type I is likely to atrophy rapidly and is not preserved by isometric contractions.

Type II Fibers (Fast-twitch Fibers)

The Type II fibers are used for explosive-type activity and generate much force over a short period of time (half the time of Type I fibers). On the whole, fast-twitch fibers have a much higher level of adenosine triphosphatase and glycolytic enzyme activity (enzymes that help break down glycogen but do not require oxygen) than do slow-twitch fibers.

There are three fast-twitch fibers presently described—Type IIa, IIab, and IIb. They differ mainly in terms of endurance.[11]

Type IIa fibers have a certain amount of endurance despite being fast and powerful, but not as much endurance as Type I. Type IIb fibers are the powerful sprint fibers that fatigue more quickly than any other type (they have very few mitochondria).[12,13] They are purely glycolytic, meaning that they can function without oxygen, but for short periods of time only. Type IIab fibers lie somewhere between Type IIa and IIb in power and endurance.

It is thought that with training, Type IIb fibers may take on some of the features of Type IIa.

If a limb is immobilized, isometric contractions may prevent atrophy of Type II fibers.

Biochemical and Microscopic Changes that May Occur with Training or Conditioning

Endurance-type training causes large increases in concentration of mitochondria and in the levels of oxidative enzymes within the muscle cells. High-intensity sprint-type training does little to evoke such changes, but may produce an increase in the glycolytic enzyme system.

Endurance training appears to be able to double the glycogen stores. In addition, adaptations occur which enable the muscle to conserve glycogen by substituting the burning of fat for energy.

The level of oxidative enzymes may be three to five times greater in muscles of trained athletes compared with untrained individuals. It has also been shown that even fast-twitch fibers can develop and enhance oxidative capacity as a result of endurance training.

Endurance training may result in an increase in the number of capillaries per muscle fiber, but seems to have little or no effect upon the cross-sectional size of the muscle fiber, whereas heavy resistance exercise (weight training) usually causes an increase in the size of the fiber and thereby the strength, but no increase in the oxidative potential of the muscle.[14,15]

GENERAL CONDITIONING PRINCIPLES

There are some common principles that apply to the development of the components of conditioning. These include:

1. *Overload.* To facilitate improvement, the system involved must be progressively and gradually challenged or placed under additional stress. Depending upon the component of conditioning being challenged, overload might be implemented by increasing the

 a. resistance
 b. repetitions or sets
 c. rate (intensity) of work or exercise
 d. duration of work or exercise

2. *Specificity.* The effects of the conditioning program are specific to the type of stress applied and to the particular system of the body that is exercised.

All of the above might be summarized in one principle, the SAID principle (Specific Adaptation to Imposed Demands). The SAID principle states that if the body is placed under stress of varying intensities and durations, it attempts to overcome the stress by adapting specifically to the imposed demands.[16] While it is important to overload or place demands on the body so that improvement may occur, the stress should not be so severe as to prevent the body from being able to cope or adapt.

TABLE 2.3   Characteristics of Skeletal Muscle Fiber Types

Fiber Type	Contraction Speed	Endurance	Oxidative[a] or Glycolytic[b]	Burns Fat and Glycogen Aerobically
I	slow	yes	oxidative	yes
IIa	fast	yes	oxidative	yes
IIab	fast	some	oxidative and glycolytic	maybe
IIb	fast	no	glycolytic	no

[a] Oxidative = the ability to use oxygen for prolonged periods to synthesize and use ATP.
[b] Glycolytic = ability to function without oxygen, though only for short periods of time.

Strength

One muscle fiber consists of many myofibrils, which in turn is made up of many thousands of sarcomeres. When the sarcomeres receive the appropriate stimulation from the nervous system, chemical reactions occur which provide energy from ATP breakdown. This results in contraction of the sarcomeres as the actin "slides" on the myocin.

For muscle growth or hypertrophy to occur, the muscle must be stressed. When repetitively subjected to high-intensity demands, the muscle will respond by increasing in size and strength.

The improvement that might occur as a result of a strength-developing program is influenced by the level of strength possessed by the individual at the onset of the program as well as by the method and intensity of the program. Strength programs can be classified according to the type of resistance that is applied to the limb (Table 2.4).

The first step in formulating an individual strength-training program is to determine the:

1. type of resistance to be used
2. amount of weight or resistance to be used
3. number of repetitions per set
4. number of sets per workout
5. number of workout sessions per week

The level of strength may be determined by using devices such as a

1. cable tensiometer
2. dynamometer
3. Cybex isokinetic dynamometer

However, the most commonly used "in-the-field" determination of the starting level of strength is the one-repetition maximum, which seems to be adequate for that purpose.

When attempting to develop strength, it is necessary to work at maximum resistance in order to maximize gains. Berger's studies found that those individuals training with four, six, and eight repetitions per set showed significantly greater gains than those who trained with two, ten, and twelve repetitions per set.[17]

DeLorme[18,19] developed a system based upon a maximum of ten repetitions (10RM):

	Resistance	**Repetitions**
First set	50% of 10 RM	10 repetitions
Second set	75% of 10 RM	10 repetitions
Third set	100% of 10 RM	10 repetitions

The specific strength-development program should be individualized and determined according to the needs of the athlete. The trainer should be familiar with the correct lifting techniques used in different types of strength-training programs (Figure 2.3).[20,21]

TABLE 2.4 Commonly Used Types of Resistance

Type of Resistance	Type of Movement	Device Used
Isometric	Muscle contraction, no movement	Any immovable object or device
Isotonic concentric eccentric	Fixed resistance, variable speed of movement Contraction with muscle shortening Contraction with muscle lengthening	Free weights Wall pulleys Guided weight apparatus (Universal Gym, Nautilus, etc.)
Isokinetic	Fixed speed, resistance accommodates to force applied (accommodative resistance)	Cybex, Orthotron

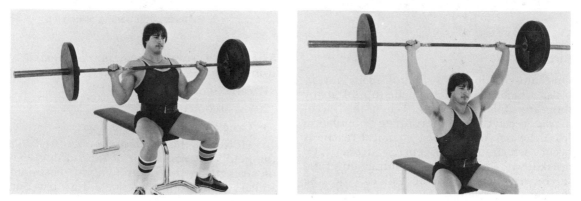

FIGURE 2.3a Seated Military Press

Beginning position: Seated, the bar in a chest-rest position. **Grip:** Pronated, with the hands placed slightly wider than the shoulders. **Technique:** Sit erect, chest high, press bar overhead until arms are outstretched, keep bar close to body, keep head up, lower bar to beginning position. **Breathing:** Inhale during the upward movement and exhale during the downward movement. **Major muscles Involved:** trapezius, serratus anterior, anterior deltoid, pectoralis major, triceps.

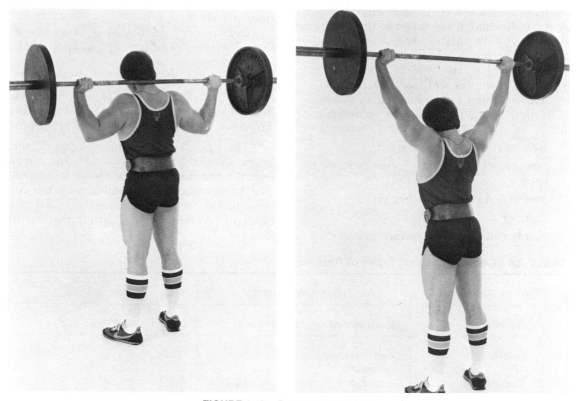

FIGURE 2.3b Press Behind Neck

Beginning position: Bar behind the head lightly touching the base of the neck. **Grip:** Pronated, with hands placed wider than the shoulders. **Technique:** Press bar overhead until arms are extended. **Breathing:** Inhale during the upward movement, and exhale during the downward movement. **Major muscles involved:** upper trapezius, middle and anterior deltoids, triceps.

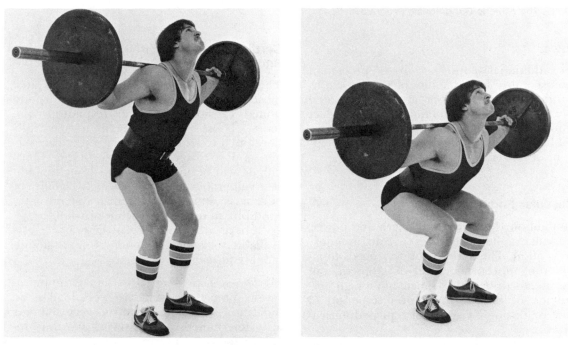

FIGURE 2.3c Squat
Beginning position: Bar resting across the shoulders, head held erect. **Grip:** Pronated, hands placed wider than the shoulders. **Technique:** Squat with control until the thighs are parallel to the floor. **Major muscles involved:** erector spinae, quadriceps, gluteus maximus, hamstrings.

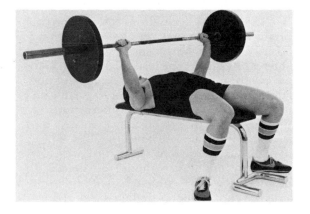

FIGURE 2.3d Bench Press (*left*)
Beginning position: Receive the bar (from spotter) while supine, head supported on the bench, back flat, and feet on floor. **Grip:** Pronated, placed slightly wider than shoulder width. **Technique:** Lower the bar to a light touch of the upper chest and pressure the bar to a lock-out position of the elbow. **Breathing:** Inhale when lower bar to the chest, exhale when press is completed. **Major muscles involved:** anterior deltoid, pectoralis major, latissimus dorsi, triceps.

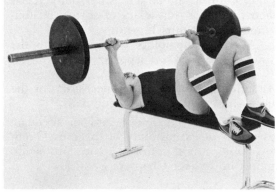

FIGURE 2.3e Bench Press Variation (*right*)
In order to prevent hyperextension and thus protect the lower back, the feet may be placed on the bench.

Power

An additional contribution to protection against injury is the ability of the muscle to contract or exert force at an accelerated speed (power may be defined as the product of force and speed). The isokinetic apparatus has been shown to be useful in the development of power.[22,23]

Muscular Endurance

In addition to muscular strength and power, muscular endurance plays a role in injury prevention. The athlete not only needs to attain the appropriate level of strength, but also needs to be able to maintain a high percentage of that strength over a period of time or through a series of repeated muscular efforts.

The general principles that apply to strength development also apply to the development of muscular endurance, so that strength-training methods can be adapted for use in muscular-endurance training with the following modifications:

1. Reduce the amount of resistance
2. Increase the rate of work
3. Increase the number of repetitions and, possibly, sets

Flexibility

Another quality of the muscular system that is important to the athlete is flexibility. It has been suggested that a lack of normal flexibility may lead to muscle strains.

Adequate flexibility is important to the athlete in at least two aspects:

1. Full range of motion is necessary for the successful execution of athletic skills.[24]
2. Normal resting length and an adequate excursion of extensibility of the muscle-tendon unit might afford some protection against injury (see Chapters 1 and 3).

Cardiovascular-Respiratory (Aerobic) Endurance

The ability of the athlete to sustain repeated muscular effort requires adequately conditioned cardiovascular and respiratory systems. These systems need to be fully developed to extract, deliver, and utilize oxygen and so prolong the time before which fatigue will occur. Fatigue can leave the athlete vulnerable to injury through inability to effectively utilize the muscular system or respond to an injury-producing situation.

There are a number of laboratory tests available for assessing the level of cardiopulmonary fitness.

1. *Step-up tests.* These tests utilize the pulse-rate response to a standard work load as an indication of fitness.[25] The recovery ability is also determined, by measuring the time required for the pulse rate to return to a predetermined percentage of the resting heart rate.

2. *Bicycle ergometer and treadmill testing.* This is used to measure the maximal oxygen uptake, the maximal rate at which oxygen can be utilized during exercise (VO_2Max).

"In-the-field testing" is more practical for the athletic trainer in assessing the cardiovascular-respiratory status of groups of athletes. Results from tests such as the Cooper twelve-minute run or the one-and-one-half-mile run can be compared to established norms;[26] but it is probably of more value for the individual to establish his or her own base line of distance or time.

The development of cardiovascular-respiratory endurance should be specific to the needs of the athlete.[25] The following variables should therefore be considered:

1. Intensity of training activity
2. Duration of workouts
3. Frequency of workouts

The *intensity* of activity can be simply determined by the response of the pulse, presuming the athlete has been adequately screened before participating in the endurance program (see Chapter 1). Utilizing the heart rate as an indicator of the effect of the activity on the athlete, the appropriate level of intensity can then be prescribed. For instance, the age-related maximal heart rate for the twenty-to-thirty-year-old is usually listed at 190 beats per minute. If it is determined that the athlete should work at 80 percent of this maximal heart rate, then the appropriate "training heart rate" for the athlete would be 152 beats per minute for at least ten to fifteen minutes at a time. This is the training heart rate for the endurance portion of the program. However, the *duration* needs to be determined by the athlete's present level of conditioning. A session of at least 30 minutes, while maintaining the pulse at a target heart rate, should produce significant endurance conditioning. The minimal number of workouts (*frequency*) that will have an effect on the athlete's endurance is two sessions of aerobic activity per week; most athletes should have at least three or four sessions per week.

Anaerobic Conditioning

While aerobic fitness is important for the prevention of fatigue, there is a need for the development of the anaerobic systems of the body. The improvement of anaerobic conditioning will depend upon the type of athletic

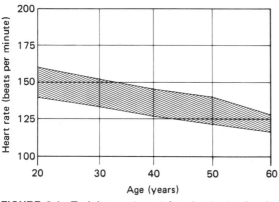

FIGURE 2.4 Training or target heart rate to develop endurance

activity in which the athlete is engaged. For instance, rapid explosive movements of short duration demand this type of conditioning in order to build up a reserve of high energy compounds and to train the system to resynthesize these compounds at a faster rate. However, the anaerobic system also needs to be developed by athletes participating in longer-duration activities, e.g., by interval training.

This discussion has been concerned with the pre-season conditioning program. However, for complete injury prevention purposes there needs to be concern for:

1. *The in-season conditioning program.* Many athletes consider that mere participation in athletic activity can effectively produce a high state of physical conditioning, and they do not realize that without a specifically planned program the various components of physical fitness can deteriorate during the season.

2. *The post-season conditioning program.* This phase of the program should identify and emphasize the areas that need special rehabilitation, and should help to maintain at an adequate level each of the components that make up the term *physical fitness*.

REFERENCES

1. Reid SE, Schiffbauer W: Role of athletic trainers in prevention, care and treatment of injuries. *Lancet* 77:83–84, 1957.
2. Gallagher JR: *Understanding Your Son's Adolescence.* Boston, Little, Brown and Company, 1951.
3. Rasch PJ: Endurance training for athletes. *J Assoc Phys Mental Rehabil* 13:182–185, 1959.
4. Thorndike A: *Athletic Injuries.* Philadelphia, Lea and Febiger, 1956.
5. Adams A: Effect of exercise on ligament strength. *Res Q* 37:163–167, 1966.
6. Falls HB, Wallis EL, Logan GA: *Foundations of Conditioning.* New York, Academic Press, 1970.
7. Kraus H: Physical conditioning and the prevention of athletic injury. American Medical Association, *Proceedings of the 7th National Conference on the Medical Aspects of Sports*, Chicago, November 30, 1966, pp. 98–103.
8. Cahill BR, Griffith EH: Effect of preseason condi-

tioning on the incidence and severity of high school football knee injuries. *Am J Sports Med* 6:180–183, 1978.

9. Gollnick PD, Hermansen L, Saltin B: The muscle biopsy: still a research tool. *Phys Sportsmed* 8:50–55, January 1980.

10. Saltin B, Henricksson E, Nygaard E, et al: Fiber types and metabolic potentials of skeletal muscles in sedentary man and endurance athletes. *Ann NY Acad Sci* 301:3–29, 1977.

11. Andersen P, Henriksson J: Training induced changes in the subgroups of human type II skeletal muscle fibres. *Acta Physiol Scand* 99:123–125, 1977.

12. Asmussen E: Muscle fatigue. *Med Sci Sports* 11:313–321, 1979.

13. Essen B, Häggmark T: Lactate concentration in type I and II muscle fibres during muscular contraction in man. *Acta Physiol Scand* 95:344–346, 1975.

14. Gollnick PD: Relationship of strength and endurance with skeletal muscle structure and metabolic potential. *Inter J Sports Med* 3:26–32, 1982.

15. Thorstensson A, Hulten B, von Döblen W, et al: Effects of strength training on enzyme activities and fiber characteristics in human skeletal muscle. *Acta Physiol Scand* 96:392–398, 1976.

16. Allman FL: *Sports Medicine*. Ryan AJ, Allman FL, editors. New York, Academic Press, 1974, p. 311.

17. Berger RA: Effect of varied weight training programs on strength. *Res Q* 33:168–181, 1962.

18. DeLorme T: Heavy resistance exercises. *Arch Phys Med Rehabil* 27:607–630, 1946.

19. DeLorme T, Watkins A: Techniques of progressive resistance exercise. *Arch Phys Med Rehabil* 29:263–273, 1948.

20. O'Shea JP: *Scientific Principles and Methods of Strength Fitness*. Reading Ma, Addison-Wesley, 1969.

21. Brady TA, Cahill BR, Bodnar LM: Weight training-related injuries in the high school athlete. *Am J Sports Med* 10:1–5, 1982.

22. Councilman JE: The importance of speed in exercise. *Scholastic Coach* 46:94–99, 1976.

23. Halling AH, Dooley JN: Importance of isokinetic power and its specificity to athletic conditions. *Athletic Training* 14:83–86, 1979.

24. Shon D, Treadway L: Developing and testing flexibility. *Phys Sportsmed* 6:137–138, October 1978.

25. Atomi Y: Effects of intensity and frequency of training on aerobic work capacity of young females. *J Sports Med Phys Fitness* 18:3–9, 1978.

26. Cooper K: *The New Aerobics*. New York, Bantam Books, 1970.

RECOMMENDED READINGS

Åstrand PO, Rodahl K: *Textbook of Work Physiology*. New York, McGraw-Hill, second edition, 1977.

Aten DW, Knight KL: Therapeutic exercise in athletic training—Principles and overview. *Athletic Training* 13:123–126, 1978.

Caldwell F: The search for strength. *Phys Sportmed* 6:83–88, January 1978.

Costill DL, Coyle WF, Fink GR, et al: Adaptations in skeletal muscle following strength training. *J Appl Physiol* 46:96–99, 1976.

Miles S: Sports fitness and its relationship to sports injuries. *Br J Sports Med* 11:46–49, 1977.

Pipes TV: Strength training modes: What's the difference? *Scholastic Coach* 46:96 and 120–124, 1977.

Shephard RJ: Aerobic versus anaerobic training for success in various athletic events. *Can J Appl Sport Sci* 3:9–15, 1978.

CHAPTER 3

The Warm-Up Period

Is the Warm-Up Necessary?

Most athletes consider the warm-up an integral part of their event. It is something that helps get their bodies and minds ready for the workout or competition. They feel that it not only helps their performance, but it also helps prevent injuries.

Most research seems to agree with these subjective impressions. It appears that an increase in the temperature within the muscles is necessary for the attainment of optimal performance, though an elevation of the core temperature is also considered an important criterion. The athlete's body tends to work more efficiently, more safely, and at a higher level when "warmed up."

Some of the advantages of the warm-up include a raised maximal oxygen intake, a reduction in the oxygen needed for a specific activity, and a reduction in the resistance of pulmonary blood flow. In addition, there is an increased rate of neuromuscular transmission and recruitment of muscle fibers, as well as activation of "neuromuscular memory" for the specific movements that are necessary for the event. From the psychological standpoint the warm-up helps the athlete to focus on the forthcoming action.

Every athlete should be encouraged to find the type of warm-up that is best suited for his or her personality and sport. Much of this may be related to subjective impressions, superstitions, the influence of coaches, or what the athletes happened to do on a particular day when they performed well. It would seem, though, that a warm-up schedule that is related to the event would be preferable, particularly if certain aspects of

the event could be practiced as part of the warm-up.

The intensity and duration of the warm-up should be governed by the event and the level of fitness of the athlete; for instance, a high-performance, well-conditioned athlete may require twenty to thirty minutes of fairly intense exercise in order to perform at his or her maximal potential. This type of warm-up would be totally inappropriate for a less-well-conditioned athlete and would result in exhaustion. For the muscle temperature to be at a satisfactory level, the rectal temperature should have increased by two degrees. If an athlete is sweating freely in normal climatic conditions, it can be assumed this temperature has been reached.

In the final analysis, it appears that there is sufficient evidence to endorse the concept of a well-thought-out and organized warm-up program as long as it is adjusted to the level and the needs of the individual athlete.

An Outline of a Warm-Up Schedule

Here is an outline of a warm-up and warm-down schedule which combines general with specific warm-up activities:

1. *Stretching.* The initial stretching should be gentle, light, and limited to the muscles that will be stressed.

2. *Jogging.* The athlete should jog or run over a distance and at a pace related to his or her degree of fitness and type of sport. This should produce sweating and an increase in the core temperature.

3. *Stretching.* Following the jogging, the athlete should stretch slowly but thoroughly.

4. *Sport-specific warm-up activities.* These should be performed next and should consist of such exercises as skill-drills incorporating the actual activities of that sport.

5. *Rest period.* In order to regain body homeostasis the athlete should relax for a period of about ten minutes before participating. During this time he or she may wish to engage in visualization of the event and positive "psyching-up" thoughts.

6. *The event.*

7. *Post-event warm-down.* Following the event, the athlete should be allowed a warm-down activity period of about three to five minutes. This has the effect of removing lactic acid and other products of metabolism from the muscles and tissues, thereby helping reduce some of the stiffness and tightness so often experienced the following day. This also allows the athlete time to settle down physically and psychologically after the outpouring of adrenalin and the excitement of the event.

8. *Stretching.* Following the warm-down period, stretching should be repeated. Many athletes find this to be mentally relaxing as well. The amount of stretching undertaken depends on the intensity and type of event.

Stretching

The type of stretching that is advocated is a slow, gentle stretch in which the athlete begins to become acquainted with the flexibility of his or her muscles. The athlete needs to be educated in this type of stretching technique. There should be no competition with other athletes, as each individual has a different amount of normal flexibility and a different potential for developing further flexibility.

The main advantages of this type of stretching are related to the athlete's increased body awareness and to learning how to relax. At the same time, it appears that the increased flexibility which is achieved also enhances performance and probably helps reduce injuries. This is particularly true for those who have tight muscles and those engaged in sporting activities that tend to produce muscle imbalances, such as long-distance running (tight hamstrings) and basketball (tight hamstrings and back muscles).

While he or she is stretching, the athlete's mind should be focused on the body as well as on slow, gentle, normal breathing. In this way the athlete begins to feel the subtleties of muscle tension, contraction, and relaxation, of which, in all likelihood, he or she was previously unaware. The athlete also learns that the body is never the same on two successive days—the degree of flexibility achieved on one day may not be repeatable on the next. This should be considered normal, and adjustments for these variabilities should be made on a day-to-day basis.

Coaches should be educated in the art of stretching, particularly with reference to encouraging the athlete's concentration on what he or she is doing at the time, and in the need to discourage competition between athletes in achieving increased flexibility. The athlete should, by concentration and experience, learn what is right for his or her particular body and thus achieve maximal results. The coach should discourage any bouncing or rapid movements and should point out muscle tensions unnoticed by the athlete. Such tensions are manifested by active muscle contractions, quivering of the muscles, a strained expression on the athlete's face, holding of the breath, or to-and-fro bouncing movements.

Ballistic stretching, or rapid bouncing, has very few good features. The basic argument against ballistic stretching is that muscles will reflexively contract when suddenly stretched. Therefore the stretch will be against a contracted muscle which (a) can injure the muscle tissue, and (b) will not produce any actual stretching of the muscle. It also has undesirable psychological features compared with the slow, static stretch. It is not advised.

In the beginning, the athlete should gently hold the stretch in a comfortable position for approximately ten to fifteen seconds. There should be no straining, no breath holding, and no feeling of pain or discomfort. In fact, it should seem easy, as if nothing is being achieved. During this stage the athlete first becomes aware of unknown tensions and inappropriate muscle contractions. For instance, while stretching the hamstrings, he or she might notice the quadriceps muscles contracting. As the athlete learns to concentrate, these inappropriate muscle contractions tend to disappear.

As the athlete becomes more experienced in the technique of stretching, the duration of the stretch should be increased to thirty seconds, and eventually up to a minute at a time. Even during these extended periods of stretching, there should be no tension or holding of the breath and no pain, though there might be some initial discomfort.

Stretching should be a pleasant, enjoyable experience. It should not be a painful, uncomfortable time spent wishing that one were doing something else. Each athlete needs to learn what stretches are most applicable to his or her particular athletic activity as well as what is necessary for his or her particular body type. Some basic stretches are shown in Figures 3.1 through 3.7.

FIGURE 3.1 Hamstring stretch To isolate the stretch to the hamstrings, keep the body erect. Move forward at the hips only. Do *not* let the head and neck come forward. Ensure that the quadriceps relax.

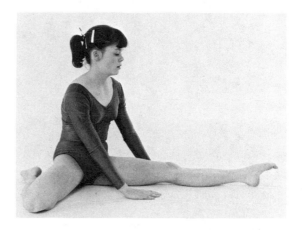

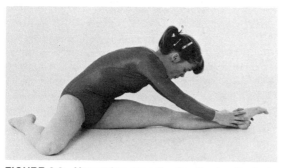

FIGURE 3.2 Hamstring stretch By allowing the body and head to come forward towards the knee, the stretch includes not only the hamstrings, but also the back.

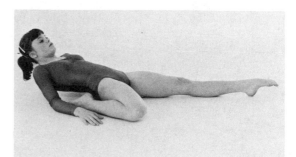

FIGURE 3.3 Quadriceps stretch This stretch should be done cautiously by athletes with medial ligament laxity or by those who have a tendency to sublux the patella.

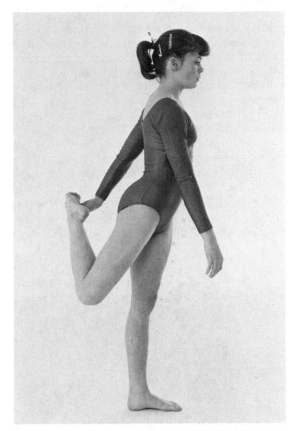

FIGURE 3.4 Quadriceps stretch The hip should be extended in order to stretch the rectus femoris muscle.

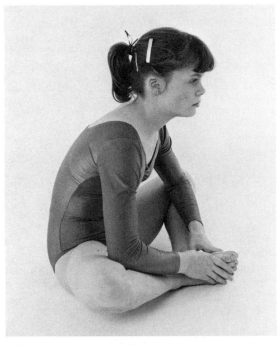

FIGURE 3.5 Groin stretch The elbows may be used to exert pressure and thus increase the stretch.

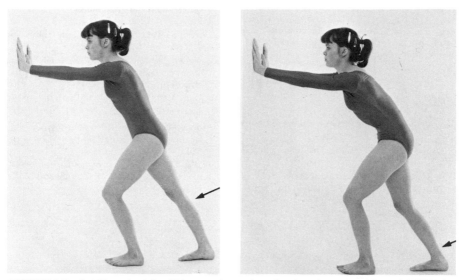

FIGURE 3.6 Achilles stretch This stretch needs to be done in two positions. **(a)** With the knee straight in order to stretch the gastrocnemius. **(b)** The knee is bent to concentrate the stretch on the soleus. *Note:* the foot should be pointing straight ahead, and the arch should be maintained and not allowed to flatten out.

Partner Stretching Using the Proprioceptive Neuromuscular Facilitation Technique

Some athletes with very tight muscles find it exceedingly difficult to relax so as to accomplish the initial stages of stretching. In order to help these athletes, a partner-stretching program may be helpful. Stretching of the hamstrings is illustrated in Figure 3.7.

The athlete lifts the leg with the knee straight until a feeling of tension is experienced in the hamstrings. This position is then held for ten seconds, following which the athlete pushes downwards with maximal effort while keeping the knee extended. The trainer provides isometric resistance. This contraction is held for five seconds, following which the hamstrings are again gently stretched by the trainer. The procedure is repeated a number of times. After three or four such repetitions, an increase in hamstring flexibility should be noticed. This technique can be performed in the same manner with other muscle groups.

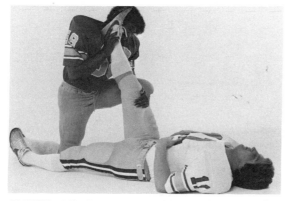

FIGURE 3.7 Partner stretching (using the PNF technique) The leg is held by the partner so the knee is straight and the hamstrings are comfortably stretched. The athlete then pushes the leg as firmly as possible against the partner's resistance, keeping the knee straight. This sequence is repeated several times.

REFERENCE

1. Surburg PR: Neuromuscular facilitation techniques in sports medicine. *Phys Sportsmed* 9:114–127, September 1981.

RECOMMENDED READINGS

Anderson B: *Stretching.* Bolinas CA, Shelter Publications, 1980.

Beaulieu JE: *Stretching for All Sports.* Pasadena, Athletic Press, 1980.

Cornelius WL, Hinson MM: The relationship between isometric contractions of hip extensors and subsequent flexibility in males. *J Sports Med Phys Fitness* 20:75–80, 1980.

Cornelius WL: Two effective flexibility methods. **Athletic Training** 16:23–25, 1981.

deVries HA: *Physiology of Exercise for Physical Education and Athletics.* Dubuque Iowa, William C. Brown Company, third edition, 1980.

Knight KL: Cryostretch for muscle spasm. In Trainer's Corner, *Phys Sportsmed* 8:129, April 1980.

Moore MA, Hutton RS: Electromyographic investigation of muscle stretching. *Med Sci Sports Exerci* 12:322–329, 1980.

Wallis EL, Logan GA: *Figure Improvement and Body Conditioning Through Exercise.* Englewood Cliffs NJ, Prentice-Hall, 1964.

CHAPTER 4

Protective and Supportive Equipment

In some sports it may be necessary to utilize protective equipment to

1. protect the athlete from injury
2. protect an injury from additional trauma

Protective Equipment

In the selection and utilization of protective equipment, the athletic trainer needs to ask the following questions:

1. Is the particular protective device or item required by the rules of the sport?

EXAMPLE: NCAA Football Rules[1] (1979), Section 4, Article 4: "All players must wear the following mandatory equipment:

   a. Soft kneepads at least a half-inch thick worn over the knee
   b. Head protectors with a secured four-point chin strap
   c. Shoulder pads, hip pads, thigh guards
   d. A single intra-oral mouth protector comprised of at least two portions: one an interocclusal portion, the other a labial portion."

2. If the protective item is required, or the decision is made to utilize the item, what standards have been established to assist the athletic trainer in the purchase of the item?

EXAMPLE: NCAA Football Rules[1] (1979), Section 4, Article 4: "All players shall wear head protectors which carry the manufacturer's or reconditioner's certification indicating satisfaction of NOCSAE* test standards."[2]

3. Have there been research studies to determine if the item of protective equipment is of value in the prevention of injuries?[3,4]

4. Is an exact fit of the protective item necessary in order to obtain adequate protection?

EXAMPLE: The fit of the suspension-type football helmet.

5. Is maintenance, repair, and storage of each item of protective equipment necessary to preserve the protective qualities of that item?

6. How important is the role of the regulation uniform in protecting the athlete? In some sports the rules require that the uniform conform to certain standards of fit, and be in good repair.

EXAMPLE: NCAA Football Rules[1] (1979), Section 4, Article 4: "If a player's jersey is so torn that it does not conform with rules 1–4–4e, he must leave the game to repair or replace the torn jersey."

7. Is it important for an athlete to develop a positive attitude in order to accept a particular item of protective equipment?

*NOCSAE: National Operating Committee on Standards for Athletic Equipment.

EXAMPLE: In wrestling, ear protectors are mandatory for collegiate competition. However, if the wrestler does not wear them during practice, he may sustain an ear injury.

8. Is there emphasis on developing a philosophy towards protective equipment which stresses the prevention of injuries and not the utilization of equipment as an offensive weapon? The increased incidence of cervical injuries in recent years is an indication of the wrong attitude taken by both coaches and players. Torg et al.[5] report that " . . . development of a protective helmet-face mask system (as used in football) has effectively protected the head and by doing so allowed it to be used as a battering ram in tackling and blocking techniques. . . . "

Fitting the Football Helmet*†

Although the modern helmet is not capable of eliminating head injuries completely, it does appear to significantly lessen their severity. Wearing an improperly fitted helmet enhances the opportunity for head injuries. Although the following comments concern the fitting of the suspension-type helmet, the same principles and testing procedures apply to fitting other types of helmets including the padded, the air, and the fluid-lined helmets.

General preparation. (See Fig. 4.1 a through h.)

1. Fit helmet at normal hair length.

2. Observe any noticeable head-shape variation such as a long oval head, a slanting

*Adapted from *Comments in Sports Medicine*.[6] Reprinted by permission of the American Medical Association.

†In this section, the player is assumed to be a male. While the majority of football players are male, it should be pointed out that a number of female football teams exist. The procedure for fitting the helmet is the same for both sexes.

forehead, a heavy brow, or an extra-large occipital bone.

3. If the helmet is a suspension type, check to make sure the knot is tied correctly.

Proper method of placing the head into the helmet.

1. Put thumbs in earholes of the helmet, and hold the helmet with fingers placed along the sides (Figure 4.1a).

2. Put the helmet directly over the head, then tilt it backward and rotate it to the front while pulling it down into position (Figures 4.1b and 4.1c).

3. Make sure the neckband is not rolled up; if it is, shift the helmet forward.

Side-to-side check.

1. Make a quick visual examination to be sure the fit is close to being correct.

2. Have the player hold his head straight forward, and try to turn the helmet on his head. The helmet should turn only slightly if the fit is correct (Figure 4.1d).

Note: The helmet on a long oval-shaped head may turn somewhat even if properly fitted, due to excessive room on each side. This can be checked by inserting the fingers inside the helmet and along the suspension and can be corrected by spacers.

Crown adjustment.

1. Check visually to see if the helmet sits about one finger-breadth above the eyebrows.

2. Exert firm pressure on the top of the helmet, and press straight down. Ask the player if he feels the top of his head against the rubber crown, or if all the pressure is across the forehead. If the latter, the helmet is too low and should be adjusted (Figure 4.1e).

3. The neckband should be snug and positioned comfortably. A loose neckband will permit the helmet to rotate forward. Al-

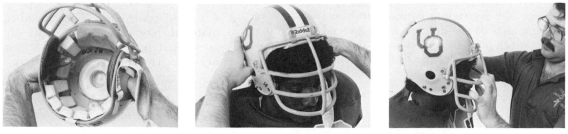

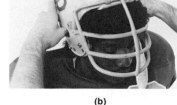

(a)   (b)   (c)

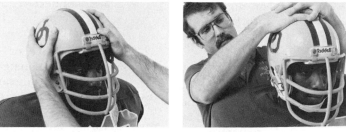

(d)   (e)

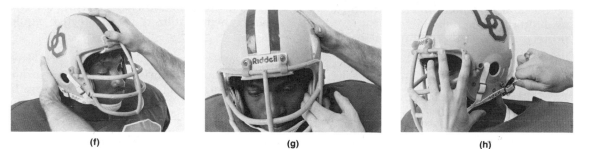

(f)   (g)   (h)

FIGURE 4.1   Fitting the football helmet

though neckbands come in ten sizes, and are fitted into proportionately sized helmets, it is possible that a player could require a non-standard size.

Back-press test for continued forehead pressure.

If a player feels undue pressure on his forehead, stand facing him and put one of your forearms on his shoulder with your hand on the back of the helmet. While the player braces his head against your hand, check the forehead clearance. The suspension should be able to slide slightly on the forehead but should not leave a large gap (Figure 4.1f).

Jaw-pad fit.

A correctly sized pad fits the jaw area snugly and prevents lateral rocking of the helmet. Pads are available in four sizes (Figure 4.1g).

Chin-strap fit.

1. Adjust the chin strap to a tight position, with equal tension on both sides. A tight chin strap facilitates dental occlusion and helps keep the helmet in its proper position (Figure 4.1h).

2. The chin strap should release under high load; it should never be "locked" on.

3. The four-point chin strap gives added support by restricting forward and backward movements of the helmet. Its enhanced safety features prevent bothersome and unnecessary lacerations over the bridge of the nose.

Final check.

1. After removing the properly fitting helmet, recheck to be sure the square knot is tight and the crownpiece is secure.

2. Enter the player's name or number in the helmet and record this information in your files. Ensure that each player always wears his own helmet.

The protective value of a football helmet is indisputable, but research has not yet produced a helmet that can fully protect the brain in a vigorous contact sport such as football. The trainer can help maximize the helmet's protective value by ensuring a perfect fit and by taking other precautions such as requiring the athlete to wear a mouth protector, develop strong neck muscles, and use proper blocking and tackling techniques.

Though the fitting of protective equipment is illustrated by using the example of a football player, the same principles apply to other contact or collision sports such as ice hockey and lacrosse.

Fabrication of Protective and Supportive Devices

The trainer should be knowledgeable and proficient in the design, fabrication, and use of various types of protective and supportive devices. Each device should be individually designed and fitted, the only limitation being the rules of the sport in which the athlete is participating and the imagination of the trainer.

Materials. The trainer should be familiar with the various available materials that are suitable for the fabrication of protective and supportive devices. These materials can be classified as follows:

1. Shock-absorbing material.

   a. *Closed-cell construction.* The closed-cell material has component cells that are closed and sealed so that air cannot pass from one cell to another.

EXAMPLE: Ensolite, which is a foam blended from nitrated rubber and PVC. The cells of PVC are filled with nitrogen.

   b. *Open-cell construction.* Open-cell material consists of component cells that are connected by passageways so that air can pass freely from one cell to another.

2. Hard dispersive or deflective material. High-impact plastic material is used mainly for the shell of headgear. This material is usually selected because of its ability to distribute the forces applied against it and to resist deformation.

3. Other materials. New materials of various consistencies and characteristics are constantly being utilized for protective equipment.

EXAMPLE: Pneumatic (air-filled) protective pads. In certain sports, rules exist regarding the type of protective equipment that can be prescribed.

EXAMPLE: NCAA Football Rules[1] (1979), Section 4, Article 5: "No hard or unyielding substances on the hand, wrist, forearm, or elbow of any player, no matter how well covered or padded. No hard or unyielding substance in thigh guards, shin guards, knee or leg braces unless such an article is covered on both sides and all of its edges are overlapped with closed-cell slow-recovery foam padding no less than one-half inch thick, or an alternate material of the same minimum thickness having similar physical properties." An example of an exception is the soft playing splint introduced by the Cleveland Clinic—a custom-made rubber splint devised to allow safe sports participation with significant hand and wrist injuries. This splint is acceptable to the NCAA for use in intercollegiate contact sports (Figure 4.2).[7,8]

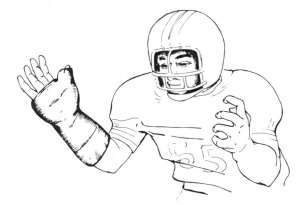

FIGURE 4.2   A soft splint for wrist and hand injuries that may be used in a game situation (Details may be obtained from the Cleveland Clinic, Section of Sports Medicine, Cleveland, Ohio.)

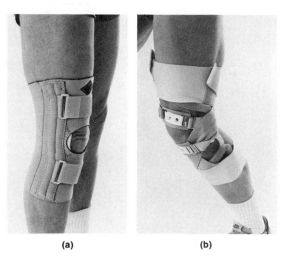

(a)   (b)

FIGURE 4.3a   A neoprene sleeve, which may incorporate a patellar stabilizing pad, or medial and lateral metal stays

FIGURE 4.3b   The Lenox Hill derotation brace is particularly useful in rotational instabilities of the knee. The brace is used following knee ligament injuries, particularly those involving the anterior cruciate ligament, which result in anteromedial and/or antrolateral rotatory instability.

The trainer should always keep in mind that protective equipment should not endanger other players, and should therefore choose materials that will protect the player from an injury without being harmful to others.

Supportive devices. There are numerous types of supportive devices available. In deciding on the appropriate device for a particular situation, the athletic trainer needs to consider the

1. anatomical area involved
2. types of material available
3. appliances available

EXAMPLE: The knee joint is an area that often needs some sort of brace or supportive device (Figure 4.3). Some of the methods for supporting this area include:

1. adhesive taping, elastic wrapping, or both (see Chapter 5)
2. elastic sleeve with or without plastic or metal supports on one or both sides, which may also be hinged
3. neoprene sleeve with or without a patellar stabilizer or pad
4. various combinations of other materials[9]

Protective devices.   Use may be made of the *donut* design, in which the padding is placed around the injury in order to transmit the force of impact to uninvolved areas. The material usually selected for construction of this pad is one of the softer materials (closed- or open-cell).

The *bubble* or *bridge* type of injury pad deflects the force or isolates the injury from additional contact. The material utilized for the shell is one of the plastics, fiberglass, or a material that can be molded or shaped into the desired form. When hardened or "cured," it forms a rigid protection.[10,11,12]

Motion-limiting devices.   The best example of a motion-limiting device is the shoulder harness. In cases of shoulder dislocation or subluxation, there may be a need to restrict excessive abduction and external rotation, and this can be achieved by applying a harness around the chest and upper arm (Figure 4.6).

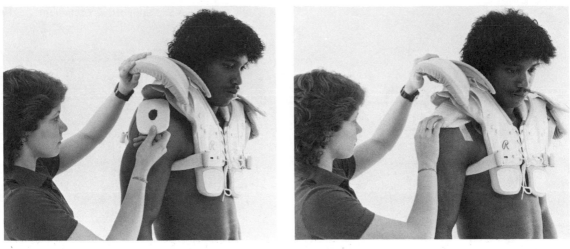

(a)   **(b)**

FIGURE 4.4   Donut pad   (a) In this example, the donut pad is used to take the pressure off a contused distal clavicle (i.e., a "shoulder pointer").   **(b)** The donut is covered with padding.

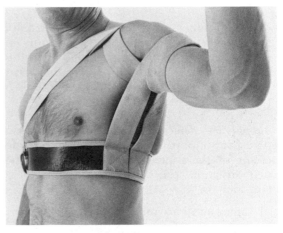

FIGURE 4.6a   West Point shoulder harness This device is used to limit abduction and external rotation of the glenohumeral joint, and thereby helps reduce the incidence of anterior subluxation and/or dislocation of the shoulder.

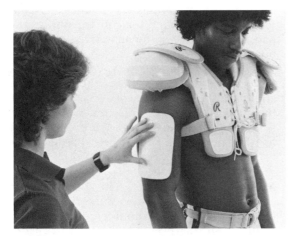

FIGURE 4.5   Lateral humeral protector This particular model is one that can easily be constructed in a training room setting from Regalite and Plastazote. These materials are heated in a convection oven and then molded to the athlete's arm.

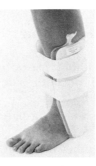

FIGURE   4.6b   The   Airsplint This is used following ankle sprains to limit inversion or eversion, yet allow plantar flexion and dorsiflexion.

Another example of a condition demanding restricted motion is that following the "pinched nerve syndrome" involving the brachial plexus, where it may be considered useful or necessary to restrict excessive movement of the cervical spine. This may be accomplished by the use of a cervical collar or by attaching restraining straps on the helmet and shoulder pads.[13]

REFERENCES

1. National Collegiate Athletic Association, *NCAA Football Rules.* Shawnee Mission Kansas, 1979.

2. Cushing D: Helmet reconditioning: Does NOCSAE ensure safety? *Phys Sportsmed* 8:101–104, October 1980.

3. Clarke KS, Powell JW: Football helmets and neurotrauma—an epidemiological overview of three seasons. *Med Sci Sports* 11:138–145, 1979.

4. Hughes JR, Wilms JH, Adams CL, et al: Football helmet evaluation based on players EEG's. *Phys Sportsmed* 5:73–77, May 1977.

5. Torg JS, Truex Jr R, Quedenfeld T, et al: National Football Head-Neck Registry—report and conclusions. *JAMA* 241:1477–1479, 1979.

6. Craig T, editor: *Comments in Sports Medicine.* Chicago, American Medical Association, 1973.

7. Bergfeld JA, Andrish JT, Weiker G, et al: *Soft Playing Splint.* In Cleveland Clinic Foundation, Section of Sports Medicine, Cleveland, Ohio.

8. Bassett III FH, Malone T, Gilchrist RA: A protective splint of silicone rubber. *Am J Sports Med* 7:358–360, 1979.

9. Palumbo Jr PM: Dynamic patellar brace: a new orthosis in the management of patellofemoral disorders. A preliminary report. *Am J Sports Med* 9:45–49, 1981.

10. Wershing CE: A specialized pad for the acromioclavicular joint. *Athletic Training* 15:103–108, 1980.

11. Rylander RC: Custom-made protective pads and heel cup. *Athletic Training* 8:169–183, 1973.

12. Michel LM: Special pads for special problems. *Athletic Training* 14:68–69, 1979.

13. Andrish JT, Bergfeld JA, Romo LR: Method for the management of cervical injuries in football. A preliminary report. *Am J Sports Med* 5:89–92, 1977.

RECOMMENDED READINGS

Black RA: The football helmet crisis. *Interscholastic Athletics* 5:10–12, 1978.

Klein FC: Facts about the much abused football helmet. *Scholastic Coach* 48:4–6, 1978.

LaCava G: Environment, equipment and prevention of sports injuries. *J Sports Med Phys Fitness* 18:1–2, 1978.

Mac Collum MS: Protecting upper extremity injuries in sports. *Phys Sportsmed* 8:59–64, July 1980.

Mueller FO: Moderator Round Table on Protective Equipment: problems and promise. *Phys Sportsmed* 4:66–73, February 1976.

Ryan, AJ: Protective equipment—boon or bane? Editorial in *Phys Sportsmed* 4:80, February 1976.

PART II

The Treatment of Athletic Injuries

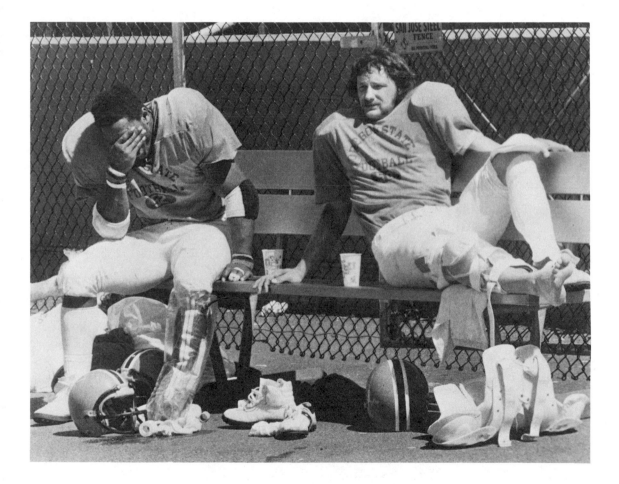

CHAPTER 5

Taping and Wrapping Techniques

Adhesive Taping

The application of adhesive taping as an athletic training tool is both an art and a science and has been developed over the years by coaches, athletic trainers, and sports medicine physicians. However, questions regarding the effectiveness of adhesive taping have not as yet been adequately answered by scientific investigation. Therefore, at this time much of the information regarding adhesive taping is strictly empirical.

Before the athletic trainer becomes involved in the techniques and procedures of taping, there are a series of questions that need to be considered:

1. Does adhesive taping actually prevent ligament sprains? Garrick and Requa[1] conducted a study in which high-top shoes plus preventive ankle taping decreased the frequency of ankle sprains in intramural basketball.[2]

2. Does adhesive taping provide support for a joint and, if so, for what period of time? There have been several studies concerned with the length of time and the degree to which adhesive taping contributes to the support of a joint. Some have shown that correct ankle taping provides significant support for only a relatively short period of time, while others indicate that it is quite effective.[3,4,5,6,7]

3. Does adhesive taping cause any adverse effects on the strength or the normal range of motion of the joint being taped? There has been some speculation that taping might result in the loss of muscular strength around the taped joint, but this idea has nev-

er been proven and does not appear to be clinically valid. Range of motion studies do not show significant impairment.[8,9]

4. Does adhesive taping enhance or restrict normal motor athletic performance (speed, agility, jumping ability, etc.)? Most studies that have investigated the effects of taping on motor performance have not found any negative results.[9,10]

5. Does adhesive taping cause an increased incidence of injury to an adjacent untaped joint? For instance, are there more knee injuries when the ankle is taped?[11,12] Garrick and Requa report that there was no increase in knee sprains in athletes who taped their ankles.[1]

6. Does adhesive taping produce any other protective effects in addition to the physical reinforcement of the normal supportive structures? There has been a study suggesting that ankle taping stimulates the peroneal muscles, resulting in earlier firing of these muscles, thereby preventing inversion ankle sprains.[10]

7. Does adhesive taping produce a physiological dependence that causes the athlete to neglect the physical conditioning aspect of prevention? This is theoretically possible, but in practice does not appear to be significant. Psychological dependence on tape after an injury does occur, but does not appear to produce any harmful effects besides being costly.

After studying the answers to the above questions, it becomes clear that more research is needed to define indications for, and effects of, taping. In particular, evidence needs to be accumulated regarding the advantage of one taping technique over another.

Taping is one of the athletic trainer's most useful tools, and he or she should develop sufficient and effective techniques. Taping skills should be developed by first acquiring the necessary background on the general principles and then proceeding on to specific techniques and variations.

General principles. The athletic trainer should:

1. Acquire a functional understanding of the normal joint and supportive structures (anatomy) and of joint movements (kinesiology)

2. Know the common mechanisms of injury as they might affect a particular joint

3. Visualize the purpose for which the adhesive taping is to be applied, that is, for full immobilization or for functional support of the joint through a particular range of motion

Guidelines for adhesive taping. The athletic trainer needs to learn to do the following:

1. Select the correct type and width of tape for the particular area in question.

2. Adequately prepare the area to be taped:
   a. Shave, clean, and dry the area to be taped if it is appropriate to do so.
   b. Utilize a suitable amount and type of tape adherent so the skin becomes "sticky." The trainer should be aware that skin sensitivity or allergic reactions to the adherent can develop, particularly to benzoin.[13,14]
   c. Use protective material (e.g., underwrap, gauze pads) between the skin and the tape in selected areas.
   d. Tape the affected part only when it is at normal body temperature—do not tape immediately after cold or hot treatments or after hydrotherapy.
   e. Be aware of skin sensitivity or an allergy to the tape itself. If this is found, apply the tape over a few layers of gauze pads or underwrap, or use nonallergenic tape.

3. Apply the tape in a smooth, firm manner, taking care not to crimp or wrinkle it, as this could interfere with the circulation, cause nerve, muscle, or tendon irritation, or result in blistering of the skin.

4. Position the joint correctly to achieve the objective or objectives of the taping procedure and at the same time permit free range of desirable and functional movements.

5. Properly tear the tape. The technique for this is to
   a. keep the tape in an extended or "stretched" position, not allowing the edge to fold over into the area of the tear
   b. use forearm movements and not finger movements when tearing the tape
   c. attempt to actually break the tape rather than tear it

6. Approach each taping procedure as an individualized problem that needs a specific taping technique for the prevention of a particular injury or the protection of an injured part.

7. Use a minimum of tape without compromising the objectives of the taping procedure.

8. Properly remove, or instruct the athlete to remove, the tape after participation is completed:
   a. Do not use excessive force or violent movements to remove the tape.

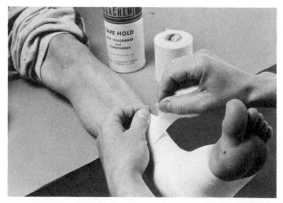

FIGURE 5.1 The technique of tearing tape

b. When cutting the tape off, use only bandage scissors or tape cutters designed for this specific purpose.

c. Utilize the proper technique with bandage scissors or tape cutters to avoid damaging the skin, letting natural concave areas of the body serve as "paths" for the cutting instrument (Figure 5.2).

9. Take proper care of the skin once the tape has been removed:

a. Clean the skin of all tape residue with soap and water, or use only those tape-removal liquids that are approved for this purpose.

b. Apply a moisturizing cream if the skin is dry.

c. Apply an antibiotic ointment if the tape has caused skin abrasions. If signs of infection or allergy develop, seek medical guidance.

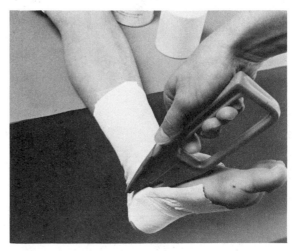

FIGURE 5.2 Using a tape cutter to remove tape

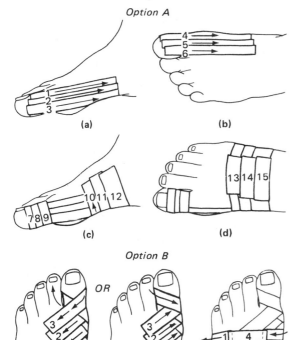

FIGURE 5.3 (*left*) **Big Toe Support**
Indications: Pain, particularly a sprain of the first metatarsophalangeal (M/P) joint. **Objectives:** To limit dorsiflexion and/or abduction of the first M/P joint. **Tape:** 2.5 cm/1 inch tape. **Taping position:** Athlete supine on taping table with foot over edge of table. The toe is placed in a "corrected" position. **Taping technique:**

Option A:
1. Longitudinal strips are placed on the superior-medial aspect of the foot. These strips extend from the mid-portion of the distal phalanx to proximal to the first metatarsal head (**a**).
2. Overlap additional longitudinal strips around to the plantar aspect of the toe and foot (**b**).
3. Secure the longitudinal strips by encircling tie-down strips around the toe and arch. *Caution*—do not apply these strips too tightly. Leave a gap on top of the foot and then bridge this gap with additional strips (**c**) and (**d**).

Option B: Half-figure-eight procedure
1. Begin the first strip on superior-medial aspect of the foot and then go between the big toe and the second toe, encircle the big toe and end on the superior aspect of the foot. These strips may be applied in a reverse direction (depending on correction needed) (**e**).
2. Continue with overlapping strips (using the same procedure as used for strip number one).
3. Secure in place as in Option A (**f**).

Note: These two procedures may be combined:
1. Apply Option A longitudinal strips.
2. Apply Option B half-figure-eight strips.
3. Secure with tie-down strips.

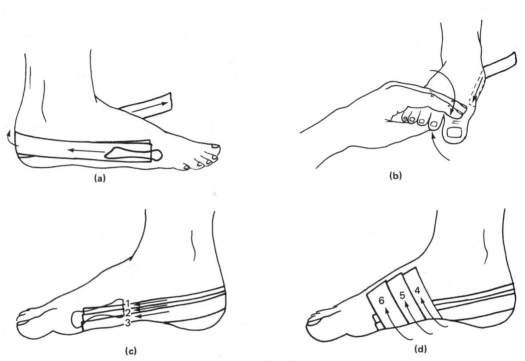

FIGURE 5.4 LowDye Taping

Indications: Medial arch strain; plantar fasciitis; excessive pronation. **Objectives:** To reduce strain on the plantar fascia and medial arch structures; to help control excessive pronation. **Tape:** 2.5 cm/1 inch tape. (Tape adhesive should also be used.) **Taping position:** Athlete sits on taping table with leg extended over the edge of the table. The foot should be relaxed. **Taping Technique:** Tape is applied to the lateral border of the foot, starting just proximal to the head of the fifth metatarsal. This tape is brought around the heel and lightly applied just proximal to the first metatarsal head (**a**). The plantar aspect of metatarsal heads 2 to 5 are supported by the thumb, and the first metatarsal head is depressed in a plantar direction by the index and middle fingers. Do *not* pronate the foot while doing this; keep the foot in a neutral position. Then secure the tape just proximal to the medial aspect of the first metatarsal head (**b**). Repeat this procedure 3 or 4 times (**c**). Then tie these strips down with circumferential strips running from the dorso-lateral aspect of the foot to the dorso-medial aspect (**d**).

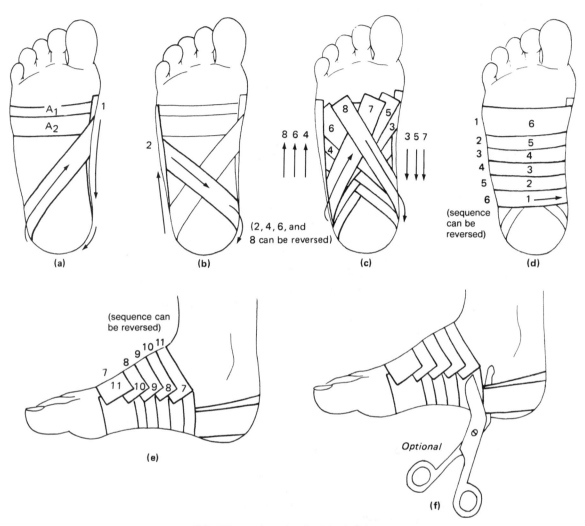

FIGURE 5.5 Longitudinal Arch Support

Indications: Plantar fasciitis; medial arch strain. **Objectives:** To reduce the tension on the plantar fascia and medial arch during the mid-support phase of gait. **Tape:** 2.5 cm/1 inch tape. **Taping position:** Athlete supine or prone on the taping table with foot over the edge. **Taping technique:** Place two anchor strips circumferentially just proximal to the metatarsal heads (apply lightly). Begin the first strip of tape on the medial side of the foot (just proximal to the head of the first metatarsal). Go behind the heel and angle the tape under the foot, crossing the longitudinal arch. Stop near the origin of this strip (**a**). Place the second strip of tape on the lateral side of the foot (just proximal to the head of the fifth metatarsal) and go under and around the heel, up the lateral side, and stop near the origin of this strip (**b**). Continue alternating strips in the same pattern until the "fan" is filled in (**c**). Tie down the entire procedure by placing circumferential strips over the previous strips by starting on the dorsolateral aspect of the foot and then continue under the arch and finish on the dorso-medial aspect of the foot. Leave a gap on the top of the foot, bridging this by placing short strips of tape across the gap (**d**) and (**e**). *Option*—Once the "tie-down" strips are in place, the heel strips may be cut and removed (**f**). This may prevent excessive tightness and/or blisters, although some of the support will be lost.

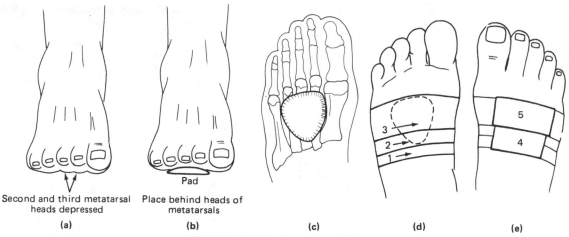

Second and third metatarsal heads depressed	Place behind heads of metatarsals			
(a)	(b)	(c)	(d)	(e)

FIGURE 5.6 Metatarsal Arch Support

Indications: Metatarsal arch pain/strain; metatarsalgia. **Objectives:** To control the metatarsal arch and the stress on the intermetatarsal ligaments (**a**). **Tape:** 2.5 cm/1 inch tape; metatarsal arch pad. **Taping position:** Athlete lies prone on the taping table with the foot extended over the end. **Fabrication of the metatarsal pad:** Oval in shape, edges bevelled, thickest portion of pad should be placed where the most pressure is required. Place pad behind the metatarsal heads (**b** and **c**). **Taping technique:** Secure the pad in place: Begin the tape on the dorso-lateral aspect of the foot and then continue under the foot and up to the dorso-medial aspect of the foot (leave a gap by encircling only two thirds of the foot) (**d**). Fill in the gap by placing several short strips of tape on top of the foot. This permits expansion of the foot when weight-bearing (**e**).

FIGURE 5.7 (*opposite*) **Ankle Taping**

Indications: Preventive ankle taping; following inversion sprains. **Objectives:** Support the lateral ligaments of the ankle without restricting functional motion. **Tape:** 3.75 cm/1½ inch tape. **Taping position:** Athlete sits on the taping table with the lower leg extended over the edge of the table. The ankle is held at right angles to the lower leg (neutral dorsi/plantar flexion), and slightly everted. **Taping technique:**

1. Place lubricated gauze pads on the instep and behind the heel. Wrap the foot and lower leg with underwrap and secure the underwrap with two anchor strips at the top (A_1 and A_2) and the bottom (B_1 and B_2). The anchor strips should overlap the underwrap and adhere to the skin (**a–c**).

2. Apply vertical or stirrup strips:

Option A: Start the first stirrup on the medial aspect of the lower leg, go under the heel and up on the lateral aspect of the foot and lower leg. Continue overlapping these stirrup strips (three to five) until the last strip is well in front of the malleolus (**d**).

Option B: Start the vertical or stirrup on the medial side of the leg and behind the malleolus; go under the foot to the lateral aspect of the foot and lower leg (angle the tape so that it comes up in front of the malleolus). Start stirrup number two on the inside of the lower leg and in front of the malleolus and end with the tape angling upwards on the lateral aspect of the lower leg. The last stirrup strip covers both the medial and lateral malleolus (no angle) (**e**).

3. Following the application of the vertical stirrups, horizontal or "horseshoe" strips are then placed around the ankle. The first strip is started low on the outside of the foot and taken behind the heel and along the medial aspect of the foot (applying the "horseshoe" strips in this manner adds some support to the long arch). Continue applying these strips in an overlapping manner until the malleolus is covered (**f**).

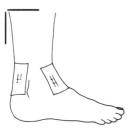

(a) Gauze pads

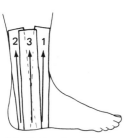

(b) Underwrap

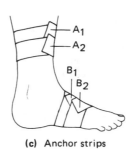

(c) Anchor strips

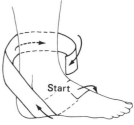

(d) Option A — Stirrups

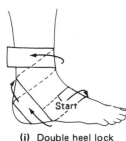

(e) Option B — Stirrups

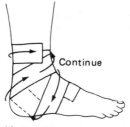

(f) Horseshoe strips

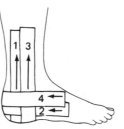

(g) Option C

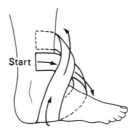

(h) Basic heel lock

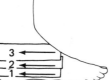

(i) Double heel lock

(j) Double heel lock, cont.

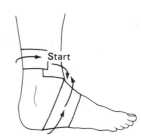

(k) Half figure-eight

(l) Figure-eight

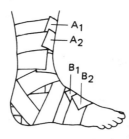

(m)

Option C: In this procedure the stirrup and "horseshoe" strips are alternated, producing a basketweave effect **(g)**.

4. A heel lock is applied by starting on the top of the instep and then taking the tape under the foot, behind the heel, and around the lower leg. Heel locks should be applied in both directions **(h–j)**. The novice "taper" can begin applying heel locks by starting the procedure on the plantar surface of the foot.

5. Half figure-eights are applied by starting on the lateral aspect of the lower leg and crossing over the instep, then going under the foot and coming up on the lateral aspect of the lower leg before being attached medially **(k)**. Several of these should be applied and they should overlap and progress down the foot. A full figure-eight is an option. This is accomplished by having the tape completely encircle the lower leg **(l and m)**.

FIGURE 5.7 Ankle Taping (*cont.*)
Ankle Taping (for Medial Support)

Indications: Following eversion sprains. **Objectives:** Protect a mild sprain of the deltoid ligament, or support medial laxity. **Taping technique:** Direction of pull on the stirrup should be reversed from that done for lateral support, i.e., apply from the lateral to the medial side with the foot in neutral position and slightly inverted. The half figure-eight should also be applied in the opposite direction.

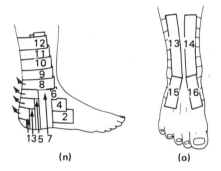

(n)   (o)

Acute Ankle Injury—Open Basketweave

Swelling frequently occurs following an ankle sprain. In order to prevent constriction of the circulation, which may happen if tape encircles the ankle, open basketweave taping should be used in the acute ankle sprain until the swelling has stabilized (**n** and **o**).

FIGURE 5.8 (*opposite*) **Ankle Wrap: Muslin Wrap**

Indications: Prevention of sprains; ankle support. **Objectives:** Generally support the structures around the ankle. **Wrap:** 5 cm/2 inch wide muslin wrap (approximately 270 cm/108 inches long). **Wrapping postion:** Same as with ankle taping. **Wrapping technique:**

Option A: Conventional method (**a–h**).

1. Start the wrap on the lateral aspect of the lower leg, encircle the leg and go over the instep. Proceed under and around the foot.
2. Next, bring the muslin up at an angle and secure an ankle lock. Then proceed around the lower leg, over the instep, and under the foot to form a heel lock on the opposite side.
3. Depending on the length of wrap, additional heel locks may be applied. Finish with figure-eight or by encircling the lower leg.
4. Secure the procedure in place by duplicating the pattern with tape, or tie down with a short piece of tape.

Option B: Pull tab method (**i–p**).

1. Start on the lateral aspect of the lower leg and bring the wrap laterally under the heel. Swing over the lateral malleolus and add a heel lock. Repeat in the opposite direction.
2. After the completion of the procedure, the "tab" may be pulled up (this will place the ankle in more of an everted position) and then tied down.

Conventional method — *Medial view*

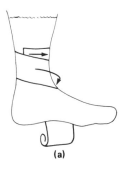
(a)

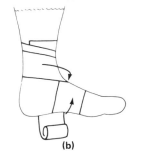
(b)

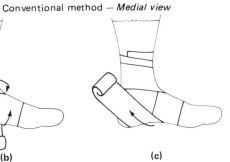
(c)

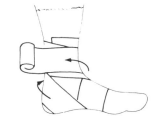
(d)

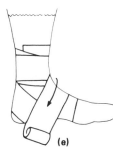
(e)

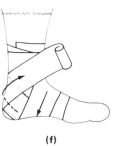
(f)

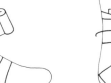
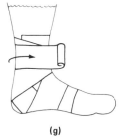
(g)

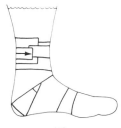
(h)

Pull tab method — *Lateral view*

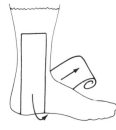
(i)

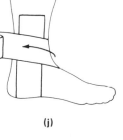
(j)

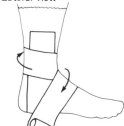
(k)

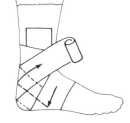
(l)

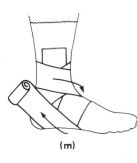
(m)

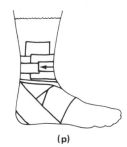
(n)

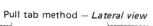
(o)

(p)

Achilles tendon taping position

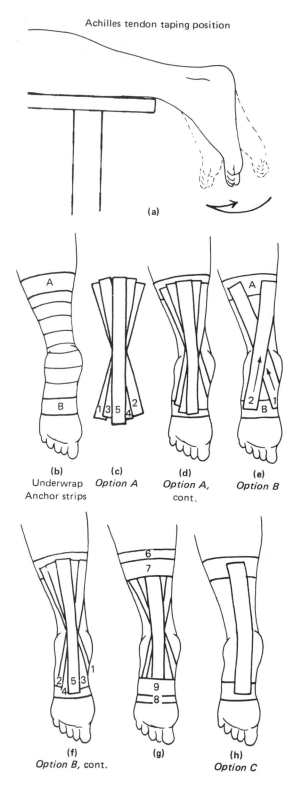

(a)

(b)
Underwrap
Anchor strips

(c)
Option A

(d)
Option A,
cont.

(e)
Option B

(f)
Option B, cont.

(g)

(h)
Option C

FIGURE 5.9 Achilles Tendon Taping
Indications: Achilles tendinitis; gastrocnemius-soleus
strain. **Objectives:** Prevent extreme dorsiflexion of the
ankle. **Tape:** 3.75 cm/1½ inch tape. **Preparation:**
Shave or clip body hair from midfoot to low-calf area if
applicable; apply tape-holding spray to the skin. **Taping position:** Prone, foot over edge of the table. The
foot should be placed midway between plantar and
dorsiflexion, or slightly plantar flexed from that position
(a). **Taping technique:**

1. Apply underwrap from midfoot to the low-calf area **(b)**.
2. Place an anchor strip at midcalf and anchor at
   midfoot. The anchor strips should overlap the
   underwrap and attach to the skin (A and B in **[b]**).
3. Secure a restraining strap from the plantar surface of
   the foot, up the posterior aspect of the lower leg.

Option A: Construct a "fan" on a table top or other
   smooth surface. Peel off and apply to the athlete.
   The individual strips of the fan should run from the
   foot to the calf in order to pull the foot into a plantar
   flexed position **(c and d)**.

Option B: Construct the "fan" directly on the athlete **(e–
   f)**.

Option C: Split a bicycle inner tube and attach **(h)**. Tie
   down as in **(g)**.

4. Tie down the "fan" with circumferential strips (numbers 6–9 in **[g]**).

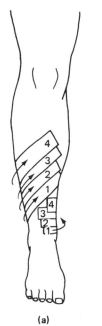 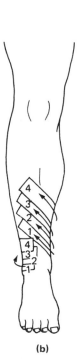

(a)   (b)

FIGURE 5.10 Taping for Shin Pain

Indications: Pain in the lower leg while running, not associated with a compartment syndrome or a stress fracture/reaction (see Chapters 9 and 21). **Objectives:** To support the lower leg musculature and reduce the symptoms. **Tape:** 3.75 cm/1 inch tape, 5 cm/2 inch elastic tape, and/or 7.5 cm/3 inch elastic wrap. **Preparation:** Shave or clip body hair from the lower leg. **Taping position:** Athlete may either stand or sit on taping table. **Taping technique:**

1. *Anterior leg symptoms.* Begin the first strip on the inside of the lower leg above the medial malleolus and apply the tape around and behind the leg, and then spiral upwards finishing on the anterior aspect of the leg. Overlap each strip of tape or wrap and apply as many strips as needed (**a**).

2. *Posteromedial leg symptoms.* Begin the first strip on the outside of the lower leg above the lateral malleolus. Apply the tape around and behind the leg, spiral upwards, and finish on the anterior aspect of the leg.

Options: Additional support may be obtained by securing the tape with elastic tape or wrap. If both anterior and posteromedial symptoms are present, a combination of the two techniques may be used. Apply alternating interlocking strips. In addition, medial arch taping or Low-Dye taping may be incorporated to help control excessive pronation (**b**).

FIGURE 5.11 (*opposite*) **Taping to Prevent Hyperextension of the Knee**
Indications: Sprained posterior capsule; strained lower hamstrings; anterior cruciate ligament laxity. **Objectives:** Prevent hyperextension of the knee. **Tape:** 3.75 cm/1½ inch tape; 5 cm/2 inch elastic tape optional. **Preparation:** Place adequate padding behind the knee (lubricated gauze pads) and then apply underwrap from the midcalf to midthigh. **Taping position:** Athlete stands on top of the taping table. Extend the knee until a strain is experienced. Allow the knee to bend slightly towards flexion. By placing a roll of tape under the heel, the knee can be kept in flexion (**a**). **Taping technique:**

Option A (**b** and **c**):
1. Secure the underwrap with anchor strips top (A_1 and A_2) and bottom (B_1 and B_2), which should adhere to the skin.
2. Construct a "fan" on the posterior aspect of the knee. Form the pattern by establishing the outer borders of the fan and then fill in the pattern.
3. The "fanned" strips of tape should run from distal to proximal.
4. Secure the fan by utilizing "tie-down" strips (either white tape or elastic tape).

Option B (**d–g**) This procedure is also utilized for cruciate ligament support:
1. Anchor strips (same as Option A).
2. Begin the first strip on the anteromedial aspect of the lower leg. Proceed below the patella, continue behind the knee, spiraling upwards to finish high on the thigh.
3. The second strip begins on the anterolateral aspect of the lower leg, runs below the patella, and spirals upwards to finish high on the opposite side of the thigh.
4. Continue with overlapping strips.
5. To finish, "tie down" the tape with white or elastic tape. Be careful not to over-tighten. If the tape is too tight around the thigh, release the tension by cutting the top posterior aspect, and then filling in the gap with short strips of tape (**h** and **i**).

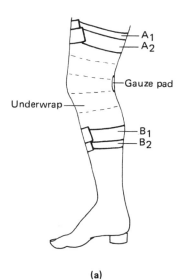

A₁
A₂

Gauze pad

Underwrap

B₁
B₂

(a)

Option A — "Fan"

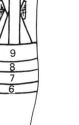

2   1

1 3 5 4 2

(b) Posterior view

Option A, cont.

1
2
3
4
5

9
8
7
6

(c) Posterior view

Option B– also for cruciate ligament support

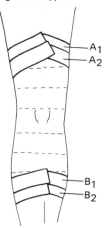

A₁
A₂

B₁
B₂

(d) Anterior view

Option B, cont.

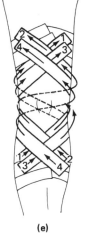

(e)

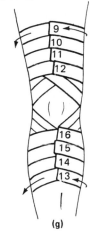

1 3 4 2
 5 7 8 6

(f)

9
10
11
12

16
15
14
13

(g)

Using tape scissors, cut a gap in the "tie–down" strips and then bridge this gap with short strips of tape.

(h) Posterior view

(i)

FIGURE 5.12 (*opposite*)   **Collateral Ligament Support**

Indications: Mild sprain of the medial or lateral collateral ligaments; supporting established laxity of one of these ligaments.   **Objectives:** Support the knee against valgus or varus stress.   **Tape:** 3.75 cm/1½ inch tape; 7.5 cm/3 inch elastic tape.   **Taping position:** Athlete stands on top of the taping table with knee slightly flexed (**a**).   **Taping technique:**

1. Wrap with underwrap from midcalf to above midthigh.
2. Secure the underwrap as shown in Figure 5.11 (hyperextended knee).
3. Begin the first strip on the anteromedial aspect of the lower leg and angle the tape up (near the inferolateral border of the patella) to high up the thigh.
4. Start the second strip on the anterolateral aspect of the lower leg and angle upwards (near inferomedial border of the patella) to high up the thigh.
5. Start the third strip near the first, and angle upwards (superomedial border of the patella) to high on the thigh.
6. Start the fourth strip near the second strip and angle upwards (near the superolateral border of the patella) to high on the thigh.
7. Continue alternating and overlapping strips of tape duplicating the pattern formed by the first four strips until the medial and lateral aspects of the knee are covered (**b** and **c**).
8. Proceed to either Option A or Option B:

Option A: Apply a "fan" on the involved side of the knee, and complete the taping (i.e., add a top layer to "tie down" the tape) (**d**).

Option B: Utilize 7.5 cm/3 inch elastic tape. Apply a modified figure-eight to reinforce the involved side of the knee. Apply an *X* procedure on the opposite side. Tie this tape down with elastic tape (**e–h**).

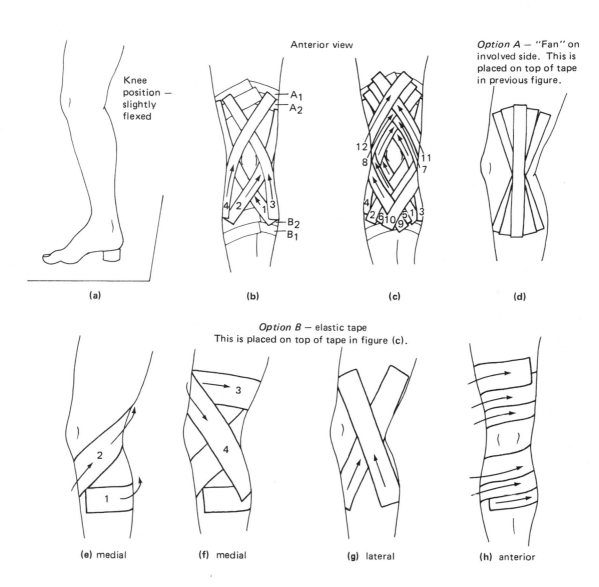

Anterior view

Knee position — slightly flexed

A₁
A₂

B₂
B₁

Option A — "Fan" on involved side. This is placed on top of tape in previous figure.

Option B — elastic tape
This is placed on top of tape in figure (c).

(a)

(b)

(c)

(d)

(e) medial

(f) medial

(g) lateral

(h) anterior

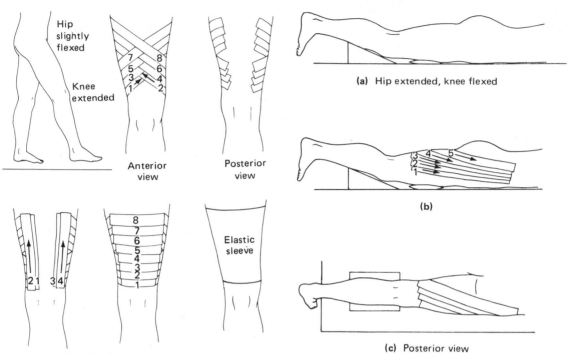

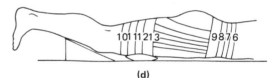

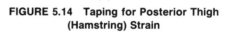

FIGURE 5.13 Taping for Anterior Thigh (Quadriceps) Strain

Indications: Strain of the quadriceps muscles; contusion of the quadriceps muscles. **Objectives:** Support the quadriceps muscle group and reduce the tensile stress on a minor strain. May also be used to support a pad to protect a quadriceps contusion. **Tape:** 7.5 cm/ 1½ inch tape. **Taping position:** Athlete stands with the hip slightly flexed and knee extended. **Taping technique:** Begin on the lateral side posteriorly and spiral up and around the leg to end on the posterior side medially. Repeat in the opposite direction. Alternate sides, producing an interweaving effect. Support the posterior edges of tape with vertical strips and fill in the gap. An elastic thigh sleeve may be worn over the tape.

FIGURE 5.14 Taping for Posterior Thigh (Hamstring) Strain

Indications: Hamstring muscle group strain, particularly biceps femoris. **Objectives:** Reduce the tensile stress on the hamstring musculature. **Preparation:** Shave or clip body hair on the posterior thigh and buttock area— if applicable. **Tape:** 3.75 cm/1 inch tape. **Taping position:** Prone, with a bolster placed beneath the lower leg so as to flex the knee. **Taping technique:** Apply strips from low down on the thigh to the iliac crest area. "Tie down" with strips; these should not completely surround the limb. The gap should then be filled in (as shown in Figure 5.13). If the strain is mainly medial, e.g., the semitendinous muscle, the tape should be applied so as to cover the medial side as well as the postero-lateral.

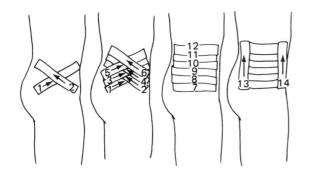

FIGURE 5.15 Taping for a "Hip Pointer"
Indications: Contusion to iliac crest area. **Objectives:** Protect the contused area; may be used in conjunction with a pad. **Preparation:** Shave or clip body hair over the involved area. **Tape:** 3.75 cm/1½ inch tape. **Taping position:** Standing erect. **Taping technique:** Interlocking strips, then cover with horizontal, overlapping layers. Secure with two vertical strips.

Internal rotation wrap

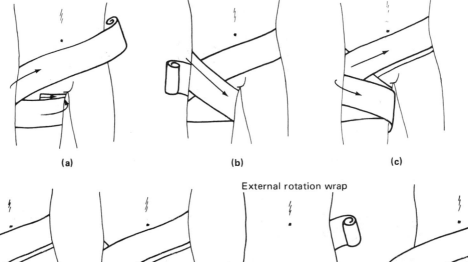

External rotation wrap

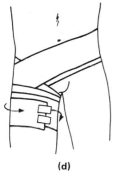

(a)　　　　　　　(b)　　　　　　　(c)

(d)　　　　(e)　　　　(f)　　　　(g)

FIGURE 5.16 A Hip Spica for a Groin Strain
Indications: Groin and lateral hip strains. **Objectives:** Allow the hip to assume a relaxed position and to functionally limit motion. **Preparation:** Shave or clip body hair over the involved area if tape is used. **Tape:** 7.5 cm/3 inch elastic tape; 3.75 cm/1½ inch tape; or 7.5 cm/3 inch elastic wrap. **Taping position:** Standing erect. **Wrapping technique:** Surround the limb and body with either elastic tape or wrap. Secure with tape. The leg should be held in internal rotation when the adductors and/or anterior groin muscles are involved (**a–e**). The external rotation spica can be applied when the tensor fasciae latae, gluteals, and posterolateral buttock musculature are symptomatic (**f** and **g**).

Taping for extension injury—**a–f**.

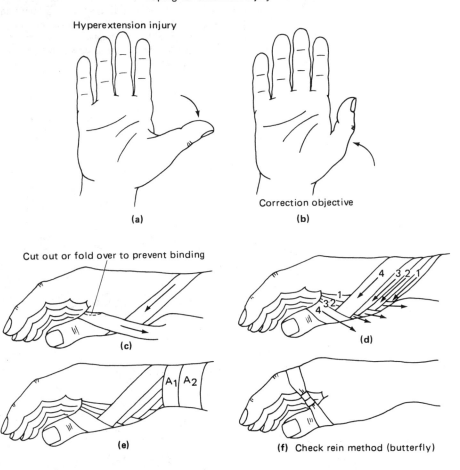

Hyperextension injury

(a)

Correction objective

(b)

Cut out or fold over to prevent binding

(c)

(d)

(e)

(f) Check rein method (butterfly)

FIGURE 5.17   Taping for Thumb Injuries (*this page and opposite*)
Indications: Abduction and/or extension sprains of the thumb. **Objectives:** Protect the involved ligaments and prevent extension and abduction during healing. **Tape:** 2.5 cm/1 inch tape. **Taping position:** See diagram. **Taping technique:** See diagram. The option of additional support may be used under the basic figure-eight arrangement. The check rein method should be incorporated (**f**), and may be used by itself after healing has occurred.

Additional support—*Option A*—**k–m**. *Option B*—**n**.

Taping for abduction injury—**g–j**.

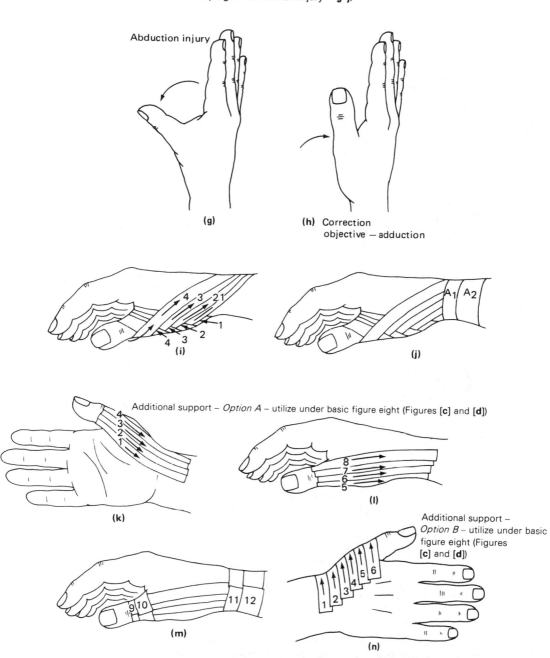

Abduction injury

(g)

(h) Correction
objective — adduction

(i)

(j)

Additional support – *Option A* – utilize under basic figure eight (Figures **[c]** and **[d]**)

(k)

(l)

Additional support –
Option B – utilize under basic
figure eight (Figures
[c] and **[d]**)

(m)

(n)

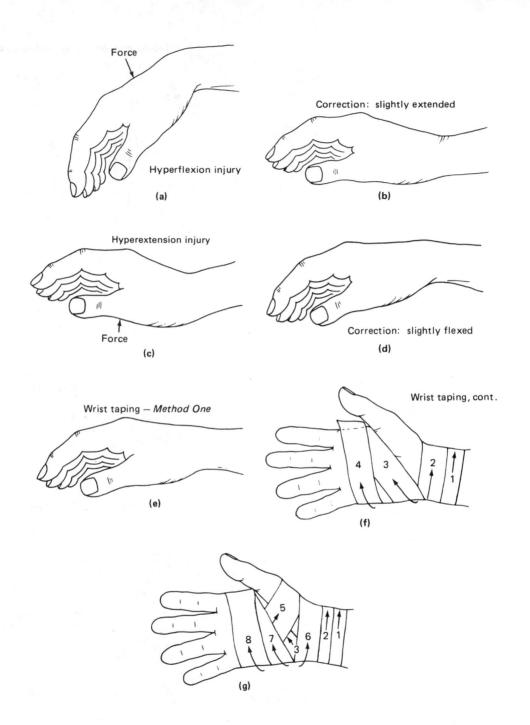

Force

Hyperflexion injury

(a)

Correction: slightly extended

(b)

Hyperextension injury

Force

(c)

Correction: slightly flexed

(d)

Wrist taping — *Method One*

(e)

Wrist taping, cont.

4 3 2 1

(f)

5
8 7 6 2 1
3

(g)

FIGURE 5.18 Taping for Wrist Injuries (*this page and opposite, top*)
Indications: Mild sprains or contusions to the wrist. **Objectives:** Limit range of motion and support the wrist. **Preparation:** Shave or clip body hair from part to be taped. **Tape:** 2.5 or 3.75 cm/1 or 1½ inch tape. **Taping position:** See diagram. **Taping technique:** See diagram. Ensure that the tape over the palm of the hand is not too tight.

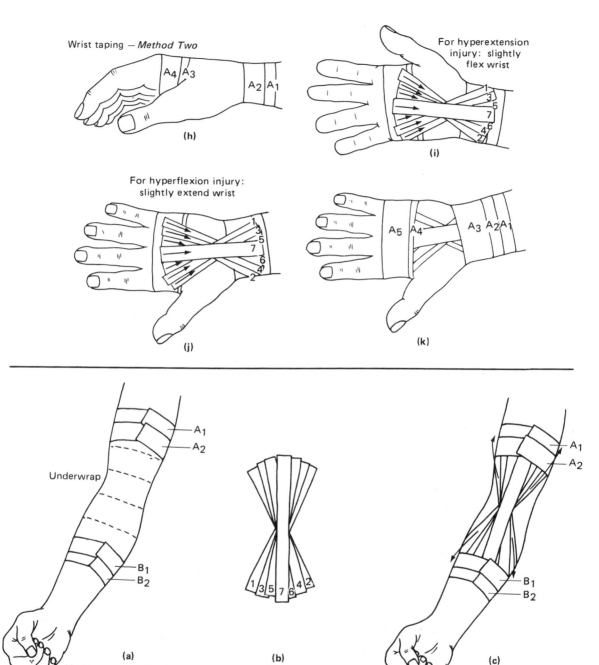

Wrist taping — *Method Two*

(h)

For hyperextension injury: slightly flex wrist

(i)

For hyperflexion injury: slightly extend wrist

(j)

(k)

Underwrap

(a)
Underwrap — optional —
use gauze pad, anchor strips

(b)
Fan

(c)

FIGURE 5.19 Taping for a Hyperextension Injury of the Elbow
Indications: Hyperextension elbow injury; mild sprain to medial collateral ligament. **Objectives:** Prevent hyperextension of the elbow. **Tape:** 3.75 cm/1½ inch tape. **Taping position:** Elbow slightly flexed; forearm neutral to slightly supinated. **Taping technique:** Apply underwrap; secure with tape above and below **(a)**. Construct a "fan" of tape **(b)** and apply to the front of the athlete's elbow. Secure with strips above and below **(c)**. The athlete should not be able to fully extend the elbow.

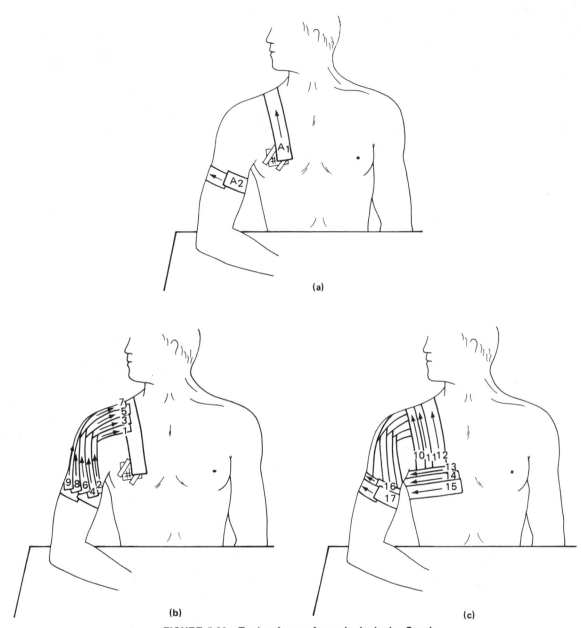

FIGURE 5.20 Taping for an Acromioclavicular Sprain

Indications: Mild strain of the shoulder musculature. **Objectives:** Support the shoulder in a nonspecific fashion. **Preparation:** Shave or clip body hair from area to be taped. **Tape:** 3.75 cm/1½ inch tape. **Taping position:** Sitting; shoulder relaxed and somewhat internally rotated. **Taping technique:** Apply a protective pad to the nipple area (**a**). An anchor strip should be applied from the scapula, over the clavicle, to (or just above) the nipple line. A second anchor is placed around the arm at the insertion of the deltoid. Interlocking strips are then applied, starting at the posterolateral aspect of the arm, crossing the shoulder to the anterior aspect of the chest (**b**). The second strip then runs from the anterior aspect of the arm to the scapular area. This alternating pattern is continued, and then tied down with strips applied over the anchors. The chest anchors are then secured (**c**).

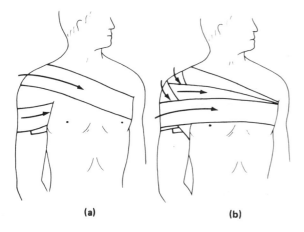

(a)   **(b)**

FIGURE 5.21 A Shoulder Spica—Using Elastic Wrap

Indications: Occasionally used in the acute management of a shoulder injury in place of a sling; may be used in the later stages of rehabilitation as a functional support. **Objectives:** Support the shoulder joint; help relax the musculature; restrict motion to a limited extent. **Preparation:** Shave or clip hair from body area to be taped. **Tape:** 7.5 cm/3 inch elastic wrap; 7.5 cm/3 inch elastic tape; or 3.75 cm/1½ inch tape. **Wrapping technique:** Apply the wrap or tape around the upper arm, then proceed across the back, under the opposite axilla, across the chest, and over the shoulder **(a)**. Repeat this a number of times, progressing down the arm **(b)**. Secure with tape.

REFERENCES

1. Garrick JG, Requa RK: Role of external support in the prevention of ankle sprains. *Med Sci Sports* 5:200–203, 1973.

2. Garrick JG: The frequency of injury, mechanism of injury, and epidemiology of ankle sprains. *Am J Sports Med* 5:241–242, 1977.

3. Malina RM, Plagenz LB, Rarick LG: Effects of exercise upon the measurable supporting strength of cloth and tape ankle wraps. *Res Q* 34:158–165, 1963.

4. Sprigings EJ, Pelton JD: An EMG analysis of the effectiveness of external ankle support during sudden ankle inversion. *Can J Appl Sport Sci* 6:72–75, 1981.

5. Rarick GL, Bigley G, Karst R, et al: The measurable support of the ankle joint by conventional methods of taping. *J Bone Joint Surg* 44A:1183–1190, 1962.

6. Laughman RK, Carr TA, Chao EY, et al: Three-dimensional kinematics of the taped ankle before and after exercise. *Am J Sports Med* 8:425–431, 1980.

7. McCluskey GM, Blackburn Jr TA, Lewis T: Prevention of ankle sprains. *Am J Sports Med* 4:151–157, 1976.

8. Fumich RM, Ellison AE, Guerin GJ, et al: The measured effect of taping on combined foot and ankle motion before and after exercise. *Am J Sports Med* 9:165–170, 1981.

9. Abdenour TE, Saville WA, White RC, et al: The effect of ankle taping upon torque and range of motion. *Athletic Training* 14:227–228, 1979.

10. Glick JM, Gordon RB, Nishimoto D: The prevention and treatment of ankle injuries. *Am J Sports Med* 4:136–141, 1976.

11. Ferguson AB: A case against ankle taping. *J Sports Med* 1:46–47, 1973.

12. Wells J: The incidence of knee injuries in relation to ankle taping. *Athletic Training* 4:10–13, 1969.

13. Ryan AJ: Taping prevents acute and repeated ankle sprains. *Phys Sportsmed* 1:40–47, November 1973.

14. Cooper DL, Fair J: Contact dermatitis, benzoin, and athletic tape. In Trainer's Corner, *Phys Sportsmed* 6:119, December 1978.

RECOMMENDED READINGS

Davies GJ: The ankle wrap—variation from the traditional. *Athletic Training* 12:194–197, 1977.

DeLacerda FG: Ankle strapping with tape. *J Sports Med Phys Fitness* 18:18, 1978.

DeLacerda FG: Effects of underwrap conditions on the supportive effectiveness of ankle strapping with tape. *J Sports Med Phys Fitness* 18:77–81, 1978.

Drake EC: The case for ankle taping. Letter to the editor. *J Sports Med* 1:45, 1973.

Emerick CE: Ankle taping: Prevention of injury or waste of time? *Athletic Training* 14:149–150 and 188, 1979.

Felder CR, McNeeley J: Ankle taping: An alternative to the basketweave. *Athletic Training* 13:152–156, 1978.

Libera D: Ankle taping, wrapping and injury prevention. *Athletic Training* 7:73–75, 1972.

Ross SE: The supportive effects of Modified Duke Simpson strapping. *Athletic Training* 13:206–210, 1978.

Simon JE: Study of comparative effectiveness of ankle taping and ankle wrapping on the prevention of ankle injuries. *Athletic Training* 4:6–7, 1969.

Stover CN: Functional semirigid support system for ankle injuries. *Phys Sportsmed* 7:71–75, May 1979.

Whitesel J, Newell SG: Modified Low-dye strapping. *Phys Sportsmed* 8:129, September 1980.

CHAPTER 6

Emergency Care and Athletic First Aid

A trainer will often be at the site of an athletic accident. He or she should therefore have the appropriate educational background and training to deal with such a situation. This includes certification in standard first aid, advanced first aid, and cardiopulmonary resuscitation. He or she should also know how to deal with the following situations in a sports environment:

1. Cardiopulmonary emergencies
2. Head and neck injuries
3. Shock
4. Internal injuries
5. Superficial bleeding
6. Fractures
7. Dislocations
8. Soft-tissue injuries

EMERGENCY CARE— LIFE-THREATENING SITUATIONS

Cardiopulmonary Emergencies

There are a variety of situations in athletics that can result in a need for cardiopulmonary resuscitation (CPR). The athletic trainer must be able to recognize the signs of respiratory failure and cardiac arrest and know how to initiate the proper CPR procedures to maintain life. These procedures should be continued until the athlete has recovered sufficiently for CPR to be safely discontinued. Transportation to the nearest hospital should then be arranged, with constant medical supervision until the athlete is placed on an advanced life-support system, or until the

athletic trainer is instructed to terminate CPR by the attending physician.

The basic steps in cardiopulmonary resuscitation consist of the following ABCs:

$$\left.\begin{array}{l} \textbf{A}\text{irway} \\ \textbf{B}\text{reathing} \end{array}\right\} = \left.\text{Artificial ventilation}\right\} = CPR$$
$$\textbf{C}\text{irculation} = \text{Artificial circulation}$$

Clearing the airway. In many cases, clearing the airway is all that is required to restore breathing. Two recommended methods of opening or clearing the airway are

1. tilting the head backward
2. forward displacement of the lower jaw

As the attending athletic trainer always needs to consider the possibility of multiple injuries, most importantly a cervical spine injury, forward displacement of the lower jaw is the most desirable method. This technique consists of the following steps:

1. Place the index fingers behind the angles of the jaw.
2. Displace the lower jaw (mandible) forward while using the thumbs to retract the lower lip.
3. Keep the cervical region stationary and not hyperextended, unless certain that there is no injury to the cervical spine.

If the aforementioned methods do not succeed in opening the airway, an oral airway (which should always be carried by the trainer during athletic practices and events) is inserted to bring the tongue forward and thereby open the respiratory passage. This

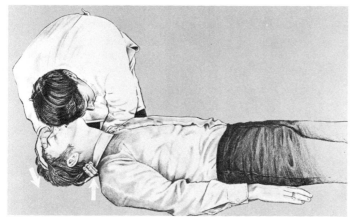

(a)

FIGURE 6.1 Cardiopulmonary resuscitation (CPR) (Figures 6–1 and 6–3 reproduced with the permission of Laerdal Medical Corp.)

(**a**) First, establish if the athlete is breathing by placing an ear over the mouth and, at the same time, observing for movement of the chest.

(**b**) The unconscious athlete. Where a neck injury cannot be excluded, the neck should *not* be hyperextended. The jaw-thrust technique should be used to open the airway.

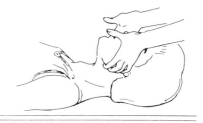

(b)

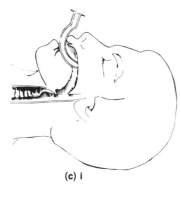

(c) i

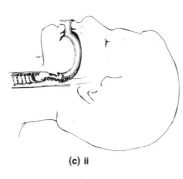

(c) ii

(**c**) (**i**) Inserting the oral airway— Insert the airway wrong way up and gently rotate once in the mouth. (**ii**) The airway has been rotated and is now in place.

(**d**) If no respiratory movement occurs, pinch off the athlete's nose and, making an airtight contact, initiate mouth-to-mouth resuscitation by blowing air into the athlete's lungs. Note movement of the chest; if this does not occur, check the airway.

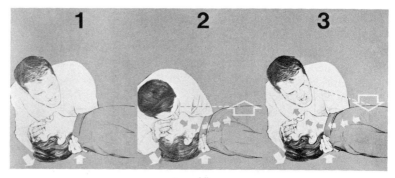

(d)

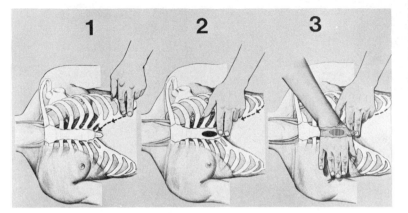

(e)

(e) If a pulse is not present, initiate external cardiac massage. Pressure should be placed only over the lower half of the sternum; no pressure should be exerted on the xiphisternum. Feel along the ribs until the xiphisternum is palpated; then place the heel of the right hand over the sternum, but not onto the xiphisternum.

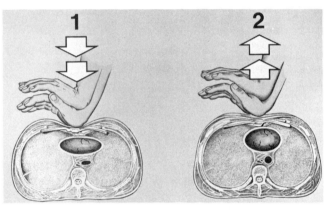

(f)

(f) Downward pressure will compress the heart between the sternum and vertebral bodies.

(g) Elbows should be kept extended, the force coming from the weight of the resuscitator. The fingers may be kept separate or locked.

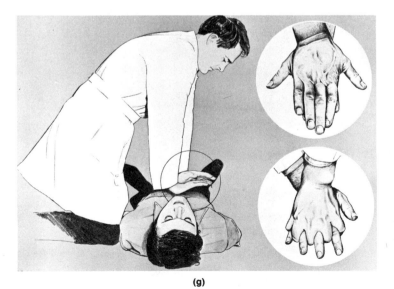

(g)

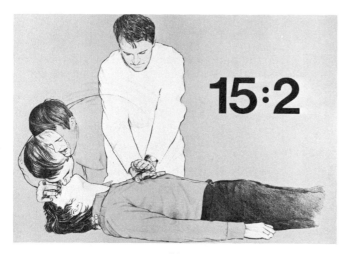

(h)

(h) If only one resuscitator is present, fifteen cardiac compressions should be followed by two breaths.

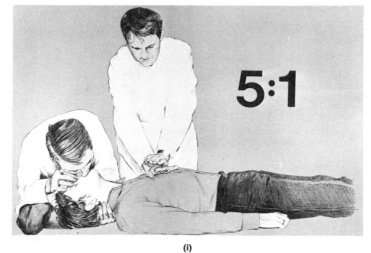

(i) If two resuscitators are available, the ratio should be five compressions to one breath. The breath should be between compressions. The timing is important to ensure that there is no delay in the cardiac resuscitation and no drop in blood pressure.

(i)

oral airway should be inserted wrong side up and, once in the mouth, gently rotated behind the tongue.

As it may be difficult to open the mouth because of a spasm of the mandibular muscles, the trainer should always have available a device such as an oral screw.

If the athlete does not promptly resume adequate respiration after clearing the airway, begin artificial ventilation. If at this time, after the airway has been cleared and artificial ventilation started, there is no pulse over the carotid artery, begin external cardiac compression immediately.

The Face Mask in Football

In football, where the face mask can interfere with the administration of CPR, a plan of action should be available to deal with the situation.[1] Remember that the helmet should not be removed until a cervical spine injury can be confidently excluded. The method of removal depends on the type of face mask:

1. If the helmet has a hinged or swing-away face mask, the trainer should use a sharp pocket knife to cut the plastic or rubber mounting and thereby release the mask (see Figure 16.17).

81

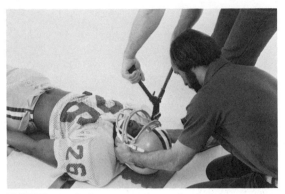

FIGURE 6.2 Bolt-cutters It may be necessary to use bolt-cutters to remove the face mask from an injured football player. Bolt-cutters should always be readily available when this type of face mask is used.

2. If the face mask is permanently fixed to the helmet by means of screws or other devices, a pair of bolt cutters is required. When this variety of face mask is in use, a suitably-sized bolt cutter should always be kept on the sidelines (Figure 6.2).

Obstruction by a Foreign Object

In athletics there is always the possibility of inhaling a foreign object. The trainer should make every effort to discourage the use of chewing gum and to educate the athlete in removing dentures or dental appliances before athletic participation. If any obstruction to the upper airway should occur, the athlete will suddenly be unable to speak or cough and will make exaggerated attempts to breathe. However, no air movement will be present. If a foreign object is suspected as being the cause of the obstruction, the trainer should deliver a series of four or five sharp blows to the spine between the scapulae. If this fails to remove the obstruction, the Heimlich maneuver should be performed. This maneuver has proven effective in removing a variety of foreign objects from the upper airway.

The Heimlich maneuver. The Heimlich maneuver consists of a series of rapid thrusts to the upper abdomen.* It is performed with the athlete in either a vertical or horizontal position.

1. With the athlete vertical—the trainer
   a. stands behind the athlete and wraps his or her arms around the athlete's waist.
   b. grasps one fist with the other hand, placing the thumb side of the fist against the athlete's abdomen between the xiphoid and the umbilicus.
   c. presses the fist into the athlete's abdomen with a quick upward thrust.

2. With the athlete horizontal (the horizontal technique is more applicable to the situation in which a cervical spine injury may exist):
   a. Put the athlete in a supine position, kneel close to the athlete's hips, or straddle the hips or one leg.
   b. Place the heel of one hand against the athlete's abdomen, between the xiphoid and the umbilicus; place the second hand on top of the first.
   c. Press the hands into the athlete's abdomen with a quick upward thrust.

In cases where the foreign object cannot be dislodged, mouth-to-mouth resuscitation may provide an adequate amount of air to maintain the victim until the obstruction is removed or a tracheotomy is performed. An alternative to a tracheotomy is the insertion of a wide-bore needle (No. 12 to No. 14 gauge) through the cricothyroid membrane into the trachea (Figure 6.3d).

Shock

The term *shock* implies a state of collapse of the cardiovascular system and constitutes a medical emergency. Every significant injury has the potential to lead to a state of shock. If this should occur, the trainer needs to realize that treating shock is the immediate pri-

*Adapted from *Emergency Care and Transportation of the Sick and Injured*, American Academy of Orthopaedic Surgeons, 2nd ed. (Chicago, 1977). Reprinted by permission of the publisher.

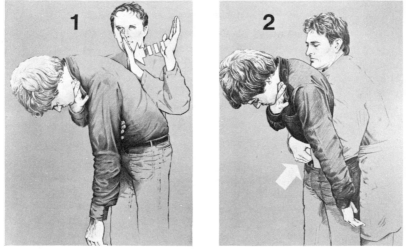

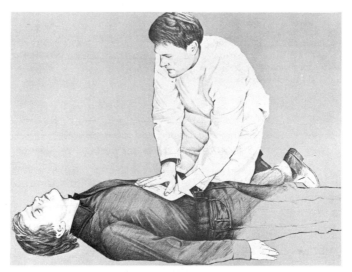

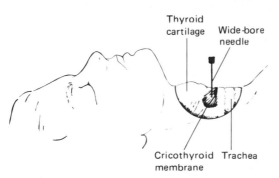

Thyroid
cartilage

Wide-bore
needle

Cricothyroid   Trachea
membrane

(d)

FIGURE 6.3 Parts (a), (b) and (c)
show the **Heimlich maneuver**. Part (d)
shows the insertion of a wide-bore needle through the crico-thyroid membrane
into the trachea.

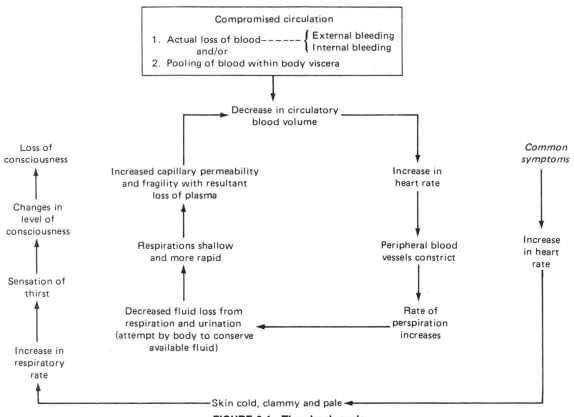

FIGURE 6.4 The shock cycle

ority and that the original injury can be treated once this problem is under control.

Shock can occur from

1. hemorrhage (internal or external)
2. pooling or stagnation of the blood flow

If the shock cycle is allowed to progress, serious and even irreversible changes may occur. The athletic trainer should attempt to prevent shock from occurring and, if it does develop, should treat it as follows:

1. If the injured athlete is conscious, respond in a confident, reassuring, and controlled manner.

2. Position the athlete correctly in view of other injuries that might be present. In general, the optimal position is *reclining with the feet higher than the head.* This position will allow available blood to perfuse the brain.

3. If bleeding is present, use the proper procedures to bring it under control.

4. Relieve or minimize the pain. For instance, if a fracture or fractures are present, adequate immobilization of the injured area will reduce the amount of pain.

5. Control heat loss, but do not actively warm the athlete, as the cutaneous blood vessels will dilate and remove much-needed blood from the vital organs.

INJURIES

Internal Injuries

The thoracic area.   An injury to the thorax may result in damage to the lungs, possibly causing a *pneumothorax* (tearing of part of the lung, leading to the accumulation of air between the lung and the chest wall), a *hemothorax* (blood between the lung and the chest wall), or both.

The athlete will be short of breath and may cough up blood. The trainer should supply oxygen, place the athlete in a comfortable position (usually a semi-reclining 45° position), and transport him or her to a medical facility.

Occasionally *contusions of the heart* will result in swelling of the pericardial sac, which will impair heart function. This is a dire emergency in which the athlete needs urgent medical attention.

The abdominal area. The most common serious abdominal injuries are (a) rupture of the spleen[2] and (b) contusion or rupture of the kidney. Other organs, such as the liver, may also be involved.

The initial signs, besides abdominal pain, are those of early shock, especially a rapid pulse and decreased blood pressure. The athlete should be placed into a supine position, with padding beneath the knees to relax the abdominal musculature, and rapidly transported to a medical facility.

Head and Neck Injuries

In many situations a head and a neck injury may occur simultaneously.

A head injury may result in intracranial bleeding, either venous or arterial. Immediate management consists of

1. assessment of the state of consciousness
2. assessment and observation of the athlete's airway, breathing, and circulation
3. a decision as to the appropriate form of management

The trainer needs to be aware that an athlete may relapse after apparently recovering and may suddenly lose consciousness. (For a complete discussion of head injuries, see Chapter 11.)

A neck injury is often associated with a head injury. When dealing with a head injury, *the trainer should assume that a neck injury is present until it is proven otherwise.* In a sport where a helmet is worn, the helmet should *not* be removed until a neck injury has been ruled out. Palpate for possible deformities of the spine and test the power and sensation in the extremities. If a neck or spinal cord injury is suspected, the head and neck should be adequately immobilized and the athlete moved only with supervision by a physician or trained personnel.

External Bleeding

In athletics, serious bleeding from superficial wounds is an uncommon but potentially significant injury. Various types of superficial wounds include:

1. *Abrasions*—The outer layer of skin is scraped or abraded away.
2. *Lacerations*—The skin and deeper tissues are cut, torn, or both.
3. *Puncture wounds*—A sharp object has deeply penetrated the skin.

When bleeding needs to be controlled, the athletic trainer can usually accomplish this by means of a dressing and direct pressure over the wound. In addition, cold can be applied (but not to the unconscious athlete) and the body part elevated if possible. If there are serious bleeding problems not controlled by the simple measures mentioned, the trainer should consider pressure to the supplying artery.

Fractures

Fractures can be

1. *Closed*—The bone is broken, but the skin is not damaged.

2. *Open (compound)*—There is an associated open wound in the area of the fracture. The fractured bone may or may not be visible.

A fracture can be caused by a number of different forces.

1. *Direct force*—The bone is broken at the site of the force.

2. *Indirect force*—Trauma is inflicted at a distance from the resulting fracture. An example of this is falling on the outstretched hand and sustaining a fracture of the clavicle.

3. *Avulsion force*—A portion of the bone is pulled off by the attached muscle, tendon, or ligament.

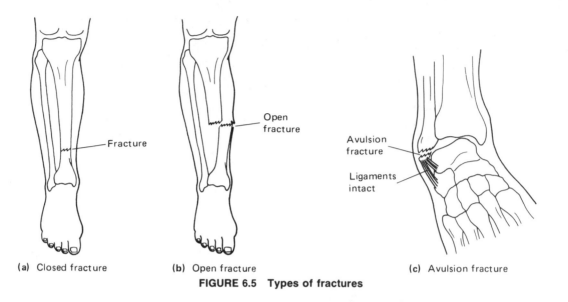

(a) Closed fracture   (b) Open fracture   (c) Avulsion fracture

FIGURE 6.5   Types of fractures

If a fracture is present, the main features are

1. unnatural mobility of the part
2. deformity
3. local tenderness over the bone
4. crepitation

The early management of a closed fracture consists of applying a splint or some form of immobilization. Immobilization will reduce the pain, protect the underlying blood vessels and nerves from further damage, and reduce the likelihood of shock.

When dealing with an open fracture, the trainer needs to cover the wound with a sterile dressing and control the bleeding. The fracture should then be immobilized and elevated if possible.

Prompt medical attention should always be obtained when a fracture is suspected.

Immobilization techniques.   There are a variety of splints that can be utilized:

1. Ordinary wooden splints, preferably padded

2. Improvised materials substituting for wooden splints (e.g., cardboard or rolled-up papers or magazines)

3. Commercially available disposable splints

4. Pneumatic or air splints (*Caution:* This type of splint should not be overinflated, as this may impair the circulation and the nerve supply to the toes or the fingers)

Guidelines for Emergency Splinting of Specific Fractures

Fracture of the humerus.

SPLINTS: Two padded wooden or improvised-material splints.

TECHNIQUE: Holding the elbow at 90°, place the shorter padded splint on inner surface of upper arm; the longer padded splint, on outer surface.

POSITION: Arm against chest, hold in position with two cravats. The forearm is supported in a narrow sling suspended from the neck.

ALTERNATIVE: Air splint.

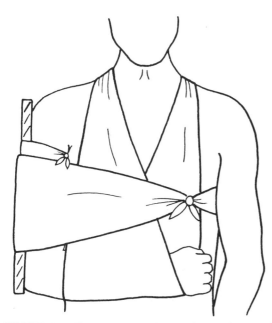

FIGURE 6.6 Emergency splinting for a fractured humerus

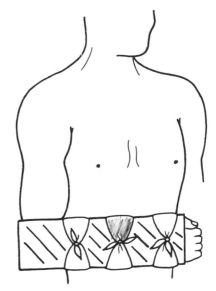

FIGURE 6.7 Emergency splinting for a fractured forearm

Fracture of the forearm.

SPLINTS: Two padded wooden splints or improvised-material splints.

TECHNIQUE: With splints in palm-down position, apply inside splint from elbow to palm; outside splint, from elbow to backs of fingers. Utilize two cravats to fix splints in place (one above and one below the fracture). Hold arm across chest with cravat sling.

ALTERNATIVE: Air splint.

Fracture of the wrist.

SPLINT: Padded wooden or folded-newspaper or magazine splint.

TECHNIQUE: Place wrist onto splint and wrap in place with bandage or elastic wrap.

SPECIAL CONSIDERATION: The trainer needs to be aware of the differential diagnosis of a suspected wrist fracture (see Chapter 15, Navicular Fracture of the Wrist).

Fracture of the hand (metacarpals).

SPLINT: Rolled bandage.

TECHNIQUE: Place rolled bandage in palm of hand and wrap in place with another rolled bandage or elastic wrap. Secure the fingers of the affected metacarpals to the adjacent fingers.

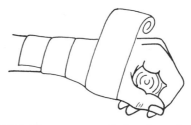

FIGURE 6.8 Emergency splinting for a fracture of the metacarpals

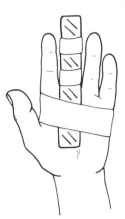

FIGURE 6.9 Emergency splinting for a fractured finger

Fracture of the fingers.

SPLINT: Padded tongue depressor or padded aluminum splint.

TECHNIQUE: Place splint from palm to past the end of the finger, and wrap loosely in place (Figure 6.9). Secure the adjacent finger or fingers to the affected finger for added support.

Fracture of the femur.

SPLINTS: Two padded wooden splints four to six inches wide, one long and one short.

TECHNIQUE: Place the longer splint on the outside (lateral) surface of the leg, extending from the axilla to the heel. The shorter splint should extend from the groin to the heel on the inside (medial) surface of the leg. Use seven to eight cravats to secure the splints in place (Figure 6.10).

Fracture of the patella.

SPLINT: Four-to-six inch well-padded wooden splint.

TECHNIQUE: The splint should reach from the buttock to below the heel. Place it under the leg and secure it by four to six cravats. The patella should be left exposed. The knee should be kept straight (extended).

Fracture of the lower leg.

SPLINTS: Two padded wooden splints four to six inches wide, one long and one short.

TECHNIQUE: Place the longer splint on the lateral surface of the leg, extending from the upper thigh to the heel. The shorter splint should extend from the groin to the heel on the medial surface of the leg. Use four to five cravats to secure the splints in place.

ALTERNATIVE: Air splint, extending from the upper thigh to the foot.

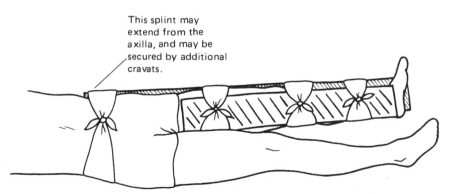

This splint may extend from the axilla, and may be secured by additional cravats.

FIGURE 6.10 Emergency splinting for a fractured femur

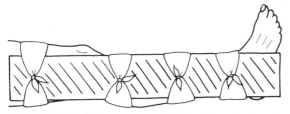

FIGURE 6.11 Emergency splinting for a fractured lower leg or ankle

Fracture near the ankle (tibia, fibula, or both).

SPLINTS: Two padded wooden splints four to six inches wide.

TECHNIQUE: Place the longer splint on the lateral surface of the leg from the upper thigh to the heel. The shorter splint extends from the groin to the heel on the inner surface of the leg. Use four to five cravats to secure the splints in place and be sure the foot is secured.

ALTERNATIVE: Air splint extending from below the knee to the foot.

Fracture of the foot (tarsals and metatarsals).

SPLINT: Padded, right-angled splint.

TECHNIQUE: Place the splint onto the posterior aspect of the lower leg and foot, extending to the ball of the foot, and secure it in place with four to five cravats.

ALTERNATIVE:

1. Ankle air splint
2. Four well-padded splints, secured so little or no movement can take place at the ankle joint

Fracture of the cervical spine.

SPLINT: Cervical spine board.

TECHNIQUE: The handling of an injury to the cervical spine is discussed in the section on neck injuries, and in the section on stretchers at the end of this chapter.

Note: An athlete with an injury to the cervical spine or evidence of cord compression should be moved only by personnel adequately trained to handle this type of injury, preferably under the supervision of a physician.

Fracture of the thoracic or the lumbar spine.

SPLINT: Long spine board.

TECHNIQUE: The handling of the thoracic or the lumbar spinal injury is discussed in the section on stretchers at the end of this chapter.

Note: An athlete with a thoracic or a lumbar fracture should be moved only by personnel adequately trained to handle this type of injury, preferably under the supervision of a physician.

Dislocations

A dislocation is a displacement of a bone from its joint and usually involves an injury to the capsule and the ligaments. Sometimes the dislocation may involve the articular surface and the tearing of muscles and tendons.

The following general symptoms and signs are associated with a dislocation:

1. Deformity of the joint (sometimes fixed or "locked" in the deformed position)
2. Pain, especially with movement
3. Inability to use the joint

The initial management of the dislocation consists of immobilizing or splinting the involved joint and extremity. Attempts to reduce the dislocation should be performed by a physician. It is important to realize that an improper or ill-advised attempt to reduce a dislocation may cause additional tearing of ligaments, muscles, or tendons, or injury to blood vessels and nerves.

Soft-Tissue Injuries

Soft-tissue injuries may be due to:

1. collisions
2. strains or sprains
3. cumulative overstress

Although most soft-tissue injuries do not fall into the life-threatening category, there is still a need to apply the correct athletic first-aid procedure to minimize the extent of the injury and effect a quick and complete recovery.

Most soft-tissue injuries are treated by the standard formula of I.C.E. plus S^2:

I. C. E. *plus* S^2

I = *ice* (cold) application

C = *compression*

E = *elevation* of the affected limb if applicable

S^2 = *stabilization* or protection of the original injury from additional trauma

    gentle *stretching* of the injured area over ice if applicable

---

FIRST AID

Ice or Cold Application

The application of cold is a very important first-aid procedure. Cold is used in the acute soft-tissue injury because it decreases the metabolism of the injured tissues, thereby reducing the need for oxygen at a time when there may be a limited amount available at the cellular level. It also limits the extent of the injury and controls the size of the hematoma. The severity of pain and spasm may also be lessened.

Various types of cold application include the following:

1. *Ice*—Place crushed ice in a double plastic bag, a wet towel, or a conventional ice bag. Use an elastic wrap that has been pre-soaked in cold water to hold the ice in position. The time schedule for the ice application depends on the type and severity of the injury, but twenty to thirty minutes every hour for the first twenty-four hours is a good rule of thumb.

2. *Chemical cold pack*—Though there are many varieties of cold packs available, their ability to lower the temperature of the deeper soft tissues is limited,[3] and their use should be restricted to emergency situations where there are no other options.

3. *Inflatable (pressure) cold devices*—Combination units may be very useful in initial and subsequent management of soft-tissue injury.

4. *Ethyl chloride and related chemical sprays*—Sprays are used in soft-tissue injury, particularly when it is accompanied by muscle spasm. These sprays must be cautiously applied because skin damage from freezing may occur.

Compression

Compression is usually accompanied by application of an elastic wrap, which can first be soaked in cold water to aid the cooling process (a dry elastic wrap has insulating properties and may counteract the effect of cold). There are a variety of commercial devices that can achieve a combination of compression and cold and may be very useful in treating the acute injury.

Elevation

Elevation is most applicable to an extremity. Where practical, the involved part should be elevated higher than the heart for much of the first twenty-four hours following injury. Again, elevation works mainly by limiting the amount of dependent edema and swelling that can occur after an injury.

Crutch Fitting

While there are a variety of crutches available, the axillary adjustable (wooden or aluminum) crutch is most commonly used. The method of adjusting or fitting the crutch to the individual includes these steps:

1. Have the athlete stand erect, place the crutch tips about six inches away from the

sides of the feet and slightly in front of the toes.

2. Adjust the length of the crutches so that two or three fingers can fit between the top of the crutch and the axilla.

3. Adjust the handgrip so as to permit the elbow to bend 25° to 30° (Figure 6.12).

Gait Instruction

While there are a number of gaits, the *three-point or featherweight-bearing* gait is the one most applicable to the athlete and most commonly used. It is important for the athlete to attempt to go through the action of a normal gait motion without actually putting weight on the affected limb. Not only does this

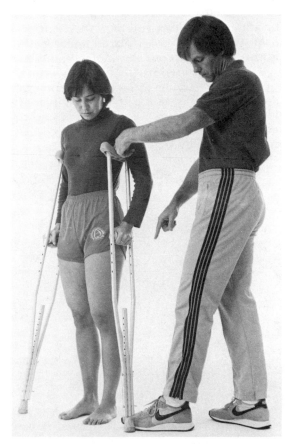

FIGURE 6.12 Fitting crutches

maintain relative flexibility of the ankle joint and Achilles tendon, but more importantly, it allows proprioceptive contact to be maintained so that the sensory system does not "switch off" the affected limb.

The three-point gait permits controlled weight bearing. The athlete should

1. place both crutches and the involved limb forward at the same time

2. push down against the handles of the crutches as his or her weight shifts forward (bringing the body forward as the hands push down). Do not allow the top of the crutches to press into the axillae. Most of the weight is taken on the crutches, but a controlled amount is taken on the affected limb. The athlete should attempt a normal heel-to-toe movement, not allowing the affected foot to be maintained in a position of plantar flexion

3. move the uninvolved foot through, and step ahead of, the crutches

If the affected limb is immobilized in a cast and no weight bearing is prescribed, the athlete should

1. move the crutches forward together, one to a position about twelve inches in front, and the other six inches to the side, of the toes

2. push down against the handles of the crutches

3. permit the body to swing through between the crutches

4. land in front of the crutches and on the heel of the uninvolved foot

5. If the involved leg is not in a cast and weight bearing is not allowed, the athlete should not plantar flex the ankle but dorsiflex the foot as the leg is brought forward, without taking any weight on that foot

Ascending stairs: First lift the healthy leg up a step, then follow with the injured leg *and* the crutches.

Descending stairs: Lower the crutches *and* the injured leg first, then follow by lowering the healthy leg.

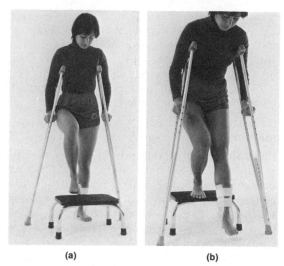

(a)   (b)

FIGURE 6.13 Crutch walking (a) Ascending stairs
(b) Descending stairs

Stretcher Use

Stretchers and spine boards should be readily available during any athletic activity, but particularly during contact and high-risk sports such as football, wrestling, rugby, lacrosse, and gymnastics.

The most commonly used stretcher is the military folding type with d-ring legs, usually known as the "Army stretcher" (Figure 6.14). Recently the scoop stretcher has become popular, because the athlete does

not have to be moved and is easily secured to the stretcher. When using this type, one must be careful not to pinch the patient or catch clothing between the halves of the stretcher as it is closed together.

Any sports medicine team needs to prepare for the emergency transportation of an athlete from the scene of play. Practice drills should be set up and a team leader appointed to be in charge of deciding the timing of the lift, the placement of the personnel, and the control of the injured part.

The stretcher is most commonly used in athletics to remove a player with an ankle or knee injury from the scene of participation to the sidelines. Placing the athlete on a stretcher is usually easily accomplished with this type of injury. The injured joint or limb should be adequately supported by the leader as the athlete is placed onto the stretcher. The athlete can either roll onto the unaffected side with the stretcher placed underneath, and then roll back onto the stretcher, the injured limb supported by the team leader; or, other players, trainers, or bystanders can help lift the player as the stretcher is placed underneath. The player is then gently lowered onto the stretcher while the injured extremity is carefully supported. If a fracture is suspected, the limb should be splinted before the player is moved. If circumstances permit, an injured knee should be placed

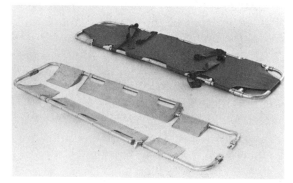

FIGURE 6.14 The Army-type stretcher (above) **and the scoop stretcher** (below)

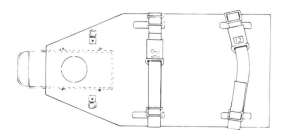

FIGURE 6.15 Cervical spine board (Modified from Joseph S. Torg, Theodore C. Quedenfeld and William Newell, "When the athlete's life is threatened," *The Physician and Sports Medicine* 3:54–67, March 1975. Reproduced by permission of the publisher, McGraw-Hill Book Company, and courtesy of William Newell, Purdue University.)

into a postoperative knee immobilizer before the athlete is placed upon the stretcher.

When moving an unconscious player, or one who is suspected of having a cervical, thoracic, or lumbar spine injury, special care needs to be taken. A short or, preferably, a long spine board is used.[4] The player is placed onto the spine board as one solid unit while the head, shoulders, pelvis, and legs are controlled under the direction of the leader (see Figure 16.17). The spine board is then placed in position and the athlete rolled back onto it and secured to it.

As mentioned, if an athlete has a cervical, thoracic, or lumbar spine injury, he or she should only be moved by personnel adequately trained to handle this type of injury, preferably under the supervision of a physician. This may mean a delay in the athletic event, but the player's health and well-being must be the prime consideration.

REFERENCES

1. Torg JS, Quedenfeld TC, Newell W: When the athlete's life is threatened. *Phys Sportsmed* 3:54–60, March 1975.
2. Hahn DB: The ruptured spleen: Implications for the athletic trainer. *Athletic Training* 13:190–191, 1978.
3. McMaster WC, Liddle S, Waugh TR: Laboratory evaluation of various cold therapy modalities. *Am J Sports Med* 6:291–294, 1978.
4. Loomis JL, Johnson A, Hochberg WJ, et al: Equipment update: Penn State's foldable rigid stretcher. *Phys Sportsmed* 7:135–136, October 1979.

RECOMMENDED READINGS

Compton R: The four "S" shoulder wrap. *Athletic Training* 12:94–96, 1977.

Moore R: Emergency medical care of athletic injuries. *Emergency* 3:184–186, 1975.

Smith WS: Esophogeal airway—an alternative to mouth-to-mouth. *Athletic Training* 14:38–39, 1979.

CHAPTER 7

Therapeutic Modalities and Procedures

INTRODUCTION

Over the years, heat in various forms (e.g., hot packs, ultrasound) has been the standard therapeutic modality. Cold is now being applied more frequently, not only for the initial treatment of the acute injury, but also for the recovery phase.

Basic Physics As It Applies To Therapeutic Modalities*

Heat. Heat is transferred from the source to the recipient by one or more of the following methods:

1. *Conduction.* The transference of heat by conduction technically involves the diffusion of energy through the collision of molecules. In order to get warm by conduction, the recipient needs to be in close contact with the source (e.g., hydrocollator pack).

2. *Convection.* Convection requires movement of the heating medium, usually warm water or air, which transfers heat by a flow from the source to the recipient.

3. *Radiation.* Heating by radiation is the transference of energy through space by means of electromagnetic waves (e.g., infrared lamp). The spectrum of radiant energy waves can be broken down into specific wave

*The athletic trainer or therapist needs to be aware of state laws regarding the prescription and administration of current therapeutic modalities and procedures.

lengths. This organization of wave lengths is referred to as the electromagnetic spectrum (Figure 7.1).

The two laws of physics that apply to radiation are:

1. *The inverse square law.* The intensity of radiation varies inversely with the square of the distance from the source.

IMPLICATION: The athletic trainer should consider the fact that when the distance from the source of the heat to the area being treated is decreased by 50%, the intensity of radiation is increased by 200%.

2. *The cosine law.* Optimal radiation is received when the source of radiation is at right angles to the area being treated.

IMPLICATION: When the angle of radiation is focused at 30° it takes double the exposure to produce the same intensity as when the angle of radiation is set at 90°.

Electricity. An electrical current is a stream of loose electrons passing along a

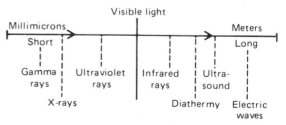

FIGURE 7.1 The electromagnetic spectrum

conductor. The two basic forms of electrical current in common use are:

Direct Current (DC), which flows in one direction only (also referred to as galvanic current)

Alternating Current (AC), which periodically reverses its direction of flow

For an understanding of the principles of electricity, there are four terms that need to be defined.

ampère (amp): $= I =$ represents the flow of charge at a rate of 1 coulomb per second past any point or through a conducting wire (3,600 coulombs equals one ampère hour).

volt: $= v =$ Joule/coulomb $=$ potential driving force for electrical conductivity:

$$v = I \cdot R$$

ohm: $= R =$ resistance of an electrical conductor, which equals $v \div I$.

watt, which equals a unit of power:

$$(I)^2 \cdot R \quad \text{or} \quad v^2 \cdot R^{-1}$$

When utilizing electrical energy for therapeutic purposes, the following effects should be noted:

1. *Thermal effects.* Almost all electrical currents cause a rise in temperature in the conductor, due to the "ohmic" resistance. This thermal effect is utilized in both shortwave and microwave diathermy because the tissue acts as the conductor.

2. *Electromagnetic effects.* This is used in muscle stimulation and transcutaneous electrical nerve stimulation.

3. *Chemical or ionic effects.* When a direct current is passed between two electrodes immersed in an electrolytic solution, the positive ions will be attracted to the negative pole and the negative ions to the positive pole (this type of effect is seldom intentionally used in athletic training).

Joule's laws. Joule's laws are applicable to the athletic trainer, because they are concerned with heating the body tissues by high-frequency electrical currents. The heat produced is directly proportional to the

1. square of the current strength
2. resistance of the conductor
3. time during which the current flows

IMPLICATION: In the use of high-frequency electrical currents for heating deep-body tissues, regulation of treatment depends upon

1. power output
2. various tissues of the human body that act as current conductors
3. treatment time

GENERAL PRINCIPLES OF THERAPEUTIC MODALITIES AND PROCEDURES

In the utilization of therapeutic modalities the athletic trainer should consider:

1. *The injury*—its type and severity and the anatomical site
2. *The modality*—indications and contra-indications
3. *Operation of the modality*—individual treatment time and its frequency, and operational procedures:
   a. warm-up
   b. safety procedures
   c. positioning of the athlete
   d. instructions to the athlete
4. *Treatment and progress records*

Any modality or procedure that is legally considered a therapeutic agent must be used on the prescription of a physician and must be administered by a licensed trainer or therapist.

The individual therapeutic modalities discussed below have, in most instances, been presented in outline form. The reader is encouraged to consult the reference list at the conclusion of this chapter for additional information.

Hydrocollator (Hot-Moist Packs)

INDICATIONS: After soft-tissue injury, such as contusions, muscle strains, and localized muscle spasms.

CONTRA-INDICATIONS AND PRECAUTIONS: Any general contra-indication to heat, specifically an impairment or deficiency in thermal sensation and thermoregulatory control.

THERAPEUTIC AND PHYSIOLOGICAL EFFECTS: Analgesic; reduction of muscle spasm; increase in surface (cutaneous and subcutaneous) circulation.

TREATMENT TECHNIQUES:

1. Set the temperature of the unit at approximately 65°C (149°F). Remove the pack from the unit and permit the excess water to drain off (handle with forceps, being careful to avoid contact with the water).

2. Place a number of dry towels between the athlete and the pack, to prevent an excessive amount of heat from reaching the skin.

3. Treatment time is usually twenty to thirty minutes.

Hydrotherapy (Whirlpool)

INDICATIONS:

1. As part of the immediate injury care, in which case a low water temperature is utilized (12.8°C [55°F]).

2. In the ongoing treatment of sprains, strains, contusions, tendinitis, and tenosynovitis. We recommend that cold temperatures be used in the majority of musculoskeletal conditions, and it is our opinion that only the occasional case needs warmer temperatures.

3. After surgery or immobilization, to help regain a range of motion.

4. As an exercise medium.

5. As a cleansing agent after removal of a cast and for skin lesions such as abrasions, blisters, and other wounds.

CONTRA-INDICATIONS AND PRECAUTIONS:

1. An electrical safety inspection should be conducted every three months by a qualified technician. A ground-fault circuit interrupter should be part of the electrical system.

2. Do not utilize warm or hot whirlpool treatment where there is hemorrhaging or swelling.

3. Be aware of the possibility of the athlete developing a heat-stress syndrome when the whirlpool is used at high temperatures for prolonged periods of time.

Advise the athlete to refrain from adjusting or turning on the device, and *never leave athletes alone* while they are being treated in a whirlpool. Make certain the level of water is well below the upper limits before turning the unit on. Thoroughly clean the tank with a disinfectant between treatments, particularly after treating open lesions.

THERAPEUTIC AND PHYSIOLOGICAL EFFECTS:

1. Sedative and analgesic action
2. Reduction of muscle spasm
3. Stimulating action on circulation (blood and lymph)

TREATMENT TECHNIQUES:

1. Select the proper size of whirlpool.
2. Select the proper water temperature:

Very cold	< 12.8°C	(< 55°F)
Cold	12.8°C to 18.3°C	(55°F to 65°F)
Tepid	26.7°C to 33.9°C	(80°F to 93°F)
Warm	33.9°C to 36.7°C	(93°F to 98°F)
Hot	> 37.2°C	(> 99°F)

The temperature selection should be influenced by

    a. indication for treatment
    b. duration since injury
    c. inflammatory-reaction state

3. Properly position the turbine so the flow is not directed at an acute lesion.

4. Treatment time is usually twenty to thirty minutes.

Diathermy

There are three different types of diathermy:

1. Longwave
2. Shortwave
3. Microwave

In the treatment of athletic injuries, shortwave and microwave diathermy are more commonly used to heat the deeper tissues. Many agree that shortwave diathermy produces a generalized heating effect, whereas the effect of microwave diathermy is more local.

The effects on the tissues are produced mainly as a result of the local increase in temperature and through reflexes associated with temperature receptors. There is increased blood flow and tissue metabolism, scar tissue may yield more easily when stretched, and tension within a musculotendinous unit may decrease, possibly as a result of decreased sensitivity of the muscle spindle to stretch.

Shortwave diathermy. Shortwave diathermy is a form of heat that uses a high-frequency electrical current to heat the deeper tissues, which it does by conversive heating, e.g., the electrical current is converted into heat within the deeper tissues without burning the intervening ones. Most shortwave diathermy machines operate at a frequency of 27.33 MHz, though other frequencies are available. The dose should be monitored by the athlete's subjective feeling of warmth.

INDICATIONS: Strains of the musculotendinous unit during the postacute stage.

CONTRA-INDICATIONS AND PRECAUTIONS: Any general contra-indication to heat, specifically nondraining infections, areas with on-

going hemorrhage, acute inflammation, limited circulation, and peripheral vascular disease. Do not use over clothing, dressings, adhesives, casts, metal implants, screws, or staples. Before applying, check the sensation of the skin. Do not use on a metal table.

THERAPEUTIC AND PHYSIOLOGICAL EFFECTS: Dilatation of blood vessels, with increased blood flow. Shortwave diathermy is both a mild sedative and an analgesic that reduces muscle spasm.

TREATMENT TECHNIQUES: Shortwave diathermy is administered either through the

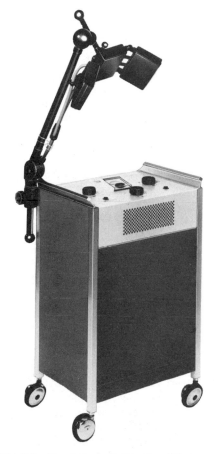

FIGURE 7.2 **Shortwave diathermy** (Photo courtesy of The Birtcher Corporation.)

application of one condensor plate on each side of the area to be treated (this produces more current density at the surface than in the deeper tissues), or by means of an induction coil which uses a magnetic field to induce a current within the tissues.

Select the method of application and place double-layered toweling between the drum and the area to be treated. Treatment time is usually twenty to thirty minutes.

EXAMPLE:

Injury: Chronic supraspinatus tendinitis, one month postinjury

Modality: Shortwave diathermy unit (hinged-drum application)

1. Set up unit and patient for treatment.

2. Instruct patient on procedure to be used.

3. Adjust unit and increase intensity until patient indicates a feeling of warmth or until the meter indicates the machine is operating within a safe range, even if the patient does not feel the warmth.

Microwave diathermy.   Microwave diathermy uses electromagnetic radiation to heat the deeper tissues by conversion. Tissues with a higher water content, such as muscle and fat, are more likely to absorb microwave energy than bone, and heat is likely to be produced at the fat-muscle interface. The depth of the tissue that is affected depends to a large extent on the frequency of the machine (900 MHz allows good tissue penetration; 2,500 MHz may only heat subcutaneous tissues).

INDICATIONS: The indications are the same as with shortwave diathermy, with the addition of selective use in trigger points (for a discussion of trigger points see sections on Neuroprobe and Cold Spray in this chapter). If a skin lesion contra-indicates hydrocollator usage, then microwave therapy may be useful.

CONTRA-INDICATIONS   AND   PRECAUTIONS: Essentially the same contra-indications as shortwave diathermy.

THERAPEUTIC AND PHYSIOLOGICAL EFFECTS: As with shortwave treatment, dilation of vessels, with increased blood and lymph flow and reduction of muscle spasm. A "beamed" or cylinder heating pattern produces deeper and more localized tissue heating.

Ultrasound

Ultrasound therapy is associated with the transference of sound waves into the body. Present-day ultrasound equipment is designed to emit waves well beyond the acoustical range, usually one megacycle (one million cycles) per second. The ultrasound waves may be interrupted or pulsed in order to reduce the heating effects.

INDICATIONS: Postacute soft-tissue trauma (sprains, strains, contusions, tendinitis, bursitis, and fibrositis), joint contracture, and scarring.

CONTRA-INDICATIONS   AND   PRECAUTIONS: An actively hemorrhaging contusion. Also, ultrasound should not be used in an area of limited vascularity that may not be able to meet the metabolic demands. Precautions should be exercised when treating near the heart, endocrine glands, central nervous system, ears and eyes, epiphyses, reproductive organs, and in an area of anesthesia.

THERAPEUTIC AND PHYSIOLOGICAL EFFECTS: Most of the therapeutic effects of ultrasound are due to the local, and often selective, increase in temperature of the tissues being treated.[1] However, other effects seem to occur and may relate to the diffusion of ions across the cell membranes under the influence of ultrasonic waves. Changes in the biochemistry of the tendon and joint capsule collagens and other items may also account for the increase in extensibility sometimes found during treatment.

TREATMENT TECHNIQUES: Treatment can be either by direct contact or by an underwater technique. The ultrasound can be pulsed, producing a mechanical effect only, or constant, which will also heat the tissues.

1. *Direct-contact technique.* This is useful over flat and smooth surfaces. Apply a coupling medium (gel) to the skin so as to transmit the sound waves from the transducer into the area in need of treatment. Hold the transducer at right angles to the skin surface and keep it constantly moving with small circular or longitudinal strokes at a speed of about one inch per second. Overlap each previous stroke by half.

Treatment time averages five to eight minutes. The minimum required treatments are three per week, but preferably it should be done daily. The prescribed dosage intensity can be adjusted while the transducer is moving. For instance:

low intensity = 0.1 to 0.8 watts per square centimeter (or five to eight total watts)

medium intensity = 0.8 to 1.5 watts per square centimeter (or eight to fifteen total watts)

high intensity = 1.5 to 3 watts per square centimeter (or over fifteen total watts)

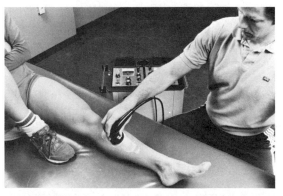

FIGURE 7.3 An ultrasound machine in use

EXAMPLE:

Injury: Hamstring muscle strain

Modality: Ultrasound

Treatment program:

a. For first twenty-four to forty-eight hours after injury, use ice, elevation, and compression (compression with ice).

b. For twenty-four to forty-eight hours from time of injury continue with above, but begin ultrasound. Start with a low dose (0.8 watts per square centimeter) that is pulsed, so a minimum of heat is produced. This dose can be increased to 1.5 watts per square centimeter over several treatments. Up to ten treatments are usually advocated.[2] The ultrasound treatment should be followed by gentle stretching and ice massage.

2. *Underwater technique.* This is used on uneven surfaces or body areas which are highly sensitive to pressure. Place the body part to be treated under water, and hold the transducer one-half to one inch from the surface. As with the direct-contact method, keep the transducer moving. Make sure the system incorporates a ground-fault circuit interrupter.

Iontophoresis

Iontophoresis is the method by which ionized medication is driven through the skin by means of an electrical current or by ultrasound. Most commonly, an ionized solution of dexamethasone (Hexadrol) in combination with a 4% viscous Xylocaine preparation is used.

INDICATIONS: Postacute soft-tissue trauma, for instance contusions, tendinitis, and strains.

CONTRA-INDICATIONS AND PRECAUTIONS: Contra-indications are as mentioned for electrical stimulation and ultrasound, and the specific medication being used.

TREATMENT TECHNIQUES: Place the medication on a special application pad. Place the pad directly over the tender area and apply current for approximately five minutes. The intensity of the current may be increased over the course of treatment. If a larger area is affected, spread the medication over this area and apply ultrasound in a dose of 1.5 watts per square centimeter for five to ten minutes at a time.

Phonophoresis

Phonophoresis is a technique whereby whole molecules of medication are driven through the skin by means of ultrasound. Experimentally it has been found that the medication, usually hydrocortisone, has reached a depth of up to six centimeters.[4]

INDICATIONS: Postacute soft-tissue trauma, for example, tendinitis, strains, contusions, and painful areas.

CONTRA-INDICATIONS AND PRECAUTIONS: The contra-indications are those listed for ultrasound and the specific medication being used. At the present the most frequent medication used for phonophoresis is hydrocortisone as a 10% cream, sometimes in conjunction with a local anesthetic agent such as Xylocaine.[3] One should therefore be aware of the possibility of suppression of the adrenal glands and the tendon-weakening effect of corticosteroids. Sensitivity to local anesthetic agents should also be noted if this preparation is used.

THERAPEUTIC AND PHYSIOLOGICAL EFFECTS: The effects are the same as those for ultrasound, plus the anti-inflammatory action of the hydrocortisone. If Xylocaine is used in combination with the hydrocortisone, a temporary local anesthetic effect on the tissues may also occur.

TREATMENT TECHNIQUES: The area should be well localized, washed thoroughly to remove skin oils, and preheated. A layer of approximately 3 to 5 millimeters of the preparation should be applied evenly to the surface. The best results appear to be with ultrasound of low intensity but longer duration, for instance 250 kilocycle frequency (though 1,000 kilocycle frequency is most commonly used in clinical practice) at a dose of 1 to 1.5 watts per square centimeter for 15 minutes.[4] Treatment time is usually 5 to 7 minutes.

For bony prominences or other irregular surfaces, use immersion therapy with the water at 33°C (91.4°F), ensuring good underwater coupling. The number of treatments recommended is from five to ten.

Electrical Muscle Stimulation

Electrotherapy modalities use either a direct or an alternating current, or a combination of the two. The current may be altered in a variety of ways.

1. Interrupted—The current is turned on and off at intervals.
2. Surging—The magnitude is slowly increased and decreased.
3. Modulation—The magnitude of a wave form is altered.

INDICATIONS: Peripheral nerve lesion involving the musculotendinous unit. Electrical muscle stimulation may help prevent, as well as treat, the muscular atrophy which occurs when a limb is immobilized.[5] It is also used in muscle re-educational programs. Muscle stimulation may also be useful in reducing swelling and pain around a joint, and for treating localized trigger points and spasms.

CONTRA-INDICATIONS AND PRECAUTIONS: Electrical stimulation is of questionable value in conditions where there is a permanently interrupted nerve pathway. The difficulty is in deciding if the nerve pathway is irreversibly damaged or not. It may therefore be justified to try electrical muscle stimulation to see if any effect is produced.

THERAPEUTIC AND PHYSIOLOGICAL EFFECTS: When a muscle is allowed to atrophy, enzy-

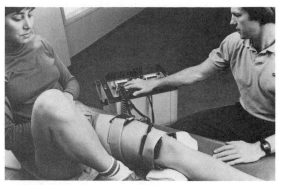

FIGURE 7.4 An electrical muscle stimulator

matic and structural changes occur. Modern muscle stimulation techniques may prevent many of these changes.

TREATMENT TECHNIQUES:

1. *Unipolar technique.* Electrodes are of unequal size and used when treating small muscles or trigger points. The active electrode is placed over the motor point of the muscle to be treated, while the dispersive electrode is placed at a point distant to the area being stimulated (usually on the same side and under the extremity).

2. *Bipolar technique.* Electrodes are of equal size and are used to exercise muscle groups or a large muscle (both active and dispersive electrodes are on the same muscle or muscle group). For instance, when treating the quadriceps muscles, the active electrode is placed over the motor point on the lower third of the thigh, while the dispersive is placed over the proximal portion of the femoral nerve. An intermittent surging current of five-seconds-on and five-seconds-off can be used. The intensity of the current can be increased as tolerated, as can the length of time, for instance, up to one-minute-on and one-minute-off.

Ultrasound and Electrical Muscle Stimulation Used Together

INDICATIONS: Postacute soft-tissue trauma, for example sprains, strains, and contusions.

CONTRA-INDICATIONS AND PRECAUTIONS: The same as described in the separate sections on ultrasound and on electrical muscle stimulation.

THERAPEUTIC AND PHYSIOLOGICAL EFFECTS: May prevent development of adhesions within healing tissues.

TREATMENT TECHNIQUES: The combination of ultrasound and muscle stimulation can be useful in certain sprains and localized muscle strains. The specific techniques are the same as those discussed in the sections on ultrasound and muscle stimulation.

EXAMPLE:

Injury: Severe hamstring muscle strain

Modality: Combination of ultrasound and muscle stimulation

Treatment program:

1. First seventy-two hours after onset of injury—cryotherapy (gentle stretching on ice)

2. Fourth and fifth days after the injury:

   a. Ultrasound (at 1.0 watts per square centimeter) plus electrical stimulation (pulsed and set at a rate of seven to eight, intensity set at six to seven). Generally a high number of contractions at a low intensity. (The numbers given here are for a Medcosonlator machine.)

   b. Two treatments per day of seven minutes each.

3. Sixth day and onward—ultrasound (1.5 watts per square centimeter for seven minutes) plus electrical stimulation (pulsed and set at six to seven, with intensity set at seven to eight). At this stage of treatment the rate of concentration begins to be decreased and the intensity increased. Continue this for fifteen minutes, then gradually modify the setting until the rate reaches four and the intensity ten.

Transcutaneous Electrical Nerve Stimulation (TENS)

INDICATIONS: Acute and chronic pain. Transcutaneous electrical nerve stimulation is used successfully in treating pain immediately after surgery or an acute injury, thereby reducing the need for pain-killing medication and allowing earlier muscle and joint function.[6,7,8] The TENS unit can be used continuously as well as intermittently in treating chronic or long-standing pain.

CONTRA-INDICATIONS AND PRECAUTIONS: The TENS should not be used over the carotid sinuses, during pregnancy, or on those with cardiac pacemakers. One should be cautious not to mask the pain of a serious or potentially serious injury just to allow the athlete to return to participation.

THERAPEUTIC AND PHYSIOLOGICAL EFFECTS: Exactly how TENS works is subject to speculation. Initially, the gate-control theory of pain was used to explain the effectiveness of its pain control.[9] It has been found that if large diameter afferent nerve fibers are electrically stimulated, pain perception decreases, perhaps by the inhibition of pain conduction through the small fibers at the dorsal horn level of the spinal cord. It is also thought that the activation of the inhibitory substantia gelatinosa cells will close the gate to the transmission of pain sensation. In addition, it is thought that chronic pain may depend upon neuroreverberating circuits and that TENS breaks these circuits by activating the descending pain-inhibiting pathways, thus decreasing the amount of pain experienced. It has recently become apparent that endorphins and enkephalins—pain-inhibiting chemicals released by the body in certain situations—are found in increased quantities, both during and after TENS treatment, and this may also explain why TENS is effective.

TREATMENT TECHNIQUES:

1. *Operation of apparatus—setting the controls.* On most pieces of apparatus it is possible to set the pulse rate, the pulse width, and the amplitude of the current. The current amplitude should be such that the athlete perceives a comfortable sensation, and there

should be no muscle twitching or contractions. There should be no discomfort with this procedure.

2. *Placement of the electrodes.* Proper electrode placement is an art based upon knowledge of the anatomical position of the dermatomes, the peripheral nerves, and the trigger points, which can only be refined by experience. Most commonly, one electrode is placed near or directly onto the site of discomfort or onto an area served by the peripheral nerve. The second electrode is placed more proximally, either along that dermatome or on a trigger-point area.

Very often the athlete will be able to distinguish an improvement in the pain sensation within the first five minutes. If the treatment session is then continued for twenty to sixty minutes, there may be a carry-over effect lasting a variable number of hours. This treatment can be repeated two or three times a day.

If no improvement is noted within fifteen minutes, however, the placement of the electrodes should be altered. This procedure should be repeated until the correct electrode placement for that particular condition and athlete is found.

EXAMPLE:

Injury: Paravertebral muscle strain with accompanying muscle spasm

Modality: Dual-channel TENS unit

Treatment program:

1. Electrode placement
   a. Lubricate electrodes with electrode gel.
   b. Choose electrode pattern, for example, *X* pattern (current directed through site).
   c. Stabilize electrodes in place with hypoallergenic tape.
2. Unit adjustment
   a. Set pulse rate 70 to 150 pps per second.

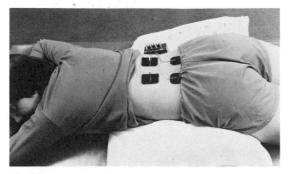

FIGURE 7.5 Transcutaneous electrical nerve stimulation for pain relief

  b. Set pulse width—the highest setting is often used initially, and then the setting is adjusted.
  c. Adjust output until patient perceives comfortable sensation under the electrodes.
  d. Adjust the output as the skin resistance decreases.

Neuroprobe

When pain syndromes develop, certain locations on the body called trigger points become sensitive to palpation or electrical stimulation. These trigger points are myofascial foci of irritation found within or just distal to the area of pain. It is a localized palpable spot of deep hypersensitivity which, when irritated, results in pain being referred to a predictable area on the skin. This area of referral may be a distance away from the trigger point.[10]

A diagnostic sign of a trigger point is a so-called jump sign. This sign is produced by accurately palpating the trigger point to produce pain in the area of referral as well as muscle contraction (or a jump) of the involved extremity. For instance, when the trigger point of the extensor carpi radialis is palpated, pain should be felt over the dorsum of the hand and the wrist should jump towards radial deviation and into extension.

Stimulation of these points by an instrument such as the Neuroprobe can often effectively reduce pain.[11]

INDICATIONS: Multitude of pain syndromes including acute or chronic pain, pre-operative and postoperative pain, neuralgias, and joint pain.

CONTRA-INDICATIONS AND PRECAUTIONS: The use of neuroprobe stimulation is contraindicated in those with pacemakers and in pregnant women, and should not be used over the carotid sinus. It is for external use only. The cause of the pain should be determined by the physician before applying the stimulation, as the treatment could mask a serious underlying condition.

THERAPEUTIC AND PHYSIOLOGICAL EFFECTS: The neuroprobe is a combination point-location and point-stimulation instrument. It determines the exact location of the trigger points, measures the pain threshold at each point, and provides the treatment stimulus which controls pain. The mode of therapy is sometimes referred to as hyperstimulation analgesia, and the technique of stimulation appears to be a reduction of pain without loss of motor control or sensory reception.

The exact means by which results are achieved are not yet completely understood, but may be attributed to the gate-control effect (see section on TENS in this chapter).

Most athletes will get some degree of immediate relief following treatment. Approximately 5% of patients, however, will experience increased pain after the initial stimulation, which then subsides after the second or third session.

TREATMENT TECHNIQUES: Select the appropriate acupuncture chart for the patient's pain problem and locate the anatomical point relative to that athlete's problem. Have the athlete hold the grounded electrode, then turn on the unit and adjust the sensitivity controls. Move the probe tip over the approximate point site. When the exact point is located, as indicated by an audible signal, begin stimulation and increase the intensity to tolerance. Repeat this on a number of other points as indicated in the individual

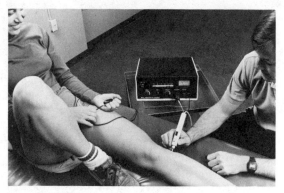

FIGURE 7.6 The neuroprobe apparatus

athlete. The usual stimulation time is sixty seconds per point.

Best results are usually obtained through a comprehensive program that includes stimulation of acupuncture points, both local and auricular, as well as appropriate use of other modalities and exercises where indicated.

Cryotherapy

When applied to the injured part, ice or cold packs result in the cooling of that part by the transfer of heat energy. Cold has been found to be a very effective modality in treating athletic injuries.[12,13,14]

INDICATIONS: Any of the typical athletic soft tissue indications, for example sprains, strains and contusions, both acute and established. Cryotherapy can also be used for relieving muscle spasm and trigger points.[15,16]

CONTRA-INDICATIONS AND PRECAUTIONS: Circulatory disturbances such as Raynaud's disease or hypersensitivity to cold. Be cautious about placing ice near or onto a superficial nerve, as this can lead to damage that results in temporary or permanent impairment of the nerve function[17] (e.g., cold damage to the peroneal nerve at the head of the fibula may result in foot drop). If left on the

skin for a prolonged period, skin damage with blister formation or frostbite may result.

THERAPEUTIC AND PHYSIOLOGICAL EFFECTS:

1. Reduction in pain through an anesthetic effect.
2. Reduction in swelling and inflammation.
3. Decrease in muscle spasm by reduction of nerve conduction and muscle spindle excitability.
4. Reduction in the metabolic and oxygen needs of the injured tissues, limiting the extent of the initial injury.[18]

TREATMENT TECHNIQUES:

1. Ice massage
   a. Freeze water in a styrofoam cup (score the top of the cup with a sharp knife as this facilitates peeling the top off. Place a toothpick or similar small piece of wood through the cup to prevent the ice from falling out as it melts).
   b. Rub the skin in circular or to-and-fro movements.
   c. Apply treatment for approximately three to ten minutes and repeat a number of times per day (Figure 7.7).
2. Immersion—Select desired water temperature:
   a. Tap water—12.8°C (53°F)
   b. Water with ice (slush)—approximately 0°C to 4°C (32°F to 39.2°F)
3. Ice packs[19,20]
   a. Use crushed or shaved ice, as this conforms more easily to the body part. Place in a double-layered disposable plastic bag.
   b. Apply treatment approximately twenty minutes per hour and repeat a number of times per day.
4. Refreezable commercial packs—follow instructions which accompany each specific make.

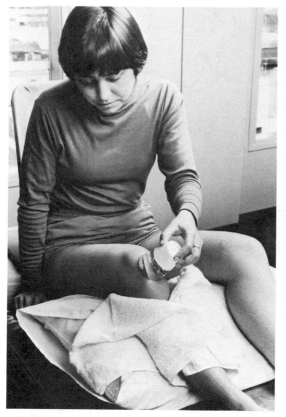

FIGURE 7.7 Ice massage to the patellar tendon

5. Evaporative cooling—ethyl chloride or FluoriMethane spray. These sprays cool by the heat-exchange effect of rapid evaporation and result in reflex muscle relaxation.[15]

For those individuals who have never experienced cryotherapy treatment, or for those who do not seem to be able to tolerate ice massage or ice immersion, begin the treatment with tap-water immersion and then progress to ice packs, ice massage, or ice immersion for short periods of time as tolerated.

Cryotherapy and Compression

INDICATIONS: Acute soft-tissue injury, especially sprains.

CONTRA-INDICATIONS AND PRECAUTIONS: As found with cryotherapy, that is, circulatory disturbances and hypersensitivity to cold. Precautions must be taken to prevent the placement of ice on a superficial nerve, and blister formation and frostbite must be avoided.

THERAPEUTIC AND PHYSIOLOGICAL EFFECTS: As with cryotherapy, reduction of pain, swelling, and muscle spasm and decrease in the metabolic and oxygen needs of the injured tissues.

TREATMENT TECHNIQUES: Ice plus a cold compression wrap. However, commercial units are available, for instance the Jobst Cryo/Temp unit (Figure 7.8).

EXAMPLE:

Injury: Moderate inversion ankle sprain

Modality: Jobst Cryo/Temp unit

Treatment program:

1. Place crushed ice into the appropriate section of the unit and fill with water.

2. Place the injured ankle into the correctly sized boot and close the zipper.

3. Turn the machine on.

4. As the bladder of the boot fills with water, add more water to the unit so there is enough to recycle through the system.

5. Set the pressure dial at 90 millimeters of mercury and the temperature at 7.4°C (45° F). The machine then applies alternating pressure.

6. Elevate the ankle during treatment, but not above the height of the unit.

7. Continue treatment for twenty to thirty minutes.

Cryokinetics (Cold and Therapeutic Exercise)

INDICATIONS: Same as cryotherapy.

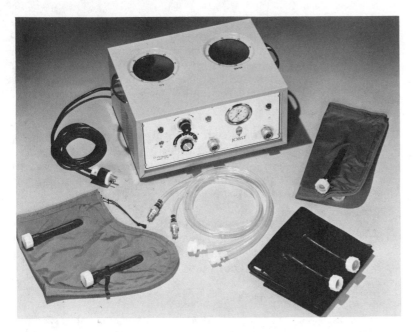

FIGURE 7.8 Intermittent cold and pressure unit (Photo courtesy of Jobst Institute, Inc.)

CONTRA-INDICATIONS AND PRECAUTIONS: Circulatory disturbance, such as with Raynaud's disease, or hypersensitivity to cold.

THERAPEUTIC AND PHYSIOLOGICAL EFFECTS: The concept of cryokinetics is to allow the injured part to be numbed by the effect of the cold, and then put through a range of normal movement and controlled exercise. Cryokinetics enhances the healing process by stimulating the circulation (through the exercise), while at the same time preventing inhibitory neural responses and allowing the surrounding tissues and muscles to return to early activity.[21]

TREATMENT TECHNIQUES: After applying cold to the injured part, begin an exercise program appropriate to that particular injury. When pain is felt, stop the exercise. Apply the cold for five to ten minutes, and repeat the cycle a number of times.

EXAMPLE:

Injury: Mild, second-degree inversion sprain involving the lateral ligaments of the ankle.

Treatment program:

1. First post-injury day
   a. Ice, compression, and elevation
   b. Gentle range-of-motion exercises
2. Second post-injury day and onward
   a. Ice for ten to twenty minutes. Then the athlete attempts a normal heel-to-toe walking gait. If this can be achieved without a limp, the athlete should continue until pain is felt. Then re-apply the ice and repeat the procedure three to five times.
   b. Perform the same routine with eversion exercises, toe-raises, and hopping.
   c. Always conclude the exercise session with ice, compression, and elevation.

Cold Spray

The technique of "spray and stretch" has been used for many years with ethyl chloride or, more recently, FluoriMethane, but it has not achieved wide recognition or popularity. However, there is no question in the minds of those who use this method that it has a place in the treatment of athletic injuries.

INDICATIONS: The spray and stretch technique is used to relieve pain arising from muscle spasm or an irritable myofascial trigger point.

CONTRA-INDICATIONS AND PRECAUTIONS: Hypersensitivity of the skin to the cold spray.

THERAPEUTIC AND PHYSIOLOGICAL EFFECTS: The concept is that a muscle in spasm produces pain regardless of the cause. In order to relieve the spasm and achieve normal resting muscle length, the cycle producing the muscle spasm must be blocked. It is thought that the effectiveness of the cold spray in relieving muscle spasm is due to the cold receptors conducting the sensation more rapidly than the pain impulses. This results in the muscle-pain impulses being blocked and the muscle spasm being relieved, which restores the normal reflex patterns, so long as the muscle is stretched during the application of the cold spray. Whatever the exact mechanism might be, the counter-irritation of cold applied in a specific way, together with stretching of the muscle, produces a reversal of muscle spasm in many cases, especially when dealing with trigger points.[10,15]

Cold spray can also be used for non-specific muscle spasm. For instance, if an athlete is subconsciously protecting an injured limb by contracting a particular muscle, this can produce intense pain in that limb without the athlete's being aware of the cause. Spraying along the muscle from origin to insertion, together with gentle stretching of the involved muscle, may produce immediate and complete relief from the discomfort of the muscle spasm.

TREATMENT TECHNIQUES: The cold spray currently being used is FluoriMethane. This spray appears to be safer and more effective than ethyl chloride. A specific technique should be carefully followed if satisfactory results are to be obtained (Figure 7.9).

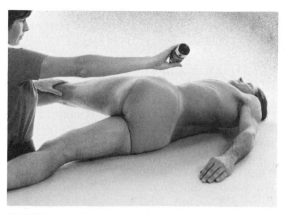

FIGURE 7.9 Spray and stretch technique as used for piriformis muscle spasm When treating an athlete, the skin should be exposed and the spray directed along the course of the piriformis muscle.

1. The muscle to be sprayed should be stretched to the point of discomfort.

2. The container is held approximately eighteen inches (45 cm) from the skin.

3. The jet stream should meet the body's surface at an angle, not perpendicularly.

4. The stream should move from the trigger point or origin of the muscle to the reference area or insertion of the muscle.

5. The speed of movement is about four inches (10 cm) per second.

6. Usually three or four parallel lines are sprayed. Movements are in one direction only and not across the muscle.

7. There should be no frosting of the skin if the technique is correctly applied.[15]

Contrast Bath (Alternating Cold and Heat)

INDICATIONS: Alternating cold and heat applications have been found useful in aiding recovery in the postacute phase, particularly after sprains of the extremities.[22]

CONTRA-INDICATIONS AND PRECAUTIONS: Peripheral vascular disease and lesions where there is active hemorrhaging (see contra-indications as described in the sections on heat and cold modalities and procedures).

THERAPEUTIC AND PHYSIOLOGICAL EFFECTS: It is thought by some that the alternate use of ice and heat may increase circulation to the injured area, thus aiding healing, reducing inflammation, and improving range of motion.

TREATMENT TECHNIQUES: Partially fill two containers: one with ice slush and one with lukewarm water (33.9°C to 36.7°C [93°F to 98°F]). The athlete first places the injured extremity in the ice slush for, say, two minutes and then immerses it in the warm water for thirty seconds. This is repeated a number of times over a ten or fifteen minute time span. The exact time for each treatment will vary with each athlete and the condition being treated. The treatment should always begin and end with the application of cold.

Paraffin Bath

INDICATIONS: Following a joint injury, particularly the smaller joints of the hands and feet.

CONTRA-INDICATIONS AND PRECAUTIONS: Any contra-indication to heat, specifically where there is active hemorrhaging or impairment of local circulation.

THERAPEUTIC AND PHYSIOLOGICAL EFFECTS: The paraffin bath is particularly useful in enhancing circulation and providing relief from pain. The cutaneous receptors are shut off from all stimuli except the warmth of the paraffin, and the insulation (layers of hardened paraffin) prevents heat loss.

TREATMENT TECHNIQUES:

1. Paraffin mixture formula—Twenty-five kilograms of solid paraffin to one liter of oil (paraffin or mineral).

2. The paraffin heating unit should be set to maintain the paraffin at a temperature of 52°C to 58°C (125.6°F to 136.4°F).

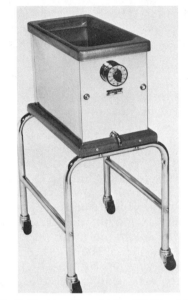

FIGURE 7.10 Paraffin bath (Photo courtesy of Thermo-Electric Co.)

3. Method of application:
   a. Paraffin dip-and-wrap method—Dip the relaxed extremity into the melted paraffin for two or three seconds, then remove it to permit air drying. Repeat this procedure six to twelve times. Cover the area with paper towels and then a cloth towel. Total treatment time is twenty to thirty minutes.

   b. Paraffin dip-and-soak method—Use the same procedure as the wrap method except that once the "glove" has been formed it is not wrapped. Instead, immerse and soak it in the liquid paraffin for fifteen to twenty minutes.

   c. Paraffin "painting"—Dip a paintbrush into the melted paraffin and apply to the body part. Repeat this procedure six to twelve times, then allow the paraffin to air dry. Total treatment time is from twenty to thirty minutes.

Infrared

INDICATIONS:

1. Soft-tissue injury after the initial inflammation has subsided.
2. Useful when the athlete cannot tolerate the pressure from, or the weight of, a hot pack or heating device.

CONTRA-INDICATIONS AND PRECAUTIONS: Infrared is generally contra-indicated for an athlete with a deficiency in heat perception.

THERAPEUTIC AND PHYSIOLOGICAL EFFECTS: A reduction in muscle spasm and an analgesic effect.

TREATMENT TECHNIQUES:

1. Luminous lamp (an eighteen-to-forty centimeter diameter lamp)
   a. If 250 watts are used, the distance should be 40 to 50 centimeters (15 to 20 inches) from the athlete.
   b. If 1,250 watts are used, the distance should be 75 to 90 centimeters (30 to 35 inches).
2. Nonluminous lamp—250 watts, set at a distance of 50 centimeters (20 inches).

The trainer should review the cosine and inverse square laws.

Ultraviolet

Objects heated to a very high temperature produce wave lengths too short to be perceived by the human eye, including ultraviolet rays. The chief artificial sources of ultraviolet radiation are electric arcs between electrodes of metals and of carbon and mercury in quartz.

Ultraviolet penetrates tissue to a very limited extent. The human skin arrests ultraviolet radiation beyond a depth of two millimeters. The many variables associated with ultraviolet (e.g., production, transference, and recipient factors) make the exact prescription and dosage of ultraviolet difficult.

INDICATIONS: Indications are limited for the athletic trainer and consist mainly of open wounds or lesions that are resistant to healing.

CONTRA-INDICATIONS AND PRECAUTIONS: Inquire if the athlete is taking any medications that might cause an increased sensitivity to ultraviolet light, e.g., a tetracycline antibiotic. Special goggles to protect the eyes should be worn at all times during the ultraviolet therapy.

THERAPEUTIC AND PHYSIOLOGICAL EFFECTS: Erythema production, bacteriocidal for certain bacteria, and photochemical reactions.

TREATMENT TECHNIQUES: Test the athlete to determine the minimal erythemal dose suitable for that individual. The specific type of apparatus will determine the exact operational procedure.

Massage

INDICATIONS: Postacute soft-tissue trauma, particularly strains.

CONTRA-INDICATIONS AND PRECAUTIONS: Acute injuries with ongoing hemorrhaging, infections, thromboses, and situations where calcification might occur with massage, for example, thigh contusion with the possibility of myositis ossificans and conditions in which the nervous system has suffered some damage.

THERAPEUTIC AND PHYSIOLOGICAL EFFECTS: The effects vary according to the specific type of massage applied. However, these effects are usually classified as either mechanical or reflexive.

TREATMENT TECHNIQUES: Determine the specific type of massage to be utilized for the particular situation and injury. Types of massage are:

1. *Effleurage*—Superficial or deep stroking movements administered with the flat of the hand and fingers:

a. *Deep massage*—Mechanical forces are applied to the deeper structures such as the muscles.

b. *Superficial massage*—No pressure is applied, so that the main effect is that of sensation rather than of mechanical force.

2. *Petrissage*—There is a kneading of the muscles. All the movement is executed by grasping or picking up the muscle tissue, then compressing, rolling, or squeezing it. The pressure is usually applied into the muscle rather than along the body surface.

3. *Tapotement*—With this technique, there is mechanical percussion with the fingers, the fingertips, the palms, or the sides of the hands to create tapping, cupping, slapping, or hacking movements.

4. *Vibration*—The hand is kept in contact with the athlete to produce a trembling, vibratory forward-and-backward movement. The direction of massage is usually distal-to-proximal—for example, in the upper extremity, from the fingers to the wrist or from the elbow to the shoulder; in the lower extremity, from the ankle to the knee or from the knee to the hip; on the back, from the buttocks to mid-scapula along the spine.

5. *Friction*—In frictional and, especially, cross-frictional massage, firm fingertip pressure is applied to or across the muscles, tendons, or both. This is a particularly useful technique for breaking down scar tissue, for example, lateral epicondylitis or rotator-cuff tendinitis.[23]

Manipulative Therapy

The use of manipulative therapy (also called mobilization therapy) is undoubtedly controversial.[24] However, this does not mean that the subject should not be explored. Exponents of manipulative therapy find athletes to be particularly good subjects, as they are prone to problems that tend to be amenable to manipulation and are less likely to have the contra-indications nonathletes might have.

For those wishing to use manipulative techniques, it is important to understand the indications, limitations, and possible dangers. Manipulation should not be undertaken without a thorough understanding of the subject and should be guided by an experienced therapist. Manipulation should not be used as a cure-all, for it can certainly be dangerous if used in the wrong circumstances.[25]

WHAT DOES MANIPULATION DO? WHY DOES IT WORK? There are many theories as to why manipulation works. One of the most acceptable and easily understood is that presented by John Mennell, M.D. as the concept of *joint play* and *joint dysfunction*.[26,27]

Joint play refers to the normal range of involuntary movement of which a joint is capable. An example that Dr. Mennell often refers to is the metacarpophalangeal joint, which has joint play in several directions. For instance, the joint can be opened by pulling the finger in a long-axis direction (long-axis extension). The phalanx can be moved anteriorly and posteriorly (this is anteroposterior glide). Also, it can be tilted either to the medial or the lateral side, as well as rotated medially or laterally. These are all normal movements of that particular joint and constitute joint play.

The theory states that if normal *joint play* is not present, pain will be experienced either in that joint or as referred pain. Pain will be felt both when the joint is moved voluntarily and when it is moved in testing for joint play. This pain is referred to as *joint dysfunction*. Stated another way, the normal range of voluntary movement depends upon the normal range of involuntary movement, i.e., joint play.

Manipulation restores normal joint play by taking the movement of that joint to its limits. If this is done in a correct manner, the pain in that joint will disappear, if due to joint dysfunction as defined above.

Athletes involved in running activities are particularly prone to joint dysfunction of the lower back and feet. Gymnasts and rowers are subject to lower-back joint dysfunction, and wrestlers to neck-joint dysfunction. Those involved in weight training often develop joint dysfunction of the wrists. Immobilization of a joint for a period of time to allow healing may result in dysfunction of that joint. All these problems may, after careful evaluation, be suitable for manipulative therapy.

Muscle spasm can follow or be associated with joint dysfunction and can make it very difficult for manipulative techniques to be employed. Muscle spasm can indeed persist after normal joint play has been restored and should be specifically treated by massage, cold spray, cryotherapy, or other suitable techniques.

BEFORE MANIPULATION IS CONSIDERED:

1. A *positive diagnosis* of joint dysfunction should be made. In order to make this diagnosis, the trainer must appreciate the extent of normal joint play for each individual and should compare the affected joint with the normal opposite joint in making this determination.

2. The *contra-indications* for manipulative therapy should be thoroughly understood. For instance, if joint or bone inflammation or disease exists, then no manipulation should take place. It is not indicated during the healing phase of ligament sprains or muscle strains; nor if there are any signs of a disc protrusion or rupture in the cervical or lumbar areas. It is therefore important to make a distinction between radiating pain, indicating a probable disc protrusion, and referred pain, which might be associated with joint dysfunction.

RULES FOR EMPLOYING MANIPULATIVE THERAPY:

1. Both patient and therapist must be completely relaxed. A patient cannot relax if there is a feeling of tension in the grip or the movements of the therapist.

2. Only one joint should be moved during each manipulation (though there are occasional exceptions to this).

3. Only one movement should be performed at each joint at a time.

4. One bone of the joint should be stabilized while the other is moved.

5. There should be very little force and no abnormal movements. Manipulation is achieved by velocity of acceleration, without any real force being applied to the movement. The joint itself should be moved through its full range of normal joint play (which is thought to be nearly always less than three millimeters).

REFERENCES

1. Lehmann JF, Stonebridge JB, deLateur BJ, et al: Temperatures in human thighs after hot pack treatment followed by ultrasound. *Arch Phys Med Rehabil* 59:472–475, 1978.

2. Reid DC, Cummings GE: Factors in selecting dosage of ultrasound. *Medical Electronics and Data* 6:52–56, 1975.

3. Moll M: A new approach to pain: Lidocaine and Decadron with ultrasound. *USAF Med Serv Dig* 30:8–11, 1979.

4. Quillen WS: Phonophoresis: A review of the literature and technique. *Athletic Training* 15:109–110, 1980.

5. Eriksson E, Häggmark T: Comparison of isometric muscle training and electrical stimulation supplementing isometric muscle training in the recovery after major knee ligament surgery. *Am J Sports Med* 7:169–171, 1979.

6. Roeser WM, Meeks LW, Venis R, et al: The use of transcutaneous nerve stimulation for pain control in athletic medicine. A preliminary report. *Am J Sports Med* 4:210–213, 1976.

7. Moore S: Transcutaneous electrical nerve stimulation (TENS) for the treatment of football injuries. *Athletic Training* 13:146 147, 1978.

8. Thorsteinsson G, Stonmington HH, Stillwell GK, et al: Transcutaneous electrical stimulation: A double blind trial of its efficiency for pain. *Arch Phys Med Rehabil* 58: 8–13, 1977.

9. Melzack R, Wall PD: Pain mechanisms: A new theory. *Science* 150:971–979, 1965.

10. Travell J, Rinzler SH: The myofascial genesis of pain. *Postgrad Med* 11:425, 1952.

11. Melzack R, Stillwell DM, Fox EJ: Trigger points and acupuncture points for pain: Correlations and implications. *Pain* 3:3–23, 1977.

12. Knight KL: Cryotherapy in sports medicine. *Relevant Topics in Athletic Training*. Ithaca NY, Movement Publications, 1978.

13. McMaster WC: A literary review on ice therapy in injuries. *Am J Sports Med* 5:124–126, 1977.

14. Olson JE, Stravino VD: A review of cryotherapy. *Phys Ther* 52:840–853, 1972.

15. Mennell J McM: The therapeutic use of cold. *J Am Osteop Assoc* 74:1146, 1975.

16. Grant AE: Massage with ice (cryokinetics) in the treatment of painful conditions of the musculoskeletal system. *Arch Phys Med Rehabil* 45:233–238, 1964.

17. Drez Jr. D, Faust DC, Evans JP: Cryotherapy and nerve palsy. *Am J Sports Med* 9:256–257, 1981.

18. Knight KL: Effects of hypothermia on inflammation and swelling. *Athletic Training* 11:7–10, 1976.

19. McMaster WC, Liddle S, Waugh TR: Laboratory evaluation of various cold therapy modalities. *Am J Sports Med* 6:291–294, 1978.

20. Lowdon B, Moore R: Determinate and nature of intramuscular temperature changes during cold therapy. *Am J Phys Med* 54:223–233, 1975.

21. Knight KL, Londeree BR: Comparison of blood flow in the ankle of uninjured subjects during therapeutic applications of heat, cold and exercise. *Med Sci Sports* 12:76–80, 1980.

22. Cooper DL, Fair J: Contrast baths and pressure treatment of ankle sprains. In Trainer's Corner, *Phys Sportsmed* 7:143, April 1979.

23. Cyriax J, Russell G: *Textbook of Orthopaedic Medicine: Treatment by Manipulation, Massage, and Injection*, Vol II, New York, Macmillan, tenth edition, 1980.

24. Schiötz EH, Cyriax J: *Manipulation, Past and Present*. London, William Heinman Medical Books Ltd, 1975.

25. Schellhas KP, Latchaw RE, Wendling LR, et al: Vertebrobasilar injuries following cervical manipulation. *JAMA* 244:1450–1453, 1980.

26. Mennell J McM: *Joint Pain*. Boston, Little Brown and Company, 1964.

27. Mennell J McM: *Back Pain*. Boston, Little Brown and Company, 1960.

RECOMMENDED READINGS

Behnke R: Cryotherapy and vasodilation. *Athletic Training* 8:136–137, 1973.

Benton LA, Baker LL, Bowman BR, et al: *Functional electrical stimulation—A practical clinical guide*. Rancho Los Amigos Rehabilitation Engineering Center, Rancho Los Amigos Hospital, 7601 East—Imperial Highway, Downey, CA., 1980.

Bonica J: Management of myofascial pain syndromes in general practice. *JAMA* 164:732–738, 1957.

Bourdillon JF: *Spinal Manipulation*. London, William Heinemann Medical Books Ltd, 1970.

Griffin JE, Karselis TC: *Physical Agents for Physical Therapists*. Springfield Ill., Charles C. Thomas, 1978.

Knight KL, Aquino J, Johannes SM: A re-examination of Lewis Cold Induced Vasodilatation—In the finger and the ankle. *Athletic Training* 15:248–250, 1980.

Knight KL, Elam JF: Rewarming of the ankle, forearm, and finger after cryotherapy: Further investigation of Lewis cold-induced vasodilation. *J Can Ath Ther Assoc* 8:15–17, 1981.

Kramer JF, Mendryk SW: Cold in the initial treatment of injuries sustained in physical activity programs. *Canadian Journal of Health, Physical Education and Recreation* 45:27–29 and 38–40, 1975.

Lehmann JF, editor: *Therapeutic Heat and Cold*. Baltimore, Williams and Wilkins, third edition, 1982.

Maigne R: *Orthopedic Medicine*. Springfield, Ill., Charles C. Thomas, 1972.

Maitland GD, Brewerton DA: *Vertebral Manipulation*. London, Butterworths, fourth edition, 1977.

Melzack R: Prolonged relief of pain by brief, intense transcutaneous electrical stimulation. *Pain* 1:357–373, 1975.

Pasila MT, Visuri T, Sundholm A: Pulsating shortwave diathermy: Value in treatment of recent ankle and foot sprains. *Arch Phys Med Rehabil* 59:383–386, 1978.

Peppard A, Riegler H: Ankle reconditioning with TNS. *Phys Sportsmed* 8:105–108, June 1980.

Peppard A, Riegler HF: Trigger-point therapy for myofascial pain. *Phys Sportsmed* 9:161–164, June 1981.

Rogoff JB, Editor: *Manipulation, Traction and Massage*. Baltimore, Williams and Wilkins, 1980.

Shriber W: *A Manual of Electrotherapy*. Philadelphia, Lea & Febiger, fourth edition, 1975.

Snedeker J, Recine V, Cortee CM: Cryotherapy and the athletic injury. *Emergency* 3:170–175, 1975.

Warren CG, Koblinski JN, Sigelmann RA: Ultrasound coupling media: Their relative bansmissivity. *Arch Phys Med Rehabil* 57:218–222, 1976.

Wilson DH: Treatment of soft tissue injuries by pulsed electrical energy. *Br Med J* 2:269–270, 1972.

Zohn DA, Mennell J McM: *Musculoskeletal Pain: Principles of Physical Diagnosis and Physical Treatment*. Boston, Little, Brown and Company, 1976.

CHAPTER 8

Injury Rehabilitation

One of the major contributions the trainer can make to the welfare of the athlete is in the area of rehabilitation. The type of rehabilitation program that is prescribed frequently determines what level of athletic participation will be possible in the future.

The quality of rehabilitation also influences the frequency of injury. An example comes from a study by the New York Public High School Athletic Association (report of 1971), which included over 61,000 high school football players. This study showed a rate of knee injury which was 15 to 17 times greater for those with previously injured knees than for players who had not sustained knee injuries. Most of those re-injured had not had adequate rehabilitation. The study recommended that any athlete with a knee injury be placed in a planned rehabilitation program under the direction of a physician. No athlete was allowed to return to varsity football without completing the program.

The West Point Military Academy study of 1969[1] pointed out that 80% of the knee injuries at the academy occurred in athletes previously injured in high school. As a result of these findings, cadets with weak thigh muscles were prohibited from participating in contact sports. They were channeled into a remedial program instead, resulting in a marked decrease in the total number of knee injuries.

GOALS OF REHABILITATION

The goals in rehabilitating an injured athlete are usually considered different from those for the general population. Vigorous, in-tense, but controlled exercise allows early return to participation, ensuring that the injured part is as optimally conditioned as possible. As Dr. Fred Allman[2] has said many times, "The goal of treatment must be restoration of function to the greatest possible degree in the shortest possible time." That means that rehabilitation should begin at the same time as treatment of the injured part. Treatment and rehabilitation should blend imperceptibly into one, as acute care and early rehabilitation can minimize the effects of the injury (see section on ankle rehabilitation in Chapter 20).

No longer does rehabilitation wait until the injured part is "healed"; rather, rehabilitation is started while healing is taking place, resulting in an earlier return to activity and perhaps an improvement in the quality of the tissue that forms during the healing process. The aim is not necessarily to speed up healing (which cannot as yet be done), but rather to do all that is possible to avoid slowing it down.[3,4]

It is necessary, however, for the rehabilitation program to be influenced by a number of factors:

1. The severity of the injury
2. The stage of tissue healing[5]
3. Type of treatment including surgery and all precautions and restrictions of the particular injury or surgical procedure affecting the rehabilitation program
4. Strength of the muscles of the limb
5. Pain on motion of the joint
6. Range of joint motion
7. Joint swelling

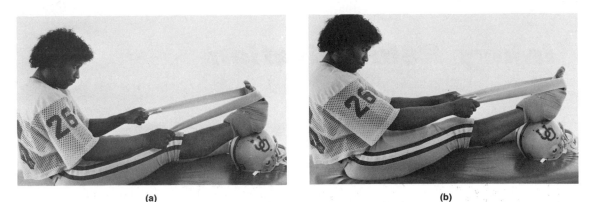

(a)   (b)

FIGURE 8.1 Acute care Rehabilitation starts at the time of acute care. An ankle sprain may be treated initially with ice, compression, elevation, as well as with dorsiflexion and plantar flexion exercises.

8. Other conditions within the joint—for example, chondromalacia of the patella

9. Demands that will be made by the sport upon the injured part

REHABILITATION PROGRAM

An individualized program that is drawn up for each athlete is a necessity. This program (rehabilitation prescription) should include how long each session should last and the number of times per week that each exercise should be performed, and should also include a long-term plan that estimates when each exercise should be used.

There are many pieces of specialized equipment on the market and these are very useful. One can use little or no equipment, however, and still obtain adequate results if the program is carefully and knowledgeably designed for a particular athlete's needs, and if the athlete is adequately motivated and supervised for the duration of the program. Having the most expensive machinery will not guarantee results if there is an inadequate program, little motivation, or poor supervision.

The program should be *progressive*, so that an increasing amount of work is performed at each session, as long as predetermined limits as well as the limits of discomfort are not exceeded. Minor injuries may be started on high-intensity, short-duration exercises initially, while more serious injuries may need to begin at a low-to-moderate intensity and then progress into the high-intensity program. Correct form with each exercise should be constantly stressed in order to maximize the results and prevent injury. There should be a definite rhythm and timing to the exercises, depending upon the type of apparatus being used.

The rehabilitation should proceed in an orderly fashion through a number of planned stages. In judging an athlete's rate of recovery and attempting to determine the timing of return to participation, factors such as functional tests and pain are used. Artificial guidelines of arbitrary time periods have limited, if any, value in modern athletic treatment as long as healing time is within physiological limits. These stages need to be individualized, but they generally include:

1. Initially, emphasis should be on cardiovascular fitness and isometric contractions, if a joint is immobilized.[6] Exercising the opposite limb may evoke a crossover reaction and maintain the muscles of the opposite limb.[7,8] If permitted, an attempt at limited motion within the confines of the immobilizer may help healing.[4,9] Muscle stimulation is also frequently used at this stage.[10]

2. When the immobilization is removed, a pain-free range of motion is regained through graded exercises, proprioceptive neuromuscular facilitation patterns (PNF),[11] transcutaneous electrical nerve stimulation (TENS), and cryotherapy. All of these techniques are used to overcome the neural inhibitions that frequently limit progress at this stage.[12] The effects of immobilization on the joint and soft tissues should always be kept in mind.[13]

3. As joint motion and flexibility return, resistance exercises can be increased. Some programs start with limited-range isotonic exercises, but others are achieving excellent and rapid results with low-resistance, moderately high-speed exercise on isokinetic machines, using submaximal intensity through a limited range of motion.

4. As strength is developed, more emphasis is placed on speed, power and endurance, circuit-training techniques, and flexibility exercises.

5. As the last step, specific skill patterns and sport-related skills are prescribed, with progressively complex drills.[14]

There are several criteria listed below that should be measured during and at the end of the rehabilitation program. Before releasing the athlete for full activity, these criteria should equal measurements obtained from the opposite uninjured side. These criteria include:

1. Strength of each muscle group

2. Power of each muscle group

3. Endurance of each muscle group

4. Balance between antagonistic muscle groups

5. Flexibility of the muscles around the joint that was rehabilitated

6. Proprioception of the injured joint and affected limb

7. Functional use of that limb in the required sport[15]

Common Mistakes

The more common mistakes are listed here so that they can be avoided:

1. Rehabilitation is often focused on a single muscle group only. After evaluation of the athlete to find out which muscles are particularly weak, all muscles of the limb need to be exercised, concentrating on those that are weaker. However, the limitations imposed by the injury or surgery should be observed.

2. Rehabilitation is seldom continued until the injured limb is found to be equal or superior to the uninjured side. The seven parameters previously mentioned need to be tested and the results documented before allowing return to participation.

3. Exercises for developing proprioception are often forgotten.

4. Postural defects and anatomical malalignment, as well as biomechanical imbalances, are frequently neglected when the rehabilitation program is developed.

5. Specific sports skills and the SAID principle (specific adaptation to imposed demands) are often not incorporated into the program. Exercises should be adapted to the specific needs of the athlete's particular position in a sport.[15]

TYPES OF EXERCISES

Isometric Exercise

An isometric contraction does not result in any movement of the joint. The contraction is often performed against a fixed resistance, and frequently is the only type of exercise that can be used, for instance, if a limb is immobilized in a cast.

Though Hettinger and Müller found considerable gains in muscle strength with the use of isometric contractions,[6] the current opinion in sports circles in the United States is that isometric exercises are probably the least effective form of strength improvement.[16] Isometrics, while useful, do not increase muscle bulk significantly, and they strengthen the muscle mainly at the joint angle at which the contraction is performed. With prolonged isometric exercise, the speed of a joint may actually be decreased, while endurance is not improved to any extent. Isometrics will not directly help improve a joint's range of motion.

To achieve the greatest benefit from isometric exercises, the joint should be at an angle which will permit the muscle to contract maximally (e.g., the quadriceps will contract maximally with the knee joint fully extended). The frequency and duration of isometric exercises depend on the state of the athlete's musculature as well as on the underlying reason for performing the exercises. For example, an athlete who has excellent quadriceps musculature, but who has the limb immobilized for a sprain of the medial collateral ligament, should be able to perform twenty quadriceps sets at maximal intensity every hour during the waking day, as well as one session each day of three quadriceps sets held for one minute. Contrast this with a case of chondromalacia patellae with poor quadriceps strength. Performing intensive quadriceps sets may actually cause a flare-up of the condition. The trainer needs to work closely with the athlete in this situation, as it may be found that contracting the quadriceps with the knee fully extended causes pain. Therefore these contractions may need to be performed initially with the knee slightly flexed. If genu recurvatum is present, the athlete needs to learn where the zero position of extension is and to perform the contractions in this position. In the beginning, an athlete with this condition may only be allowed to perform two or three quadriceps sets at 50% to 70% of intensity, each lasting five seconds, three times a day. If this does not cause pain, the intensity and number of contractions can then be increased. This example again emphasizes the need for an individualized program for each athlete.

Isometric contraction force can be measured with a strain-gauge device or on isokinetic machines.

Isotonic Exercise

Isotonic means that a joint is moved through a range of motion against the resistance of a fixed weight. This weight may be a sandbag, a weighted boot, an N–K table, a Universal Gym, or other similar machines. Isotonics is a simple and easily accessible form of exercise which was developed by DeLorme as progressive resistance exercise (PRE).[17,18] His formula is to first determine the maximum weight that can be lifted more than eight but less than twelve times (this equals ten repetitions maximum). Three sets of ten repetitions are then performed at 50%, 75%, and 100% of the ten-repetition maximum, which is determined once weekly and adjusted accordingly.

A variation on this is the Oxford technique, in which the weight is taken off rather than added on (e.g., sets of 100%, 75%, and 50%). This method is probably less effective and is seldom used in sports medicine.

To achieve a rapid increase in strength, the muscle group needs to be subjected to loads which will cause momentary failure. This high-intensity work is mandatory to rehabilitation techniques in sports medicine, in order to develop the muscles as fully as possible in the shortest time. For this reason, DeLorme's PRE program has been modified to include daily adjustments (the DAPRE technique[19]—see section on knee rehabilitation, p. 353).

Isotonic exercise consists of concentric and eccentric work. *Concentric* (or positive) *work* occurs when the muscle shortens as the weight is lifted; *eccentric* (or negative) *work* occurs when the muscle lengthens while the weight is being lowered.[20] Eccentric work appears to effect a greater gain in strength, but is also more stressful, often resulting in muscle soreness and, in the case of the knee, an overload on the patella.

It is often possible to lower a much heavier weight than can be lifted, and this knowledge can be utilized in a variation of the standard exercise, whereby the athlete lifts the weight with two legs and then lowers with the affected leg only (Figure 8.2).

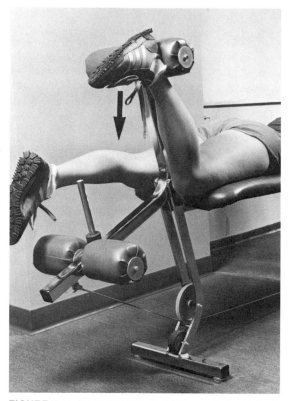

FIGURE 8.2 Isotonic exercise To maximize isotonic resistance, the weight is lifted with two legs and then lowered with only one leg.

Isotonic exercise produces improvement by developing tension within the muscle. More tension is developed at a slow, controlled rate of movement—for example, lifting to a count of three, holding for two counts, lowering to four counts. Much of the effect may be lost due to the ballistic movement of the weight if the procedure is done too rapidly.

There are disadvantages to isotonic exercise:

1. When using isotonic exercise in knee rehabilitation, the patellofemoral joint is subjected to reactive forces which may cause pain and even articular cartilage injury or degeneration.

2. The amount of weight is fixed and usually determined by the "sticking point" or weakest part of the range of motion of the lift. This means that, except for this point, the muscles moving the weight are working at below-maximum intensity. For this reason, in particular, weight-machine manufacturers have produced an isotonic machine which will vary the resistance to correspond to the changes in muscle strength throughout the range of motion—*variable-resistance* isotonic exercise machines. Such machines include the Nautilus and DVR Universal. Whether these actually result in greater gains in strength is subject to much controversy, with each manufacturer claiming spectacular results. There is also the question of the ability of the muscles developed by these machines to transfer the strength gains into a sport-specific activity. In summary, these machines appear to be an advance on the standard isotonic machines, but how much better they may be awaits further investigation (Figures 8.3 and 8.4).

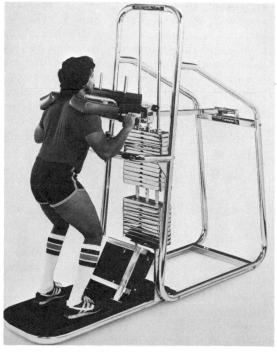

FIGURE 8.3 An example of a Universal DVR (variable resistance) isotonic machine

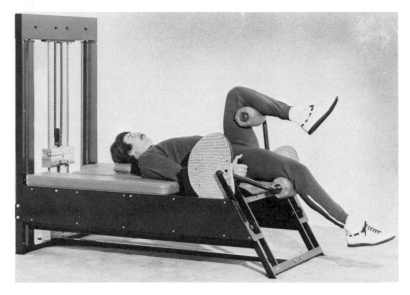

FIGURE 8.4 Nautilus hip and back machine Variable resistance isotonics

Isokinetic Exercise

Isokinetic exercise is an *accommodating variable resistance*, in which the speed of motion is set and the resistance accommodates to match the force applied. This is a relatively new form of rehabilitation made popular by the Cybex and the Orthotron machines, and has gained increasing acceptance over the past few years.[21] The possible speed settings range from 0° per second to 300° per second. Strength is usually developed between 60° per second and 120° per second; and power, at 180° per second. However, clinical evidence is being accumulated to show that strength and power gains are also excellent at faster speeds, possibly due to an increase in muscle recruitment. Endurance may also be developed at the faster speeds. One technique is to attempt to perform as many flexion/extension movements as possible (or whatever movement is appropriate) in a set time, for instance, one minute (see section on knee rehabilitation. p. 358).

One of the advantages of using isokinetic exercise is the visual readout possible with these machines, which not only helps the trainer evaluate progress, but also seems to act as a powerful psychological stimulus for the athlete. Also, as an appropriate resistance is applied throughout the range of motion, the athlete can reduce the force at the point of pain. In addition, a condition such as chondromalacia patellae or lateral epicondylitis of the elbow which, when painful, is often difficult to treat by means of isotonic exercise, frequently responds to high-speed isokinetic exercise.

A definite disadvantage of the isokinetic machines is their cost. This limits usage to a fraction of those who could benefit from the advantages of isokinetics. The isokinetic machines are also potentially dangerous when used in an uncontrolled manner on joints that are not stable. For instance, anterolateral rotatory instability can be produced if too vigorous a contraction is attempted through the last 30° of extension in a knee lacking an intact anterior cruciate ligament. In addition, chondromalacia patellae can be aggravated by high torque at slow speed.

SPECIAL FORMS OF EXERCISE

Manual Resistance

Manual resistance is a form of exercise in which the trainer should develop a special skill. When properly done it falls under the category of accommodative variable resistance, with the trainer adjusting the speed of movement and resistance to that best suited to the athlete's needs at the particular moment, which will vary according to the stage of rehabilitation and the state of fatigue. Almost any movement can be performed, and manual resistance can exercise patterns of movement that cannot be duplicated on machines (Figure 8.5).

Proprioceptive Neuromuscular Facilitation

Proprioceptive neuromuscular facilitation,[22] or PNF as it is commonly called, consists of a group of techniques that have been used with increasing frequency in sports medicine in recent years. It is based on stimulating proprioceptors such as the muscle spindles, the Golgi tendon organs, the pacinian corpuscles, and the free nerve endings to promote a response applicable to the rehabilitation of muscle function. If properly administered, PNF increases the motor (efferent) activity by stimulation of the proprioceptors.

The techniques most commonly used in sports medicine are the contract-relax exercise and the spiral-diagonal pattern.

1. The *contract-relax technique*[23,24] is used to increase the flexibility of a tight muscle group, for instance, the hamstrings (see Chapter 3).

2. The *spiral-diagonal pattern* is usually used to rehabilitate weak muscle groups and improve specific muscle patterns. The muscles are initially placed under maximal stress. Appropriate manual resistance is then applied to maintain facilitory stretch and afferent input, as well as to recruit the weaker muscles through the effort of the stronger ones. This recruitment of the weaker muscles by "irradiation" from the selected repetitive motion of the stronger muscles requires an intimate knowledge of the technique to correctly select appropriate patterns of movement for each chain of muscles. The movement ends with the muscles maximally shortened, to allow each muscle to go through the fullest possible length change and range of motion. A balance of tension needs to be maintained between the antagonist and the agonist, so that reciprocal relaxation of the antagonists occurs, with facilitation of the weaker muscle group by the stronger. Selection of appropriate patterns of movement is made for each chain of muscles.

With increasing knowledge and experience in the use of these techniques in sports

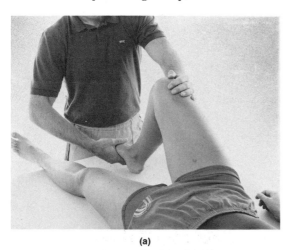

(a)

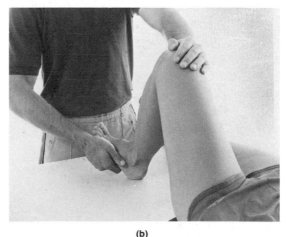

(b)

FIGURE 8.5 Manual resistance exercises The trainer should learn to apply the correct resistance for each individual athlete and injury. These illustrations demonstrate resistance to (a) inversion and (b) eversion of the ankle.

medicine, it is predicted they will be used more frequently, particularly in conjunction with progressive resistance and isokinetic exercise (Figure 8.6).

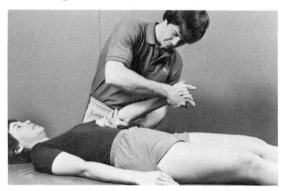

(a)

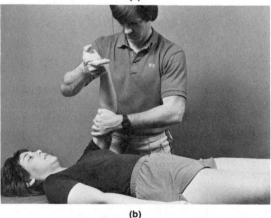

(b)

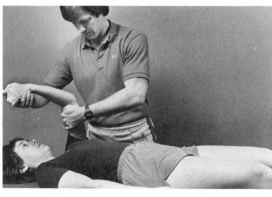

(c)

FIGURE 8.6 Proprioceptive neuromuscular facilitation This sequence demonstrates a pattern that is used in shoulder rehabilitation.

Elasticized Rubber Tubing (Surgical Tubing)

Rubber tubing is available in different thicknesses and can therefore provide a variety of resistances, which permits a type of resistive exercise to be done in almost any setting. Almost any muscle of the extremities or the back can be exercised by adjusting the direction of the pull (Figure 8.7).

An interesting technique that has been developed uses high-speed motion through a particular plane to place localized stress on a muscle. When performed in this manner until the onset of fatigue, a recruitment of muscle fibers appears to occur, resulting in immediate improvement in the function of the muscle. There may also be some gains in strength.

Circuit Training

When the athlete is nearing full recovery, all muscle systems can be placed under maximal stress by incorporating a circuit into the rehabilitation program. Such a circuit may incorporate thirty repetitions on the isotonic knee flexion/extension machine, followed immediately by high-speed knee flexion/extension on an isokinetic machine, performed submaximally until the thigh muscles

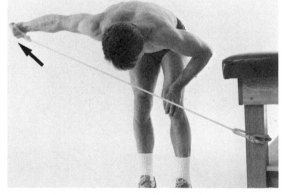

FIGURE 8.7 Elasticized rubber tubing (surgical tubing) This simple exercise technique is one of the most useful and practical ways to exercise individual muscles as well as groups of muscles. This illustration demonstrates the exercise for the posterior deltoid muscle.

burn from fatigue (elasticized rubber tubing may be substituted). This is then followed by a one-minute isometric contraction of the quadriceps. The circuit is repeated as many times as possible without a break.[25] This type of training can be adapted to almost any major joint of the extremities.

SPORT-SPECIFIC SKILLS

No rehabilitation program is complete until the athlete is graduated back into a specific sport and has developed the ability to perform the movements required by this sport. The athlete can be helped with exercises and skills that are an integral part of the sport. These exercises should become increasingly complex as the rehabilitation program progresses and should be performed for some time before return to actual participation.

THE PRESCRIPTION OF REHABILITATION PROGRAMS

In order to help those who are unfamiliar with the prescription of rehabilitation programs, a short summary of some common conditions follows. This outline shows the progression of an exercise prescription program. Many details obviously need to be filled in. Do not forget: Each athlete is different, and each program needs to be individualized.

1. *A mild second-degree sprain of the lateral ligaments of the ankle.* Following the initial treatment of ice, compression, and elevation and the start of the cardiovascular fitness program, the ankle exercise program may consist of:
   a. Initially—isometric eversion, followed by isotonic and isokinetic exercises and stretching of the Achilles tendon
   b. Eventually—proprioception exercises, hopping, and running figure eights
   c. Additional work on the entire extremity
   d. Specific return-to-sport exercises and activities

2. *A mild second-degree medial collateral ligament sprain of the knee.*
   a. Initially—quadriceps and hamstring isometric exercises, followed by isotonic and isokinetic exercises and stationary cycling
   b. Hamstring stretching exercises and strengthening of the other muscle groups
   c. Internal tibial rotation, abduction, toe raises, and work on the hip stabilizers
   d. Hopping and stationary running, followed by stair-running
   e. Eventually—figure eights, cariocas, and other functional exercises

3. *Following a surgical repair of an anterior shoulder dislocation.*
   a. Initially—isometric internal rotation followed by isotonic and isokinetic exercises
   b. Later—exercises for the deltoid, the rotator-cuff, and the trapezius muscles
   c. Eventually—arm hanging, pull-ups, and pegboard climbs

4. *Rotator-cuff impingement under the coracoacromial arch*, for instance in an athlete who does much throwing.
   a. Initially—gentle exercise, with gradually increasing intensity. At first, pendulum circles and isometric exercises for the trapezius, the latissimus dorsi, the deltoid, and the rotator-cuff muscle groups.
   b. Progression into isokinetic followed by isotonic exercises and elasticized tubing exercises.
   c. Eventually—throwing exercises following the FUNGO routine (see Chapter 14).

REFERENCES

1. Abbott HG, Kress JB: Preconditioning in the prevention of knee injuries. *Arch Phys Med Rehabil* 50:326–333, 1969.
2. Allman FL: *Sports Medicine.* Ryan AJ, Allman FL, editors. New York, Academic Press, 1974.

3. Leach RE: The prevention and rehabilitation of soft tissue injuries. *Int J Sports Med* 3:18–20, 1982.

4. Dehne E, Torp RP: Treatment of joint injuries by immediate mobilization: Based upon the spinal adaptation concept. *Clin Orthop* 77:218–232, 1971.

5. Paulos L, Noyes FR, Grood E, et al: Knee rehabilitation after anterior cruciate ligament reconstruction and repair. *Am J Sports Med* 9:140–149, 1981.

6. Hettinger ERT, Müller EA: Influence of training and of inactivity on muscle strength. *Arch Phys Med* 51:449–462, 1970.

7. Hellebrandt FA: Cross education: Ipsilateral and contralateral effects of unimanual training. *J Appl Physiol* 4:136–144, 1951.

8. Hellebrandt FA, Waterland JC: Indirect learning. The influence of unimanual exercise on related muscle groups of the same and the opposite side. *Am J Phys Med* 41:45–55, 1962.

9. Tipton CM, Matthes RO, Maynard JA, et al: The influence of physical activity on ligaments and tendons. *Med Sci Sports* 7:165–175, 1975.

10. Eriksson E, Häggmark T: Comparison of isometric muscle training and electrical stimulation supplementing isometric muscle training in the recovery after major knee ligament surgery. *Am J Sports Med* 7:169–171, 1979.

11. Hauglum P: Techniques of PNF in athletic training. *Athletic Training* 10:44–45, 1975.

12. Aten DW, Knight KL: Therapeutic exercise in athletic training—principles and overview. *Athletic Training* 13:123–126, 1978.

13. Sargeant A, Davies CTM, Edwards RHT, et al: Functional and structural changes after disuse of human muscle. *Clin Sci Mol Med* 52:337–342, 1977.

14. Yamamoto SK, Hartman CW, Feagin Jr JA, et al: Functional rehabilitation of the knee. A preliminary study. *J Sports Med* 3:288–291, 1975.

15. Allman FL: *Sports Medicine*. Ryan AJ, Allman FL, editors. New York, Academic Press, 1974, p. 311.

16. Steadman JR: Rehabilitation of athletic injuries. *Am J Sports Med* 7:147–149, 1979.

17. DeLorme TL: Restoration of muscle power by heavy resistance exercises. *J Bone Joint Surg* 27:645–667, 1945.

18. DeLorme TL, Watkins AL: Techniques of progressive resistance exercise. *Arch Phys Med* 29:263–273, 1948.

19. Knight KL: Knee rehabilitation by the daily adjustable progressive resistive exercise technique. *Am J Sports Med* 7:336–337, 1979.

20. Komi PV, Buskirk ER: Effect of eccentric and concentric muscle conditioning of tension and electrical activity of human muscle. *Ergonomics* 15:417–434, 1972.

21. Hinson MN: Isokinetics: A clarification. *Res Q* 5:3035, 1979.

22. Knot M, Voss D: *Proprioceptive Neuromuscular Facilitation: Patterns and Techniques*. New York, Harper and Row, 1968.

23. Tanigwa MC: Comparison of the hold-relax procedure and passive mobilization on increasing muscle length. *Phys Ther* 52:725–735, 1972.

24. Rogers JL: PNF: A new way to improve flexibility. (Proprioceptive Neuromuscular Facilitation) *Track Technique* 74:2345–2347, 1978.

25. Steadman JR: Rehabilitation after knee ligament surgery. *Am J Sports Med* 8:294–296, 1980.

RECOMMENDED READINGS

Clarke DH: Adaptation in strength and muscular endurance resulting from exercise. *Exerc Sport Sci Rev* 1:73–102, 1973.

Eriksson E: Sports injuries of the knee ligaments: Their diagnosis, treatment, rehabilitation and prevention. *Med Sci Sports* 8:133–144, 1976.

Kraus H: Evaluation and treatment of muscle function in athletic injury. *Am J Surg* 98:353–362, 1959.

Krejci V, Koch P: *Muscle and Tendon Injuries in Athletes*. New York, Stuttgart, Thieme, 1979.

Pipes TV, Wilmore JH: Isokinetic versus isotonic strength training in adult men. *Med Sci Sports* 7:262–274, 1975.

Smith M, Melton P: Isokinetic versus isotonic variable-resistance training. *Am J Sports Med* 9:275–279, 1981.

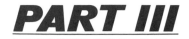

PART III

Specific Athletic Injuries and Related Problems

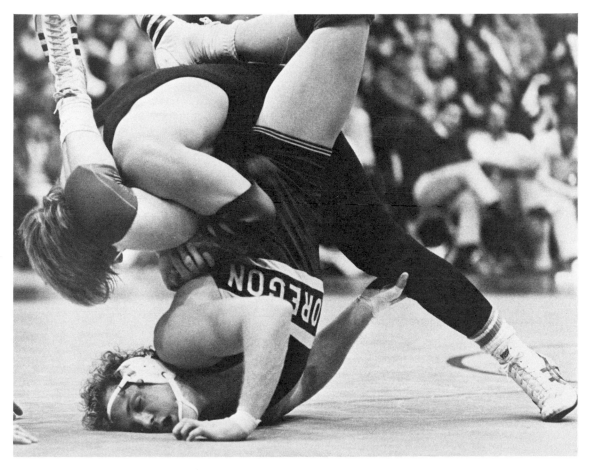

Photo by Mike Shields

CHAPTER 9

Inflammation, Microtrauma, and Stress-Related Injuries

Modern sports place intense demands on the recovery and restorative powers of the body. The present-day athlete is asked to do far more training and to subject his or her body to more stress than ever before. Very often, however, we find that the adaptive and healing processes have not kept pace with the imposed demands, resulting in overuse injuries which are frequently difficult and frustrating to treat.

This chapter discusses the process of inflammation as it applies to acute and chronic overuse injuries, the concept of microtrauma, and, finally, the stress-related injuries of bone.

THE INFLAMMATORY AND HEALING PROCESS

It is important to realize that the body's initial reaction to an injury is similar to its reaction to an infection. This reaction is termed inflammation and may manifest macroscopically (such as after an acute injury) or at a microscopic level, with the latter occurring particularly in chronic overuse conditions.

The trauma, or initial lesion, leads to an increase of the friction that occurs between moving tissues as well as to a release of chemical mediators, both of which may start the inflammatory process.[1] This process may present macroscopically with a number of signs, particularly (a) pain, (b) swelling, and (c) redness and warmth. However, microtrauma may not present with any of these signs, particularly during the early stages,

even though the inflammation is proceeding at the microscopic level.

1. *Pain.* The pain is thought to be due to a combination of factors acting in a vicious circle. For instance, the trauma itself may stimulate the pain receptors. Pain may also result from cell anoxia, because of interference with the blood supply, due to damage suffered by the capillaries at the time of the injury.

Oxygen and nutrients are essential for cellular survival, and their lack releases chemical substances such as bradykinin and prostaglandin, further aggravating the pain.

2. *Swelling.* The swelling originates from a number of sources. There is bleeding from the torn arteries, veins, and capillaries. Damaged cells fail to retain intracellular fluid, losing it to the extracellular compartment. As more cells succumb to anoxia, more fluid leaks out. The increased protein in the extracellular fluid raises the osmotic pressure of the extracellular compartment surrounding the site of the injury. Therefore fluid is drawn out of the cells, which are alive but functioning suboptimally. If the limb is held in a dependent position, gravity adds yet another factor that may increase the swelling.

3. *Redness and warmth.* The redness and warmth are indications of an increase in the blood supply to the injured area, which occurs once the healing process is initiated. This may also result from the release of his-

tamine, serotonin, bradykinin, and prostaglandin by the injured tissues and inflammatory cells.

The purpose of the inflammatory process is to heal the injured tissues. In order to clarify the process of inflammation and healing, it has been defined in three stages: (1) cellular response, (2) regeneration, and (3) remodeling.

1. *Cellular response.* The cellular response results in mast cells, macrophages, and granulocytes invading the traumatized area. These cells can survive under anaerobic conditions and are therefore suited to working in an area lacking oxygen. The mast cells release histamine and serotonin, while the granulocytes release prostaglandin. This in turn produces a vasodilatory effect on the surrounding blood vessels and leads to the stimulation of several humoral factors or systems, including the fibrinolytic system, the clotting system, the complement system, and the kinin system (Figure 9.1).

2. *Regeneration.* After the cellular response, the body initiates mechanisms with which it attempts to regenerate the damaged tissue. The body's potential for regeneration is somewhat limited, however, and usually a

less specialized tissue or form of *collagen* is produced. The first step in the regenerative phase is to remove the debris that results from the trauma, as well as the cells that have succumbed from anoxia. The granulocytes and macrophages accomplish this for, as mentioned, they can survive under relatively anaerobic conditions. The next stage is for capillaries to be formed in order to bring oxygen and nutrients (amino acids, sugars, vitamins, and enzymes) into the damaged area. Thus, endothelial cells regenerate, leading to the proliferation of capillary buds, which connect to form a new capillary system.

Fibroblasts then become active, and this in turn leads to collagen production. This can begin once there is sufficient oxygen at the cellular level, as the manufacture of collagen takes place in the ribosomes of the reticulum, which requires oxygen. Three polypeptide chains are formed when proline is hydroxylated by the enzyme prolinehydroxylase, together with vitamin C, into hydroxyproline. Glycine is also added. These chains, which consist of about a thousand amino acids each, are coiled into a spiral. Three of these chains then join, forming a triple helix. The triple helix configuration adds strength to the collagen, as does cross-linkage, which occurs by the joining of aldehydes produced from lysine (Figures 9.2 and 9.3).

At the same time as the collagen is being produced, it is being broken down by the lytic process of the enzyme collagenase, which is produced by macrophages and granulocytes. This occurs particularly during the first two weeks following the injury. For adequate healing to occur, there should be a balance between the synthesis and breakdown of collagen, but as less energy is needed for the lytic process, more breakdown than synthesis may occur initially. This means that during the first two weeks after an injury the tissues may have a decreased tensile strength. The healing tissues are then reinforced by ground substance which adds strength and defines the type of collagen that will eventually develop.

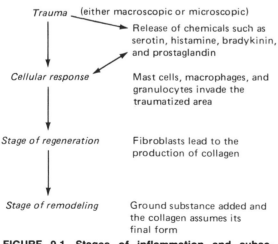

Trauma __ (either macroscopic or microscopic)

Release of chemicals such as serotin, histamine, bradykinin, and prostaglandin

Cellular response — Mast cells, macrophages, and granulocytes invade the traumatized area

Stage of regeneration — Fibroblasts lead to the production of collagen

Stage of remodeling — Ground substance added and the collagen assumes its final form

FIGURE 9.1 Stages of inflammation and subsequent healing

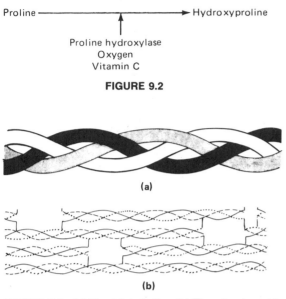

Proline ⟶ Hydroxyproline

Proline hydroxylase
Oxygen
Vitamin C

FIGURE 9.2

(a)

(b)

FIGURE 9.3 **(a) The triple helix** **(b) The structure of collagen** Triple helix plus cross linkages

3. Remodeling. The injured tissues next undergo remodeling, which can take up to one year to complete in the case of major tissue disruption.[2] The remodeling stage blends in with the latter part of the regeneration stage, which means that motion of the injured tissues will influence their structure when they are healed. This is one reason why it is necessary to consider using controlled motion during the recovery stage. If a limb is completely immobilized during the recovery process, the tissues may emerge fully healed but poorly adapted functionally, with little chance for change, particularly if the immobilization has been prolonged. Another reason for encouraging controlled motion is that any adhesions that develop will be flexible and will thus allow the tissues to move easily on each other. Caution should be observed during the first two weeks, as mentioned previously, as the tensile strength of the tissues may be markedly reduced.

Tissue constriction. One of the problems related particularly to inflammation from chronic overuse stress is that of constriction of the tissues by the healing process. If this occurs, it will not only affect the movement of tissues on each other, but will also control the amount of blood (and therefore oxygen) that is available to the tissues, especially during high-demand situations.[3] This hypoxia may explain the occurrence of pain after an injury has apparently healed. Tissue constriction can result from repetitive stress, which leads to microtrauma and an inflammatory reaction, or it can be due to adhesion formation following a period of immobilization.

Electrical polarity. One aspect of tissue healing that has recently been explored relates to the effects of electrical polarity on the cell. It is thought that cells may become depolarized as a result of an injury, and that this may be one factor that influences the rate of healing. Using specific electrical repolarization and magnetic stimulation techniques may affect the polarity of the cell's membranes, producing conditions favorable to the healing process. The application of this concept is still in the experimental stage, but it does add another exciting dimension to our understanding of the effects of tissue trauma and the healing process.

MICROTRAUMA

Constant repetitive maximal stressing of the body day after day leads not only to adaptive changes which enhance performance, but also to changes in some athletes which result in pathological microscopic lesions involving the tendon, or the junction of muscle and tendon or tendon and bone. These pathological changes result from an inflammatory response to the microtrauma of repeated stress and lead to edema and hemorrhage, followed by the invasion of inflammatory cells. If this reaction is not reversed at an early stage, the permanent organization of fibrin and the formation of adhesions and scar tissue may follow. This in turn may lead to constant pain both during and after activity. An example of this is patellar tendinitis, which results from the repetitive stress of jumping and landing and leads to an inflammatory response to microtrauma at the attachment of the patellar tendon to the patella.[4,5]

The microtraumatic lesion appears to be an individual reaction in particular athletes, with some being more disposed to develop the problem than others, even though they may all be engaged in the same activity.

SYMPTOMS: The inflammatory response to microtrauma can be divided into phases according to the severity of the symptoms.

Phase I. Pain *after* activity only

Phase II. Pain *during and after* activity, with no significant functional disability

Phase III. Pain during and after activity *with* significant functional disability

Phase IV. Pain *all the time*, with significant functional disability

TREATMENT: Discussing the concept of microtrauma with the athlete is important so that he or she has a clear understanding of the condition and the prognosis, and is thereby more inclined to cooperate in the treatment program.

Phases I and II:

1. Modification of the athlete's activity, if possible

2. Removal of any aggravating exercises

3. Ice massage or heat before activity, depending on which modality is more comfortable for the athlete

4. Ice and ice massage after activity

5. Accessory supports according to the area involved (e.g., patellar neoprene support and/or in-shoe orthotic devices)

6. Strengthening exercises of the muscles involved, so long as these exercises do not aggravate the condition

7. Anti-inflammatory medication (e.g., aspirin, Naprosyn, or Motrin)

8. Physical therapy modalities (e.g., high-voltage galvanic stimulation and transcutaneous electrical nerve stimulation)

Phase III:

1. Modification of activity, ice massage both before and after activity, and the treatment modalities mentioned for Phases I and II

2. More powerful anti-inflammatory medications (e.g., Butazolidin or Tandearil) for short periods of time (one or two weeks)

3. Intralesional cortisone injections in the more refractory cases once or twice only, if at all

Phase IV: Surgery in selected cases

STRESS REACTIONS AND STRESS FRACTURES

If an overuse condition affects the bones rather than the soft tissues, a stress fracture or a pre-stress fracture (a "stress reaction") can result. Stress fractures are among the most common athletic injuries and should always be considered when an athlete complains of pain related to bone, particularly if the pain is aggravated by activity and relieved by rest. The trainer needs to maintain a high index of suspicion for this condition in order to make an early diagnosis and apply the correct treatment, thereby decreasing the morbidity and complication rate.

The term *stress reaction* is used to describe a condition in which microfractures of the bone are present.[6] Some of these microfractures will heal if the athlete decreases the intensity of the causative activities. However, if the force on the bone is increased, an actual stress fracture may result (see the discussion of tibial stress reaction on p. 433).

It is becoming apparent that the diagnosis of a stress fracture is increasing in frequency. Part of this is due to earlier detection both clinically and by utilization of procedures such as the bone scan, but part may also be due to an actual increase in fractures because of greater athletic participation by the general public.

ETIOLOGY: A stress fracture will occur if the forces applied repetitively to a bone exceed the structural strength of the bone. Though most stress fractures are related to impact forces associated with weight bearing, others are not (such as the fractured humerus of the ball thrower or javelin thrower). The factors that seem to be most clearly associated with the development of stress fractures are:

1. Muscle forces acting across the bone

2. Repetitiveness of the activity

The muscle forces, or torque, across the bone may stress that bone if an imbalance between antagonistic muscles exists.[7] In addition, though muscles may be rapidly strengthened by a particular activity, bone is thought to adapt and strengthen at a much slower rate and is thus subjected to forces for which it is not ready. Initially, as mentioned, microfractures may occur and in some cases may progress to become complete fractures.

Types of stress fractures. There are four basic types of stress fractures (see Figure 9.5):

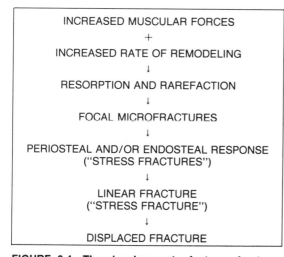

```
INCREASED MUSCULAR FORCES
            +
INCREASED RATE OF REMODELING
            ↓
  RESORPTION AND RAREFACTION
            ↓
      FOCAL MICROFRACTURES
            ↓
PERIOSTEAL AND/OR ENDOSTEAL RESPONSE
      ("STRESS FRACTURES")
            ↓
        LINEAR FRACTURE
       ("STRESS FRACTURE")
            ↓
      DISPLACED FRACTURE
```

FIGURE 9.4 The development of stress fractures (Adapted from C. L. Stanitski et al., "On the nature of stress fractures," *American Journal of Sports Medicine* 6:391–396, 1978. Reprinted by permission.)

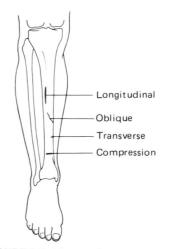

FIGURE 9.5 Types of stress fractures

1. Oblique fracture—the most common variety

2. Compression fracture

3. Transverse fracture—the most dangerous because it can displace

4. Longitudinal fracture—very rare

Bones most frequently affected. Almost any bone in the body can be affected by a stress fracture. In athletes, the ones most commonly affected (Figure 9.6) are the following:

1. Tibia—either the upper third or the junction of the mid-third and lower thirds. Occurs particularly in running activities.

2. Fibula—usually the lower third. Occurs mostly in running athletes.

3. Metatarsal shaft—especially the second through fourth. Can result from marching, walking, running, or jumping.

4. Calcaneus.

5. Femur—either the lower third or the femoral neck. These are serious fractures which can displace if not adequately treated.

6. Pars interarticularis of the lumbar vertebrae—stress fractures in this area can result in spondylolysis. These fractures are particularly common in gymnasts and football linemen.

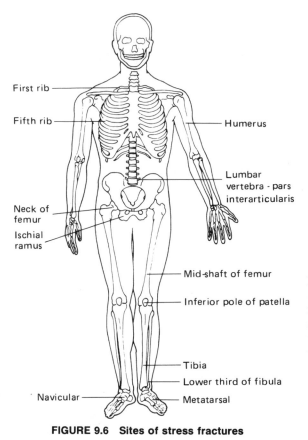

First rib
Fifth rib
Humerus
Lumbar vertebra - pars interarticularis
Neck of femur
Ischial ramus
Mid-shaft of femur
Inferior pole of patella
Tibia
Lower third of fibula
Navicular
Metatarsal

FIGURE 9.6   Sites of stress fractures

7. Rib fractures—especially the first rib in weight lifters and the eighth rib in tennis players.

8. Humerus—oblique-spiral fractures of the midshaft of the humerus have been recorded in throwing sports.

SYMPTOMS AND SIGNS: The athlete complains of pain which initially occurs during the activity and is relieved by rest, though occasionally a stress fracture will present with sudden acute pain. In the next stage the pain continues for hours, perhaps through the night, or it might become worse during the night (pain that becomes worse at night is highly suggestive of bone pain). Swelling may occur, particularly after activity.

Localized tenderness with or without

swelling is almost always present over the fracture (Figure 9.7). Percussion is often very painful and should be performed gently. One may also percuss away from the affected area. For example, with a suspected stress fracture of the tibia, percussing the heel may produce pain in the area of the fracture.

The tuning-fork test may help to add weight to the presumptive diagnosis of a stress fracture. With this test a vibrating tuning fork with a flat base is placed onto the tender area. If discomfort or pain is felt (which is not present when the unaffected limb is tested), it is suggestive of a stress fracture. While this test is not always positive, it is seldom positive without a stress fracture being present (Figure 9.9).

X-RAYS: It is important to realize that a stress fracture may not be visible on ordinary X-rays for two to eight weeks after symptoms commence. It is therefore important to X-ray the painful area again if symptoms persist, or to obtain a bone scan.

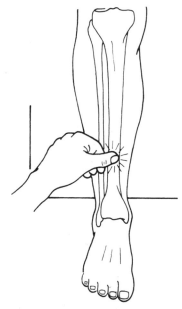

FIGURE 9.7   Localized tenderness is highly suggestive of a stress fracture

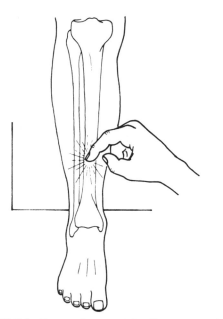

FIGURE 9.8 Percussion used to diagnose a stress fracture

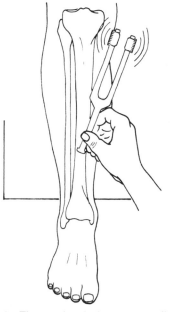

FIGURE 9.9 The tuning-fork test to diagnose a stress fracture

The first signs on ordinary X-rays are rarefaction of bone, a hairline fracture, a thin layer of callus along the periosteum, or all three. In the compression-stress fracture, a dense sclerotic line appears in the substance of the bone. The dangerous transverse variety has a clear fracture line running at right angles to the bone shaft which may appear to involve only part of one cortex, but the weakness usually extends right across the shaft (Figure 9.10).

BONE SCAN: A radioactive-labeled substance (technetium–99m) is taken up by metabolically active bone. This produces the increased uptake or "hot spot" of a positive bone scan and can be seen within the first few days of the symptoms presenting.[8,9,10,11] The *stress reaction state* may produce a "hazy" bone scan (see tibial stress reaction, p. 433) (Figure 9.12).

COMPLICATIONS: The most serious complication involves displacement of a complete stress fracture. This is particularly dangerous when it occurs through the neck of the femur, as avascular necrosis may follow.

Occasionally, nonunion of a stress fracture occurs, necessitating surgery and possibly bone grafting. Some stress fractures require a long period of relative inactivity to heal completely and may recur after apparent healing.

TREATMENT: Rest is the basic treatment for stress fractures, but each case has to be evaluated on its own merits. For instance, it is frequently permissible for the athlete to continue participation while suffering from a stress fracture of the third or fourth metatarsal shaft as long as a special in-shoe modification is used. However, the individual with a stress fracture at a site such as the femur should not be permitted to continue with athletic activity until the fracture has healed.[12,13]

Resumption of training should be graduated so that enough time is allowed for adequate bone adaptation to take place. If training is resumed too rapidly, the symptoms will frequently recur.

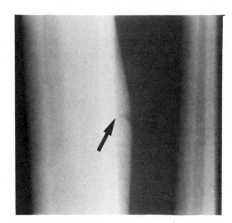

FIGURE 9.10 Transverse fracture of the anterior crest of the tibia

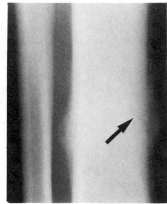

FIGURE 9.11 A stress fracture at six weeks Note the callus indicating that healing is taking place.

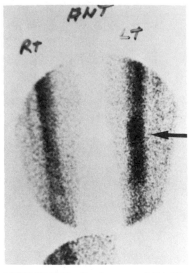

FIGURE 9.12 Bone scan of the tibiae A "hot spot," signifying a stress fracture, can be seen.

REFERENCES

1. van der Meulen JCH: Present state of knowledge on processes of healing in collagen structures. *Int J Sports Med* 3:4–8, 1982.
2. Paulos L, Noyes FR, Grood E, et al: Knee rehabilitation after anterior cruciate ligament reconstruction and repair. *Am J Sports Med* 9:140–149, 1981.
3. Kvist M, Järvinen M: Clinical, histochemical and biochemical features in repair of muscle and tendon injuries. *Int J Sports Med* 3:12–14, 1982.
4. Williams JGP: Wear and tear injuries in athletes —an overview. *Br J Sports Med* 12:211–214, 1979.
5. Blazina ME, Kerlan RK, Jobe FW, et al: Jumper's knee. *Orthop Clin North Am* 4:665–678, 1973.
6. Jackson DW: Shin splints: common, painful, and confusing. *Consultant* 16:75, 1976.
7. Devas M: *Stress Fractures.* London, Churchill Livingstone, 1975, pp 224–227.
8. Geslien GE, Thrall JH, Espinosa JL: Early detection of stress fractures using 99m Tc-polyphosphate. *Radiology* 121:683–687, 1976.
9. Prather JL, Nusynowitz ML, Snowdy HA, et al: Scintigraphic findings in stress fractures. *J Bone Joint Surg* 59A:869–874, 1977.
10. Daffner RH: Stress fractures: Current concepts. *Skeletal Radiol* 2:221–229, 1978.
11. Garrick JG: Presentation, 43rd American Academy of Orthopedic Surgeons, New Orleans, Louisiana, February 1976.
12. Kaltsas D-S: Stress fractures of the femoral neck in young adults. *J Bone Joint Surg* 63B:33–37, 1981.
13. Todd RC, Freeman MAR, Pirie CJ: Isolated trabecular fatigue fractures in the femoral head. *J Bone Joint Surg* 54B:723–728, 1972.

RECOMMENDED READINGS

Belkin SC: Stress fractures in athletes. Symposium on sports injuries. *Orthop Clin North Am* 11:735–741, 1980.

Fordham SD: Stress fracture affects variety of exercisers. *Phys Sportsmed* 4:79–82, November 1976.

Latshaw RF, Kantner TR, Kalenak A, et al: A pelvic stress fracture in a female jogger. A case report. *Am J Sports Med* 9:54–56, 1981.

Morris JM, Blickenstaff LD: *Fatigue Fractures: A Clinical Study.* Springfield Ill., Charles C Thomas Company, 1967.

Orava, S, Puranen J, Ala-Ketola L: Stress fractures caused by physical exercise. *Acta Orthop Scand* 49:19–27, 1978.

Stanitski CL, McMaster JH, Scranton PE: On the nature of stress fractures. *Am J Sports Med* 6:391–396, 1978.

Taunton JE, Clement DB, Webber D: Lower extremity stress fractures in athletes. *Phys Sportsmed* 9:77–86, January 1981.

Woo SLY, Kuei SC, Amiel D, et al: The effects of prolonged physical training on the properties of long bone: A study of Wolff's law. *J Bone Joint Surg* 63A:780–787, 1981.

CHAPTER 10

Epiphyseal Injuries

Adolescents and pre-adolescents are subject to a special group of injuries because their bones have not yet matured. These injuries, which affect the growth centers, should be known to the trainer who is involved in the health care of the young athlete.

Pre-adolescence is defined as the time from childhood until the onset of secondary sex characteristics, whereas adolescence is considered to begin after secondary sex characteristics appear and to continue until there is skeletal maturity.

The highest incidence of epiphyseal injuries occurs in twelve- to fourteen-year-olds, with boys being injured more frequently than girls.

Physiology of bone growth. The growth center (Figure 10.1) consists of three main parts:

1. Epiphysis, in which a secondary center of ossification may form
2. Growth plate (or physis)
3. Metaphysis

Epiphyses may be divided into pressure or traction epiphyses. Pressure epiphyses relate to the longitudinal growth of long bones and are found at the ends of the bones. Traction epiphyses, or *apophyses*, are located at the attachment of certain tendon's to the bones, for example, the patellar tendon's attachment to the tibia, and the medial epicondylar epiphysis from which originate the forearm flexor muscles of the humerus.

The growth plate consists of four layers of cartilaginous cells. The first lies adjacent to the epiphysis and is called the resting layer. The cells of the resting layer increase in number (proliferate) and form the second layer, the zone of proliferating cells. These cells then form columns (columnate) and increase in size (hypertrophy). This zone of hypertrophied cells in turn becomes calcified (zone of provisional calcification) and, finally, ossified (Figure 10.2). The zone of hyper-

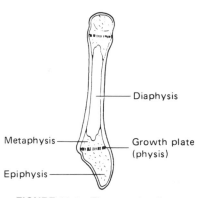

FIGURE 10.1   The growing bone

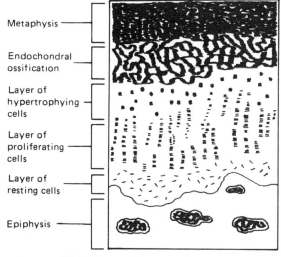

Metaphysis

Endochondral ossification

Layer of hypertrophying cells

Layer of proliferating cells

Layer of resting cells

Epiphysis

FIGURE 10.2   The growth plate

trophying cells is the weakest part of the growth plate and is the area through which separation usually occurs in the event of an injury. Fortunately this does not usually interfere with the blood supply or the zone of resting cartilage cells, so that growth is not disturbed.

Prevention of epiphyseal injuries. Though epiphyseal injuries occur in organized sports, they are more likely to happen during unorganized play activity.[1] For instance, only 15% of fractures of the distal femoral epiphyseal plate were found to result from organized athletic participation.

In order to reduce to a minimum the number of epiphyseal and other injuries that do occur in organized athletics, certain points should be remembered.

1. If an athlete suffers an injury or illness that results in muscular atrophy or loss of tone, he or she should be placed on a program of rehabilitation exercises before being allowed to return to a competitive environment.

2. The adolescent may be more likely to suffer epiphyseal injuries during certain developmental stages (e.g., "growth spurts") particularly if involved in contact sports.

3. There are adolescents who should be encouraged to take up activities other than contact sports, for example, the obese Fröhlich-like adolescent or the tall, thin, rapidly growing youth who is uncoordinated and has poor muscle development. These youths should be re-examined when their bodies have matured and at that time it should be determined whether they are better able to withstand the forces of contact-sport participation.

4. Heavily muscled or more mature adolescents should not be allowed to compete in contact sports with those who are smaller and relatively immature in their development, because this exposes the smaller athletes to a higher rate of injury. Contact sports should be organized so that weight, size, and strength are taken into consideration. In an attempt to reduce the injury rate, the New York Public High School Association devised a program that grouped adolescents on the basis of physical fitness, skills, and physical maturity. This program has apparently resulted in a 50% reduction of the injury rate.

Classification of epiphyseal injuries. The most frequently used classification is that developed by Salter and Harris,[2] which divides the injuries into five types—type I producing the least damage to the epiphysis and type V being the most serious (Figure 10.3).

The most common types of epiphyseal fractures seen in athletes are type I and type II. It has often been stated that the epiphyseal plate is the weakest link in the tendon-bone chain. Some studies have shown that the capsule and ligaments around joints are between two to five times stronger than the growth plate. This means that an injury that would result in ligament damage in an adult leads to an epiphyseal injury in a child (Table 10.1).

Treatment of epiphyseal injuries.

1. Type I or type II epiphyseal injuries, in which minimal separation is present and no remodeling necessary, need only be immobilized for about three weeks, followed by a period of rehabilitation.

2. Type I or II, where there is slightly more separation or where remodeling is necessary, should be immobilized for about six weeks, followed by a gradual rehabilitation program before return to participation.

3. Type III, IV, or V injuries include an osseous component in the injury and thus are slower to heal than when the growth plate alone is injured. Adolescents with these injuries should be off contact and collision sports for at least one year. If the involved epiphysis is related to a weight-bearing joint, the athlete should not participate in running or jogging activities for at least one year, but he or she can swim. At the end of the year, the athlete should be re-assessed with regard to further participation.

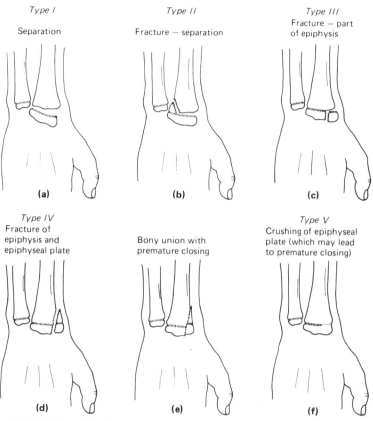

Type I

Separation

(a)

Type II

Fracture — separation

(b)

Type III

Fracture — part
of epiphysis

(c)

Type IV
Fracture of
epiphysis and
epiphyseal plate

(d)

Bony union with
premature closing

(e)

Type V
Crushing of epiphyseal
plate (which may lead
to premature closing)

(f)

FIGURE 10.3   The Salter-Harris classification of epiphyseal fractures

Complications and prognoses of epiphyseal injuries. Injuries to the growth plate may have a number of possible effects, though the majority do not result in interference with bony growth. Significant growth distur-bance occurs in approximately 10% of epiphyseal injuries. This relatively low figure is due to the fact that most fractures occur through the zone of hypertrophying cells or of provisional calcification, neither of which interferes with blood vessels supplying the epiphyseal cells.

The complication rate depends on the bone involved, the extent of the damage to the epiphyseal plate, and the degree of maturity reached by that epiphysis. In some cases, a temporary increase in the growth of the bone is produced, but this does not usually result in any deformity.

Most type I, II, and III injuries have a good prognosis as long as the epiphyseal blood supply remains intact. Type IV has a relatively poor prognosis, particularly if the epiphyseal plate is not perfectly realigned.

TABLE 10.1   Adolescent and Pre-adolescent Injuries

1. An adolescent or pre-adolescent is much more likely to sustain an injury to the growth plate than to suffer a ligamentous injury.
2. The growth plate is the weakest link in the chain involving the muscles, tendons, ligaments, and bone.
3. Any injury or "sprain" around a joint in a growing child should be considered an epiphyseal injury until proven otherwise.

Type V injuries are associated with crushing of the epiphysis and therefore have the poorest prognosis, but fortunately this injury accounts for only about 2% of all epiphyseal fractures.

In the small number of cases in which the growth plate closes, bony growth is disturbed. If the whole epiphysis is affected, one limb will be shorter than the other, though this deformity does not produce any angulation. If the bone involved is one of a pair (e.g., the ulna and the radius or the tibia and the fibula), shortening of one bone will result in the development of a deformity of the related joint. On the other hand, if only part of the epiphyseal plate closes while the other part continues to grow, an angulation of the limb will result.

Overuse injuries of the growth plate.
The growth plate may also be injured by an overuse type of stress.[3] Though this is not a common injury, it is nevertheless an area of concern as more and more adolescents and pre-adolescents subject themselves to intense training techniques.[4,5]

X-ray changes are seen in stress fractures of the proximal humeral epiphyses in baseball players[6]; ischial crest epiphyses[7] and proximal tibial epiphyses stress fractures in runners[8]; and stress changes to the distal radial epiphyses in gymnasts (Figure 10.4).

X-RAY EXAMINATION: It should be remembered that usually very little change shows on the X-rays, even though the epiphysis has been injured. The epiphysis can be displaced at the moment of injury and then return to the normal anatomical position. Comparison X-rays of the opposite extremity should be taken. Slight widening or irregularity of the growth plate may be noted, but often the only way to prove that an epiphyseal fracture has occurred is to perform stress X-rays (usually under anesthesia) and note if this results in any opening of the growth plate. Stress X-rays should be performed in certain areas, such as around the knee joint, especially with injuries to the distal femoral epiphysis (Figure 10.5).

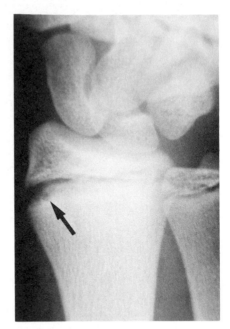

FIGURE 10.4 Stress changes of the distal radial epiphysis as seen in gymnasts (compare with Figure 1.8). Some of the changes include widening and irregularity of the epiphyseal plate.

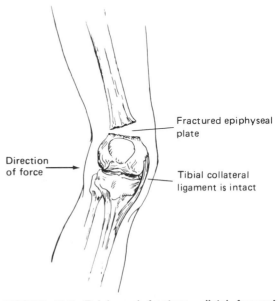

Fractured epiphyseal plate

Direction of force

Tibial collateral ligament is intact

FIGURE 10.5 Epiphyseal fracture—distal femoral epiphysis This injury may result from a valgus force (as illustrated).

Which epiphyses are most commonly injured? The epiphyses most likely to be injured in athletic participation are the:

1. Distal radial epiphysis (wrist injuries)
2. Distal tibial and fibular epiphyses (ankle injuries)
3. Distal femoral epiphysis (knee injuries)
4. Distal and proximal humeral epiphyses (including the medial epicondylar epiphysis of the humerus, which is particularly at risk in young pitchers)
5. Phalangeal epiphysis (finger injuries)

SPECIFIC AREAS

The Wrist

The *distal radial epiphyseal plate* may be injured by a fall on the hand of an outstretched arm. All "sprains" of the wrist in the adolescent and the pre-adolescent should therefore be examined with this possibility in mind and referred for X-ray examination (see section on wrist injuries, p. 232).

The Ankle Joint

The *distal fibular and tibial epiphyseal plates* are commonly injured, usually due to an inversion plantar flexion injury to the ankle (though sometimes they are injured by an eversion force). A high index of suspicion is necessary to avoid missing the diagnosis and calling the injury a "sprain." It is therefore important that all ankle sprains be evaluated not only clinically but also by X-rays.[9]

The Knee Joint

A valgus force applied to the lateral side of the knee is likely to result in a sprain of the medial collateral ligament in an adult, whereas in the growing athlete the growth plate is more commonly injured. It is not unusual for a sixteen-year-old to have open epiphyses which will take the force of the injury rather than tear the ligaments.[10] This is because the capsule and the ligaments surrounding the joint are two to five times stronger than the growth plate. Also, the anatomy of the ligamentous attachment is important. At the knee, the collateral ligaments are attached below the distal femoral epiphysis, while the proximal tibial epiphysis is above the ligament, thus making the distal femoral epiphysis more susceptible to injury. In a pre-adolescent, ligamentous and meniscal injuries are relatively rare.

The symptoms and signs of an epiphyseal knee injury may be very similar or even identical to a knee ligament injury. Obtaining a complete series of X-rays (including valgus-stress views) before making a definitive diagnosis is often important (see Figure 10.5). As with any knee ligament injury, examine for damage to the popliteal artery or nerve (particularly with proximal tibial epiphyseal injuries).

If the adolescent presents with pain around the knee, but no specific knee injury is found, remember that a hip or back problem may be the cause of the pain. For instance, a slipped capital femoral epiphysis or Perthes disease of the hip may present with knee pain without hip pain.

The Elbow Joint

1. *The medial epicondylar epiphysis* of the elbow may be avulsed in a Little League baseball pitcher.[11,12,13] There may be a history of pain with a particular pitch, or the symptoms may come on gradually. Tenderness is localized to the medial epicondylar epiphysis, and swelling may be present. Extension of the elbow may be limited and valgus stress may produce pain, as may forced resistance to wrist flexion. The epiphysis is usually minimally avulsed, but occasionally may slip into the elbow joint (special X-ray views of both elbows may be necessary).

2. *The proximal radial epiphysis.* The head of the radius may be injured by a fall on the outstretched hand, and a type II injury to the radial head may be produced by compression against the capitulum of the humer-us.[14] The head of the radius may also be injured in a posterior dislocation of the elbow.

Chronic stress such as occurs in baseball pitching or in gymnastics can produce traumatic osteochondrosis of the capitulum and the articular surface of the radial head[15] (see section on throwing injuries of the shoulder and the elbow, p. 211).

The Hip Joint

A slipped capital femoral epiphysis occurs in young teen-agers, most frequently in males who have a Fröhlich-type disposition with large quantities of subcutaneous fat and delayed secondary sex characteristics. As mentioned, this condition may present with pain either in the hip or in the knee; *there may be no pain in the hip at all—the only complaint being vague knee pain.*

Diagnosis is made from X-rays, where the displacement of the capital femoral epiphysis can be seen (Figure 10.6).

Treatment is usually by surgical correction.

The hip should always be examined in any adolescent or pre-adolescent who presents with knee pain without an obvious cause.

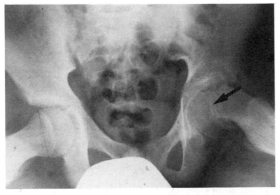

FIGURE 10.6   Slipped capital femoral epiphysis

OTHER EPIPHYSEAL PROBLEMS

Pain at the Tibial Tubercle (Osgood-Schlatter Disease)

Osgood-Schlatter is not a disease but rather a group of conditions involving the tibial tubercle epiphysis, the most common of which are discussed next.

1. *Traction epiphysitis.* Traction epiphysitis implies separation of a portion of the cartilaginous apophysis from the proximal tibial epiphysis, due to stress at the insertion of the patellar tendon (an apophysis is a non–weight-bearing epiphysis). The onset of this condition is often related to a particular episode, but it may develop spontaneously over a period of time. Some clinicians feel it may be related to a growth spurt.

SYMPTOMS AND SIGNS: Athletic participation is usually impaired by pain, which may occur both during and after activity. There may be swelling over the tibial tubercle, and a lump is often visible, palpable, or both. Tenderness is localized to the tibial tubercle area and the distal patellar tendon.

Bilateral X-rays of the tibial tubercles may show some sclerosis or a moth-eaten appearance of the proximal tibial epiphysis, which is considered by some to be indicative of a stress fracture.

TREATMENT: Traction epiphysitis is usually treated by decreasing the activity level to one of comfort and by commencing rehabilitation exercises, particularly quadriceps-strengthening exercises with the leg fully extended, hamstring-stretching exercises, and ice massage to the tibial tubercle. A gradual increase in activity is then permitted. Some physicians may elect to inject corticosteroids to dampen down the inflammatory response, though this form of treatment is not generally recommended.

2. *Tendinitis at the insertion of the patellar tendon.*

Tenderness is localized to the distal patellar tendon, and it may be difficult to differentiate tendinitis of the patellar tendon from traction epiphysitis. The bursa between the patellar tendon and the tibia may be inflamed; other symptoms and signs may be very similar. However, there are usually no abnormal findings on X-ray examination.

TREATMENT: Activity, particularly jumping, may need to be decreased for a period of time, during which the quadriceps muscle should be strengthened with isometric exercises and the hamstrings stretched. Ice massage should be applied frequently to the tender area. Mild oral anti-inflammatory medication can be used, and though corticosteroid injections are used on occasion, this should be done with discretion and the utmost caution.

3. *Formation of patellar tendon ossicle(s).*

Ossicles usually occur in the older adolescent. The symptoms are often magnified by an activity such as excessive jumping or

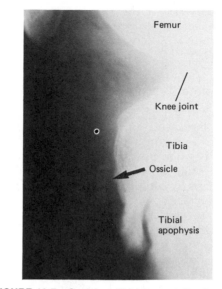

FIGURE 10.7   Ossicle within the patellar tendon

squatting (e.g., in a baseball catcher). The diagnosis is based on X-ray examination (Figure 10.7).

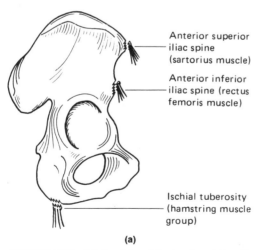

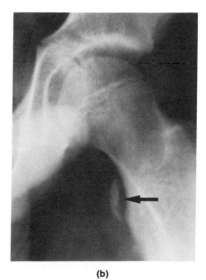

FIGURE 10.8   (a) Avulsion injuries involving the pelvic apophyses (lateral view of right pelvis) **(b) Avulsion fracture of the lesser trochanter from excessive traction of the iliopsoas muscle**

TREATMENT: If the ossicles are considered the cause of the presenting symptoms, surgical removal is necessary, often with excellent results.[16]

Complete Avulsion of the Epiphysis of the Tibial Tubercle

Complete avulsion is a dramatic injury and occurs as a result of a sudden deceleration, such as when a basketball player comes to a rapid stop or a long jumper lands. The epiphysis is pulled upward by the contracting quadriceps; the fracture may extend right through into the knee joint.[17]

This injury may occur with the same mechanism as that which would cause an anterior cruciate ligament tear in an adult and should be considered in the differential diagnosis of a large knee hemarthrosis in an adolescent.

Other Avulsion Injuries Involving Apophyses

Avulsion fractures may occur at the

1. anterior superior iliac spine at the origin of the sartorius muscle
2. anterior inferior iliac spine at the origin of the rectus femoris
3. ischial tuberosity at the origin of the hamstring group (Figure 10.8)
4. lesser trochanter at the insertion of the iliopsoas.

REFERENCES

1. Larson RL: Epiphyseal injuries in the adolescent athlete. *Orthop Clin North Am* 4:839–851, 1973.
2. Salter RB, Harris WR: Injuries involved in the epiphyseal plate. *J Bone Joint Surg* 45A:587–622, 1963.
3. Orava S, Saarela J: Exertion injuries to young athletes. *Am J Sports Med* 6:68–74, 1980.
4. Godshall RW, Hansen CA, Rising DC: Stress fractures through the distal femoral epiphysis in athletes. A previously unreported entity. *Am J Sports Med* 9:114–116, 1981.
5. Hunter LY, O'Connor GA: Traction apophysitis of the olecranon. A case report. *Am J Sports Med* 8:51–52, 1980.
6. Cahill BR, Tullos HS, Fair RH: Little league shoulder. *J Sports Med* 11:150–153, 1974.
7. Clancy WG, Foltz AS: Iliac apophysitis and stress fractures in adolescent runners. *Am J Sports Med* 4:214–218, 1976.
8. Cahill BR: Stress fracture of the proximal tibial epiphysis: A case report. *Am J Sports Med* 5:186–187, 1977.
9. Goldberg VM, Aadalen R: Distal tibial epiphyseal injuries: The role of athletics in 53 cases. *Am J Sports Med* 6:263–268, 1978.
10. Salter RB: Epiphyseal plate injuries in the adolescent knee. In *The Injured Adolescent Knee*, edited by Kennedy JC. Baltimore, Williams and Wilkins, 1979, pp 77–102.
11. Tullos HS, King JW: Lesions of the pitching arm in adolescents. *JAMA* 22:264–271, 1972.
12. Lipscomb AB: Baseball pitching injuries in growing athletes. *J Sports Med* 3:25–34, 1975.
13. Francis R, Bunch T, Chandler B: Little league elbow: A decade later. *Phys Sportsmed* 6:88–89, April 1978.
14. Micheli LJ, Santore R, Stanitski CL: Epiphyseal fractures of the elbow in children. *Am Family Physician* 22:107–116, 1980.
15. Brown R, Blazina ME, Kerlan RK, et al: Osteochondritis of the capitellum. *J Sports Med* 2:27–46, 1974.
16. Mital MA, Matza RA, Cohen J: The so-called unresolved Osgood-Schlatter lesion. A concept based on fifteen surgically treated lesions. *J Bone Joint Surg* 62A:732–739, 1980.
17. Ogden JA, Tross RB, Murphy MJ: Fractures of the tibial tuberosity in adolescents. *J Bone Joint Surg* 62A:205–215, 1980.

RECOMMENDED READINGS

Butler JE, Eggert AW: Fracture of the iliac crest apophysis. An unusual hip pointer. Brief communications. *J Sports Med* 3:192–193, 1975.

DeHaven KE: Athletic injuries in adolescents. *Pediatr Ann* 7:96–119, 1976.

Ogden JA: The development and growth of the musculoskeletal system. In *The Scientific Basis of Orthopaedics*. Albright JA, Brand RA, editors. New York, Appleton-Century-Crofts, 1979, pp 41–103.

Pappas A: The osteochondroses. *Pediatr Clin North Am* 14:549–570, 1967.

Wilkins KE: The uniqueness of the young athlete: Musculoskeletal injuries. *Am J Sports Med* 8:377–382, 1980.

CHAPTER 11

Head and Face Injuries

ANATOMY

The skull is covered by the scalp on the outside, and it protects the brain on the inside. Between the skull and brain are three layers of tissue: the dura mater, the arachnoid, and the pia mater. In order to understand the various bleeding problems that can occur after a head injury, it is necessary to have a basic knowledge of the anatomy of these three layers.

1. *The dura mater.* The dura mater lies under the skull and is a thick fibrous membrane which encloses the various venous sinuses, for instance, the superior sagittal sinus.

2. *The arachnoid.* Under the dura mater lies the arachnoid. This layer is crossed by bridging cerebral veins. Between the dura mater and the arachnoid is a potential space called the *subdural space.*

3. *The pia mater.* The pia mater is a thin tissue enclosing the brain. Between the pia mater and the arachnoid is the *subarachnoid space,* in which flows the cerebral spinal fluid. Here are found the major arterial blood vessels and bridging cerebral veins.

The brain is supplied by two arterial systems:

1. Internal carotid arteries anteriorly

2. Vertebral arteries posteriorly

These link up on the undersurface of the brain to form the circle of Willis.

An important artery that can be injured in head trauma is the *middle meningeal artery,* which crosses through the skull above the ear.

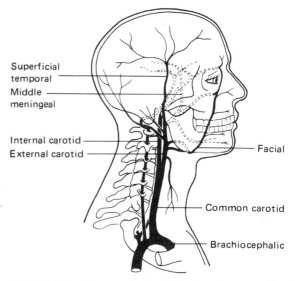

FIGURE 11.2 Blood supply of the head and neck (Modified from Jacob and Francone, *Structure and Function in Man*, published by W.B. Saunders Co., Philadelphia.)

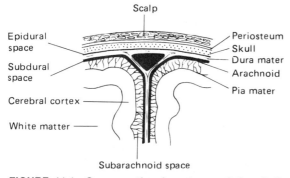

FIGURE 11.1 Cross-sectional anatomy of the skull and meninges

INJURIES TO THE HEAD

The effects of a head injury depend on the amount of damage to the brain and its surrounding structures. A blow to the head, as when a basketball player falls and strikes his or her head against the floor, can lead to a superficial *contusion* of the scalp in one athlete, while in another it may lead to a rapidly fatal intracranial hemorrhage. The possibility of developing a serious condition after a simple contusion should therefore not be forgotten. A blow to the head can lead to

1. scalp hematoma
2. fracture of the skull
3. concussion
4. cerebral edema
5. intracranial bleeding

Scalp Hematoma

A scalp hematoma is a collection of blood within the layers of the scalp superficial to the skull. Treatment with ice is usually sufficient unless there is also a laceration of the scalp. If there is any suggestion of a skull fracture, the athlete should be referred for X-rays.

Skull Fracture

The presence of a fracture indicates that a very forceful injury has occurred, and brain damage or injury to the surrounding structures must be carefully excluded. It should be realized, however, that serious or fatal intracranial injuries can occur in the absence of a fracture.

A fracture in the area of the middle meningeal artery has the potential to damage that artery and may result in the development of an extradural hematoma. Any fracture that occurs within the anatomical area of the middle meningeal artery should be very closely observed for the development of symptoms or signs suggestive of intracranial bleeding.

An additional danger from a skull fracture is the introduction of bacteria through the laceration and fracture site into the intracranial cavity, which can result in septic meningitis. Also, a depressed fracture can injure the brain substance, leading to future scarring and possible epilepsy.

Concussion

Concussion is defined as "a clinical syndrome characterized by immediate and transient impairment of neural function, such as alteration of consciousness, disturbance of vision, equilibrium, etc., due to mechanical forces."[1] The term "concussion," therefore, no longer requires the patient to have had a complete loss of consciousness, and is a diagnosis made only in retrospect—after there has been a return to the normal level of consciousness. It is possible for an athlete to appear normal following a blow to the head, but later to lapse into unconsciousness from an extradural hemorrhage. For this reason, it is important that an athlete not be left alone after suffering what appears to be a concussion, as a relapse into unconsciousness may occur.

Concussion is classified according to the length of time of unconsciousness, and the symptoms and signs (see Table 11.3, p. 147).

1. *First-degree concussion.* No actual loss of consciousness occurs, only a blurring of consciousness lasting less than ten to twenty seconds. Minimal or no symptoms or signs are present.

2. *Second-degree concussion.* A blurring or loss of consciousness occurs, lasting from twenty seconds to one or two minutes. Minimal-to-moderate symptoms and signs are found.

3. *Third-degree concussion.* There is loss of consciousness lasting two or more minutes.

Cerebral Edema

A fairly frequent and sometimes alarming complication of a blow to the head is the development of cerebral edema. In this condition there is an increase in pressure inside the skull, probably due to an increase in the amount of cerebrospinal fluid and, possibly, the occurrence of a self-limited intracranial bleed. The symptoms and signs of a rise in intracranial pressure may be present (see Table 11.1).

Intracranial Bleeding

Intracranial bleeding is a life-threatening situation which needs to be rapidly evaluated and diagnosed. Depending on the anatomical layer effected, bleeding may occur in the

1. extradural space
2. subdural space
3. subarachnoid space

Extradural hemorrhage.   If the middle meningeal artery is damaged, bleeding will occur between the skull and the dura. This represents arterial bleeding, which leads to rapid compression of the brainstem and will be fatal unless the pressure is relieved and the bleeding stopped.

The classic history is that of a blow to the head followed by a temporary loss of consciousness. The athlete then recovers and appears to be normal. This is sometimes referred to as the "lucid interval." This lucid interval may last for a few minutes or up to an hour or two, following which the athlete

may lapse into lethargy or become unconscious, or may suffer a seizure and then rapidly deteriorate unless treated. In some cases, the lucid interval may not occur. The athlete may never recover from the initial loss of consciousness. Or there might not be an initial loss of consciousness at all, only a momentary stunning as a result of a blow to the head.

An extradural hemorrhage is one of the true emergencies in which seconds or minutes are vital in determining whether the athlete will succumb or survive.

Subdural hemorrhage.   Bleeding occurs in the subdural space as a result of tearing of the bridging cerebral veins which run from the cerebral cortex to the dural sinuses (Figure 11.4).

In an *acute* subdural hemorrhage, the athlete is knocked out and seldom regains consciousness. In a *subacute* subdural hemorrhage, there may or may not be loss of consciousness, and the indications that this injury has occurred may not be present for a number of hours or even days.

A *chronic* subdural hematoma is a rare condition which follows trauma to the head. This results in a relatively small amount of bleeding which becomes surrounded by a semipermeable membrane that attracts tissue fluid by osmotic pressure. The fluid passes through the membrane, increasing the size of the hematoma. This process may continue for a number of months as the brain adapts to the gradually increasing pressure.

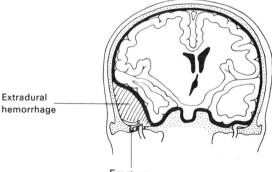

FIGURE 11.3 An extradural hemorrhage due to a skull fracture and damage to the middle meningeal artery

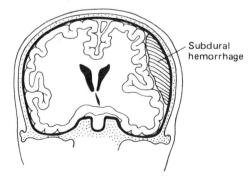

FIGURE 11.4 A subdural hemorrhage

Subarachnoid hemorrhage. A subarachnoid hemorrhage in an athlete is usually due to a rupture of a congenital aneurysm (an aneurysm is an abnormal dilation of one of the arteries). This is a not infrequent cause of sudden death in young people, and while it may occur in athletic activities, it is probably unrelated.

A subarachnoid hemorrhage may also occur in conjunction with diffuse cerebral damage resulting from a serious head injury. This type of injury implies severe impairment in cerebral function.

EVALUATION

Evaluation Following a Head Injury

There are a number of different symptoms, signs, and tests which should be used to evaluate the seriousness of a particular head injury:

1. *Headache.* This is a fairly constant finding following a blow to the head and indicates all is not as it should be. The athlete should not be allowed to return to participation until the headache has completely cleared.

2. *Nausea and vomiting.* An increase in intracerebral pressure stimulates the reflex onset of nausea and vomiting. This sign indicates that a fairly significant increase in cerebrospinal fluid pressure has occurred.

3. *Amnesia.* A loss of memory frequently occurs following a blow to the head. Start by asking the athlete simple questions (i.e., score, date, what he or she ate earlier that

TABLE 11.1 Symptoms and Signs of Increasing Intacerebral Pressure

1. Persistent and/or increasing headache
2. Nausea and/or vomiting
3. Slowing of the pulse below the athlete's norm
4. Increase in systolic blood pressure while diastolic pressure decreases
5. Pupil irregularity

day). If these are easily answered, ask more complicated questions related to the athletic event. For instance, in football the reserve quarterback can be asked to question the injured athlete about plays.

Amnesia may vary with time. An athlete who has received a blow to the head may have full recollection of the blow and other events immediately afterwards, and may be able to answer questions clearly, and yet fifteen minutes later, the same questions may produce a totally different response, with amnesia for recent events being the most obvious.

4. *The 100-minus-7 test.* This is a useful procedure to determine ability for concentrated thought. The athlete is asked to subtract seven from one hundred, then seven from that answer, and to continue in that manner as rapidly as possible.

5. *The pupils.* The pupils should be carefully evaluated and compared. Note their size, equality, and reaction to light. An extradural hematoma may compress one side of the brain, resulting in an enlarged pupil on the side of the hematoma. (Note, however, that some people normally have one pupil that is larger than the other.)

6. *Eye movements (nystagmus).* Nystagmus is the occurrence of rapidly oscillating movements of the eyes. It is most easily observed when the athlete is asked to look to the side while keeping the head still. This test is a sensitive indicator that all is not right with cerebral function. If nystagmus is present, it is advisable to keep the athlete out of participation.

7. *Finger/nose coordination test.* The athlete is asked to place his or her finger alternatively on the examiner's finger and then on his or her own nose. The examiner's finger is moved to a different position each time. Again, if not performed satisfactorily, it is an indication that the athlete should not be allowed to resume playing.

8. *Romberg's test.* The athlete is asked to stand with the feet together and the arms

held out at 90° of forward flexion. Closure of the eyes should not result in any loss of posture, and the athlete should not sway excessively. The test can be made more sensitive by asking the athlete to perform the same maneuver, standing on the heads of the metatarsals.

9. *Heel/toe walking.* The athlete should be able to accomplish this test easily.

10. *The pulse.* A slowing of the pulse below that which is normal for the athlete may be an indication of an increase in intracerebral pressure.

11. *Blood pressure.* Another indication of possible increasing cerebrospinal-fluid pressure is an increase in systolic blood pressure with a decrease in diastolic pressure. Blood pressure should therefore be monitored over a period of time.

12. *Respiratory difficulty.* Complete cessation or difficulty with respiration may occur following a head or neck injury (Table 11.2). This is one reason why a trainer should always carry an oral airway during any athletic practice or event.

13. *Leakage of cerebrospinal fluid.* If a fracture of the cribriform plate occurs, cerebrospinal fluid may leak from the nose. This may be diagnosed by testing the fluid with a urine Multistix (or similar "stix" with a glucose indicator). If glucose is present in the discharge, it strongly suggests the fluid is cerebrospinal.

A fracture of the base of the skull may result in bleeding or leakage of cerebrospinal fluid from the ear. If the eardrum is not perforated, the buildup of blood behind the eardrum can be observed.

14. *Loss of emotional control.* Loss of emotional control or irrational behavior may indicate a disturbance of normal cerebral function and should preclude the athlete's returning to play.

15. *Papilledema.* Examination of the fundus with an ophthalmoscope may reveal blurring of the medial margins of the optic disk. This can indicate early papilledema—an impor-

tant sign of an increase in intracerebral pressure.

On-Field Evaluation and Management of the Unconscious Athlete

Any unconscious athlete should be assumed to have a *neck injury* in addition to any head injury.

1. Check the airway and if impaired:
   a. Cut face mask with bolt cutters or similar tool (if applicable).
   b. Do not remove helmet (if applicable).
   c. Stabilize head and neck.
   d. Do not hyperextend neck but bring jaw forward.
   e. Insert airway and supply oxygen.

2. Check the pulse—if not present, commence CPR with the head and neck stabilized.

3. Check the blood pressure.

4. Check the pupils.

5. Remove from the field on a spine board. The head and neck *must be stabilized.* If in any doubt, obtain help from specially trained EMTs (emergency medical technicians) before removing the athlete from the field.

If there are signs of an *extradural hemorrhage*, for instance, unconsciousness with a dilated pupil on one side and paralysis of the

TABLE 11.2   Cessation of Breathing Resulting from Injury to the Head or Neck

Cessation of breathing may occur with or without cardiac arrest. Noncardiac causes include:

1. *A direct head-on contact injury* which results in (a) impingement of the vascular supply to the brain stem and (b) brain stem contusion, or (c) both.

2. *Impingement of the cord above* C4–5 (a C4–5 lesion will result in the ability to breathe abdominally only; a lesion above this will lead to complete cessation of respiration).

3. *Ruptured intervertebral disc* (C3–4).

opposite side of the body, transport the athlete to a hospital as rapidly as possible. If it is just as quick for the ambulance to be summoned to remove and transport the athlete from the field to the hospital, then this should be done. If you have to remove and transport the athlete yourself, ensure that he or she is removed from the field on a spine board with the neck stabilized, and if possible supply oxygen. While the athlete is being transported, a responsible person should be sent to telephone the emergency room at the hospital, informing them an athlete with a potentially serious head injury is en route.

Sideline Examination of a "Minor" Concussion

An athlete who has had a "minor" episode of concussion, or who has been dazed, needs a neurological evaluation. Start the examination by asking the athlete simple questions to check for amnesia. Proceed onto the 100-minus-7 test, look for nystagmus, test finger-to-nose coordination, and perform Romberg's test. Check the pupils, monitor the pulse, and, if necessary, the blood pressure. Always examine the neck to ensure no injury has occurred.

If there was only a momentary blurring of consciousness, no amnesia, and all the sideline tests are normal, the athlete may return to participation but should be observed while in action and then be re-examined at the end of the event. If there is any question as to the athlete's coordination, ability to concentrate, or emotional stability, he or she should be removed from the event immediately.

If the athlete has blurring or loss of consciousness lasting from twenty seconds to one or two minutes, return to participation should not be allowed that day. He or she should be under constant surveillance during the initial postconcussion period (see the "lucid interval" of the extradural hemorrhage, p. 143). The athlete should be carefully examined and observed on the sideline and then placed under medical care for the following eighteen to twenty-four hours. Thereafter, the athlete should be examined on a daily basis and should not be allowed to return to participation until the headache has disappeared and the neurological examination shows a complete return to normal.[2]

LACERATIONS OF FACE AND SCALP

Lacerations of the Scalp

Scalp lacerations frequently bleed copiously. The initial bleeding can usually be controlled by pressure from a sterile dressing. The wound should be kept covered and clean until it can be sutured.

Lacerations of the Eyebrow

Lacerations of the eyebrow may bleed freely but are relatively easy to temporarily tape with Steri-Strips. Ice and compression can be applied over the strips. If the athlete wishes to resume participation, he or she may be permitted to do so providing the laceration does not affect the eye itself. If bleeding recurs, the athlete should be withdrawn from participation until the wound is sutured but can frequently return soon after suturing, depending on the circumstances.

Lacerations of the Central Portion of the Face

Almost any laceration on the central portion of the face should be carefully sutured for an acceptable cosmetic result. This should be done within a few hours of the injury, not the next day.

Immediate treatment consists of either Steri-Strips or a pad. Ice should be used to reduce the swelling. With this type of laceration, it is preferable to keep the athlete out of further participation until the wound has healed.

Some lacerations do not need to be sutured, and can be treated satisfactorily with Steri-Strips. A decision as to the necessity

TABLE 11.3   Classification and Management of the Unconscious Athlete

	First-Degree Concussion	Second-Degree Concussion	Third-Degree Concussion
Period of unconsciousness	No actual loss of consciousness ("dinged" or "bell-rung") but blurring of consciousness lasting less than 10–20 seconds	Blurring or loss of consciousness lasting from 20 seconds to 1–2 minutes	Loss of consciousness lasting 2 or more minutes
On-field management	Check for neck injury. The athlete, when recovered, can walk off the field if no neck injury is present.	Check for neck injury. The athlete, when recovered, can walk off the field if no injury is present.	See p. 145.
Off-field examination			
Symptoms	No amnesia No headache No nausea	Headache and amnesia often present.	
Signs	No positive signs on neurologic testing and examination. Athlete should be fully oriented and emotionally in control.	Confusion and disorientation. May have some neurologic signs, e.g., nystagmus.	
Return to participation	If all the above criteria are present, and if the diagnosis is a first-degree concussion, athlete may return to game.	No return to game	No return to game
Management	Observe frequently during the game and re-examine afterward.	Observe frequently during game while athlete sits on the sideline. Hospitalize for observation for 24 hours.	Hospitalize immediately for observation and treatment.
Time off from practice and competition	If headache, nausea, amnesia or other signs develop later, athlete should be off contact for 2 days after this clears.	Usually three to five days, longer if necessary; each case should be evaluated individually.	One season[a]
Disqualifying factors	If repeatedly suffers "dings," particularly with minor trauma, carefully evaluate status with regard to contact participation.	More than two episodes in a season disqualifies athlete for the rest of that season. Each athlete should be individually evaluated with regard to further participation in contact sports.	Two or three third-degree concussions in a career should preclude athlete from further participation in contact sports.

[a]The New York State Athletic Commission has stated that every boxer knocked unconscious must be kept out for 90 days. In addition, full neurological examinations must be performed, including EEG's and CAT scans.

for suturing should preferably be made by a physician, but if the wound is linear and is superficial, so that it does not gape, and a satisfactory approximation of the wound can be made with the application of Steri-Strips, then this may be an alternative to suturing. Continue use of the Steri-Strips until the wound is completely healed, which is usually five to seven days for a face laceration.

After a facial wound has healed, it is necessary to continue protecting it with Steri-Strips if there is continued participation in contact sports. Protection should be continued for at least another seven days.

FACIAL FRACTURES

Fracture of the Jaw

Following a blow to the jaw, there is frequently intense pain, making it difficult to determine if a fracture is present. The following points may help in deciding:

1. Ask the athlete to open and close his or her mouth. Note any asymmetry in movement.

2. Ask the athlete to bite, and note any malocclusion.

3. Feel for any irregularity along the jaw, both when it is at rest and when it is being opened and closed.

If a fracture is suspected, the athlete should be referred for X-rays and specialized treatment.

Fracture of the Maxilla or Sinuses

A fracture to the maxilla, the sinuses, or both usually occurs from a direct blow. Tenderness is present over the injured area, and diffuse swelling may occur. The examiner should palpate for a "step-off" fracture and should test for hypesthesia in the distribution of the infra-orbital nerve beneath the eye and along the side of the nose.

On occasion, nose blowing will cause a swelling to appear around the eye. This is very suggestive of a fracture of the maxilla or ethmoid sinus. The athlete should be sent for X-rays and a specialist's evaluation.

DENTAL INJURIES

Prevention

Dental injuries can occur in almost any contact activity, and often result in permanent damage. Mouth guards and preventive dental appliances have become increasingly accepted as important pieces of equipment and should be worn by athletes in both practice and game situations for sports such as football, ice hockey, rugby, boxing, and wrestling.[3]

Mouth guards vary from inexpensive plastics that are heat-molded to conform to the athlete's dental pattern (Figure 11.5), to those that are custom-made. The latter are particularly useful for athletes who have to be able to communicate clearly during the game, e.g., quarterbacks in football.

The use of mouth guards has not only dramatically reduced the incidence of dental

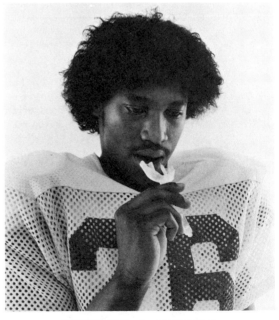

FIGURE 11.5   A mouth guard

injuries, but has been shown to lessen the incidence of concussion. The mechanism of this effect is thought to relate to the shock absorbency characteristics of the mouth guard, which decreases the force with which the jaw snaps shut on head impact.[4,5]

Dislocated Tooth

When a tooth has been knocked out it should, if possible, be reimplanted immediately. If this proves impossible, the tooth should be placed in a cloth moistened with water or saline. The athlete should be transported to a dentist within the first half hour after injury so that a formal reimplantation can be performed. Any attempts to reimplant the tooth after twenty-four hours have a poor success rate, as root resorption frequently occurs.

Fractured Tooth

Fractures may occur through the enamel, or through the dentine and the enamel, or they may include the pulp.

Fractures through the enamel produce minimal symptoms. Fluids should be kept off the tooth if this causes any sensitivity. The tooth can later be smoothed down with satisfactory results.

If the fracture extends through the dentine as well, there is increased sensitivity to heat, cold, and fluids. If the symptoms are severe, an injection of a local anesthetic near the root of the tooth can be performed by a dentist or physician to decrease the symptoms. The tooth can then be covered with temporary or permanent filling material.

Severe pain and a marked increase in sensitivity occur with exposure of the pulp. Again, a local anesthetic may relieve symptoms temporarily, but this type of injury will usually require a root-canal filling.

Loose Tooth

In cases where there is no actual displacement, just minimal loosening of the tooth, a precautionary X-ray should be taken at a con-

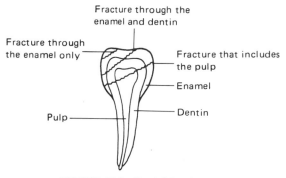

FIGURE 11.6   Dental fractures

venient time. The athlete should be warned not to bite with the tooth for at least one to two weeks.

If the tooth is displaced two millimeters or more, it should be pushed back with the finger into its anatomical position. The athlete should then be referred immediately to a dentist, so the loose tooth can be stabilized.

Fractured Crown

This is not always an emergency, as very often the crown will be situated over a dead tooth and therefore sensitivity will not be increased. If the tooth is not dead, the crown should be replaced as soon as possible.

Artificial Plates

Removable artificial plates should *not* be kept in the mouth either during practice or competition, as they are liable to be broken, resulting in some pieces being accidently swallowed, inhaled, or lodged in the gum or palate.

TABLE 11.4

Cases That Need Immediate Referral
1. The tooth is knocked out or dislodged
2. The tooth is displaced by 2 mm or more
3. A fractured crown where the tooth is still alive

EYE INJURIES

Our eyes are among our most precious organs, but they are taken quite casually by many athletes even though they are exposed to potential trauma. In sports such as racquetball and squash, serious injuries and permanent damage can easily be prevented by the use of eye protectors[6,7] (see Figure 11.7). It is strongly recommended that no athlete be allowed to participate in racquetball or squash without wearing eye protectors.[8,9]

Contusions to the Lids

As the tissues surrounding the lids are very loose, they permit a large amount of swelling to occur. The eye can rapidly become closed by swollen lids. The possibility of an underlying orbital fracture should be considered.

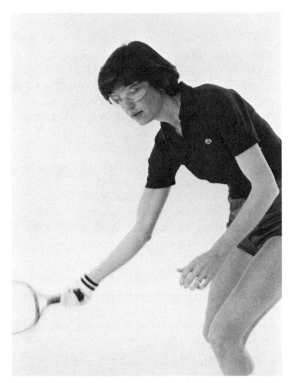

FIGURE 11.7 An eye protector should be used for racquetball and squash.

EXAMINATION: When initially examining an athlete with a swollen lid, it is important to try to assess the function and condition of the underlying eye. Visual acuity should be tested and the results recorded. Then, with the athlete lying supine, the lids should be very gently retracted. The eyes should then be inspected for obvious abnormalities. The pupils should be equal, regular, and reactive to light; eye movements should be full, unrestricted, and symmetrical. Fluorescin dye can be instilled in order to exclude or identify corneal abrasions. The athlete should then sit up, and the anterior chamber should be inspected for any evidence of bleeding. This will appear as a layer of blood with a meniscus (see Figure 11.10).

TREATMENT: Ice should not be applied in the form of a heavy ice pack. Rather, the use of specially made cold packs for eyes is recommended, or else crushed ice or cold water in a latex surgical glove which is placed on the affected eye. If there is any doubt about the condition of the eye, the athlete should be referred immediately for ophthalmologic consultation. No medication should be instilled into the eye by a trainer.

Levator Injury

The levator palpebrae superioris muscle elevates the upper lid. If a finger is jammed

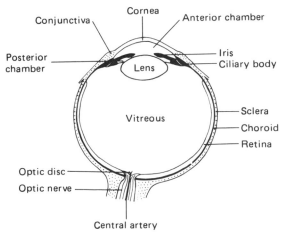

FIGURE 11.8 The anatomy of the eye

into the eye, the muscle can be damaged. If there is difficulty in opening the eye after a few days of ice treatment, patching, and rest, a specialist's opinion should be sought.

Corneal Abrasions

The athlete will complain of pain, a gritty feeling, or the sensation of a foreign body being present. A drop or two of local anesthetic solution will make the athlete feel more comfortable and permit an adequate examination. A foreign body should be sought on the cornea, and if not present, the upper lid should then be everted (if there is not too much swelling) so the conjunctiva can be adequately inspected. A corneal abrasion can best be seen by applying a strip impregnated with fluorescin dye, which will outline the area of abrasion by staining it a deep yellow. Corneal abrasions usually heal rapidly when adequately treated. The eye should be placed at rest by applying a patch, and mydriatric and antibiotic drops should be used as indicated. The patch must be tight enough to prevent opening of the lid under it, and the tape applied in a manner that will not permit it to become loose when the athlete chews food. Analgesics may be required.

Occasionally a complication such as iritis will develop, which should be referred immediately to an ophthalmologist. The first symptom of iritis is often photophobia (avoidance of bright light) and an increase in pain and redness of the eye.

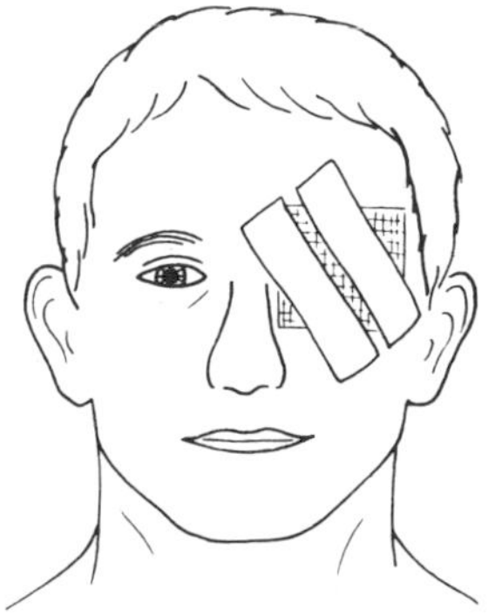

Subconjunctival Hematoma

A condition causing the athlete a considerable amount of anxiety is subconjunctival hematoma. It is a harmless condition occurring as a result of the spontaneous rupture of a small blood vessel. One can usually detect the posterior margin of the hematoma, which helps confirm the diagnosis. No treatment besides reassurance is necessary.

Injury to the Lens or Iris

Lens or iris injuries can be seen by inspecting the pupil, which may be irregular, dilated or constricted. Expert consultation should be sought immediately.

Hemorrhage into the Anterior Chamber

An anterior-chamber hemorrhage usually results from blunt trauma. Observe if a meniscus of blood is present (see Figure 11.10). Visual acuity may be reduced. The mainstay of treatment is rest. Patches may be needed on both eyes. The ophthalmologist should determine the length of time such immobilization is necessary. Secondary hemorrhage may occur if the athlete returns to participation too soon, the danger period being three to seven days after the injury. If this occurs, it could lead to permanent impairment of vision.

Hemorrhage into the Posterior Chamber

Posterior-chamber bleeding may present with a visual defect. It may be painful but is often painless. If there is considerable bleeding within the globe, the "red reflex" will be lost (normally, when a light is shown into the eye, the retina is seen through the pupil

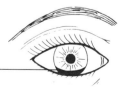

Meniscus of blood
within anterior chamber

FIGURE 11.9 An eye patch

FIGURE 11.10 Anterior chamber hemorrhage

as a red area). Bleeding into the posterior chamber is a serious injury. It should immediately be referred for specific diagnosis and treatment.

Detached Retina

Patients frequently describe the occurrence of a detached retina with phrases like "a curtain fell in front of my eye" or "multiple lights flashed on and off," or mention the appearance of "floaters" (this is caused by the retina tearing across a blood vessel). Such a history should make the trainer aware of the possibility of a detached retina, which might occur days or weeks after the traumatic event. The athlete should immediately be referred to an ophthalmologist.

NASAL INJURIES

Bleeding

Because of the copious blood supply of the nasal mucosa, bleeding is often a problem, particularly in sports such as wrestling. In most cases the bleeding is easily handled by manual compression and application of ice. However, in situations where the athlete has to return to participation, a plug of cotton will temporarily help the bleeding (it is important to remember to remove the cotton once the bleeding has stopped). If this does not suffice, adrenalin in the concentration of 1:1,000 solution can be applied to the cotton before inserting. This encourages vasoconstriction. Should the bleeding persist in spite of manual pressure and the application of ice, the athlete should be referred to an emergency room for examination and possible packing.

Septal Hematoma

A hematoma of the septum can develop quite insidiously following a blow to the nose. The first indication may be difficulty in breathing through one of the nostrils. This condition can lead to infection and destruc-

tion of the nasal cartilage. Spreading of the infection to the brain, with the development of a brain abscess, is a rare but serious complication.

Once a septal hematoma is diagnosed, it should be drained and antibiotics prescribed if necessary. It is important for the athlete to avoid contact activities for a few days after the injury, to minimize the risks of infection and the recurrence of the hematoma. If the athlete is participating in a contact sport, a facial mask should be worn to prevent further nasal trauma for seven to ten days.

Nasal Fractures

If a nasal fracture is suspected, one should look for bony deviation, which can be done visually if the athlete is seen before swelling has developed. Simple observation by the examiner as well as the athlete can often accurately assess the need for treatment. The examiner should also inspect the nose with the athlete supine, observing the athlete from behind, along the bridge of the nose. If there is any question as to whether a fracture exists, the athlete should be referred for a specialist's opinion. The immediate application of ice may help to reduce any swelling.

A nose that is deformed as a result of a number of injuries is probably best repaired by plastic surgery after the athlete is finished with his or her competitive athletic career.

EAR INJURIES

Hematoma of the Pinna ("Cauliflower Ear")

Injuries to the pinna resulting in a cauliflower ear were notorious in past years. They are the result of contact sports and are still to be found in professional boxers, rugby players, and wrestlers who do not wear ear protectors.

A cauliflower ear is the end result of one or more episodes of trauma to the pinna, which results in subperichondral hemorrhage with pressure or infection destroying the underlying cartilage. This results in a progressively increasing distortion of the pinnal shape.[10]

PREVENTION: Any athlete at risk should wear an adequate protective device designed for that sport. In rugby the positions most frequently associated with cauliflower ears are the front-row forwards, the locks, and the eighth man. Wrestling without an ear protector should not be permitted. It is important for the athlete to be sure the protector fits adequately, as friction between the protector and the ear can itself cause a hematoma. Should the hematoma occur, complications can be prevented by adequate treatment performed under aseptic conditions.

TREATMENT: Once the earlobe becomes traumatized, it should be packed with ice and a moderate amount of compression applied. If a hematoma develops, it should be drained under aseptic conditions at the earliest convenient time. A compressive dressing of a material such as cotton soaked in flexible collodion can be used[11] (see Figure 11.11). Compression should be continued for a few hours after drainage. The dressing should be kept in place for at least five days, to allow adequate healing to occur. If swelling recurs, this same procedure is repeated. Restricting the athlete's activity is not considered necessary unless a complication ensues.

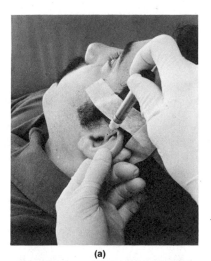

(a)

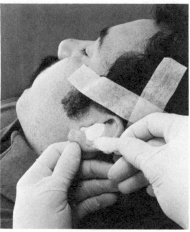

(b)

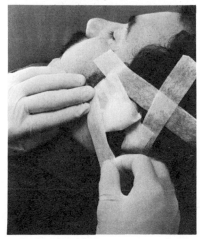

(c)

FIGURE 11.11   Draining an ear hematoma
(a) After thoroughly cleaning the pinna with an alcohol or Betadine solution, drain the hematoma with a narrow-bore needle. This should be done using strict aseptic technique.   (b) The external auditory meatus is plugged with a dry piece of cotton. Strips of cotton are then soaked in collodion and applied in layers to the pinna. (c) Paper tape is used to maintain pressure on the cotton strips. These are left in place for 3 to 5 days, after which the cotton, collodion and tape are reapplied if necessary.

Rupture of the Eardrum

Rupture of the eardrum (tympanic membrane) results from a direct blow to the ear, which causes a sudden violent increase in the pressure within the external auditory canal. Such a blow may occur from a soccer ball hitting the side of the head, from a slap of the hand against the pinna, or from falling when water skiing. It may also occur as a result of barotrauma from diving.

SYMPTOMS AND SIGNS: The athlete presents with a history of the incident and describes an intense pain, followed by hearing loss and, in some cases, severe dizziness and nausea. A small amount of bleeding from the external auditory meatus may be present. On inspecting the drum with an otoscope the diagnosis is readily apparent.

TREATMENT: Most small ruptures will heal spontaneously, but it is important that the athlete understand that water should not be allowed to enter the external auditory meatus until the drum has completely healed. If the rupture is large or persists, it may have to be repaired surgically or a graft may have to be inserted. Auditory testing should be repeated.

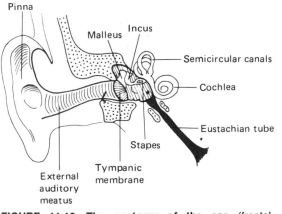

FIGURE 11.12 The anatomy of the ear (frontal cross-section)

Ear and Sinus Barotrauma in Diving

One of the reasons the ear is often affected by diving is that there is an increase in pressure of 14.7 pounds (one atmosphere) for every 33 feet of descent. This increase in pressure may damage the middle ear and sinus cavities unless there is continuous equalization of the pressure between the cavities and the exterior.

PREVENTION:

1. *Adequate diving instruction.* This is a must. Prior to any diving attempt, the student diver should acquire the ability to perform the Valsalva maneuver (the nose and mouth are held closed, an attempt is made to explosively blow out air). This will open the eustachian tubes so the pressure within the pharynx, the middle ear, and the sinuses is equalized. With experience, divers may be able to equalize pressure simply by yawning or swallowing. In addition, the novice diver must learn how to ascend and how to deal with panic situations that arise.

2. *Physical examination of a diving candidate.* This exam should include the cardiovascular and respiratory systems but, most importantly, it should include a thorough evaluation of the otolaryngological structures, including

a. inspection of the tympanic membranes
b. having the diving candidate attempt to perform the Valsalva maneuver while the examiner observes movement of the tympanic membrane
c. inspection of the external canal with particular reference to otitis externa, osteomas, and cerumen
d. inspection of the position of the nasal septum, particularly with regard to hypertrophy of the turbinates
e. inspection of the nasopharynx, especially the area of the eustachian tube orifices

If there is chronic sinusitis, this should be controlled. Any hearing loss should be appropriately recorded and individually assessed. A profound unilateral hearing loss probably contra-indicates diving, to prevent damage to the good ear. Any tendency to vertigo (e.g., active Menière's disease) or a perforated eardrum is a contra-indication to diving.

SYMPTOMS AND SIGNS: An inexperienced diver, or one who has a nasopharyngeal problem such as an infection or allergy, might find it impossible to equalize the pressure, resulting in damage to the tympanic membrane or sinuses. A reverse external ear barotrauma is sometimes possible to get when a plug of wax or an earplug blocks the external auditory canal and results in the tympanic membrane extending outward. A rebound phenomenon after use of a vaso-constrictor may cause the eustachian tube to become blocked, thereby preventing equalization of pressure while ascending.

If the pressure is sufficient to cause rupture of the tympanic membrane, the effects of cold water on the labyrinth may lead to dizziness, disorientation, nausea, and vomiting, which, in a diving situation, can be life threatening.[12] Rupture of the round window can lead to permanent loss of hearing and vertigo.

TREATMENT: *Mild* cases, which show a reddening of the tympanic membranes with or without slight hemorrhage within the drum, should be treated with vasoconstrictors, decongestants, or both. Diving should be prohibited until the symptoms have disappeared and the eardrum appears normal. This usually takes five to seven days.[13,14]

In *severe* cases, the drum may or may not be ruptured, but there is free blood in the middle ear. This requires the use of systemic antibiotics, oral vasoconstrictors, decongestants, and a topical nasal decongestant (avoid antihistamines).

Traumatic perforation of the tympanic membrane should be referred to an otolaryngologist.

Damage to the sinuses may cause hemorrhage, marked edema of the mucosa, or extravasation of fluid. Secondary infection may occur unless adequate drainage is established. Occasionally surgical drainage is required.

External Auditory Canal— "Swimmer's Ear" (Otitis Externa)

Swimmer's ear is a bacterial or fungal infection involving the lining of the external auditory canal and occurs frequently in those who neglect to adequately dry the canal.

PREVENTION: The best protection is to ensure that the swimmer dries the external auditory canal after each workout. This may be achieved by shaking the head to the side or by using a hair dryer. The use of a cotton-tipped applicator is not recommended. The instillation of a few drops of VōSol or 1% boric-acid solution (5.0 grams boric acid and 70% ethyl alcohol made up to 500 milliliters) three or four times a week may help retain the normal acid conditions of the external auditory canal and therefore prevent infection.

SYMPTOMS AND SIGNS: The athlete presents with an itching or intensely painful ear that may or may not be discharging. Pus and debris are easily seen through the otoscope. Local pressure around the external auditory meatus or pulling on the pinna will cause pain. If left untreated, the infection may spread to the middle ear and cause disturbances of balance as well as hearing.

TREATMENT: A special wick can be inserted for twenty-four to forty-eight hours and antibiotic or steroid drops used. Alternatively, Burrow's Solution (aluminum acetate) can be used initially to decrease swelling. When the swelling and pain have subsided, the ear canal should be cleared of debris. Eardrops containing alcohol or boric acid and an antibiotic should be used as necessary.

REFERENCES

1. Committee on Head Injury Nomenclature of the Congress of Neurological Surgeons: Glossary of head injury including some definitions of injury of the cervical spine. *Clin Neurosurg* 12:388, 1966.
2. Blazina ME, Carlson GJ, Drake EC: Head injuries in athletics. *J Sports Med* 2:51–56, 1974.
3. Schwartz R, Novich MM: The athlete's mouthpiece. *Am J Sports Med* 8:357–359, 1980.
4. Hickey JC, Morris AL, Carlson LD, et al: The relation of mouth protectors to cranial pressure and deformation. *JADA* 74:735, 1967.
5. Stenger JM, Lawson EA, Wright JM, et al: Mouthguards: Protection against shock to head, neck, and teeth. *JADA* 69:273, 1964.
6. Bishop PJ, Kozey J, Caldwell G: Performance of eye protectors for squash and racquetball. *Phys Sportsmed* 10:62–69, March 1982.
7. Easterbrook M: Eye protection for squash and racquetball players. *Phys Sportsmed* 9:79–82, February 1981.
8. Easterbrook M: Eye injuries in racket sports: A continuing problem. *Phys Sportsmed* 9:91–101, January 1981.
9. Easterbrook M: Eye injuries in squash and racquetball players: An update. *Phys Sportsmed* 10:47–56, March 1982.
10. Eichel BS, Bray DA: Management of hematoma of the wrestler's ear. *Phys Sportsmed* 6:87–90, November 1978.
11. Stuteville OH, Janda C, Pandya NJ: Treating the injured ear to prevent a "cauliflower ear." *Plastic and Reconstructive Surgery* 44:310–312, 1969.
12. Pipkin G: Caloric labyrinthitis: A cause of drowning. A case report of a swimmer who survived through self-rescue. *Am J Sports Med* 7:260–261, 1979.
13. Strauss MB, Cantrell RW: Ear and sinus barotrauma in diving. *Phys Sportsmed* 8:38–43, August 1974.
14. MacFie DD: ENT problems in diving. *Med Serv J Can* 20:845–861, 1964.

RECOMMENDED READINGS

Behnke AR, Austin LF: Introduction to scuba diving. *J Sports Med* 2:276–290, 1974.

Blyth CS, Schindler RD: *Forty-eighth Annual Survey of Football Fatalities 1931–1979*. National Collegiate Athletic Association and American Football Coaches Association 1980.

Downs JR: Facial trauma in intercollegiate and junior hockey. *Phys Sportsmed* 7:88–92, February 1979.

Mueller FO, Blyth CS: Catastophic head and neck injuries. *Phys Sportmed* 7:71–74, October 1979.

Reid SE, Epstein HM, Louis MW: Brain trauma inside a football helmet. *Phys Sportsmed* 2:32–35, August 1974.

Schneider RC: *Head and Neck Injuries in Football*. Baltimore, Williams and Wilkins Company, 1973.

Torg JS, editor: *Athletic Injuries to the Head, Neck, and Face*. Philadelphia, Lea and Febiger, 1982.

Torg JS, Truex Jr R, Quedenfeld T, et al: National Football Head-Neck Registry—report and conclusions. *JAMA* 241:1477–1479, 1979.

Travell J: Temporomandibular joint dysfunction—Temporomandibular joint pain referred from muscles of the head and neck. *J Prosthet Dent* 10:745, 1960.

CHAPTER 12

Shoulder Girdle Injuries

FUNCTIONAL ANATOMY

Because the shoulder girdle is designed to allow maximum mobility, there is a compromise in the degree of structural stability. In addition, there is only one point at which the shoulder girdle is attached to the skeletal system—at the sternoclavicular joint.

Bones

The bones of the shoulder girdle include

1. clavicle
2. scapula
3. humerus

1. *The clavicle.* The clavicle prevents the shoulder from dropping across the chest and thus helps in maintaining the distance be-

tween the upper arm and the sternum. It is concave posteriorly in its proximal two-thirds and concave anteriorly in its distal third. The weakest point of the clavicle is at the junction of the middle and outer thirds, and this is the area where fractures frequently occur.

The clavicle is attached to the sternum by a group of strong ligaments:

1. The sternoclavicular
2. The costoclavicular (attaching the clavicle to the first rib)

At the outer end of the clavicle, the main ligaments holding it in place are the coracoclavicular ligaments, made up of the

1. trapezoid
2. conoid

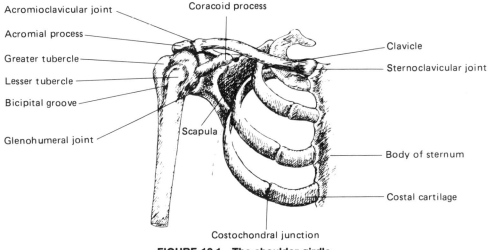

Acromioclavicular joint
Acromial process
Greater tubercle
Lesser tubercle
Bicipital groove
Glenohumeral joint
Coracoid process
Clavicle
Sternoclavicular joint
Scapula
Body of sternum
Costal cartilage
Costochondral junction

FIGURE 12.1 The shoulder girdle

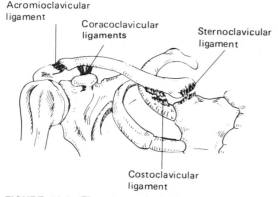

FIGURE 12.2 The sternoclavicular and costoclavicular ligaments showing a complete sprain of these ligments

There is also a weak ligament linking the distal end of the clavicle to the acromion process (the capsular or acromioclavicular ligament). If the ligaments holding the distal end of the clavicle are damaged, the clavicle will be displaced in a cephalad direction.

2. *The scapula.* The scapula (or shoulder blade) lies flat against the posterior chest wall, and its movements are closely integrated with those of the shoulder. To it are attached numerous important muscles. Some of the more important structures include the

1. acromion process
2. coracoid process

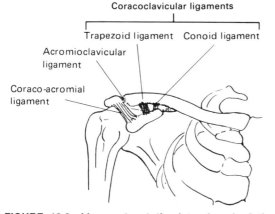

FIGURE 12.3 Ligaments at the lateral end of the clavicle

3. glenoid fossa
4. spine of the scapula

Between the acromion process and the coracoid process is a thick band of ligamentlike tissue called the coraco-acromial ligament. The coraco-acromial ligament and the acromion make up the coraco-acromial arch. The coraco-acromial ligament may cause impingement of the structures running beneath it, particularly in an athlete who uses the shoulder frequently (such as a baseball player or swimmer). The structure most frequently pinched under the arch is the supraspinatus tendon.

The glenoid fossa is lined by the labrum, a fibrocartilaginous rim which helps to deepen the glenoid fossa and thereby increase the stability of the glenohumeral joint.

3. *The humerus.* The head of the humerus fits into the glenoid fossa. Other landmarks on the proximal humerus include the greater tuberosity (to which the supraspinatus tendon is attached) and the lesser tuberosity (to which the subscapularis muscle is attached). The tendon of the long head of the biceps runs in a special groove (the bicipital) which lies between the lesser and greater tuberosities, and the transverse humeral ligament helps to prevent the biceps tendon from slipping out of the groove.

The glenohumeral joint is secured largely by a thick capsule composed of a number

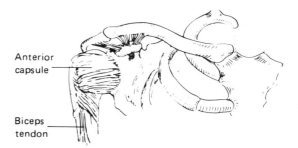

FIGURE 12.4 The glenohumeral joint and anterior capsule

of ligaments and is designed to allow the upper limb to move through an extensive range of movement. These ligaments, particularly the inferior glenohumeral ligament, can be torn with an antero-inferior dislocation of the shoulder. Incompetency of the capsule can result in recurrent subluxation or dislocation of the shoulder joint.[1]

Muscles

The main muscles associated with the shoulder girdle include the following:

1. *The trapezius.* This is a triangular muscle which covers the neck and shoulder. It arises from the occiput and the spines of the cervical and thoracic vertebrae and inserts into the posterior border of the outer third of the clavicle as well as into part of the acromion process and spine of the scapula. The insertion of this muscle into the clavicle varies in extent—in some individuals it may reach as far as the middle of the clavicle and on occasion may even blend with the posterior edge of the sternocleidomastoideus muscle. The trapezius helps to stabilize the scapula during movements of the upper limb.

2. *The latissimus dorsi.* This is a large triangular muscle which covers the lumbar region and the lower half of the thoracic area. It inserts into the upper third of the humerus. Before its insertion it wraps around the lower border of the teres major muscle, and as a result the lowest fibers are inserted highest into the humerus while the highest fibers pass into the lowest end of the tendon. The latissimus dorsi helps form the posterior fold of the axilla. Its actions are mainly those of adduction, extension, and internal rotation of the humerus, but it also acts with the pectoralis major and teres major to help depress the raised arm against resistance.

3. *The pectoralis major.* The pectoralis major is a thick muscle covering the upper and front part of the chest. It arises from the medial half of the clavicle, from the sternum, from the cartilages of the ribs, and from the aponeurosis of the external oblique muscle. It inserts into the upper third of the humerus and gives off an expansion which covers the bicipital groove. Its main actions are those of adduction and internal rotation of the humerus. When the arm is extended, the pectoralis major draws it forward and medially. When the arm is flexed, the clavicular portion of the pectoralis major acts with the anterior fibers of the deltoid. When the arms are used for movement, such as climbing,

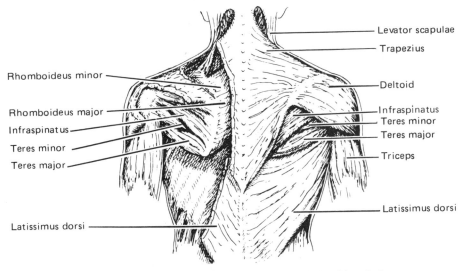

FIGURE 12.5 Muscles of the upper back and shoulder girdle

the muscle helps draw the trunk forward and upward.

4. *The serratus anterior.* This muscle lies between the ribs and the scapula and inserts into the costal surface of the medial border of the scapula. When the serratus anterior acts with the pectoralis minor muscle, it helps draw the scapula forward, and is the main muscle concerned with pushing and punching movements. It assists the trapezius in rotating the scapula forward around the chest wall and is therefore important in raising the arm above the head. During the action of abduction, the serratus anterior works together with other muscles that are inserted into the scapula to help steady the scapula and allow the deltoid to abduct the humerus. If the serratus anterior is paralyzed from damage to the long thoracic nerve, it will be unable to hold the scapula against the chest wall. If the athlete is asked to push the arm forward into protrusion, the inner border of the scapula will "wing," especially in its lower two-thirds.

5. *The deltoid.* This muscle covers the shoulder joint and gives it its smooth, rounded contour. The deltoid arises from the lateral third of the clavicle as well as from the acromion process and the spine of the scapula. It inserts by means of a thick tendon into the lateral side of the shaft of the humerus. It has three portions: anterior, middle, and posterior.

The actions of the deltoid muscle are numerous. It may act with the pectoralis major to bring the arm forward and to internally rotate the humerus. In combination with the latissimus dorsi and the teres major, it extends the arm backward. Together with the supraspinatus, it raises the arm from the side. While the deltoid is abducting the arm, the scapula is being rotated by the serratus anterior and the trapezius muscles. As this is happening, the head of the humerus is prevented from moving upward by the downward pull of the subscapularis, the infraspinatus, and the teres minor.

The axillary nerve supplies the deltoid muscle. If this nerve is damaged, the deltoid will atrophy. This can be seen when the rounded contour of the normal side is compared with the flattening of the shoulder and the prominence of the acromion process on the affected side.

6. *The rotator cuff.* The rotator cuff consists of the following muscles:

1. supraspinatus
2. infraspinatus
3. teres minor
4. subscapularis

1. The *supraspinatus* arises from the supraspinous fossa and passes under the acromion to form a tendon which inserts into the most superior portion of the greater tubercle of the humerus. It is separated from the acromion process, the coraco-acromial ligament, and the deltoid muscle by the subacromial bursa.

2. The *infraspinatus* arises from the infraspinous fossa on the scapula and inserts as a tendon into the middle portion of the greater tubercle of the humerus.

3. The *teres minor* arises from the upper two-thirds of the lateral border of the scapula on its dorsal surface. It inserts into the lowermost portion of the greater tubercle of the humerus, below the insertion of the infraspinatus.

4. The *subscapularis* is a large triangular muscle which arises from the subscapular fossa and is inserted into the lesser tubercle of the humerus.

The most important action of the rotator cuff muscles is to stabilize the head of the humerus in the glenoid. For instance, during abduction the subscapularis, the infraspinatus, and the teres minor counteract the strong pull of the deltoid and the supraspinatus, to enable the arm to be abducted away from the body. Otherwise the deltoid and the supraspinatus would tend to elevate the head of the humerus instead of abducting the arm. (The initiation of abduction is one of the main functions of the supraspinatus.) The supraspinatus also acts as an internal rotator of the humerus when the arm is hanging next to the side, while the infraspinatus and the teres minor, together with the posterior fibers of the deltoid muscle, externally rotate the humerus. (These are the only external rotators of the humerus.)

7. *The biceps.* The biceps has two heads:

1. The *short head* arises from the coracoid process.

2. The *long head* originates from the glenoid labrum at the superior aspect of the glenoid cavity within the shoulder joint. It then arches over the head of the humerus and descends into the bicipital groove. The groove is covered by the transverse humeral ligament and by the tendon of the pectoralis major muscle.

Insertion is by means of a single tendon into the tuberosity of the radius. The main action of the biceps is to supinate the forearm. It also flexes the elbow and has a weak effect on forward flexion of the shoulder joint. The long head can exert some downward pressure on the upper end of the humerus and in this way may prevent the head of the humerus from moving upward as the deltoid muscle contracts.

8. *The triceps.* The triceps muscle is situated on the back of the upper arm and has three heads.

1. The *long head* arises from the glenoid on the scapula.

2. The *lateral head* arises from the posterior surface and the lateral border of the humerus.

3. The *medial head* arises from the posterior surface of the humerus below the radial groove.

The three heads blend together to form a tendon, which inserts into the olecranon on the ulna. The long head of the triceps helps form two spaces as it travels between the teres minor and the teres major muscles. One of these spaces is the "quadrangular space," bounded by the subscapularis and the teres minor above, the teres major below, the long head of the triceps medially, and the humerus laterally. This space contains the posterior circumflexed humeral vessels and the axillary nerve. Both of these are important, for if they are damaged or compressed in this space, they cause pain and incapacity of the shoulder joint.

The main function of the triceps is that of extension of the forearm and the arm. When the arm is extended, the long head also assists in extending the shoulder and adducting it.

Nerves and Arteries

The brachial plexus and the brachial artery run in close proximity to the shoulder joint and can be damaged in an injury of the shoulder girdle, such as an anterior dislocation of the humerus or a posteriorly displaced fracture of the clavicle. When an injury involves the shoulder girdle, it is therefore important to check the blood and nerve supply to the upper limb. The dermatome areas (that is, the areas of skin supplied by a particular nerve root) should be noted (Figure 12.7).

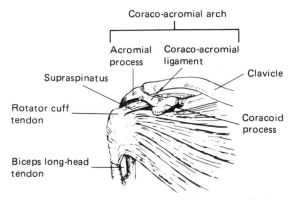

FIGURE 12.6 The relationship of the supraspinatus (and rotator cuff) to the coraco-acromial ligament

TABLE 12.1   Main Action of Muscles around the Shoulder Girdle

Movement	Main Muscles Involved
Flexion	Deltoid (anterior portion) Coracobrachialis Pectoralis major (clavicular portion)
Extension	Latissimus dorsi Teres major Deltoid (posterior portion)
Abduction	Deltoid (middle portion) Supraspinatus Serratus anterior (helps steady scapula; allows deltoid to function)
Adduction	Pectoralis major Latissimus dorsi
External rotators	Infraspinatus Teres minor (Deltoid—posterior portion)
Internal rotators	Subscapularis Pectoralis major Latissimus dorsi Teres major (Deltoid—anterior portion)
Depresses raised arm against resistance	Pectoralis major Latissimus dorsi Teres major
Arm abducted with the head of the humerus prevented from moving upwards by:	Subscapularis Infraspinatus Teres minor Biceps—long head
Scapula stabilization	Trapezius Serratus anterior Rhomboids
Scapula protraction (reaching and punching)	Trapezius Serratus anterior Rhomboids
Scapula retraction (pulling scapulae toward each other)	Rhomboid major Rhomboid minor
Elevation of scapulae (shoulder shrugs)	Trapezius Levator scapulae

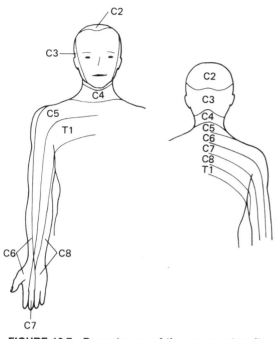

FIGURE 12.7 Dermatomes of the upper extremity

EVALUATION PROCEDURES

1. *Observe* the athlete.
   a. From the *front* (Figure 12.8), note
      1. general posture
      2. prominence of the sternoclavicular joint (subluxation)
      3. deformity of the shaft of the clavicle (fracture)
      4. prominence of the distal clavicle and the acromioclavicular joint (shoulder separation or a shoulder pointer)
      5. wasting of the deltoid muscle (axillary nerve lesion)
   b. From the *side*, note
      1. alignment of the cervical and thoracic spines
      2. swelling over the front of the shoulder joint
      3. position of the acromioclavicular joint
   c. From *behind*, note
      1. posture of the head and neck

2. muscle atrophy—particularly the deltoid and supraspinatus
3. position of movement of the scapula

2. Ask athlete to *point* with one finger to the area of pain.
3. *Palpate* for
   a. skin temperature (warmth suggests inflammation)
   b. tenderness (avoiding painful area until last)
      1. sternoclavicular joint
      2. clavicle
      3. acromioclavicular joint
      4. biceps tendon, long head
      5. under acromion process
      6. greater tuberosity of humerus
      7. anterior capsule
      8. posterior capsule
      9. posterior glenoid
      10. scapula
      11. trapezius and rhomboid muscles, and trigger points in the area of these muscles
4. Examine the following areas first, as they may refer pain to the shoulder:
   a. Cervical spine (see p. 254)
   b. Thoracic outlet (see section on thoracic outlet syndrome, p. 189)
   c. Temporomandibular joint:
      1. Observe range of motion.
      2. Observe symmetry of mouth opening and closing.
      3. Palpate for tenderness, swelling, and clicking of the joint.
5. *Check skin sensation* of the shoulder and arm and feel the distal pulses.
6. *Check active range of motion* of the shoulder—performed by the athlete (Table 12.2 and Figure 12.9).
7. *Check active range of motion*—performed against resistance. The same movements are performed, this time against isometric manual resistance provided by the examiner. Note if any weakness is present, and observe the position of the arm and the location of the pain.

Observing the athlete from the front

Note: General posture

Sternoclavicular joint

Clavicle

Distal clavicle and acromioclavicular joint

Deltoid muscle

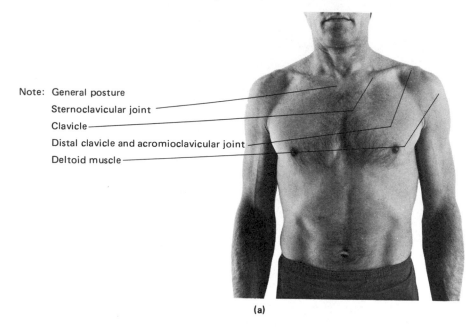

(a)

Observing the athlete from behind

Note: Alignment of the head and neck

Any muscle atrophy, especially the deltoid
and supraspinatus

The position and movement of the scapula

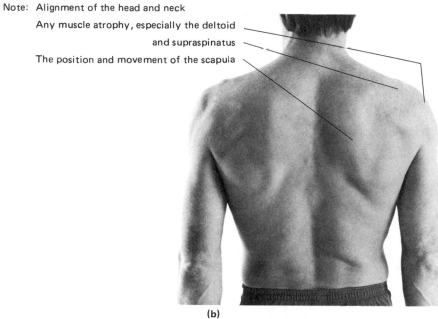

(b)

FIGURE 12.8 (a) **Observing the athlete from the front** (b) **Observing the athlete from behind**

TABLE 12.2 Movement of the Arm at the Shoulder

The following are the main movements of the shoulder girdle that need to be tested (Figure 12.9). Note range as well as smoothness of motion at the glenohumeral, acromioclavicular, and sternoclavicular joints, as well as scapulothoracic action.

1. Forward flexion
2. Backward extension
3. Abduction—observe the scapulohumeral rhythm from behind
4. Adduction
5. Internal rotation with arm at side
6. External rotation with arm at side
7. External rotation with arm in abduction
8. Internal rotation with arm in abduction
9. Horizontal extension with arm in abduction
10. Horizontal flexion with arm in abduction—try to place the hand on the opposite shoulder
11. Internal rotation posteriorly—attempt to touch the opposite scapula
12. Protraction and retraction
13. Shoulder shrugs
14. Perform the particular movement that causes pain, or is thought to be associated with the condition, e.g., a tennis serve or a baseball pitch

8. *Check passive range of motion*—feel for the quality of the end point in the range of motion and for any clicks or pops.

9. *Test for stability* of the

a. Glenohumeral joint (this is the *apprehension sign*)—The arm is placed at 90° of abduction in an externally rotated position (Figure 12.10). Pressure is then exerted in an anterior direction while the shoulder is externally rotated. Immediate discomfort and apprehension may be experienced by the athlete if the glenohumeral joint is unstable in an anterior and inferior direction. The deltoid muscle will also contract reflexively. Pain may be experienced along the inferior rim.

A variation of this test is to place the athlete's arm at 90° of abduction. The elbow is supported on the examiner's shoulder and the examiner's cupped hands are placed over the proximal humerus. The muscles surrounding the shoulder should be relaxed while the examiner directs a downward force on the proximal humerus. The humerus will displace in an inferior direction if laxity is present.

A further variation of the apprehension test may be used for a backstroke swimmer, as described in Chapter 22.

To detect apprehension when the humerus is forced posteriorly, have the athlete stand with arms at the side; the shoulder girdle is stabilized by the examiner and pressure is exerted in a posterior direction against the humeral head.

Another method to detect posterior instability is to have the athlete lying supine with the shoulder at 90° of forward flexion and internally rotated. Posteriorly directed pressure is then applied against the elbow in an attempt to sublux the humerus posteriorly.

b. Acromioclavicular joint—Stability may be tested by placing cupped hands over the acromioclavicular joint.[2] One palm is placed on the anterior aspect of the clavicle, while the other is placed over the spine of the scapula. The hands are then squeezed together, which causes a "glide" motion through the acromioclavicular joint and may demonstrate abnormal laxity or produce pain.

c. Sternoclavicular joint—Stability of the sternoclavicular joint should be tested mainly in the anteroposterior direction. Care should be exercised in grasping the proximal clavicle, as this may be uncomfortable for the

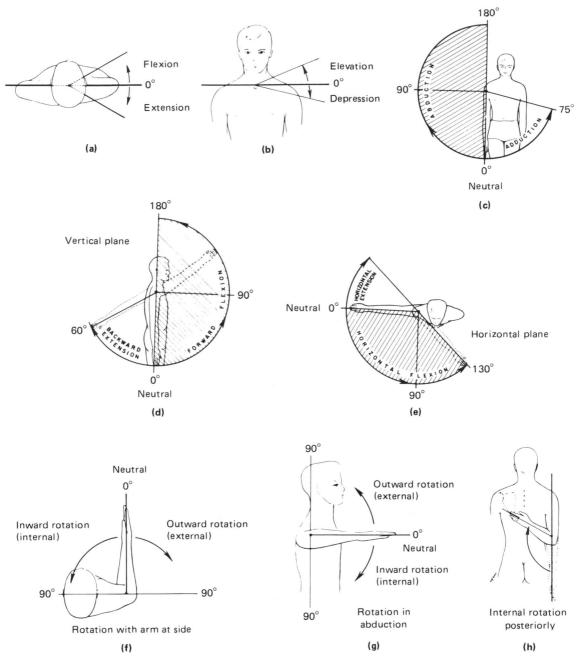

FIGURE 12.9 Shoulder joint—range of motion (Reproduced with permission of the American Academy of Orthopaedic Surgeons)

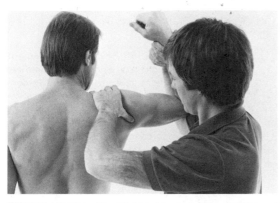

FIGURE 12.10a Examining for anterior stability of the glenohumeral joint The arm is externally rotated while an anteriorly directed force is applied to the posterior aspect of the humeral head.

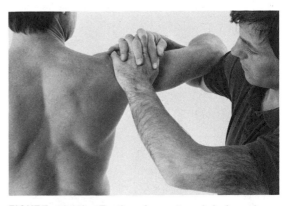

FIGURE 12.10b Testing for antero-inferior glenohumeral instability The deltoid muscles should be completely relaxed as a downward force is applied to the proximal humerus.

athlete. Abnormal motion or pain should be noted.

10. *Demonstrate impingement signs.* There are two methods of demonstrating impingement of the humerus, supraspinatus, and biceps tendons against the inferior surface of the acromion and coraco-acromial ligament:

a. Bring the arm into the extreme of forward flexion, with the forearm held in supination. If pain is experienced when the arm is brought to

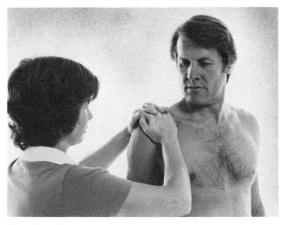

FIGURE 12.11 Testing for acromioclavicular joint stability A squeezing action may demonstrate abnormal motion or produce pain.

maximum forward flexion against resistance, a positive impingement sign is present.[3]

b. An alternative method is to have the athlete hold the arm at 90° of flexion in internal rotation and pronation. The elbow is stabilized and the forearm brought rapidly downward, which attempts to force the forearm into maximal internal rotation and brings the head of the humerus sharply up against the inferior aspect of the acromion. Pain that is localized to the area of the coraco-acromial arch is indicative of impingement (Figure 12.12).[4]

11. *Muscle testing.* Test individual muscle groups to locate any weakness (see Figure 1.6).

12. *Test nerve functions:*

a. Axillary nerve—Loss of sensation over the lateral aspect of the upper arm (Figure 12.13), as well as weakness and lack of tone of the anterior and middle deltoids during abduction, indicates an axillary nerve lesion.

b. Long thoracic nerve—Test for "winging" of the scapula (paralysis of the serratus anterior muscle) by

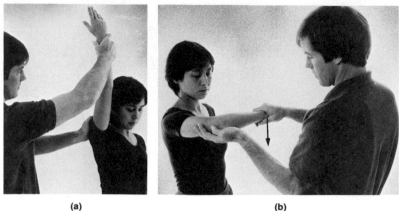

(a)   (b)

FIGURE 12.12 Impingement signs (a) Bring the arm into extreme forward elevation (flexion) with the humerus in external rotation (the forearm in supination). (b) The elbow is stabilized as the forearm is forced downward, bringing the shoulder into internal rotation. The head of the humerus is thus forced against the acromion and the coraco-acromial arch.

TABLE 12.3   Manual Muscle Testing

The following tests localize the strain to the particular muscle group tested, and comparison of the two extremities helps detect weaknesses (see p. 20).[6]

1. Arm at 90° of abduction, full external rotation and supination, force directed downward (*anterior deltoid*)

2. As above, but with some internal rotation and palm facing downward (*middle deltoid*)

3. As above, with full internal rotation and palm facing backward (*posterior deltoid*)

4. Arm at the side, elbow at 90°, force directed toward midline (*teres minor*)

5. Arm at 90° of abduction, elbow bent, force directed downward (*infraspinatus*)

6. Arm at 90° of abduction, force directed upward (*subscapularis*)

7. Resistance to initiation of abduction (*supraspinatus*)

8. Arm at 90° of abduction, 60° of horizontal flexion, full internal rotation, force directed downward (*supraspinatus*)

9. Resistance to shoulder shrugs (*trapezius*)

10. Arm at 90° of flexion, palm facing downward, force directed downward (*serratus anterior*)

11. Hand on hip, elbow at 90°, force directed forward on the elbow (*rhomboids*)

having the athlete resist downward pressure against the arm when held at 90° of flexion (Figure 12.14).[5] An alternative is the "climb-the-wall" test.

c. Dorsal scapular nerve (to the rhomboids)—Test for partial winging of the scapula when the shoulder is extended in a slightly abducted position against resistance; or, with the hand on the waist, the elbow is forced forwards (Figure 12.15).

d. Suprascapular nerve (to the supraspinatus and infraspinatus)—Test by initiating abduction against resistance (supraspinatus) and by resisting external rotation (infraspinatus).

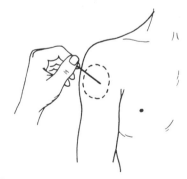

FIGURE 12.13 Sensation loss over lateral side of upper arm from an axillary nerve lesion

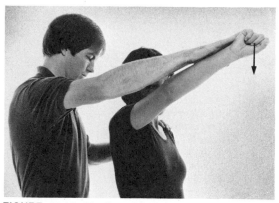

FIGURE 12.14 Testing the long thoracic nerve If the long thoracic nerve is damaged, the serratus anterior muscle will cease to function, resulting in winging of the scapula.

The trainer should be aware that pain may be referred to the shoulder from irritation of the diaphragm due to free gas or blood, from infection, and from cardiac ischemia or gallstones.

Table 12.4 is designed to help differenti-

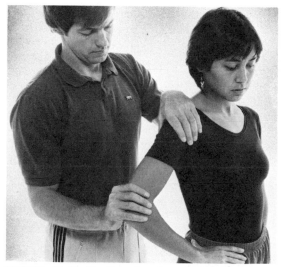

FIGURE 12.15 Testing the dorsal scapular nerve, which supplies the rhomboid muscles The athlete resists the forward force on the elbow, while the trainer observes contraction of the rhomboids and partial winging of the scapula.

ate the common shoulder conditions that may present during an athletic event.

PREVENTION OF SHOULDER INJURIES

1. *Falling technique.* Perhaps the most important preventive measure is for the athlete to learn how to fall correctly. This technique should be developed until it becomes a habit. The athlete should learn not to fall on the outstretched arm or the point of the shoulder, but rather to roll over so as to absorb the shock of impact. Falling down flat and hard is bound to cause an injury. Most people, however, fall incorrectly, and the correct techniques have to be developed by practicing falling drills. Coaches and trainers should be educated in the importance of this type of drill, particularly for athletes engaged in contact sports.

2. *Shoulder pad placement.* In football, incorrect fitting of the shoulder pads may be responsible for the occasional acromioclavicular dislocation seen in this sport. Not tying the jersey down, or cutting the sleeves, are other predisposing factors because they allow the shoulder pads to slip out of position and expose the acromioclavicular joint to possible injury.

3. *Tackling technique.* Shoulder dislocations are most frequently encountered through poor tackling technique, particularly when the arm is abducted and externally rotated while trying to stop the ballcarrier. The danger of this form of tackling should be constantly stressed so that it will not be attempted.

4. *Muscle development.* It is imperative, particularly in contact sports, that the musculature around the shoulders be strengthened to protect the shoulder girdle. This applies especially to the larger muscle groups such as the trapezius, the deltoid, the subscapularis, and the latissimus dorsi.

TABLE 12.4   On-field Examination of Acute Shoulder Injuries

Examination Procedure	Possibilities Examiner Should Consider

I.   Symptoms
  1. Pain and/or burning around shoulder area, initially diffuse.
  2. Weakness of arm and shoulder girdle.
  3. Arm just hangs down, or is supported with opposite arm.
	Acromioclavicular joint separation.
	Shoulder dislocation.
	Fractured clavicle.
	Brachial plexus lesion.
	Rotator-cuff tear.
	Biceps subluxation.
	Fractured humerus.

II. Ask athlete to point out tender area (this is often very difficult for the athlete to do initially).	

III.   *Observe* and then *palpate* gently:
  1. Sternoclavicular joint
  2. Clavicle, midshaft
  3. Clavicle, outer end
  4. Acromioclavicular joint
  5. Contour of shoulder
  6. Rest of shoulder and upper arm
	Sprain/dislocation.
	Fracture.
	Pointer or acromioclavicular separation.
	Acromioclavicular separation.
	Shoulder subluxation or dislocation.
	Fractured humerus.

IV.   If all above are negative, *palpate more firmly* over:
  1. Anterior capsule
  2. Biceps
  3. Lateral to and under acromion process
  4. Posterior capsule
  5. Greater and lesser tuberosities of humerus
	Shoulder subluxation.
	Subluxation of long head of biceps.
	Supraspinatus (rotator-cuff) tear.
	Posterior dislocation or anterior subluxation.
	Avulsion fracture; greater tuberosity (supraspinatus insertion) or lesser tuberosity (subscapularis insertion).

V.   *Range of motion*
Check shoulder through full range of active motion.
Then test range of motion against resistance.
	If athlete can't bring arm across chest (adduction and internal rotation) an anterior dislocation is probably present.
	If athlete can't abduct and externally rotate, a rotator-cuff (and deltoid) injury or posterior dislocation is probably present.
	Weakness of flexion and abduction may mean:
	  1. Muscle strain, e.g., supraspinatus strain
	  2. Brachial plexus lesion
	  3. Localized nerve lesion, e.g., axillary nerve
	  4. Inhibition due to pain

TABLE 12.4   On-field Examination of Acute Shoulder Injuries (*cont.*)

Examination Procedure	Possibilities Examiner Should Consider
VI. Check sensation over neck, shoulder, and arm.	Possible neck injury.
VII. If all above are negative, examine for tenderness over brachial plexus, neck musculature, and posterior spinous process of cervical vertebrae.	
VIII. If all the above are negative: 1. Test for subluxation of shoulder—apprehension sign. 2. Put neck through full range of motion, then full range of motion against resistance; also, compression test. 3. Test power of each muscle group of the arm.	

5. *Warm-up techniques.* In throwing activities (as well as in sports such as gymnastics, tennis, and swimming) it is important to perform a gradual warm-up program before undertaking vigorous activity. Minor injuries which occur before adequate warm-up has taken place tend to plague participants of these sports because of the repetitive nature of the shoulder-girdle motion. Included in warm-up is an adequate stretching program. This should be a slow, relaxed type of stretching that keeps the stretch well within the limits of discomfort.

6. *Throwing technique.* A large percentage of injuries in the throwing sports occur because of incorrect technique. This predisposing factor needs to be corrected as early as possible in an athlete's career so as to prevent permanent injury.

INJURIES

Injuries to the Sternoclavicular Joint

Sprains and dislocations. The most common injury to the sternoclavicular joint is a sprain, which occurs particularly in such activities as football and wrestling, when the athlete falls on his or her side with the opposition on top. This drives the shoulder forward and inward, applying a force to the clavicle which can disrupt the costoclavicular and the sternoclavicular ligaments (Figure 12.2). If the force is severe enough, a third-degree tearing of the ligaments can occur, resulting in a *dislocation* of the sternoclavicular joint. The proximal end of the clavicle may be forced medially, upward and forward, commonly resulting in swelling and deformity over the sternoclavicular joint on the side involved.

On occasion, however, the force may drive the clavicle backward (a posterior dislocation). This will produce little in the way of deformity, but may cause a great deal of distress if the clavicle impinges on the trachea and interferes with breathing. If this happens, the athlete may find that it is more comfortable to sit forward than to lie down. A posterior dislocation is also dangerous because it can rupture the underlying blood vessels.

Treatment consists of ice application, an arm sling, and anti-inflammatory medication if necessary. If the instability is severe, a plaster-of-Paris, figure-eight bandage should be used. In some cases, if reduction cannot be maintained, open reduction with fixation may be necessary.

Fractures of the Shaft of the Clavicle

A fracture of the clavicular shaft is a common injury, particularly in the child or adolescent. It usually occurs from a fall on the outstretched arm or on the point of the shoulder, less commonly from a direct blow. Most fractures occur in the middle third. Displacement is due to the muscle pull—the proximal portion is pulled superiorly in relation to the distal fragment.

In most cases the diagnosis is obvious, with a visible and palpable deformity that is accompanied by marked ecchymosis and pain. In some cases, such as the pre-adolescent with a greenstick fracture, a deformity may not occur and pain and swelling may be the only signs. If the initial X-rays are negative but pain and tenderness persist, X-rays should be repeated, because a fracture may not show up for a week or two after the initial injury.

Treatment consists of ice and a figure-eight bandage to support the shoulders and pull them backward.

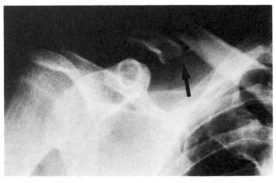

FIGURE 12.16   X-ray—fracture of the clavicle

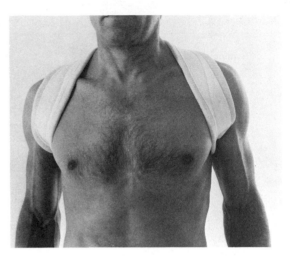

FIGURE 12.17   Figure-eight support used for treating a fractured clavicle

Contusions to the Outer End of the Clavicle ("Shoulder Pointer")

Contusions to the outer end of the clavicle are frequent and painful injuries. It is most important to be sure that one is not dealing with an acromioclavicular joint injury.

SYMPTOMS AND SIGNS: The symptoms are usually localized to the distal end of the clavicle, but may radiate into the trapezius muscle on that side. Swelling and tenderness are localized to the area of the distal clavicle and do not involve the acromioclavicular joint. There may be some tenderness and spasm of the trapezius muscle. Careful palpation should be made, to ensure that neither the acromioclavicular joint nor the coracoclavicular ligament is involved. There should be no instability of the clavicle either on clinical examination or on X-rays.

X-RAYS: These should be taken in order to exclude a fracture of the distal clavicle or a separation of the acromioclavicular joint.

TREATMENT: Ice immediately. Early use of anti-inflammatory medication is beneficial. An injection of local anesthetic containing a

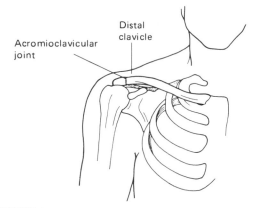

FIGURE 12.18 A contusion to the distal end of the clavicle will produce localized tenderness. If there is tenderness over the acromioclavicular joint, a sprain of this joint should be suspected.

cortisone preparation and hyaluronidase is particularly useful to reduce pain and tenderness. A pad can be used to protect the area (a donut pad should be fashioned and placed over the tender area). Progressive exercises of the shoulder, particularly of the trapezius muscle, should be instituted to prevent any atrophy from occurring.

COMPLICATIONS: Long-term complications may occur, particularly when the athlete is inadequately treated. Progressive calcification around the distal end of the clavicle can cause a painful deformity. Osteophyte formation and degeneration of the acromioclavicular joint can also occur, necessitating excision of the distal clavicle. Osteolysis of the distal clavicle is an uncommon condition but one which can occur as a result of a contusion to the distal clavicle.

Osteolysis of the Distal Clavicle

Osteolysis of the distal clavicle is a relatively rare condition in which a portion of the distal clavicle may resorb. The diagnosis is made by X-ray visualization of the distal clavicle.

ETIOLOGY: The exact etiological mechanism is poorly understood. Osteolysis of the distal clavicle usually develops following:

1. A relatively minor injury to the distal clavicle such as a first-degree or a mild second-degree acromioclavicular joint sprain or contusion to the distal clavicle.
2. Repeated minor traumata such as happen to weight lifters, gymnasts, ice-hockey players, and judo exponents.
3. A severe injury to the acromioclavicular joint or distal clavicle—much less common than the preceding two causes.

SYMPTOMS AND SIGNS: Pain in the region of the acromioclavicular joint and limitation of extreme shoulder motion appear to be the predominant symptoms. Enlargement of the soft tissue around the distal clavicle can be observed. This lump is often very tender to the touch.

X-RAYS: It usually takes a minimum of two to three weeks for the X-ray changes to appear after the initial acute injury. However, in cases of repetitive minor trauma, symptoms may be present for some weeks or months before the changes appear on the X-ray. The earliest changes are sclerosis or cystic degeneration in the distal clavicle, followed by frank osteolysis.

COURSE: Some cases resolve spontaneously, though this is uncommon if the athlete continues to participate.

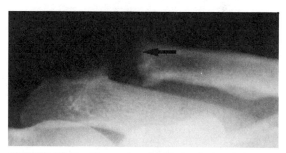

FIGURE 12.19 X-ray showing osteolysis of the distal clavicle Note the "moth-eaten" clavicle, as well as the widening of the acromioclavicular joint.

TREATMENT: Athletes such as weight lifters and gymnasts find their effectiveness limited. It appears at this time that rest for a period of six months or more is needed to allow the lesion to heal so that return to participation may be pain free.

Corticosteroid injections have not been reported to be beneficial but may be tried. Surgical removal of the distal clavicle (distal to the coracoclavicular ligament) may be necessary in cases that are resistant to conservative treatment. This surgery has been successful in selected cases.

Acromioclavicular Joint Sprains ("Shoulder Separations")

The acromioclavicular joint is a relatively unstable joint which is easily disrupted. A separation implies a sprain of the ligaments supporting the acromioclavicular joint. These ligaments are discussed under anatomy (Figure 12.3).

MECHANISM OF INJURY:

1. The athlete falls on the point of the shoulder, forcing the acromion and the coracoid processes downward. This is the commonest mechanism of injury.

2. The athlete falls on the outstretched hand, transmitting the force up the arm and through the acromioclavicular joint.

3. The athlete falls on the outstretched hand which is at right angles to the body. Contact is then made by the opposition against the shoulder, forcing the shoulder forward on the fixed arm.

4. In some sports, such as ice hockey, the acromioclavicular joint frequently gives rise to chronic symptoms.[7] The injury seems to be due to the indirect forces on the shoulder which are part of that sport.

SYMPTOMS AND SIGNS: The arm and the shoulder usually droop on the side of the injury. Severe pain accompanies most acromioclavicular sprains, but localization by the athlete is often vague. Tenderness is more specific, located directly over the acromioclavicular joint. There may also be tenderness along the clavicle and at the attachments of the trapezius and the deltoid muscles. In very severe sprains there may be tenderness over the coracoclavicular ligaments as well.

The athlete should be observed from the front, from the side, and from behind. The

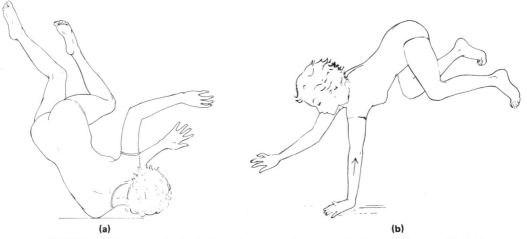

(a)   (b)

FIGURE 12.20 Acromioclavicular joint separation—mechanisms of injury (a) Falling on the point of the shoulder (b) Falling on the hand of an outstretched arm This mechanism is nonspecific, and may result in an injury to one or more structures from the wrist to the clavicle.

clavicle may ride above the level of the acromion process. This can be accentuated by gentle downward traction on the arm. One should also gently mobilize the clavicle while palpating over the acromioclavicular joint, in order to observe if any excessive motion is present (see pp. 165 and 167).

X-RAYS: Anteroposterior X-rays of the acromioclavicular joint should be taken to exclude fractures of the clavicle, acromion, coracoid, or humerus. Stress views of both shoulders should then be taken with the athlete standing. Weights are suspended from the wrists in order to apply traction through the arms to the acromioclavicular joint. A second-degree separation may show a slight elevation of the clavicle relative to the acromion process, and a slight increase in the distance between the coracoid process

and the clavicle. In the severe third-degree separation, the clavicle rides high above the acromion process and there is a wide gap between the coracoid process and the clavicle, compared with the opposite side.[8]

If one suspects a rare posterior dislocation of the clavicle (i.e., the clavicle moves in a posterior direction and not upward), then the Alexander view[9] should be taken (this is a shoulder-forward position with the shoulder against the X-ray plate).[10]

DIFFERENTIAL DIAGNOSIS: It is important to differentiate acromioclavicular joint lesions from contusions to the distal end of the clavicle ("shoulder pointer"). A shoulder pointer implies a contusion only—there is no ligamentous involvement. The main differentiating feature is the area of tenderness. In the shoulder pointer there is no tenderness over

TABLE 12.5   Findings in an Acromioclavicular-Joint Sprain

Degree of Sprain	Pathology	Clinical Findings
First-Degree	Sprain of the acromioclavicular ligament or capsule. Coracoclavicular ligament intact.	Tenderness and swelling over the acromioclavicular joint only. Minimal limitation of shoulder's range of motion. Clavicle stable when moved. No elevation of the clavicle.
Second-Degree	Severe sprain of the acromioclavicular ligament. Partial sprain or stretching of the coracoclavicular ligament.	Tenderness over the acromioclavicular joint (2+). Swelling over the acromioclavicular joint (2+). Some tenderness over the coracoclavicular ligaments. Shoulder motion considerably limited due to pain. Slight elevation of the clavicle relative to the acromion process.
Third-Degree	Complete tearing of the acromioclavicular and coracoclavicular ligaments. There is often damage to the deltoid and trapezius muscles.	The athlete supports the arm, as the symptoms are markedly increased when the arm hangs. Tenderness 3+. Swelling 3+. Obvious elevation of the clavicle relative to the acromion process.

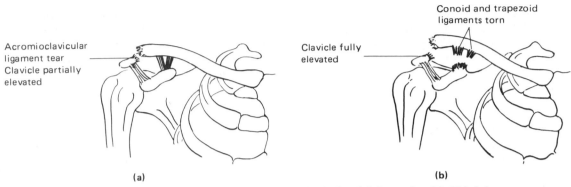

Acromioclavicular
ligament tear
Clavicle partially
elevated

(a)

Conoid and trapezoid
ligaments torn

Clavicle fully
elevated

(b)

FIGURE 12.21   (a) Second-degree acromioclavicular joint sprain   (b) Third-degree acromioclavicular joint sprain

the acromioclavicular joint. However, it is not uncommon to have a combination of the two injuries (i.e., an acromioclavicular joint sprain plus a contusion to the distal end of the clavicle).

TREATMENT:

1. *First-degree separation*: Ice and analgesics, perhaps anti-inflammatory medication, and a sling should be initially applied. This is followed by rehabilitation exercises which should rapidly return shoulder function to normal. A donut pad is placed over the acromioclavicular joint when the athlete participates in contact sports.

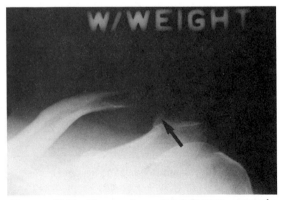

Figure 12.22 X-ray of a third-degree acromioclavicular sprain Note the clavicle riding above the level of the acromion process, and the widening of the space between the coracoid process and the clavicle, as well as between the acromion and the clavicle.

2. *Second-degree separation*: This needs to be immobilized for a period of time depending on the severity of the lesion, but usually for three to four weeks. One of the best methods of immobilization is the Kenny Howard sling. The athlete is supplied with two slings so that he or she can shower with the sling in place. The clean sling is applied while the elbow is supported on a table, so as to prevent distraction of the acromioclavicular joint. The sling that was removed is then laundered and is used the following day. The cycle is repeated daily. Sometimes the sling will need to be tightened more than once a day, but should not be removed or adjusted without the elbow being supported.

3. *Third-degree separation*:
   a. *Conservative treatment*: If the clavicle can be reduced and is easily held in place, a Kenny Howard sling can be satisfactorily used. It is applied for a period of six to eight weeks.
   b. *Surgical treatment*: There are numerous surgical procedures.
   c. *Alternative method*: It must be mentioned that some sports medicine physicians feel it is unnecessary to immobilize or repair acromioclavicular separations.[11] These physicians attempt to reduce the dislocation and then start active movement using an overhead exercise apparatus. When this motion can be accom-

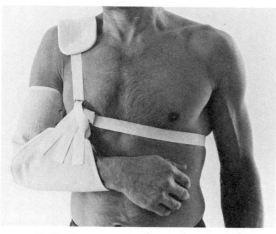

FIGURE 12.23 The Kenny Howard sling

plished comfortably, further rehabilitation exercises are progressively instituted. The athletes are then permitted to return to their activities with padding placed over the joint. Modifications of the shoulder pads are made on football players so that the forces are borne on the chest rather than the point of the shoulder. Muscle-strengthening exercises (with particular emphasis on the trapezius, deltoid, and biceps) are continued until the two arms have equal power through a full range of motion. Physicians using this method claim equally good long-term results as compared to other methods of treatment, and they point out that athletes treated this way are usually able to return to participation much earlier than those who have had conservative or surgical treatment. Even if the functional results are good, there is a definite cosmetic deformity as a result of the clavicle protruding above the acromion process. It should be emphasized that this form of treatment is not generally accepted at this time.

COMPLICATIONS:

1. Pain, disability, and decrease in the range of shoulder motion may occasionally be troublesome complications. They are particularly common following first- and second-degree separations.[12,13,14]

2. Degenerative changes may involve the acromion, resulting in spur formation which leads not only to pain in the acromioclavicular joint but to an impingement syndrome involving the rotator cuff.

3. Soft-tissue calcification can also develop over the distal clavicle and render this area painful for a period of time.

4. Osteolysis of the distal clavicle can occur.

5. Cosmetic deformity from an unreduced separation consists of an unsightly bulge over the clavicle.

REHABILITATION: Rehabilitation exercises for the entire shoulder-girdle muscle complex should be continued until pre-injury power, strength, endurance, and flexibility are obtained (see section on shoulder rehabilitation, p. 192).

TABLE 12.6 Dislocation of the Glenohumeral Joint (Shoulder Dislocation)

1. *Anterior dislocation* (98%)
   (1) antero-inferior ⎱ May end up in a subcoracoid (most
   (2) inferior ⎰ common) or subglenoid position.
2. *Posterior dislocation* (2%)
   (1) subacromial (other positions have rarely been reported).

Anterior Dislocation of the Glenohumeral Joint

This is the most common type of shoulder dislocation.

MECHANISM OF INJURY: The arm is externally rotated, abducted, and, usually, elevated. The force pushes the arm beyond the limits of the capsule and ligaments surrounding the glenohumeral joint. The greater tuberosity is levered against the acromion process and the coraco-acromial ligament. This tears the inferior glenohumeral ligament, the anterior capsule, and perhaps the labrum. The humeral head slips out, commonly in an antero-inferior direction; when the arm is dropped to the side, the head usually comes to rest under the coracoid process.[15]

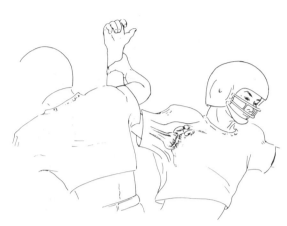

FIGURE 12.24 Mechanism of an anterior dislocation The arm is forced into extension, abduction and external rotation

TABLE 12.7   Anterior Dislocation—Antero-inferior Type (Most Common)

Severity	Sprain of Anterior Capsule and Ligaments	Subluxation of the Humerus	Dislocation
Glenohumeral movement	Arm abducted and externally rotated. Greater tuberosity forced against acromion.	Head of humerus levered partially out of glenoid.	Humerus slips out of glenoid in an anterior and inferior direction. Usually locates under the coracoid process (subcoracoid) or under the anterior aspect of the glenoid (subglenoid).
Tissue damage	Partial tearing of the anterior and inferior capsule and ligaments with a variable decrease in tensile strength.	More complete tearing. Serious decrease in tensile strength. Rotator-cuff may be damaged.	Severe stretching and tearing. Limited or no tensile strength. Rotator-cuff may be damaged or torn.
Common complications	If laxity is present after healing, subluxation may occur.	Repeated subluxations with limitation of function. Compression and/or avulsion of greater tuberosity.	Repeated dislocations from progressively less force. Fracture of the greater tuberosity. Rotator-cuff injury or tear. Nerve damage. Axillary artery damage.

    increasing severity

SYMPTOMS: The athlete usually knows that the shoulder has dislocated and is very alarmed and apprehensive. There is intense pain with the initial dislocation (though recurrent dislocations may be much less painful). There may be tingling and numbness down the arm to the hand.

SIGNS: Immediate recognition of an anterior dislocation is often possible, due to the characteristic position of the athlete's arm. Once the clothes are removed, note the

1. sharp contour of the affected limb in comparison with the smooth deltoid outline on the opposite side
2. prominent acromion process
3. humeral head beneath the coracoid process
4. resistance by the athlete to any attempt to adduct or internally rotate the arm (i.e., the arm cannot be brought across the chest)

Always examine:

1. Sensation of the
   a. lateral arm (axillary nerve)
   b. radial aspect of the forearm (musculocutaneous nerve)
   c. remainder of the arm, forearm, and hand (other brachial plexus nerves)
2. Strength (this may be difficult to examine due to pain) of the
   a. forearm pronation and supination (C6)
   b. wrist flexion and extension (C6 and C7)
   c. finger flexion and extension (C7 and C8)
   d. finger abduction and adduction (T1)
3. Radial pulse
4. Peripheral circulation to the fingernails. To check this, the nails should be lightly squeezed, which produces a whiteness of the nail bed. When the pressure is released, an almost immediate return to normal nail color takes place if the circulation is normal; however, if the microcirculation is impaired, there will be a lag before this occurs.

X-RAYS: An anterior dislocation is usually easy to see on the anteroposterior view. Additional views may be necessary to clearly define some of the fractures accompanying a dislocation.

Some authorities state that an arthrogram should be performed following a dislocation. They point out that there is an ever-constant threat of a rotator cuff tear occurring in conjunction with an initial dislocation.[16]

COMPLICATIONS:

1. Damage to the nerves around the glenohumeral joint, in particular the axillary nerve (which supplies the deltoid muscle) and the musculocutaneous or ulnar nerve.

2. Rotator cuff tears—may occur especially in conjunction with an inferior type of anterior dislocation, even in a young athlete.

3. Fractures of the humeral head and glenoid—relatively frequent in the older athlete. The greater tuberosity is the area most commonly fractured, due to its shearing against the acromion process and the coracoacromial ligament.

REDUCTION: The ideal time to reduce a shoulder dislocation is immediately after it has occurred. If there is a delay before the shoulder is reduced, pain and involuntary muscle spasm can make reduction difficult and necessitate a general anesthetic. Reduction should be done by a physician. An evaluation of the neurological and vascular structures should be performed and recorded before the reduction. If possible, X-rays should be taken before reduction is attempted; post-reduction X-rays should always be taken.

TECHNIQUES OF REDUCTION:

1. *Modified Hippocratic method.* This is the preferred technique (Figure 12.25). The athlete lies supine. The arm is held at between 30° and 45° of abduction. Countertraction is applied by means of a swathe around the upper thorax, the pull being in the opposite direction to the traction on the affected arm. The affected arm is very gently pulled in its longitudinal axis, while the patient is reas-

sured and encouraged to relax. The traction should be very gentle, with a slow increase in the amount of force exerted. It should be steady and held for approximately sixty seconds. In most cases the arm will be felt to slip back into the glenoid fossa as the athlete relaxes. The arm should then be turned into internal rotation and held in place across the chest.

2. *Hippocratic method.* If countertraction is not possible, then place an unshod foot against the chest wall (not in the axilla). Apply the same technique of gentle traction while encouraging the patient to relax.

3. *Kocher's maneuver.* If the aforementioned methods do not work, a modified Kocher's maneuver can be performed by a physician who is skilled and experienced in using this technique. There have been complications when the Kocher's maneuver has been used in a forceful manner by an unskilled person.

The arm is gently externally rotated while traction is applied in the long axis of the humerus. This usually results in the humeral head slipping back into the glenoid. As this is felt to occur, the arm is then brought into a slightly adducted and internally rotated position, which should complete the reduction.

POST-REDUCTION IMMOBILIZATION: A post-reduction check of the neurological and vascular structures should be routinely performed. The arm should be held against the side, internally rotated, and maintained in this position by means of a sling and swathe. No abduction or external rotation should be allowed (Figure 12.26). Analgesics and anti-inflammatory medication can be used as indicated. Ice should be used immediately afterward and continued for the first few days.

TREATMENT: The standard treatment for an anterior dislocation of the shoulder in an athlete may be summarized as:

1. Three to four weeks of immobilization, followed by rehabilitation
2. Return to participation when the shoulder is rehabilitated

It has been said that if the shoulder is immobilized for three to four weeks following the initial dislocation, the chances of a repeat dislocation are very small.[17] Not all agree on this point, as some sports medicine physicians do not consider that this form of

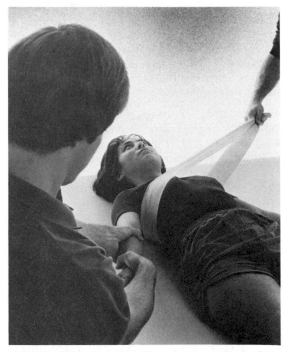

FIGURE 12.25 Modified Hippocratic method of reducing an anterior dislocation of the shoulder Gentle traction is applied along the long axis of the arm, while counter-traction is applied in the opposite direction by means of a swathe. The main emphasis during this maneuver is on helping the athlete to relax, and on the gentleness of the traction.

TABLE 12.8 Complications That Can Occur from Reducing a Dislocated Shoulder

1. Damage to one or more of the underlying nerves
2. Axillary artery damage
3. Fractures of the humerus and/or glenoid or epiphyseal damage

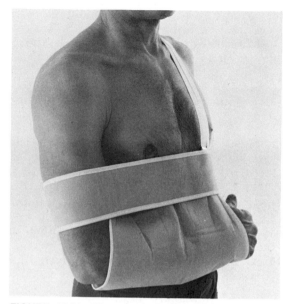

FIGURE 12.26 The arm is immobilized across the chest in a sling and swathe.

treatment necessarily influences later shoulder stability. For this reason, the following alternative programs of treatment have been suggested and are under investigation:

1. Reduction of the dislocation, followed by early surgery[18] (after an arthrogram and possibly an arthroscopic examination). This is considered a radical approach but may have some merit in certain types of athletes.

2. Immobilization until the shoulder is asymptomatic (usually ten days to three weeks), and then initiation of a vigorous but controlled rehabilitation program. The role of an extensive rehabilitation program should not be underestimated. Return to participation is permitted only when the shoulder is fully rehabilitated.

While the injured shoulder is immobilized, the athlete can still perform the following exercises under supervision:

1. Handgrip and forearm exercises (pronation and supination, flexion and extension of the elbow)

2. Isometric abduction and adduction with the arm at the side

3. Isometric internal and external rotation with the arm held in internal rotation

4. Isotonic internal rotation from 45° to 90° of internal rotation

When movement of the shoulder is permitted, the initial exercises are pendulum and internal-rotation exercises. Abduction and external rotation are attempted only when sufficient healing has taken place to allow these movements (see rehabilitation of the shoulder, p. 192).

Recurrent Anterior Dislocation of the Shoulder

If the anterior capsule and inferior glenohumeral ligaments have been badly stretched after an anterior dislocation, the stability of the shoulder is decreased. If the labrum is torn it is unlikely to heal. In addition, if rehabilitation is inadequate, this will increase the chances of a recurrent problem.

TREATMENT: Because recurrent dislocations signify that the anterior supporting structures (the anterior capsule, the inferior glenohumeral ligaments, and the subscapularis muscle) are not functioning adequately, there does not seem much point in suggesting that the athlete with an acute but recurrent dislocation be immobilized for a period of three to six weeks. A more practical approach is to

1. immobilize while symptoms are present

2. rehabilitate vigorously soon after the injury

3. assess the athlete for possible surgery only after complete rehabilitation has been attempted

SURGICAL PROCEDURES: Commonly used surgical procedures include the Putti-Platt and the Bankart operations,[19] which reinforce the anterior capsule and increase the efficiency of the subscapularis muscle, and the Bristow operation,[20,21] in which a portion of the coracoid process is removed and placed at the anterior glenoid.

Recurrent Anterior Subluxation of the Shoulder

Subluxation of the shoulder implies a partial dislocation of the humeral head. This is most commonly in an anterior direction and occurs when the athlete's arm is in a position of abduction and external rotation, or during the follow-through phases of throwing.

PATHOLOGY: Most frequently, the anterior capsule is stretched or detached, allowing the humeral head to slip forward when a certain point of abduction and external rotation is reached.

SYMPTOMS: A good history is vital in helping make the diagnosis of a subluxing shoulder. For instance, a backstroke swimmer doing a turn or a wrestler having his arm forced into an abducted, externally rotated position may convey the story of having become apprehensive at that particular moment as he felt the shoulder slip out of place. Often, however, the chief symptoms are limited to:

1. Poorly defined pain
2. A vague feeling of instability with certain actions

SIGNS: There is a full range of movement without pain when the arm is moved both actively and passively. Tenderness may be found at the

1. insertion of the inferior glenohumeral ligament anteriorly
2. origin of the ligament posteriorly (Figure 12.27)

The most important test is the *apprehension sign* (see Figures 12.10 and 12.11). This tests for laxity of the anterior capsule, the inferior glenohumeral ligament, or both. A positive apprehension sign, together with tenderness anteriorly, posteriorly, or both, is highly suggestive of a shoulder subluxation.[22,23,24]

X-RAYS: The routine radiographs of the shoulder (anteroposterior, internal and external rotation views) are usually normal in the subluxing shoulder. The technique that demonstrates the lesions associated with a shoulder subluxation is the West Point view —a modified axillary view.[25] This shows up the antero-inferior lip of the glenoid, the area commonly traumatized, which may show:

1. A chip fracture off the antero-inferior rim of the glenoid. This is a most significant X-ray finding (Figure 12.28).

2. Calcification within the anterior capsule.

3. Hill-Sach's lesion. This is a defect of the humeral head caused by compression of the head against the glenoid as the humerus subluxes (the Hill-Sach's defect can also be occasionally seen by taking an anteroposterior view with the arm in internal rotation).[26]

TREATMENT:

Conservative: Conservative treatment in the form of vigorous, controlled rehabilitation should be attempted before surgery is suggested (see shoulder rehabilitation,

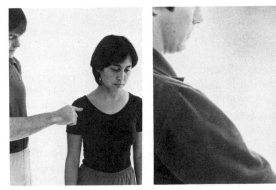

FIGURE 12.27 Recurrent anterior subluxation of the shoulder Areas where tenderness is frequently elicited anteriorly and posteriorly

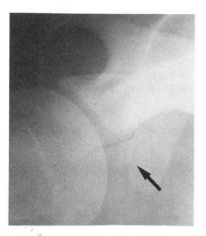

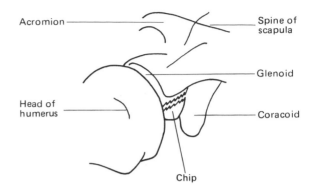

FIGURE 12.28 **West Point view of the shoulder** This view demonstrates a large chip off the glenoid, strongly suggesting that an anterior subluxation has occurred.

p. 192). If the athlete desires to continue activity in spite of the disability, a self-adjusting elastic support (e.g., the West Point harness, Figure 4.6) can be used.[27] This allows a fairly wide range of movement but prevents full external rotation and abduction.

Surgical: The surgical repair is similar to that used in the anterior dislocation. With improvement in the quality of rehabilitation programs, surgical treatment may need to be performed less frequently than previously.

Posterior Dislocation of the Glenohumeral Joint

A posterior dislocation is a rare lesion in the athlete, accounting for less than 2% of shoulder dislocations. However, the diagnosis of a posterior dislocation is often missed on the initial examination. When examining an injured shoulder, always consider the possibility of a posterior dislocation.

MECHANISM OF INJURY: The force drives the humeral head backward while the arm is in flexion (usually below 90°) and internal rotation. The head slips out posteriorly and comes to rest under the acromion process.

SYMPTOMS: Symptoms consist of generalized shoulder pain and inability to externally rotate or abduct the arm. In contrast to the

anterior dislocation, the athlete with a posterior dislocation might not realize that his or her shoulder is actually dislocated.

SIGNS:

1. The arm is held across the front of the chest.
2. There is flattening of the anterior shoulder when viewed from the side.
3. There is a bulge posteriorly when viewed from above.
4. The coracoid process is prominent.
5. The athlete cannot externally rotate or abduct the arm.
6. The athlete finds that, as the arm is held in internal rotation, on elevating it he or she cannot supinate the hand.

X-RAYS:

1. Anteroposterior views may look normal.
2. Axillary and tangential views will reveal the diagnosis.
3. If a fracture of the lesser tuberosity is present, a diagnosis of a posterior dislocation should be considered until disproven.

COMPLICATIONS:

1. Fracture of the lesser tuberosity of the humerus
2. Comminuted intra-articular fracture of the proximal humerus

REDUCTION:

1. Longitudinal forward traction with the elbow bent
2. Downward pressure on the humeral head
3. Adduction of the arm, then external rotation, followed by internal rotation[28]

IMMOBILIZATION: Immobilization is from four to six weeks in slight abduction and external rotation.

Recurrent Posterior Dislocation and Subluxation

This is an unusual condition which may not occur as infrequently as was previously thought. It is more commonly seen in those with loose ligaments, and on occasion may be combined with anterior instability (the so-called "global instability").[29] If recurrent subluxation occurs posteriorly, the posterior glenoid lip may indent the humeral head.

TREATMENT: Initially, treatment is by attempted rehabilitation of the posterior shoulder musculature. Surgery is occasionally necessary.[30]

Voluntary or Habitual Dislocators

There are some individuals who are able to voluntarily dislocate their shoulders either anteriorly or posteriorly. Others find that their shoulders slip out of joint with very little provocation and without an initial injury. These conditions may be due to

1. congenital malformations of the glenoid fossa, the labrum, or the humeral head
2. excessive laxity of the structures around the glenohumeral joint

3. ability of the individual to dissociate some of the muscles of the rotator cuff from the others, so that voluntary contraction of part of the rotator cuff moves the humeral head into a subluxed or dislocated position, while the counteracting forces of the other muscles of the rotator cuff are not called into play.

Voluntary subluxation or dislocation in either direction (i.e., anteriorly or posteriorly) is a difficult condition to treat. It may be associated with psychiatric problems in some cases.

Impingement of the Rotator Cuff

Rotator cuff impingement is an important and common lesion in the athlete. The lesion consists of the rotator cuff tendons (especially the supraspinatus tendon) and the tendon of the long head of the biceps being squeezed against the anterior edge of the acromion and the coraco-acromial ligament.

ANATOMY: Transversing the gap between the coracoid and the acromial processes is the coraco-acromial ligament, which forms an arch over the humeral head. Beneath this arch runs the supraspinatus tendon and the intra-articular portion of the tendon of the long head of the biceps. Between the acromion process and the supraspinatus tendon lies the subacromial bursa. When the arm is abducted, elevated, or externally rotated, the supraspinatus tendon falls under the coraco-acromial arch and may in certain instances be impinged against it (Figure 12.29).

ETIOLOGY:

1. *Chronic microtrauma.* Repetitive use of the arm and shoulder (such as in baseball pitching, freestyle and butterfly swimming, or playing tennis) can result in microscopic damage to the tissues under the coraco-acromial arch.[31] This leads to edema and hemorrhage with compromise in the space available. A vicious circle of impingement-

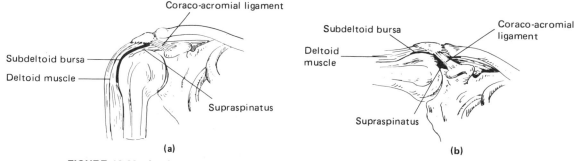

FIGURE 12.29 Impingement of the rotator cuff (a) With the arm at the side there is no impingement under the coraco-acromial arch. (b) With the arm in abduction, the space beneath the coraco-acromial arch is reduced.

swelling-muscle dysfunction-further impingement may perpetuate the problem. The supraspinatus tendon is usually the first structure involved.

2. *Vascular impairment.* In sports such as swimming, particularly in the butterfly, where the swimmer is required to rotate the arm on the shoulder many hundreds, if not thousands, of times a day, there may be interference with the blood supply to the supraspinatus tendon. This can result in a localized area of necrosis of the supraspinatus tendon, which in turn can lead to edema and an inflammatory reaction.[32]

3. *Partial tear of the rotator cuff*, particularly the supraspinatus tendon. This has the same results as vascular impairment.

4. *Previous trauma.* Previous trauma to the acromion process or acromioclavicular joint (e.g., a previous acromioclavicular separation) can cause distortion of the acromion process and reduce the space available under the arch.

SYMPTOMS:

1. The principal symptom is pain, which is often elicited by activities such as bringing the arm through the acceleration phase of the throwing motion, when the arm is whipped rapidly from external to internal rotation, as when hitting an overhead smash or serve in tennis, or in butterfly swimming. The pain is usually localized to the superolateral aspect of the shoulder, in the area just lateral or anterior to the acromion process. However, the pain may be more diffuse, particularly if there is involvement of the tendon of the long head of the biceps or if there is a more generalized inflammatory response to microtrauma.

2. A snapping feeling or sensation may occur when the arm is brought from an external to an internally rotated position or when the arm is abducted between 70° and 120°.

SIGNS:

1. Tenderness is usually vague *except* when the arm is passively abducted to 45° and pressure is exerted under the acromion process. When this is done, localized tenderness is often found. Pain may also be elicited when the arm is passively extended and the supraspinatus tendon palpated anteriorly.[33]

2. Pain is experienced when the arm is actively abducted between 70° and 120°.

3. The impingement sign may be present (see examination of the shoulder, p. 167).

4. There may or may not be atrophy of the muscles around the shoulder.

5. Evidence of biceps tendinitis may also be present.

FURTHER INVESTIGATIONS:

1. Injection of a local anesthetic under the coraco-acromial arch abolishes the impingement sign if the pain is due to rotator cuff impingement.

2. X-rays of the shoulder are usually normal.

3. A subacromial bursogram.[34]

4. An arthrogram should be performed to exclude a complete tear of the rotator cuff.

TREATMENT OF STAGE I: (See "phases" in section on microtrauma, p. 128)

Conservative:

1. Decreased activity (limitation of external rotation and abduction) or total rest of the involved shoulder.

2. Ice therapy, including ice massage.

3. Gentle stretching exercises (see "stretching" in shoulder rehabilitation section, p. 198).

4. Anti-inflammatory medications, if indicated.

5. Consultation with the coach about altering the technique of the athlete's arm motion.

6. Other conservative forms of treatment such as ultrasound and TENS.

7. Vigorous and complete rehabilitation of all the muscles around the shoulder once the signs of inflammation have settled down. This should especially include using the isokinetic apparatus for the anterior and the posterior deltoids and the external rotators. Appropriate elastic-tubing exercises should also be performed (see shoulder rehabilitation, p. 197). Cortisone injections are not generally advised, but may be used on occasion.

Surgical: If the athlete does not improve with conservative treatment, a suitable period of inactivity, and an intense rehabilitation program, division of the coraco-acromial ligament may be indicated.[31]

TREATMENT OF STAGES II AND III: Conservative therapy and intensive rehabilitation should be attempted before considering surgical release of the coraco-acromial ligament.

Tear of the Rotator Cuff

A tear of the rotator cuff may be partial or complete. The partial tear may have very similar clinical features to the impingement syndrome and, as mentioned, may indeed be a cause of that syndrome. Complete tears are rare under 30 years of age, but do occur.

A rotator cuff tear results from an acute shoulder injury. It most frequently involves the supraspinatus tendon, but it may also include the infraspinatus and the tendon of the long head of the biceps.

SIGNS: The signs may be very similar to the impingement syndrome.

1. Tenderness may be present at the insertion of the supraspinatus tendon into the greater tuberosity of the humerus. More commonly, localized tenderness is found under the coraco-acromial arch when the arm is passively abducted at 45° and pressure is applied under the arch, or if the arm is extended and pressure applied anteriorly over the supraspinatus insertion. On occasion, tenderness is also present over the biceps long head or around the acromioclavicular joint.

2. Pain is experienced on abducting the arm between 70° and 120° (this may be one of the causes of the painful arc syndrome).

3. Supraspinatus crepitus may be felt as the arm is actively abducted.

4. Impingement signs may or may not be present (Figure 12.12). Their absence may be used to differentiate this from the impingement syndrome.

5. Wasting or poor contraction of the supraspinatus may be observed when the athlete is viewed from above and from behind.

6. An athlete who has a complete tear may not be able to abduct the arm against even minimal resistance.

Note: It is possible for a muscular athlete to have a partial tear of the rotator cuff and yet be able to actively initiate abduction even against resistance without too much pain or difficulty. In addition, no muscle weakness may be elicited unless specific muscle tests are performed and the shoulder muscles are fatigued by repetitive testing.

FURTHER INVESTIGATIONS:

1. If the impingement sign is present, it may be relieved by a local anesthetic injected under the coraco-acromial arch.

2. X-rays of the shoulder are usually normal.

3. An arthrogram may be useful in making the diagnosis.

TREATMENT:

Conservative: The initial treatment can be conservative if the exact severity of a partial tear is in question.

1. Place the affected arm in a sling.

2. Use ice therapy and anti-inflammatory medication.

3. Limit external rotation and abduction for a period of time, depending upon the severity of the condition.

This should be followed by

1. rehabilitation exercises

2. gentle stretching

3. cortisone injections—These are not advised, but are used on occasion.

Surgical: If the arthrogram shows leakage of dye, surgical repair is indicated.[35] If the arthrogram is negative and the symptoms do not clear up within a reasonable period of time (this period of time will vary from athlete to athlete and from sport to sport), surgical exploration should be performed with the idea of releasing the impingement and repairing any tear.

Subluxation of the Tendon of the Long Head of the Biceps

Subluxation of the tendon of the long head of the biceps is another cause of shoulder pain, although a relatively infrequent one.

ANATOMY: The tendon of the long head of the biceps enters the bicipital groove below the humeral head and becomes intra-articular before attaching to the glenoid. The bicipital groove is formed by the lesser tuberosity medially and the greater tuberosity laterally. The roof is formed by the transverse humeral ligament. The tendon does not actually slide in the groove; rather, the groove slides over the tendon. This occurs particularly when the arm is moved from internal to external rotation and back again from external to internal rotation.

PATHOLOGY: There are usually a number of factors which together allow the biceps tendon to sublux. There may be an initial forceful injury (usually with the arm resisting abduction and external rotation), which may cause the transverse humeral ligament to become stretched, permitting subluxation of the tendon. Repetitive movement, such as throwing, may further aggravate the ligament laxity.

The shape of the groove is considered by some to predispose to the development of the condition in a particular athlete.[37] If the medial aspect of the groove (the lesser tuberosity) is flat, the groove will be shallow and the tendon may easily sublux toward the medial side.

In its course over the humeral head, the biceps tendon is angulated approximately 30° medially, so that tightening of the biceps, together with external rotation of the arm, tends to cause the tendon to bowstring toward the medial side. Most subluxations are thought to occur in the medial direction, but some cases of lateral subluxation have been noted.

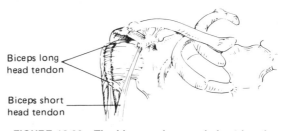

Biceps long head tendon

Biceps short head tendon

FIGURE 12.30 The biceps—long and short heads

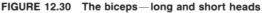

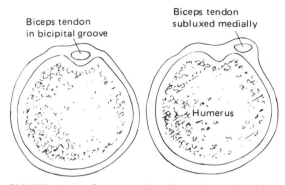

Biceps tendon in bicipital groove

Biceps tendon subluxed medially

Humerus

FIGURE 12.31 Cross-section through proximal humerus

SYMPTOMS: Most symptoms are associated with pain and a snapping sensation, particularly when the arm is rapidly moved from internal to external rotation. This pain is followed by a dull ache, which persists for the next few hours or days. Crepitus may be noted on moving the arm.

SIGNS: Tenderness is located over the bicipital groove. This area of tenderness will be observed to move laterally as the arm is externally rotated. Other areas around the anterosuperior aspect of the shoulder may also be tender, due to inflammation spreading out to include the rotator cuff and the proximal portion of the biceps muscle.

There are various clinical tests which may induce subluxation and may help with the diagnosis. Some of these are designed to bowstring the biceps tendon over the medial wall of the bicipital groove.

1. Yergason's test—The affected arm is held with the elbow at 90° and against the chest wall. Against resistance, the shoulder is externally rotated, the elbow flexed, and the forearm supinated, while downward traction is applied to the elbow.[36] The examiner palpates the tendon in the bicipital groove in order to detect subluxation of the tendon. Pain is produced by either subluxation or biceps tendinitis.

2. With the elbow at the side, and flexed to 90°, supinating from a pronated position

against resistance may cause pain over the biceps tendon. This may also be due to biceps tendinitis.

3. Gilcrest's sign—The athlete raises the weight of a light dumbbell with elbow extended to above the head, then lowers the arm to a position of 90° of abduction while supinating the forearm and externally rotating the shoulder.[2] This may elicit subluxation of the tendon from the bicipital groove and cause discomfort.

4. With the shoulder at 90° of abduction and the elbow extended, the forearm is pronated and supinated against resistance. The tendon may be felt to snap out of the groove.

5. The affected arm is passively abducted and externally rotated. The arm is turned into internal rotation and then back to external rotation while the bicipital groove is palpated for instability of the tendon.

TREATMENT:

Conservative: Conservative treatment should initially be tried in order to decrease inflammation and allow the tissues to heal in a functional position. If significant functional incapacity, swelling and tenderness are present, the arm should be splinted for a week or two in order to allow healing to occur. Ice should be applied, and anti-inflammatory medication used as indicated. A progressive rehabilitation program should then be prescribed.

Surgical: In the chronic case where conservative therapy has been tried but throwing has become nearly impossible, surgical intervention should be considered.[37] The operation consists of removal of the long head from the glenoid and suturing of the tendon into the bicipital groove. Good results from this procedure have been reported.

DIFFERENTIAL DIAGNOSES:

Biceps tenosynovitis. This often occurs in conjunction with a subluxing long-head tendon and is the result of the subluxation.

When it occurs by itself, there is no history of snapping, nor will the biceps rotation tests be positive for a subluxation (though they may be painful). Crepitus may be felt.

Biceps tendinitis.   Biceps tendinitis can occur if the groove is narrow. There is often an area of degeneration within the tendon which can lead to complete rupture of the tendon. Signs may be similar to those of biceps long-head subluxation and tenosynovitis.

Tear of the rotator cuff with extension into the biceps tendon.   A tear may result in tenderness over the bicipital groove and in pain on attempting some of the tests mentioned earlier.

Coraco-acromial arch impingement syndrome. The biceps tendon may bear the brunt of the impingement, so that most of the tenderness is present over the bicipital groove, and a snap may be felt when the arm is externally rotated or brought from an externally rotated to an internally rotated position. This snap is due to the impingement of the biceps tendon under the coraco-acromial arch. Impingement signs should be positive.

Subluxation of the glenohumeral joint.   This may produce a history similar to subluxation of the long head of the biceps, because the athlete is unable to describe exactly what anatomical structure is subluxing. The apprehension sign should be positive in a subluxing shoulder, and the tenderness should be over the bicipital groove. With external rotation, the area of tenderness should not move to the lateral side as it does with a biceps tendon problem. Subluxation of the glenohumeral joint is by far the more common condition.

Thoracic Outlet Syndrome

The name *thoracic outlet syndrome* implies compression of the neurovascular components that travel from the neck through the thoracic outlet area and supply the upper extremity.

ETIOLOGY: Many etiologies have been associated with this syndrome. The commonest include:

1. Compression of the neurovascular bundle between the anterior and middle scalene muscles.

2. Compression between the first rib and the clavicle (costoclavicular syndrome).

3. Abnormalities of the first rib.

4. Compression under the pectoralis minor muscle.

5. Compression under a cervical rib.

6. Poor posture with sagging shoulders. However, it is rare to find a thoracic outlet syndrome in tennis players and pitchers, many of whom have a dominant shoulder that sags but also have excellent muscle tone.

7. Other etiologies such as fascial fusion of muscles.

8. A combination of two or more of the above.

PATHOMECHANICS: There is compression of the neurovascular bundle, affecting particularly the inferior portion of the brachial plexus, most commonly in the distribution of the ulnar nerve, and occasionally, the median nerve.

SYMPTOMS: The symptoms may include burning and numbness of the shoulder, the inner side of the arm, the forearm, and the hand. This usually follows a pattern corresponding to a dermatome. However, on occasion pain may be localized to the shoulder, elbow, or forearm region alone.[38]

SIGNS: There may be some decrease in sensation as well as atrophy and weakness of the muscles supplied by the involved nerves. A number of tests aimed at decreasing the pulse and reproducing the symptoms are used.

1. *Adson's maneuver*—Tests for compression of the neurovascular bundle between the anterior and middle scalene muscles. The arm

is held at the side and slightly abducted and extended. The athlete looks to the side being tested, slightly extends the neck, and takes a deep breath and holds it for ten seconds. There is some downward traction of the arm while the pulse is being observed.

2. *Hyperflexion-abduction test*—The arm is held in full flexion and abduction, and the neck is somewhat extended. The arm is supinated. Obliteration of the pulse and reproduction of pain suggest tightness of the pectoralis minor muscle.

3. *Test for the costoclavicular syndrome*—Done with the athlete sitting with shoulders pulled backward and downward. The arm is in 30° of abduction and extended.

INVESTIGATIONS: Tests include (a) an X-ray of the neck to detect the presence of a cervical rib, (b) nerve conduction studies, and, in particular, (c) a Doppler blood-flow sensor with the head and the arms in different positions.

TREATMENT: Most cases respond to a program of exercise therapy designed to relieve tension on the structures involved.[38,39,40] This program should be individualized according to the etiology. Following are some exercises that may be generally useful:

1. Athlete supine, hands behind head, elbows in front of face. As the athlete inhales, elbows are drawn slowly apart and lateral to the head. As the athlete exhales, elbows are brought back together. This can be performed against manual resistance.

2. Serratus anterior exercise—Shoulder protraction using dumbbells, barbells, or the Universal Gym.

3. Mid-trapezius exercise—Athlete prone, arm abducted 90° at the shoulders, elbows bent 90° over the edge of a table. Athlete holds a dumbbell in each hand and lifts the weights and the elbows straight upward, keeping the elbows bent so the scapulae approximate each other.

4. Erector spinae strengthening—Athlete prone, back extended, and shoulders pulled backward.

5. Lower trapezius exercise—Athlete prone, forearm and elbow lifted upward to hyperflexed position of the shoulder.

6. Pectoralis stretching—Athlete standing in a corner, leaning forward with feet firmly planted, stabilizing body with elbows against the wall and bringing chest forward toward the corner.

7. Upper trapezius exercises or shoulder elevation—This can be done using a barbell for resistance.

8. In addition, passive or active stretching of the pectoralis minor and the scalene muscles, as well as cross-frictional massage, may be useful.

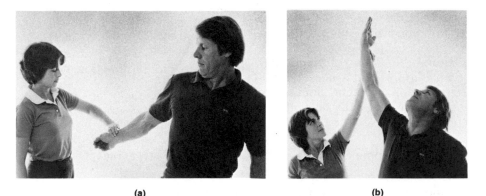

(a) (b)

FIGURE 12.32 (a) **Adson's maneuver** (b) **Hyperflexion-abduction test with the neck in extension**

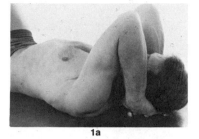

1a

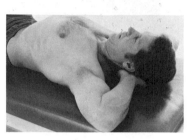

1b

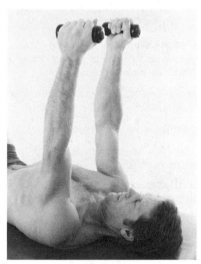

2

3

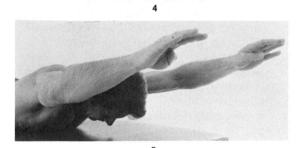

4

5

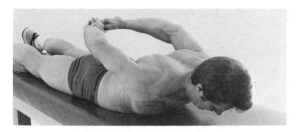

6

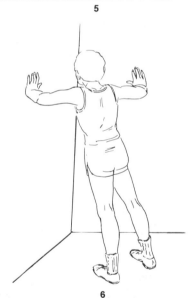

7

8

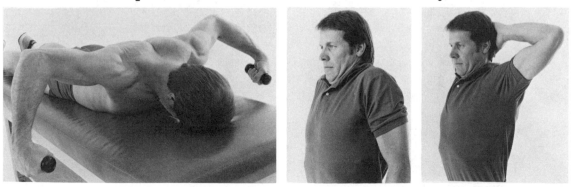

FIGURE 12.33

SHOULDER REHABILITATION

The shoulder has a far wider range of movement than any other joint, which means that a rehabilitation program can be quite complicated. For this reason, rehabilitation programs for a number of different shoulder conditions are described here.

The one generalization that can be made is that, if the shoulder is immobilized, it is much more likely to become stiff and lose motion than most other joints. It is therefore necessary to ensure that an adequate range of motion is achieved and maintained early in the program, while at the same time strengthening all the muscles around the shoulder joint.

General Outline of Exercises

1. *Isometric exercises.* Using the opposite hand as resistance, the athlete performs isometrics at different angles throughout the range of motion.

1. *Elbow*—Flexion, extension; supination, pronation.

2. *Shoulder*—Internal rotation, external rotation; abduction, adduction; flexion, depression (Figure 12.34).

3. *Squeezing ball*—Starting in the position of abduction-external rotation, the athlete squeezes the ball and holds. Then he or she moves in the direction of internal rotation-adduction and repeats the contraction at different points along this path of motion (Figure 12.35).

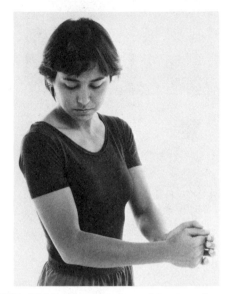

FIGURE 12.34 Shoulder isometric exercises The affected arm (right) contracts against the resistance of the left. No actual motion occurs.

4. *Scapular retraction*—Shoulder blades are pulled together.

2. *Range-of-motion exercises.*

1. Hand behind the back; hand behind the neck; hand on opposite shoulder.

2. Wand exercises—Standing or lying supine, the athlete brings arms over and behind the head (Figure 12.36).

3. Fingers climbing up the wall (Figure 12.37).

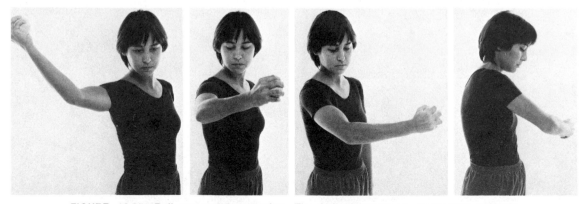

FIGURE 12.35 Ball squeezing exercise The ball is squeezed, contracting muscles throughout the arm and the shoulder. Four different isometric positions are used.

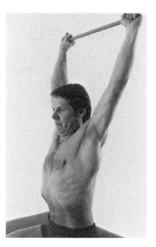

FIGURE 12.36   Range-of-motion exercise—using wand

3. *Codman's exercises.*

1. Pendulum—clockwise and counterclockwise (Figure 12.38).
2. Horizontal adduction and abduction
3. Horizontal flexion and depression
4. Protraction from horizontal position (punching) (Figure 12.39)

4. *Kerlan's shoulder exercises.*[41]

1. Codman's pendulum—clockwise and counterclockwise

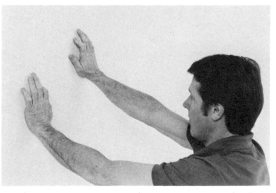

FIGURE 12.37   Finger-climbing-up-wall to increase the shoulder range of motion

2. Forward punch, pull back (Figure 12.40)
3. Shoulder shrugs

5. *Elastic tubing exercises.*

1. Horizontal motion—flexion, extension; abduction, adduction; internal rotation, external rotation (Figure 12.41)

2. Standing on tubing—curls, reverse curls, rowing, triceps, military press, abduction

3. Standing, arm at side—internal rotation, external rotation

4. Variations as needed

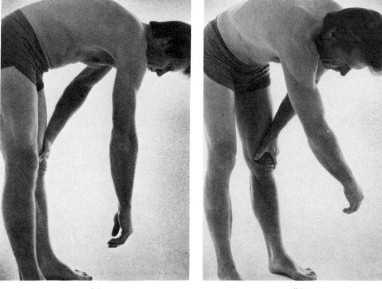

FIGURE 12.38 Codman's pendulum exercise (a) The arm should be allowed to relax and hang freely. The motion, small circles that slowly increase in size, should be gravity-assisted. (b) Abduction and adduction motions should also be performed.

(a)   (b)

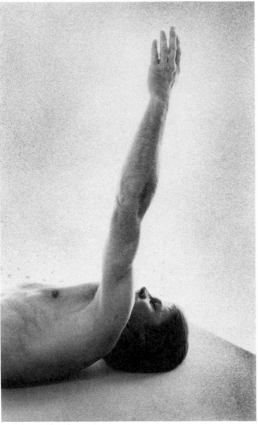

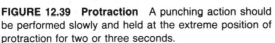

FIGURE 12.39 Protraction A punching action should be performed slowly and held at the extreme position of protraction for two or three seconds.

6. *Wall pulley exercises (e.g., MiniGym or wall weights).*

1. Internal rotation, external rotation

2. Flexion, depression in horizontal position

3. Abduction, adduction

7. *Free weight exercises—dumbbells.*

1. Elbow—curls, rowing

2. Shoulder—internal rotation

    a. Flies—standing

        1. Bending forward with arm vertical (Figure 12.42)

        2. Prone on abdomen

        3. Lying supine

        4. Sitting at 45° angle

    b. Shoulder shrugs

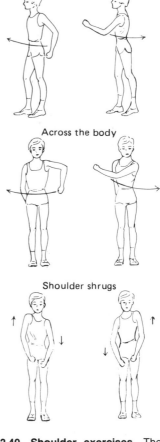

FIGURE 12.40 Shoulder exercises These may be performed free-standing, or by using resistance such as elastic tubing. (From R.K. Kerlan, F.W. Jobe, M.E. Blazina et al., "Throwing injuries of the shoulder and elbow in adults," *Current Practice in Orthopaedic Surgery* 6:41–58, 1975.)

8. *Isotonic exercises (e.g., with Universal Gym or various Nautilus shoulder machines).* Bench press, military press, lateral pulls, shoulder shrugs, curls, reverse curls, rowing, horizontal adduction and abduction.

9. *Isokinetic exercises (with the Cybex).* Flexion, depression, abduction and adduction, internal and external rotation, curls, triceps extension, horizontal adduction and abduction, and variations of these (Figure 12.43).

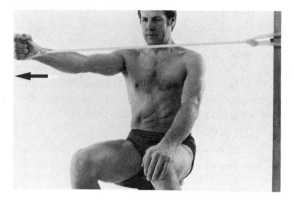
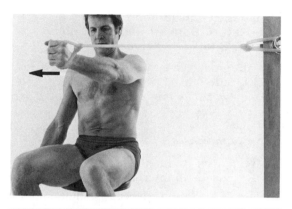
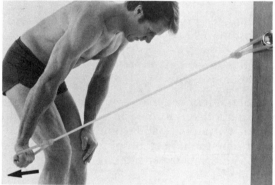

FIGURE 12.41 Elasticized tubing exercises A few examples of the many possible exercises are shown above and at right.

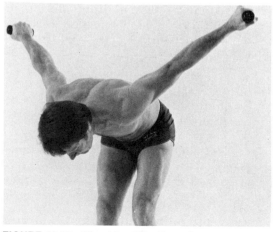

FIGURE 12.42 Shoulder "flies"—using dumbbells

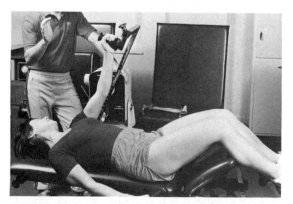

FIGURE 12.43 Isokinetic exercise (Cybex) Limited-range flexion/extension is demonstrated. The trainer/therapist controls the range of motion manually.

Shoulder Rehabilitation Following a Putti-Platt or Bankart Repair for an Anterior Shoulder Dislocation

This program can also be used in a modified, speeded-up form in cases of *anterior shoulder subluxation* or a *conservatively treated anterior dislocation.*

1. *One to three weeks postoperative.*

1. Keep arm in a sling and swath held against the side in internal rotation.

2. Use TENS and muscle stimulation as necessary.

3. Initiate isometrics—elbow flexion and extension, pronation and supination.

2. *Three to four weeks postoperative.* Continue the above, plus

1. Shoulder isometrics—internal and external rotation (performed in a position of full internal rotation), abduction and adduction (performed in a position of full internal rotation with arm against side), retraction (shoulders pulled back)

2. Codman's pendulum—small circles, clockwise and counterclockwise

3. Squeezing tennis ball (or similar), elbow at 90°, isometrics with shoulder internally rotated 45°, 60°, and 90°

4. Light dumbbells—curl, reverse curl; supination, pronation; wrist extension, side-to-side

5. Electrical muscle stimulation

3. *Four to five weeks postoperative.* Arm should be kept in a sling between workout sessions.

1. Wider range of active motion—hand behind neck; hand behind back.

2. Codman's pendulum—with light weights and increasingly larger circles; lying supine, flexion, depression, horizontal abduction and adduction, punch (scapular protraction). Athlete should not force, but move gently.

3. Isometrics—elbow at 90° and at side, abduction, external rotation.

4. Squeezing tennis ball—exercise starts in position of slight abduction and external rotation and moves across body toward adduction and internal rotation. Progressively change the starting position so that it is in slightly more abduction each time. When full abduction is reached, start to increase the amount of rotation (see Figure 12.35).

5. Wall pulley:
   a. Horizontal adduction
   b. Internal rotation with arm at side, then 90° abduction
   c. Limited flexion and depression

4. *Five to six weeks postoperative.*

1. Range of motion—Continue with above, plus:
   a. Wand—athlete lying supine, brings wand over head
   b. Fingers climbing up the wall
   c. Reaching for ceiling

2. Isometrics—add flexion at 80° to 90°, depression at 80° to 90°, abduction at 80° to 90°

3. Isokinetics—through limited-arc of motion at speeds of 180° per second and greater, emphasizing internal rotation

5. *Six to nine weeks postoperative.*

1. Free dumbbells:
   a. Curls, triceps, rowing
   b. Lying supine—flies
   c. Standing—flies to front (flexion to 90°) flies to side (abduction to 90°)
   d. Shoulder shrugs

2. Wall pulley:
   a. Internal rotation, elbow at side
   b. External rotation, elbow at side (limited)
   c. Internal rotation, elbow at 90°
   d. Horizontal flexion and depression
   e. Horizontal abduction and adduction

3. Isokinetic exercises—more extensive range of motion, multiple positions

4. Isotonic exercises (Universal Gym):
   a. Bench press—Athlete starts with arm in full extension and does shoulder

protraction, gradually building up weight to a maximum before lowering to a starting position of greater elbow flexion. Lock the machine so elbow flexion is limited to desired height (Figure 12.44).

    b. "Lat pulls"
    c. Rowing curls
    d. Military press
    e. Shoulder shrugs (with bench-press apparatus)

6. *Nine-weeks-plus postoperative*

1. Isokinetics—multiple positions

2. Isotonic exercises (with Universal Gym)—increased weights and decreased reps. Also use various Nautilus shoulder machines, if available, when full range of motion and at least 70% of strength are present.

3. Elastic tubing—entire range of tubing exercises can be performed, adapting to individual muscle needs, but emphasizing internal rotators.

Rehabilitation Exercises for an Acromioclavicular Separation[42]

1. Full range of isometrics—flexion and extension, abduction and adduction, internal and external rotation, elbow flexion and extension, supination and pronation.

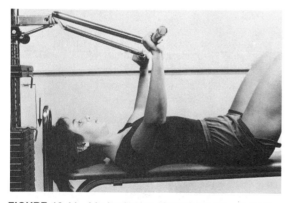

FIGURE 12.44 Limited-range bench press Note the pin which controls the range of descent of the weight stack. The position of the pin can be altered as a greater range of motion against resistance is allowed.

2. General exercises:
    a. Codman's pendulum—clockwise and counterclockwise.
    b. Tennis ball squeezing—through range of motion from abduction-external rotation to adduction-internal rotation.
    c. Weights and dumbbells—elbow flexion and extension, supination and pronation; wrist flexion and extension; flies lying prone, lying supine; bench press; punch.
    d. Wall pulley—flexion and extension, abduction and adduction, internal and external rotation.

3. Elastic tubing—to exercise specific muscle weaknesses.

4. Shoulder shrugs.

5. General shoulder exercises:
    a. Isotonic exercises on Universal Gym or Nautilus
    b. Isokinetic exercises with Cybex or Orthotron

6. Throwing, punching bag.

Rehabilitation Exercises for Overuse and Impingement Syndromes

1. General exercises with weights, pulleys, or elastic tubing
    a. Codman's pendulum
    b. Sawing action
    c. Shoulder shrugs

2. Test for specific muscle weaknesses.

3. Isokinetic exercises (with Cybex or Orthotron), especially high-speed from 180° to 300° per second. Various positions, depending on specific muscle weaknesses. No pain should be felt when doing these exercises; if slight pain is elicited, the use of TENS and muscle stimulation should be considered.

4. General shoulder improvement with isotonics (with Universal Gym or Nautilus) or free weights—as long as these do not cause pain.

5. Stretching:
    a. General
    b. Specific

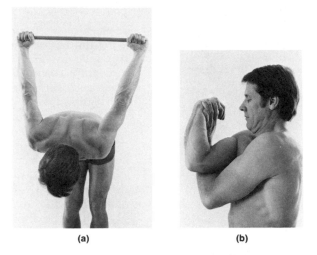

(a)   (b)

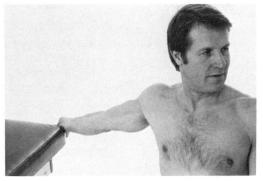

(c)

FIGURE 12.45 Some shoulder stretching exercises
(a) The wand stretch   (b) A stretch for the external rotators
(c) Stretching the anterior deltoid and other anterior shoulder structures

REFERENCES

1. Turkel SP, Panio MW, Marshall JL, et al: Stabilizing mechanisms preventing anterior dislocation of the glenohumeral joint. *J Bone Joint Surg* 63A:1208–1217, 1981.

2. Davies GJ, Gould JA, Larson RL: Functional examination of the shoulder girdle. *Phys Sportsmed* 9:82–102, June 1981.

3. Neer CS, Welsh RP: The shoulder in sport. *Orthop Clin North Am* 8:583–591, 1977.

4. Hawkins RJ, Kennedy JC: Impingement syndrome in athletics. *Am J Sports Med* 8:151–158, 1980.

5. Gregg JR, Labosky D, Harty M, et al: Serratus anterior paralysis in the young athlete. *J Bone Joint Surg* 61A:825–832, 1979.

6. Kendall HO, Kendall FP, Wadsworth GE: *Muscles, Testing and Function.* Baltimore, Williams and Wilkins, second edition, 1971.

7. Norfray JF, Tremaine MJ, Groves HC, et al: The clavicle in hockey. *Am J Sports Med* 5:275–280, 1977.

8. Allman FL: Fractures and ligamentous injuries of the clavicle and its articulation. *J Bone Joint Surg* 49A:774–784, 1967.

9. Alexander OM: Radiography of the acromioclavicular articulation. *Med Radiogr Photogr* 30:34–39, 1954.

10. Waldrop JI, Norwood LA, Alvarez RG: Lateral roentgenographic projections of the acromioclavicular joint. *Am J Sports Med* 9:337–341, 1981.

11. Glick JM, Milburn LJ, Haggerty JF, et al: Dislocated acromioclavicular joint. Follow-up study of 35 unreduced acromioclavicular dislocations. *Am J Sports Med* 5:264–270, 1977.

12. Bergfeld JA, Andrish JT, Clancy WG: Evaluation of the acromioclavicular joint following first- and second-degree sprains. *Am J Sports Med* 6:153–159, 1978.

13. Cox JS: The fate of the acromioclavicular joint in athletic injuries. *Am J Sports Med* 9:50–53, 1981.

14. Park JP, Arnold JA, Coker TP, et al: Treatment of acromioclavicular separations. A retrospective study. *Am J Sports Med* 8:251–256, 1980.

15. De Palma AF, Flannery GF: Acute anterior dislocation of the shoulder. *J Sports Med* 1:6–15, 1973.

16. Bateman JE: Cuff tears in athletes. *Orthop Clin North Am* 4:721–745, 1973.

17. Rowe CR: Prognosis in dislocations of the shoulder. *J Bone Joint Surg* 38A:957–977, 1956.

18. Rockwood Jr, CA: Dislocations about the shoulder. In *Fractures,* edited by Rockwood Jr, CA, Green DP. Philadelphia, Lippincott, 1975, p 656.

19. Rowe CR, Patel D, Southmayd WW: The Bankart procedure: A long term end result study. *J Bone Joint Surg* 60A:1–16, 1978.

20. Lombardo SJ, Kerlan RK, Jobe FW, et al: The modified Bristow procedure for recurrent dislocation of the shoulder. *J Bone Joint Surg* 58A:256–261, 1976.

21. Hill JA, Lombardo SJ, Kerlan RK: The modified Bristow-Helfet procedure for recurrent anterior shoulder subluxations and dislocations. *Am J Sports Med* 9:283–287, 1981.

22. Rowe CR, Zarins B: Recurrent transient subluxation of the shoulder. *J Bone Joint Surg* 63A:863–872, 1981.

23. Blazina ME, Satzman JS: Recurrent anterior subluxation of the shoulder in athletics—A distinct entity. In Proceedings of the American Academy of Orthopaedic Surgeons. *J Bone Joint Surg* 51A:1037–1038, 1969.

24. Hastings DE, Coughlin LP: Recurrent subluxation of the glenohumeral joint. *Am J Sports Med* 9:352–355, 1981.

25. Rokous JR, Feagin JA, Abbott HG: Modified axillary roentgenogram. *Clin Orthop* 82:84–86, 1972.

26. Hill HA, Sachs MD: The grooved defect of the humeral head. A frequently recognized complication of dislocations of the shoulder. *Radiology* 35:690, 1940.

27. Feagin JA: Elastic arm-torso harness. *J Sports Med* 2:99–101, 1974.

28. Connolly JF, editor: De Palma's *The Management of Fractures and Dislocations.* Philadelphia, WB Saunders, Vol I, third edition, 1981, p 634.

29. Neer CS, Foster CR: Inferior capsular shift for involuntary inferior and multidirectional instability of the shoulder. A preliminary report. *J Bone Joint Surg* 62A:897–908, 1980.

30. Tibone JE, Prietto C, Jobe FW, et al: Staple capsulorrhaphy for recurrent posterior shoulder dislocation. *Am J Sports Med* 9:135–139, 1981.

31. Jackson DW: Chronic rotator cuff impingement in the throwing athlete. *Am J Sports Med* 4:231–240, 1976.

32. Rathbun JB, Macnab I: The microvascular pattern of the rotator cuff. *J Bone Joint Surg* 52B:540–553, 1970.

33. Hoppenfeld S: *Physical Examination of the Spine and Extremities.* New York, Appleton-Century-Crofts, 1976, p 12.

34. Strizak AM, Danzig L, Jackson DW, et al: Subacromial bursography. An anatomical and clinical study. *J Bone Joint Surg* 64A:196–201, 1982.

35. Nixon JE, DiStefano V: Rupture of the rotator cuff. *Orthop Clin North Am* 6:423–447, 1975.

36. Hoppenfeld S: *Physical Examination of the Spine and Extremities.* New York, Appleton-Century-Crofts, 1976, p 32.

37. O'Donoghue DH: Subluxing biceps tendon in the athlete. *J Sports Med* 1:20–29, 1973.

38. Strukel RJ, Garrick JG: Thoracic outlet compression in athletes. A report of four cases. *Am J Sports Med* 6:35–39, 1978.

39. Britt LP: Nonoperative treatment of the thoracic outlet syndrome symptoms. *Clin Orthop Rel Res* 51:45–48, 1967.

40. Smith KF: The thoracic outlet syndrome: A protocol of treatment. *J Orthop Sports Phys Ther* 1:89–99, 1979.

41. Kerlan RK, Jobe FW, Blazina ME, et al: Throwing injuries of the shoulder and elbow in adults. *Curr Pract Orthop Surg* 6:49, 1975.

42. Johnson B: Treatment and rehabilitation of a complete acromioclavicular separation. *Athletic Training* 14:218–223, 1979.

RECOMMENDED READINGS

Bateman JE: *The Shoulder and Neck.* Philadelphia, WB Saunders, 1972.

Booth Jr, RE, Marvel Jr, JP: Differential diagnosis of shoulder pain. *Orthop Clin North Am* 6:353–379, 1975.

Clancy WG, editor: Symposium on shoulder problems in overhead-overuse sports. *Am J Sports Med* 7:138, 1979.

Voss D, Knot M, Kobat H: The application of neuromuscular facilitation in the treatment of shoulder disabilities. *Phys Ther Rev* 33:536–541, 1953.

CHAPTER 13

Arm and Elbow Joint Injuries

FUNCTIONAL ANATOMY

Bones

On the anteroposterior view of the elbow, note the following structures:

1. *The epicondyles.*

   1. Medial epicondyle—to which are attached the wrist flexor muscles

   2. Lateral epicondyle—to which are attached the wrist extensor muscles

2. *The joint.* The articular portion of the distal humerus is divided into two areas:

   1. Trochlear—articulates with the trochlear notch of the ulna

   2. Capitulum—articulates with the head of the radius

On the lateral view, note the following:

1. *The humerus.*

   1. Olecranon fossa

   2. Anterior and posterior fat pads

2. *The ulna.*

   1. Olecranon—fits into the olecranon fossa

   2. Trochlear notch

   3. Coronoid process

   4. Radial notch—articulates with the head of the radius

3. *The radius.*

   1. Radial head—the articular surface of the

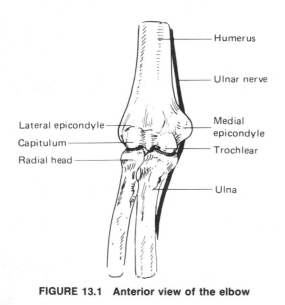

FIGURE 13.1 Anterior view of the elbow

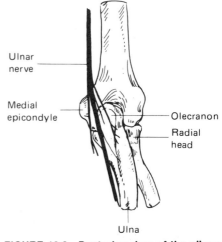

FIGURE 13.2 Posterior view of the elbow

200

radial head is slightly concave and allows pronation and supination of the forearm.

2. Radial tuberosity—the biceps tendon attaches to this.

Ligaments

1. *The medial collateral ligament.* This ligament consists of the following three portions:

1. Anterior band—running from the medial epicondyle of the humerus to the medial aspect of the coronoid process of the ulna.

2. Posterior band of the medial collateral ligament—connecting the medial epicondyle with the medial olecranon.

3. Oblique band of the medial collateral ligament—does not cross the joint but runs between the olecranon and coronoid process; it is not important in stability of the elbow joint.

In athletics, the elbow is often forced into a valgus position, which puts a strain on the medial collateral ligament. The ligaments are tight when the elbow is in full extension and the olecranon "locks" into the olecranon fossa. When the elbow moves from 10° to 60°, the medial collateral ligament is relatively lax and unstable and can easily be stressed. Most injuries take place when the arm is in this vulnerable position.[1] On reaching 90° of flexion, the ligament once more tightens and stabilizes the elbow (see Figure 14.4).

2. *The ligaments on the lateral aspect.* The ligaments on the lateral aspect of the elbow consist of two portions.

1. *Annular ligament* completely surrounds the radial head with a firm ring and thus holds the radial head against the radial notch of the ulna.

2. *Lateral collateral ligament* extends from just behind the lateral epicondyle on the humerus and blends into the annular ligament. It is a relatively weak ligament.

Muscles

1. *Muscles originating above the elbow.*

1. *Biceps brachii:* Long head—From the upper margin of the glenoid rim to the tuberosity of the radius. *Short head*—From the coracoid process to the tuberosity of the radius. *Function*: Flexes the elbow joint, supinates the forearm.

2. *Brachialis:* From the lower half of the anterior of the humerus to the tuberosity of the ulna and the coronoid process. *Function*: Flexes the elbow joint.

3. *Triceps: Long head*—From the axillary border of the scapula. *Lateral head*—From the lateral and posterior surfaces of the shaft of the humerus. *Medial head*—From the posterior surface of the shaft of the humerus below the lateral head. The three heads insert into the olecranon of the ulna. *Function*: Extends the elbow joint.

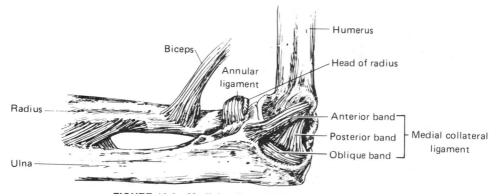

FIGURE 13.3 Medial collateral ligament of the elbow

4. *Anconeus*: From the posterior aspect of the lateral epicondyle of the humerus to the olecranon and the dorsal surface of the ulna. *Function*: Extends the elbow.

5. *Brachioradialis*: From the supracondylar ridge of the humerus to the coronoid process of the ulna. *Function*: Flexes the elbow.

2. *Muscles on the medial aspect of the elbow.*

1. *Flexor carpi radialis*: From the medial epicondyle of the humerus to the base of the second and third metacarpals. *Function*: Flexes and abducts the wrist.

2. *Flexor carpi ulnaris*: From the medial epicondyle of the humerus and the upper two-thirds of the ulna into the pisiform bone. *Function*: Flexes and abducts the wrist.

3. *Palmaris longus*: From the medial epicondyle of the humerus to the transverse carpal ligament and the palmar aponeurosis. *Function*: Flexes the wrist.

4. *Pronator teres*: From the medial epicondyle of the humerus and the coronoid process of the ulna to the middle of the radial shaft. *Function*: Pronates the forearm.

3. *Muscles on the lateral side of the elbow.*

1. *Extensor carpi radialis longus and brevis*: From the lateral epicondyle and the supra-

condylar ridge of the humerus to the base of the second and third metacarpals. *Function*: Extends and abducts the wrist.

2. *Extensor carpi ulnaris*: From the lateral epicondyle of the humerus to the common extensor tendon sheath. *Function*: Extends the wrist and fingers.

3. *Supinator*: From the lateral epicondyle of the humerus and the radial ligament of the elbow to the proximal shaft of the radius. *Function*: Supinates the forearm.

Movements

1. *The radio-ulnar-humeral joint.* The movement of this joint is limited solely to extension and flexion. In full extension the joint is stable, but with flexion the joint is dependent upon the ligaments for stability.

2. *The radio-ulnar joint.* The proximal radio-ulnar joint allows for pronation and supination of the forearm and hand. This movement takes place between the radial head and the radial notch of the ulna, and allows for about 140° of movement. If rotation of the humerus is also included, movements up to 360° can be achieved.

INJURIES ABOVE THE ELBOW JOINT

Exostoses of the Mid-humerus

The lateral aspect of the mid-humerus is very vulnerable to direct blows because the bone is close to the surface and receives little protection from muscle. There are two conditions that arise from contusions to this area. They have, however, totally different prognoses.

1. *An exostosis involving the lateral aspect of the humerus ("linebacker's arm" or "tackler's exostosis").* The exostosis results from repeated contusions to the outer aspect of the mid-humerus, with development of a hematoma and subsequent calcification. This calcification is usually in the form of a spur, which can be palpated on

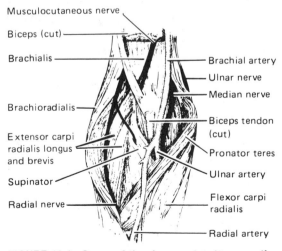

Musculocutaneous nerve

Biceps (cut)

Brachialis

Brachioradialis

Extensor carpi radialis longus and brevis

Supinator

Radial nerve

Brachial artery

Ulnar nerve

Median nerve

Biceps tendon (cut)

Pronator teres

Ulnar artery

Flexor carpi radialis

Radial artery

FIGURE 13.4 Some of the deeper structures on the front of the elbow

the lateral aspect of the humerus but seldom interferes with arm function even though it may be very tender when repeatedly contused.

TREATMENT:

Preventive: Wearing a pad or protector over the vulnerable area when playing a sport such as football can help prevent the hematoma. Once the contusion has occurred, it should be iced and compressed and an anti-inflammatory medication commenced. Repeated contusions to the area should be avoided by making sure adequate protection is worn (see Figure 4.5).

Definitive: Treatment is aimed at preventing further contusions to the area, because once calcification has formed, symptoms are rare unless there is repeated trauma. Surgical excision of the calcification is seldom necessary, but when it is, it should not be performed until the calcification is mature, usually in twelve to eighteen months.[2,3]

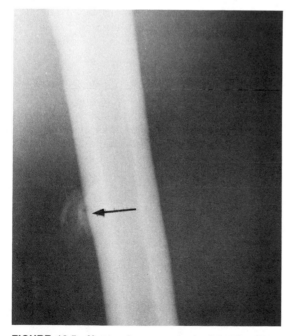

FIGURE 13.5   X-ray of an exostosis, lateral aspect, humerus This calcific spur can often be palpated, and should be protected in contact activities (see Figure 4.5).

2. *An exostosis or calcification involving the anterolateral aspect of the arm and the brachialis muscle.* This exostosis, which results from a contusion to the anterior rather than the lateral aspect of the upper arm, is a much more serious condition, because calcification involving the brachialis muscle can result in limited extension of the elbow.

The treatment of ice and anti-inflammatory medication should be supplemented by splinting the elbow. No forced movements of the brachialis should be allowed until the symptoms have subsided. At that time active range of motion can begin, but there should be no forcing of extension or passive movements.

Return to participation should be allowed only after symptoms have completely subsided. The arm should be protected from further contusions. Again, if surgical treatment is necessary, which it seldom is, it should not be contemplated until the calcification has fully matured.

Supracondylar Fracture

A child under twelve years of age who falls and complains of pain around the elbow should be suspected of having a supracondylar fracture. In many cases the deformity and diagnosis are obvious, but it may sometimes appear to be a dislocated elbow because the olecranon and distal humerus are displaced backward. It is therefore important to make no attempt at reduction of an apparently dislocated elbow until the diagnosis is confirmed. The forward displacement of the proximal humeral shaft, which occurs with most supracondylar fractures, endangers the blood vessels and nerves— this is the most serious immediate complication.

TREATMENT: The arm is splinted in a comfortable position and ice applied. The nerve supply to the hand must be examined, particularly the median nerve, and the radial pulse and peripheral circulation to the nail beds must be closely monitored. This fracture should be referred immediately for orthopedic consultation.

A supracondylar fracture results in very rapid swelling, which may compress the blood vessels around the elbow. If there is interference with the circulation, necrosis of the forearm muscles can result, which in turn can lead to Volkmann's ischemic contracture. This contracture is a permanent deformity that leaves the child with a useless limb. The supracondylar fracture must therefore be treated with the utmost care and urgency.

INJURIES AROUND THE ELBOW JOINT

Strain of the Medial Flexor-Pronator Muscles

A strain of the flexor-pronator muscle group commonly results from a valgus force (i.e., during a wrestling match or football scrimmage) or a noncontact injury (i.e., as in javelin, baseball or softball throwing). Frequently this injury occurs together with a medial collateral ligament sprain.

SYMPTOMS: Pain is present on the medial side of the elbow, particularly when the wrist is flexed and the forearm pronated.

SIGNS: Some swelling may be noted in the flexor muscles or over the medial epicondyle. Tenderness is present on the medial epicondyle or along the course of the muscles. The main finding is pain when resisting forced flexion of the wrist and pronation of the forearm. The pain is localized to the involved muscle, usually at the medial epicondyle or the musculotendinous junction just distal to the elbow (Figure 13.6). The ulnar nerve may also be injured; therefore it is necessary to check for sensation or power changes in the little and ring fingers.

SEVERITY:

First-degree strain—Only a few muscle fibers have been microscopically torn and rapid healing is to be expected.

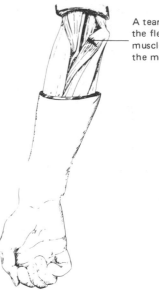

A tear (strain) of the flexor–pronator muscle group near the medial epicondyle

FIGURE 13.6   Strain of the flexor-pronator muscle group

Second-degree strain—More muscle fibers are involved, or the attachment of the tendon to the medial epicondyle may be partially avulsed. This can prolong recovery, with possible recurrence of the condition if it does not heal adequately.

Third-degree strain—A third-degree strain implies a complete tearing of the muscle or a complete avulsion of the tendon from the medial epicondyle. An additional variation is an avulsion fracture of the medial epicondyle with the tendon remaining intact.

TREATMENT:

Initial: Ice, splinting of the elbow and possibly the wrist, and early prescription of analgesics and anti-inflammatory medication.

Definitive:

First-degree strain—Icing and gentle stretching of the involved muscle group. Strengthening exercises should follow as soon as symptoms permit. Physical modalities such as ultrasound and muscle stimulation may be useful.

Second-degree strain—The elbow should be splinted until symptoms subside. Anti-inflammatory medications and physical modalities can be used. The musculature should be rehabilitated before allowing return to participation.

Third-degree strain—A decision should be made as to the advisability of surgical intervention. If the medial epicondyle is avulsed, it should be replaced to ensure pain-free function of the elbow (particularly in throwing sports). If surgery is not performed, the elbow and wrist should be immobilized for at least four to six weeks. The muscles should then be thoroughly rehabilitated.

Sprain of the Medial Collateral Ligament

The medial collateral ligament of the elbow can be injured by a

1. valgus force
2. hyperextension force

1. Valgus force. A valgus force can occur in a contact sport such as wrestling or in a noncontact activity such as javelin throwing, when done incorrectly. In addition to the ligament being injured, the flexor-pronator muscles of the forearm, as well as the ulnar nerve, may also be involved. Most of these injuries occur when a force is applied to the elbow when it is flexed at approximately 30° to 60°.

SIGNS: Tenderness and swelling are usually present over the medial side of the elbow joint, and posteromedially if the posterior band is involved.

Stability of the elbow joint should be tested by placing a valgus force on the elbow when it is bent to between 15° and 30° (Figure 13.8).[4] The elbow is normally lax in this position. The amount of laxity should be compared with that of the normal side. If the athlete cannot relax the musculature due to pain, the injured area can be anesthetized and retested.

Stress X-rays are taken with the athlete supine and the shoulder abducted and externally rotated to 90°. The humerus is supported by the table, but the forearm is allowed to hang in a valgus position at about 45° of flexion.[1] The X-ray is taken in this po-

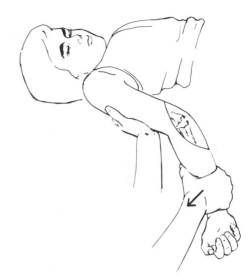

FIGURE 13.7 Valgus stress test for the medial collateral ligament of the elbow

sition. No further stress besides gravity is necessary to demonstrate an opening of the joint if a third-degree sprain is present. Comparison views should always be taken.

2. Hyperextension injuries. A partial or complete dislocation of the elbow can result from a hyperextension injury. The complete dislocation may reduce spontaneously. Frequently the athlete will give a history of having felt the elbow slip out of place and then pop back. This type of injury can damage the capsule, the ligaments, and the muscle attachments around the elbow and the arm.

SYMPTOMS AND SIGNS: There is considerable pain around the elbow both medially and laterally, and the athlete is usually very apprehensive. Swelling occurs soon after the injury and tenderness may be diffuse. Applying valgus stress is frequently very painful and is resisted by the athlete. Nerve function and the integrity of the vascular system should be checked. X-rays need to be taken to exclude the possibility of fractures or dislocations, and valgus stress used to detect any opening of the medial side of the joint, as previously described.

TREATMENT:

Immediate: The elbow should be inspected for bony deformity or dislocation. Ice should be applied around the elbow and the arm splinted, to relieve the muscle spasm that invariably accompanies such an injury. Analgesics and anti-inflammatory medication can be commenced.

Definitive: Most sprains of the medial collateral ligament are treated conservatively.

First-degree sprain—Following the initial treatment, the elbow should be iced and moved through a full range by active muscle contraction in a cold whirlpool. Isometric, followed by isotonic and isokinetic, exercises can be commenced immediately. Rehabilitation to strengthen all the musculature of the shoulder, elbow, and forearm should be continued for two to four weeks.

Second-degree sprain—A posterior splint should be used until the symptoms have subsided, followed by range of motion utilizing a cold whirlpool. Isometric exercises can be started immediately, and isotonic and isokinetic resistance can be used when symptoms permit. The length of time of immobilization depends on the severity of the sprain and the type of sport in which the athlete is participating. For instance, it is possible for a wrestler to wrestle fairly soon after a moderately severe hyperextension injury if the elbow is adequately taped to prevent extension through the final 20°. On the other hand, the javelin thrower may take many weeks to recover sufficiently and rehabilitate enough to be able to return to throwing activities.

Third-degree sprain—A complete tear of the medial collateral ligament often occurs in conjunction with dislocation of the elbow. The elbow should be splinted with posterior and anterior splints initially (to allow for swelling), followed by a cast with the elbow at 90° of flexion. This cast is retained for three to six weeks. Surgery is occasionally required.

During this time, isometric contractions are performed every hour. When the cast is removed, active range-of-motion and strengthening exercises should commence. The athlete should not return to participation until normal strength has been regained throughout the affected arm.

Limitation of motion is not an uncommon occurrence following severe sprains, particularly limitation of extension. One should never try to achieve full range of motion by forced passive movements. All this will do is encourage the formation of more scar tissue and possibly calcification. The only movements permitted are active ones (i.e., movements performed by the athlete using the muscles of the affected arm only).

Rehabilitation following a sprain of the medial collateral ligament.

1. *While immobilized*: Isometric as well as limited isokinetic and isotonic exercises can be started. The isometric contraction should include setting the biceps, triceps, pronators and supinators, lateral and medial wrist flexors, and wrist and finger extensors. Squeezing a tennis ball is a useful exercise. Shoulder exercises, particularly range-of-motion and isometric, should not be forgotten. Muscle stimulation and transcutaneous electrical nerve stimulation (TENS) can begin soon after the injury.

2. *While partially immobilized*: Partial immobilization means that the athlete can remove the immobilizing device under the direction and control of the trainer, but he or she should wear it at all other times.

Active range-of-motion exercises in a cold whirlpool can begin early in the rehabilitation process, as can isokinetic exercises (limited-arc elbow flexion and extension, pronation and supination, and wrist flexion and extension). Manual-resistance exercises may also be useful.

Strength may be increased before a full range of motion has been achieved. Isokinetic exercise should be combined with isotonic strengthening using dumbbells for curls, triceps extensions, and abduction of the arm with the elbow in different degrees of flexion.

3. *When immobilization is discontinued*. Adduction of the arm and the use of elastic tubing

should be undertaken only when there has been sufficient healing of the medial collateral ligament to permit such movement. Wrist and shoulder strengthening should be continued and increased. Finally, curls, upright rowing, military and bench presses, pull-ups and dips should be performed with progressively increased resistance.

Dislocation of the Elbow

Most dislocations in athletes are due to a hyperextension force and consist of posterior, and often lateral, displacement of the ulna and the radius on the humerus. Fractures are frequently found (Figure 13.8). In the case of a dislocated elbow, one can assume there has been damage to the medial collateral ligament, the anterior capsule, and the brachialis muscle.

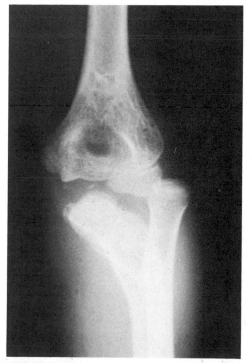

FIGURE 13.8 X-ray of a fracture-dislocation of the elbow

SYMPTOMS AND SIGNS: The athlete usually has intense pain and is often aware that the elbow has dislocated. Swelling is frequently rapid. The elbow cannot be extended and the olecranon is prominent posteriorly, with the forearm appearing to be shortened. Palpation of the elbow usually confirms the diagnosis clinically.

IMMEDIATE COMPLICATIONS: The following complications should be looked for:

1. Vascular impairment—check the
   a. radial pulse
   b. peripheral circulation, by compressing the nail beds and noting the return of normal color

2. Nerve damage—in particular, examine for signs of median nerve impairment. Examine sensation over the palm, the thumb, the index finger, and the middle fingers, and note the ability to contract the abductor pollicis brevis by resisting forced abduction.

TREATMENT AT THE SCENE OF THE INJURY:

1. A dislocated elbow should be regarded as an emergency. Apply ice immediately and splint the arm.

2. Check the vascular and the neurological status of the hand.

3. Transport the athlete immediately for definitive orthopedic care and X-rays.

POST-REDUCTION TREATMENT: The arm is usually immobilized for a number of weeks, depending on the severity of the bony and soft-tissue injuries. However, isometric setting of the forearm muscles, the biceps, and the triceps can begin soon after reduction is complete.

When mobilization of the arm is permitted, those in charge should instruct the athlete not to allow any passive movement of the elbow. All movements should be done *actively by the athlete*, using the affected arm only (the other arm should not be allowed to help move the affected arm). Isometric exercises can be started, followed by isokinetic flexion-extension and pronation-supination exercises and light isotonic exercises. However, all movements and exercises should be done within the limits of comfort; the elbow should never be forced beyond the pain-free range.

COMPLICATIONS:

1. The most serious long-term complication of a dislocated elbow is *myositis ossificans* and calcification of the soft tissues around the elbow, which limits normal elbow movement. This can be prevented to some extent by early and gentle reduction and avoidance of any passive motion of the elbow joint during rehabilitation.

2. Limitation of full elbow motion can result from the formation of scar tissue.

3. Ulnar nerve injury or entrapment is caused by scar tissue or irritation by bony spurs.

Injuries to the Ulnar Nerve

The ulnar nerve runs a course that exposes it to a variety of injuries. It can be

1. contused by a direct blow
2. stretched by a valgus force to the elbow
3. entrapped in scar tissue following trauma to the elbow
4. irritated by bony spurs

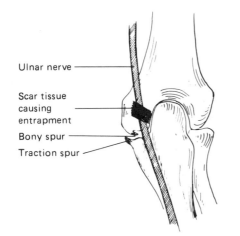

Ulnar nerve

Scar tissue causing entrapment

Bony spur

Traction spur

FIGURE 13.9   Some conditions that affect the ulnar nerve

SYMPTOMS AND SIGNS: Pain in the elbow may or may not be present. The cardinal symptoms of an ulnar nerve injury are tingling and burning of the little finger and the ulnar half of the ring finger. In chronic cases, the muscles of the hand will atrophy as many are supplied by the ulnar nerve.

To test for motor function of the ulnar nerve, place a thin sheet of cardboard between the ring finger and the little finger. This is easily removed if an ulnar nerve lesion is present. Sensation impairment can be determined by a pinprick test over the little finger and the ulnar half of the ring finger (see Figures 15.12 and 15.13).

TREATMENT: If ulnar nerve symptoms or signs persist after an injury or recur with repetitive use of the arm, the athlete should be referred for nerve conduction studies and an opinion on removing the ulnar nerve from its bony canal and transposing it to the anterior aspect of the medial side of the elbow.[5] This procedure is usually successful, provided permanent changes have not occurred within the ulnar nerve.

Olecranon Bursitis

The olecranon bursa lies between the skin and the posterior aspect of the proximal ulna. Acute swelling may follow a contusion. The swelling may be either from bleeding or from the outpouring of fluid into the bursal sac.

MODES OF PRESENTATION:

1. No symptoms may be present besides the swelling, which may not interfere with the athlete's activities.

2. The bursa may become inflamed and extremely tender to the touch, particularly after an acute contusion.

3. The bursa may become infected.

PREVENTION: Athletes who are constantly falling on their elbows (e.g., football wide receivers) should wear elbow pads to protect themselves from contusions to the olecranon bursa. This applies particularly to those who play on an artificial surface. A neoprene (wetsuit material) elbow sleeve has been developed for this purpose.[6]

TREATMENT: An ice pack should be applied to the tender area and firmly held in place with an elastic wrap. The ice should be applied for thirty minutes every hour for the first twenty-four hours. Anti-inflammatory medication should be started immediately.

If there is considerable swelling and tenderness, the olecranon bursa should be drained under sterile conditions and the fluid cultured and a long-acting local anesthetic injected. Ice, compression, and anti-inflammatory medication should be continued. Antibiotics should be used if an infection is suspected. The athlete may be allowed to return to participation as long as the elbow is adequately protected from further contusions. In most cases this protection should be continued for the remainder of the season.

In *chronic olecranon bursitis* a long-acting

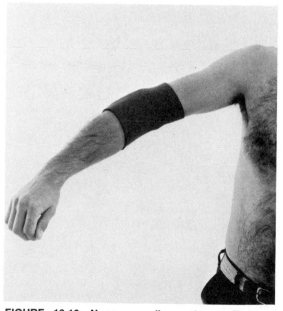

FIGURE 13.10 Neoprene elbow sleeve The pad helps protect the olecranon.

corticosteroid preparation can be injected into the bursa after it is drained—provided there is no infection. It may be necessary to surgically remove the bursa if it becomes chronically inflamed or is continuously painful.

Fracture of the Head of the Radius

A fracture of the head of the radius commonly occurs from a fall on the hand of an outstretched arm. Occasionally, however, the radial head is fractured as a result of a severe valgus force which tears the medial collateral ligament and places compression and shearing stress on the radial head.

SYMPTOMS AND SIGNS: Pain is the main symptom, and it is frequently poorly localized. There may be some swelling lateral to the olecranon. Flexion and extension may or may not be limited, but pronation and supination are usually very painful and cannot be adequately performed. Tenderness is found directly over the head of the radius (gentle palpation is all that is necessary). In the absence of other injuries, complications of the nerves or blood vessels seldom occur.

TREATMENT:

Initial: Ice and splinting of the arm to prevent muscle spasm; analgesics and anti-inflammatory medication can be started immediately. The athlete should be referred for X-rays—frequently multiple views need to be taken to demonstrate the fracture.

Definitive: Most cases of fracture of the radial head are minimally displaced and can

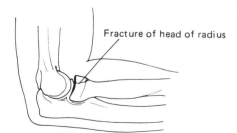

Fracture of head of radius

FIGURE 13.11 Fracture of head of radius

be treated with a sling or posterior splint for three to four weeks to relieve symptoms. If more severely displaced, an opinion on surgery should be obtained.

PROGNOSIS: If normal anatomic alignment of the radial head is not achieved, limitation to pronation, supination, or both may result. Otherwise the prognosis should be excellent.

REFERENCES

1. Woods GW, Tullos HS: Elbow instability and medial epicondyle fractures. *Am J Sports Med* 5:23–30, 1977.
2. Diamond PE, McMaster JH: Tackler's exostosis. *J Sports Med* 3:238–242, 1975.
3. Huss CD, Puhl JJ: Myositis ossificans of the upperarm. *Am J Sports Med* 8:419–424, 1980.
4. Norwood LA, Shook JA, Andrews JR: Acute medial elbow ruptures. *Am J Sports Med* 9:16–19, 1981.
5. Kerlan RK, Jobe FW, Blazina ME, et al: Throwing injuries of the shoulder and elbow in adults. *Curr Pract Orthop Surg* 6:41–58, 1975.
6. Larson RL, Osternig LR: Traumatic bursitis and artificial turf. *J Sports Med* 2:183–188, 1974.

RECOMMENDED READINGS

Halpern AA, Nagel DA: Compartment syndrome of the forearm: Early recognition using tissue pressure measurements. *J Hand Surg* 4:258–263, 1979.

Hartz CR, Linscheid RL, Gramse RR, et al: The pronator teres syndrome: Compressive neuropathy of the median nerve. *J Bone Joint Surg* 63A:885–890, 1981.

Priest JD, Weise DJ: Elbow injury in women's gymnastics. *Am J Sports Med* 9:288–295, 1981.

CHAPTER 14

Throwing and Tennis Injuries to the Shoulder and Elbow

INTRODUCTION

Acute and chronic overuse injuries to the throwing arm are frequent in athletes engaged in a throwing activity. The best example of this is the professional baseball pitcher, but injuries are also found in the pre-adolescent and adolescent Little League competitor.[1,2,3,4]

In order to understand the various injuries that occur, it is necessary to be familiar with the throwing action as well as with the changes that occur in the throwing arm. The throwing action is divided into four phases.[5]

1. Windup (cocking phase)
2. Acceleration—stage I
3. Acceleration—stage II
4. Follow-through

Changes That Can Occur in the Arm of a Pitcher

With constant, repetitive throwing, the dominant arm undergoes hypertrophy not only of the muscles, but of the bones as well. This hypertrophy is selective in that not all components are equally involved.

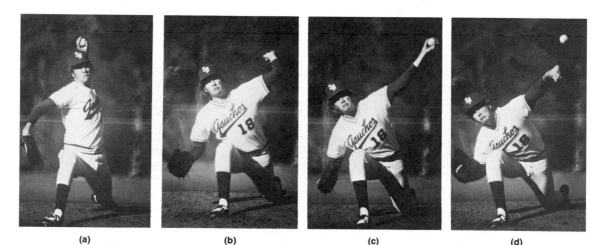

| (a) | (b) | (c) | (d) |

FIGURE 14.1 The mechanism of throwing (a) The late wind-up phase (b) The early acceleration phase (stage I); note the external rotation of the shoulder and valgus stress on the elbow joint (c) The late acceleration phase (stage II); the arm is being vigorously moved towards internal rotation (d) The follow-through; note the extension of the elbow and pronation of the forearm.

TABLE 14.1 The Mechanism of Throwing

Shoulder and Arm Movements	Primary Muscles Involved	Stress Involved
Phase I. Windup (cocking phase) *Shoulder* is abducted to 90°, hyperextended with extreme external rotation. *Scapula* is clamped against the chest wall and slightly elevated. *Wrist* is extended.	Posterior deltoid Infraspinatus Teres minor Trapezius Serratus anterior	1. Anterior capsule. The head of the humerus is forced forward. If the anterior capsule is tight (such as in a professional pitcher) and the head of the humerus is forced against the posterior glenoid, an injury to the posterior glenoid (such as the Bennett lesion) may result. 2. At the end of the windup there is stress at the origin of the anterior deltoid and the pectoralis insertion. The tendon of the long head of the biceps is also placed under tension and may sublux.
Phase II. Acceleration (Stage I) As the pitcher strides forward, the body and shoulder are brought forward while the arm and forearm are left behind.	Pectoralis major and the deltoid bring the humerus forward.	Valgus stress to the medial elbow (e.g., the medial epicondyle may be avulsed or the medial ligament torn).
Phase III. Acceleration (Stage II) This is the stage when most injuries seem to occur. The humerus is whipped from external to internal rotation; the wrist is snapped from an extended to a flexed position, to give added speed to the throw.	Pectoralis major and latissimus dorsi are the main internal rotators, together with the subscapularis. The forearm flexors vigorously contract.	1. Tremendous stress is exerted on the latissimus dorsi and pectoralis major at their insertion into the humerus. 2. Rotational injuries to the humeral shaft and epiphysis can occur, producing a stress fracture. 3. The supraspinatus may be irritated by impingement under the coraco-acromial arch during the time that the arm is rapidly brought forward and rotated from external to internal rotation. 4. The forearm flexor muscles pull on the medial epicondyle.
Phase IV. Follow-through The body's weight is firmly transferred onto the front foot. The speed of movement continually increases from the trunk to the hand, putting a considerable pull on the glenohumeral joint The elbow becomes extended; the forearm may pronate, particularly in the professional pitcher. The amount of pronation or supination depends on the type of pitch.	Subscapularis, in combination with the pectoralis major and the latissimus dorsi. Triceps. Forearm flexors, pronator teres, or supinator and biceps.	1. The posterior capsule and posterior deltoid origin become stressed. 2. The antero-inferior region is stressed by the action of the subscapularis as it turns the humerus into internal rotation. 3. The long head of the biceps is stressed at its origin on the glenoid, especially when a curve ball is thrown. 4. The glenohumeral joint may be "pulled open" by an excessively forceful pitch, i.e., subluxation may occur.

Muscular hypertrophy. The main muscles of the throwing arm that undergo hypertrophy are the pectoralis major and the latissimus dorsi. These act as powerful internal rotators of the throwing arm. The flexor muscles of the wrist and fingers also hypertrophy considerably, as can easily be seen by comparing the upper forearms.

Bony hypertrophy. There is hypertrophy of all the bones of the upper limb on the dominant side, particularly the humerus.[6] A stress reaction can occur in the mid-humerus. With hypertrophy of the humerus, there is a relative decrease in the size of the olecranon. This results in an inability of the professional pitcher to fully extend the dominant arm, because the olecranon jams into the olecranon fossa. There is also an increase in the carrying angle in longtime pitchers.[7]

Range of movement. As mentioned, extension of the elbow may be limited. Shoulder range of movement increases, in that the pitching arm may be able to externally rotate more than it can internally rotate. This results in the internal rotation becoming in-

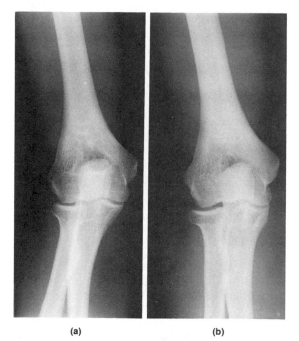

(a)   (b)

FIGURE 14.2 Humeral hypertrophy in response to exercise X-rays of the elbows of a 23-year-old right-handed tennis player who started playing at the age of nine **(a)** AP view of the left arm **(b)** AP view of the right arm

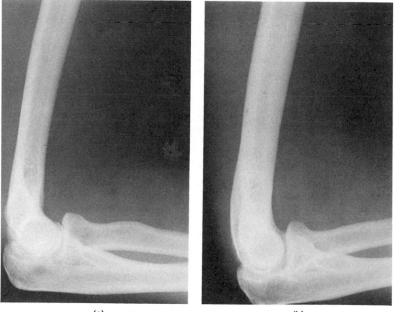

(a)   (b)

FIGURE 14.3 (a) Lateral view of the left arm (b) Lateral view of the right arm The changes are typical of those that occur in the baseball pitcher, as well as the tennis player. (From H.H. Jones, J.D. Priest, W.C. Hayes et al., "Humeral hypertrophy in response to exercise," *The Journal of Bone and Joint Surgery* 59-A:2:204–208, 1977. Illustrations reproduced with the kind permission of the authors and the publisher.)

creasingly more effective, and it allows a greater acceleration in arm motion and an increase in the velocity of ball release.

Prevention of Shoulder and Elbow Injuries in Throwing Sports

Flexibility.   Flexibility should be tested in all those engaged in a throwing sport, focusing on external rotation and extension of the shoulder. Slow, static stretching exercises should be performed on a year-round basis. As has been pointed out, an increase in the amount of external rotation leads to an increase in the velocity of the pitching arm and a decrease in stress on the structures around the elbow and shoulder.

Strength.   Any muscle weakness should be identified and corrected in the preseason using weight training, isokinetic exercise or elastic tubing. Overuse injuries around the shoulder are often thought to result from muscle imbalance, which produces a distortion of the normal movement of the humeral head in the glenoid, causing overload stress and possible impingement under the coracoacromial arch. To prevent this, each muscle should be specifically tested and any weakness corrected before symptoms develop (see section on muscle testing, pp. 20 and 22).

Technique.   The correct throwing technique can dramatically alter the stress applied to the shoulder and the medial aspect of the elbow. When major-league pitchers are studied in high-speed movies, a surprisingly similar series of pitching mechanics is seen. Athletes should be taught the overhead or three-quarter arm action rather than the sidearm action, which often produces elbow symptoms.[8] With a vertical position of the arm, the elbow is almost fully extended at the time of ball release, which decreases stress on the elbow and shoulder. Whipping and/or snapping of the pitching elbow and forearm, particularly with the sidearm action, increases speed but also increases stress on the elbow and forearm.

If the body "opens up" too soon (i.e., the body gets too far ahead of the arm), there is increased stress on the arm. A good pitching coach should observe and correct this before symptoms appear.

Extension of the nonpitching arm and a too early lifting of the back foot off the ground results in an imbalance in body mechanics. It may also indicate a technique problem elsewhere which needs correction.

The Little League Pitcher

The importance of limiting the number of throws to prevent excessive elbow stress to the ununited epiphyses and growing bones has been a frequently discussed subject over the past decade, and rules and regulations are now in force in the different Little Leagues. The Little League coach should stress to the players not only the importance of limiting the number of pitches during organized practice, but also the danger of excessive throwing in unorganized and sandlot situations. The number of curve balls pitched should also be limited.

The technique of the Little League pitcher should not differ from that of the professional pitcher, and the correct arm mechanics should be stressed. The coach should use discretion as to the frequency and length of time each player is allowed to pitch. It is important that both younger and older pitchers be brought along slowly.

Routine Care of the Throwing Arm

The following program was developed by Frank Jobe, M.D., and William Buhler, trainer of the Los Angeles Dodgers.[9] Such a program helps prevent many of the injuries which occur from incorrect and inadequate arm care.

1. Gently stretch and massage the elbow and shoulder before any throwing.

2. Perform the throwing action without the ball.

3. Start with gentle throwing, wearing a warm-up jacket.

4. Gradually increase the velocity of the throw.

5. After throwing, replace the warm-up jacket, perform gentle stretching, and allow a period of time to cool down.

6. Apply ice to the arm and shoulder or place in an ice whirlpool for thirty minutes.

SHOULDER PROBLEMS RESULTING FROM THROWING

To understand overuse injuries of the shoulder from throwing, two basic concepts should be kept in mind:

1. The concept of microtrauma, with resulting chronic inflammation of the affected tissues

2. The concept that specific muscle weakness or dysfunction can result in a less than optimal glenohumeral motion, which in turn can produce overuse or microtrauma to other structures

The various conditions affecting the shoulder are discussed under the following headings:

1. Anterior symptoms and signs
2. Posterior symptoms and signs
3. Combinations
4. Generalized symptoms and signs
5. Proximal humerus

1. Anterior symptoms and signs. Some of the conditions that should be considered when a pitcher presents with symptoms related to the anterior aspect of the shoulder include the following:

1. *Biceps tenosynovitis.* The tenderness is localized over the long head of the biceps. It moves from the anterior part of the shoulder medially when the arm is internally rotated and laterally when the arm is externally rotated.

2. *Tendinitis of the pectoralis major, latissimus dorsi or subscapularis muscles.* Symptoms of involvement of these structures are usually present at the beginning of the acceleration phase, since they are the main internal rotators of the shoulder.[10]

3. *Subluxation of the tendon of the long head of the biceps.* Usually presents when the arm is drawn back into external rotation at the beginning of the acceleration phase. This is a rare injury.

4. *Impingement of the rotator cuff.* Symptoms of this condition usually present when the arm is whipped from an externally to an internally rotated position (this occurs during the second stage of the acceleration phase).[11]

5. *Anterior subluxation of the glenohumeral joint, resulting in shoulder instability.* This is usually felt during the follow-through phase.

6. *Subdeltoid bursitis.* This is an inflammatory reaction to microtrauma occurring over a long period of time. It occurs particularly in pitchers who have poor mechanics, tend to be overachievers and go on pitching in spite of pain. Adhesions develop within the subdeltoid and subacromial bursae that keep the rotator cuff from gliding smoothly under the acromion process and coraco-acromial ligament. The pain occurs mainly during the acceleration and early follow-through phases.

The tenderness is felt over the long head of the biceps, but it remains persistently anterior despite internal and external rotation of the humerus. Symptoms are reproduced when manual resistance is applied to the arm during the acceleration and early follow-through phases.

7. *Partial or complete tears of the rotator cuff* (see p. 186).

8. *Miscellaneous conditions.* These include such conditions as fracture of the coracoid process, stress fracture of the first rib, fracture of the anterior lip of the glenoid, and fracture of the acromion process. They may all present with anterior shoulder symptoms and signs.

2. Posterior symptoms and signs.

1. *Posterior cuff strain.* This is a vague diagnosis. However, the pain is noted during the windup phase, during the follow-through

phase, or both. Tenderness is usually present over the posterior glenoid. Some of these cases show changes of the posterior glenoid on X-rays (the so-called Bennett lesion) which may be associated with tears of the glenoid labrum.[12]

2. *Subscapular bursitis*. This is thought to occur on occasion. It is the opinion of the authors that the primary lesion in the posterior group is a muscle imbalance or weakness, usually involving the posterior portion of the deltoid, the external rotators (infraspinatus and teres minor), or both. Weaknesses involving these muscles should be sought in the preseason in every baseball player and corrected before the player is permitted to throw hard.

3. *Combinations.* Anterior and posterior symptoms may co-exist.

4. *Generalized symptoms and signs.* This is usually the end stage of an inflammatory response to microtrauma and results in a poorly localized "adhesive capsulitis."

5. *Proximal humerus.* Conditions involving the proximal humerus are rare, but they do occur. Stress fractures of the humeral shaft have been reported,[13,3] as well as stress fractures in the proximal humeral epiphysis in pre-adolescent and adolescent athletes. In these cases, tenderness is present over the affected area. X-rays should always be taken; these may show a stress fracture or widening of the epiphysis.

TREATMENT OF OVERUSE PROBLEMS AROUND THE SHOULDER

The treatment of overuse problems around the shoulder in the throwing athlete is, on the whole, unsatisfactory. It is therefore important when dealing with a pitcher to keep the following in mind.

Prevention is the key to handling shoulder problems, and each of the points mentioned under the section on prevention should be diligently followed. Flexibility should be maintained, any sign of specific muscle weakness should be sought, and technical faults should be corrected.

The first sign of shoulder discomfort should alert the athlete and his or her coach and medical advisors to the possibility of a developing problem. At that stage the player should be treated vigorously, and on no account should he or she throw while there is pain. If the player does continue throwing, one of the conditions described can easily develop.

Once taken off throwing, the athlete should be treated with ice therapy, ultrasound, transcutaneous electrical nerve stimulation (TENS), anti-inflammatory medication, and gentle stretching exercises. If there is no pain at rest, strengthening exercises should be commenced. Kerlan's shoulder exercises[9] can be used without resistance, and then elastic tubing added (see rehabilitation, p. 192). Any specific muscle weakness should be corrected, then a general strengthening program for the shoulder muscles can be undertaken. The fungo routine for throwing should be performed before the athlete starts to pitch again (see Table 14.2).

TABLE 14.2 Fungo Routine

1. Make long, easy throws from the deepest portion of the outfield with the ball just getting back to the FUNGO hitter. Perform for thirty minutes on two consecutive days, then rest the arm for a day.
2. Make stronger throws from the middle of the outfield, getting the ball back on five or six bounces. Perform for thirty minutes on two consecutive days, then rest for a day.
3. Make strong, crisp throws from the short outfield with a relatively straight trajectory so that the ball bounces once on the way back to the FUNGO hitter. Perform for thirty minutes on two consecutive days, then rest for a day.
4. Return to the mound or other normal position for usual activities.

Source: "Throwing Injuries of the Shoulder and Elbow in Adults," R. K. Kerlan and others, *Current Practice in Orthopedic Surgery* 6:41–58, 1975. Reprinted by permission.

An athlete who has suffered from an injury to the throwing arm should treat it for potential recurrence. The arm should be slowly and gently warmed up. Gentle stretching exercises should be performed regularly and the arm iced down after any workout.

Local injections of corticosteroids should be used infrequently and their number limited. Surgery is reserved for the chronic case or when there is a specific indication.

ELBOW PROBLEMS RESULTING FROM THROWING

Most elbow problems result from valgus overload (Figure 14.4), which causes excessive stress on the medial side of the joint while compressing the lateral side. The elbow of the Little League athlete is particularly susceptible to damage.[1,2,4,14] Special attention should be focused on the technique of the pitcher and the number of pitches thrown.

Problems arising around the elbow are divided into anatomical areas.

1. Medial lesions
2. Lateral lesions
3. Posterior lesions
4. Combinations
5. Generalized pain

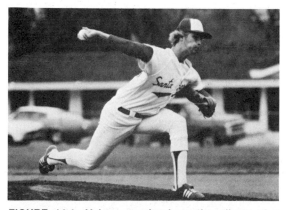

FIGURE 14.4 Valgus overload on the elbow of a pitcher (Note the degree of external rotation of the shoulder)

1. *Medial lesions.*

1. *Acute lesions.*

   a. Epicondylitis: Refers to tenderness over the medial epicondyle resulting from a strain of the origin of the medial wrist-flexor muscle group.

   b. Medial epicondyle avulsion fracture: Results from an excessive force of contraction of the medial wrist-flexor muscles.

   c. Medial ligament sprain: Palpating along the medial ligament produces pain, particularly over the medial joint line. The ligaments should be stressed at 30° to 45° of flexion. No instability will be found unless the ligaments have been completely torn. If there is a partial tear, pain will be produced with valgus stress.

   d. Flexor muscle strain: Produces pain near the elbow when active wrist flexion is resisted. Local tenderness is usually present at the musculo-tendinous junction just distal to the elbow.

   e. Ulnar nerve subluxation: Produces a sudden electric shock, like pain shooting down the forearm to the ring finger and the little finger. Tingling and numbness may also be present.

2. *Chronic conditions.*

   a. Ulnar neuritis: The pain is localized in the elbow area, and there is tenderness over the ulnar nerve. This condition may be provoked by a fracture of a traction spur.

   b. Ulnar nerve entrapment: Scar tissue formation around the ulnar nerve can cause this condition, which produces pain, numbness, tingling, and muscle weakness of the ring finger and the little finger, as well as wasting of the small muscles of the hand.[15]

   c. Soft-tissue calcification: This is an X-ray diagnosis. A number of different types of soft-tissue calcifications have been noted.

      1. Traction spur from the ulna re-

sults from a constant repetitive valgus stress pulling on the capsule attached to the ulna at the joint line. This traction spur can be symptomless in many pitchers and may not cause any discomfort unless it fractures.

2. "Stalagmite" is a buildup of calcium along the medial capsular attachment to the proximal ulna. It is probably secondary to an inflammatory response to microtrauma from valgus overload.

3. Calcification of the flexor muscle mass may occur adjacent to the medial epicondyle of the humerus. It is thought to be caused by microtearing of the muscle fibers, particularly when associated with fast- or curve-ball throwing.

d. Miscellaneous conditions: These include inflammation of the medial capsule, the pronator teres muscle, the interosseous membrane and a medial forearm compartment compression syndrome. The formation of an ossicle or an incomplete fusion of the medial epiphysis may also give rise to problems.

3. *The Little League player.* This athlete's problems are related to unfused epiphyses and immature bones. Injury to the epiphysis of the medial epicondyle of the humerus is the most common problem of the Little Leaguer. This epiphysis is usually the last epiphyseal center around the elbow to close. It is also one of the weakest and therefore easy to injure.

Pain and tenderness over the medial epicondylar epiphysis are the presenting symptoms. X-rays should always be taken of *both* elbows to determine if an avulsion of the epiphysis has occurred. The results are graded as follows:

Grade I: No X-ray changes, minimal symptoms

Grade II: No X-ray changes or less than 5 mm displacement of the epiphysis on the X-ray, more severe symptoms

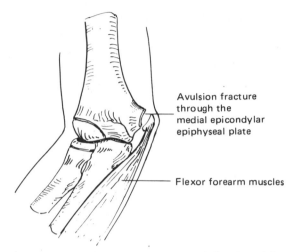

FIGURE 14.5 Avulsion of the medial epicondylar epiphysis, as may occur from pitching

Grade III: Displacement on the X-ray greater than 5 mm—these should be treated surgically

2. *Lateral lesions.* These result from compression overload on the lateral side of the joint.

1. *The adult pitcher.*

a. Lateral epicondylitis: Results from excessive or incorrect use of the wrist extensor muscles, usually in those who throw a "screw ball" or a fast ball with marked pronation of the forearm

b. Avascular necrosis: An area of dead or necrotic bone of the capitulum, with adjacent calcification

c. Loose bodies within the joint on the lateral side: Probably the result of avascular necrosis of the capitulum or radial head

2. *The Little League player.* Though injury to the lateral compartment rarely occurs in the younger athlete, when it does it results in the tragedy of a permanently damaged elbow joint.[14] The following lesions have been described (Figure 14.6):

a. Osteochondritis dissecans of the capitulum: This area of dead bone may

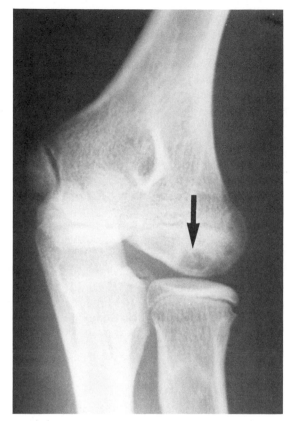

FIGURE 14.6 X-ray—osteochondritis dissecans of the capitulum Note the cystic changes within the bone, and the irregular joint margin.

displace, forming a loose body within the joint. This condition results in an incongruous joint surface and the possible onset of osteoarthritis.

b. Ostcochondrosis of the radial head: This is the same lesion, occurring in the proximal radial epiphysis.

c. Proximal radial epiphyseal compression and angulation: This epiphysis usually fuses at about age fourteen or later. If damaged, limitation of elbow extension, pronation, and supination can result. It is one of the most serious elbow injuries.

It was mentioned previously that the professional pitcher can develop a limitation to full extension because of the relative increase in size of the olecranon as compared to the olecranon fossa. *An adolescent does not have the limitation of extension that is found in the professional pitcher.* If limitation to extension is found, pathology around the elbow joint must be excluded by a thorough clinical and X-ray evaluation.

3. *Posterior lesions (result from an extensor overload).*

1. *Loose bodies.* These are probably formed by the jamming of the olecranon into the olecranon fossa.

2. *Osteochondral fracture of the middle of the trochlear notch.* This usually occurs on one particular pitch, when the elbow is rapidly extended while the valgus stress is continued. Severe pain and a "crunch" are usually felt.

3. *Hyperextension sprain.* This may include the medial ligament as well as the biceps tendon.

4. *Triceps strain.*

5. *Stress fracture of the olecranon* (rare).

4. *Combination medial and posterior lesions.*

5. *Generalized pain.* This is usually a late complication due to either osteoarthritis with general calcific debris or myositis ossificans.

TREATMENT OF ELBOW INJURIES RESULTING FROM THROWING

The concepts of microtrauma and muscle imbalance should again be stressed, along with the importance of preventing an injury or treating it early and vigorously should it occur.

The standard treatment of ice and immobilization applies to most injuries. This treatment is continued for a period of time as dictated by the severity of the injury. A sling should be used whenever necessary. Anti-inflammatory medication should be used judiciously.

Following the athlete's recovery from the initial symptoms, the elbow, wrist, and shoulder joints should be strengthened and stretched. All muscle groups should be tested for flexibility and strength, to discover any latent weakness.

In treating medial epicondylar conditions of the Little League thrower, the importance of an adequate period of rest cannot be overemphasized. Not only should this athlete be off throwing for quite a few weeks, but a gradual buildup in the number and speed of the throws should be carefully supervised before return to full activity.

In chronic conditions involving the ulnar nerve, it is possible to surgically release or relocate the nerve.[15,16] This is a relatively minor procedure producing good results, providing the ulnar nerve is undamaged. Surgery for soft-tissue calcification or a loose body is also a relatively successful procedure in selected cases. Most other surgical procedures around the elbow of the professional pitcher produce unpredictable results and are avoided whenever possible. In chronic conditions resistant to other forms of therapy, a limited number of local corticosteroid injections can be used with care.

ELBOW AND SHOULDER INJURIES FROM TENNIS

The elbow, and to a lesser extent the shoulder, are notoriously susceptible to injury in tennis players.

INCIDENCE:

1. *Lateral epicondyle.* Involvement of the lateral epicondyle occurs commonly in the "club player," especially the one who plays frequently and for long periods of time, who is competitive, and who has a poor technique, particularly on the backhand. In addition, these players are usually over thirty-five years of age.[17,18] The condition also affects the adult beginner, who invariably has a poor technique and an insufficient musculature.[19]

The expert tennis player is not excluded from lateral epicondylitis, but suffers from it far less frequently than the less proficient club player. In the expert, however, symptoms are related to both the backhand and the forehand and are probably associated with overuse and muscle imbalances rather than faulty technique.[20]

2. *Medial side of the elbow.* The medial side of the elbow is the site of injuries commonly found in the expert player who hits a hard American twist serve.

PATHOLOGY:

1. *Lateral side.* The symptoms on the lateral side of the elbow are invariably localized to the lateral epicondyle at the extensor aponeurosis (this consists of the extensor communis and extensor carpi radialis mus-

TABLE 14.3   Elbow Injuries in Tennis Players

Medial Side of Elbow	Stroke Involved	Presumed Predisposing Factors	Lateral Side of Elbow	Stroke Involved	Presumed Predisposing Factors
70% of expert males with elbow problems	Serve	American twist serve	30% of expert males with elbow problems	Forehand and/or backhand	Overuse
50% of expert females with elbow problems	Serve	Force of serve relative to musculature	50% of expert females with elbow problems	Forehand and/or backhand	Overuse
25% of club players with elbow problems	? Serve		75% of club players with elbow problems	Backhand	Technique, muscle weakness

cles). Changes found at surgery in those who have suffered from this condition for a long time include fissuring and tears of the underside of the musculotendinous junction of the wrist extensor muscles.[21,22] Occasionally calcific deposits are found in the tendon. Very seldom does a complete rupture occur.

2. *Medial side.* Medial symptoms are related to one of two areas:

    a. Medial epicondyle—to which are attached the wrist and the finger flexor muscles, the pronator teres, and the medial ligament. Repetitive forces in this area lead to changes of the medial epicondyle and the coranoid process and calcification in the medial soft tissues.

    b. Cubital tunnel—the flexor carpi ulnaris arises from this area, and it is thought that constant repetitive straining of the muscle attachment gives rise to symptoms here. In experienced players, bony changes such as spurring of the coranoid process have been found. In contrast with baseball players, the ulnar nerve itself is rarely involved.

MECHANISM OF INJURY:

1. *Lateral side.* The lateral epicondyle appears particularly prone to injury in activities that overuse the forearm muscles. These muscles frequently have relatively inadequate strength, power, endurance, and flexibility. Add to this the poor technique of the average club player, particularly with regard to the backhand (Figure 14.7). A number of factors relating to technique have been implicated, including the "leading-elbow-backhand syndrome," off-center ball contact, poor timing, poor body-weight transfer, and poor use of the forearm muscles.

2. *Medial side.* As mentioned, medial symptoms occur mainly in the expert player and seem to be related to the action of the serve. Surveys show that males are predominantly affected, the implication being that the injury

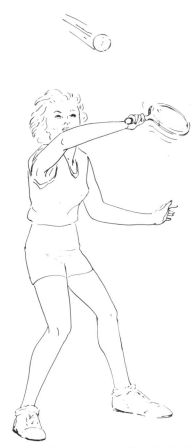

FIGURE 14.7 The "leading-elbow" backhand A mistimed shot with the arm in this position may produce microtrauma to the muscles and tendons attached to the lateral epicondyle.

is stress related, since males tend to serve harder than females. This stress may be magnified by a defect in technique, such as spinning the ball excessively during the American twist serve, where maximum pronation, ulnar deviation, and wrist flexion put a considerable strain on the medial epicondylar structures.

SYMPTOMS AND SIGNS: Symptoms usually develop insidiously and tend to become progressively worse. Occasionally they originate from one single stroke, particularly a mistimed shot.

Tenderness is localized precisely to the attachment of the extensor aponeurosis to the lateral epicondyle (Figure 14.8). On the medial side, the exact site depends on the area involved. There is very seldom swelling or ecchymosis. Weakness of the extensor muscles on the lateral side, and one of the flexor and pronator muscles on the medial side, may be found. This is due either to actual muscle weakness or to weakness related to the discomfort of the condition. Frequently weakness of one of the shoulder muscle groups is found. A decrease in wrist flexibility, particularly flexion, is often present (Figure 14.9). Spasm of the extensor carpi radialis muscles is frequently related to lateral epicondylar symptoms.

TREATMENT:

1. *The acute case.* Initial treatment consists of ice packs, resting the arm in a sling, avoidance of tennis activity for a number of days (depending on the severity of the condition), and anti-inflammatory medication in the form of aspirin (or phenylbutazone in more severe cases).

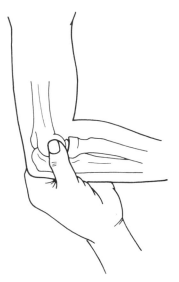

FIGURE 14.8 Lateral epicondylitis Tenderness is localized to one specific area of the lateral epicondyle.

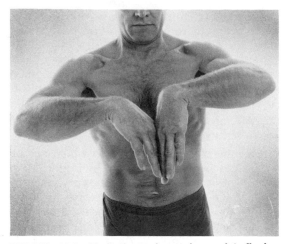

FIGURE 14.9 Limitation of passive wrist flexion due to tightness and spasm of the extensor carpi radialis muscles

2. *The chronic case.*

   a. *Before playing:* One hour before playing, apply ice or heat, depending on which modality seems to offer the best results for the particular athlete. Massage the tender area and the surrounding muscles. Half an hour before playing, the athlete takes two aspirin. Before going onto the court, the athlete does calisthenic exercises to raise the body temperature; stretching exercises (which will be outlined) for the extensor muscle groups; and shadow-playing, hitting forehands, backhands, and serves without the ball. On the court, he or she hits forehands only for five minutes before attempting any backhands.

   b. *On-court modifications:*

      1. Average club players need, in most cases, to improve their *technique of hitting a backhand;* in particular, the "leading elbow" should be eliminated. A good coach can do more than medical personnel to help prevent lateral epicondylitis in a tennis player.

Some players benefit from a change from the standard one-handed to a two-handed backhand which takes the strain off the muscles and therefore off the lateral epicondyle.

2. The *racquet* can be changed to one that produces little vibration up the forearm, particularly when the ball is hit off center. A racquet with a large "sweet spot" may also be advantageous. A lighter rather than a heavier racquet is usually better.

3. A smaller *grip size* is usually recommended, but it is more important to get the right size for any particular player.

4. The *strings of the racquet* should be 16-gauge gut, strung at the correct tension for that particular racquet, in most cases in the area of 50–52 pounds. Very tightly strung racquets are usually dangerous for the less accomplished player, as the forces of vibration are conducted up the arm when the ball is hit off center.

5. A *slower ball and slower court* have the advantage of producing fewer mistimed shots and less force in racquet-ball contact.

c. *Muscle strength*: Together with the change of backhand technique, improvement of muscular strength is probably the most important change that the average tennis player can make. Muscle-strengthening exercises should affect the shoulder girdle, the wrist extensor muscles, and the finger extensor muscles. These exercises are outlined on p. 224.

d. *Flexibility*: Improving the flexibility of the wrist and elbow may improve the symptoms of lateral epicondylitis. Ice massage applied to the stretched muscle may help to relieve symptoms and muscle spasm (Figure 14.10).

e. *Elbow band*: The elbow band is a 2½" (6 cm) nonelastic band worn just below the elbow. The counterforce of the band is thought to disseminate the forces of muscle contraction over a wider area and help decrease the strain on the lateral epicondyle (Figure 14.11).

Numerous other devices and braces (including a neoprene elbow sleeve) are on the market and seem to succeed in reducing symptoms in some players.

f. *Physical therapy*: Physical therapy procedures such as ultrasound with hy-

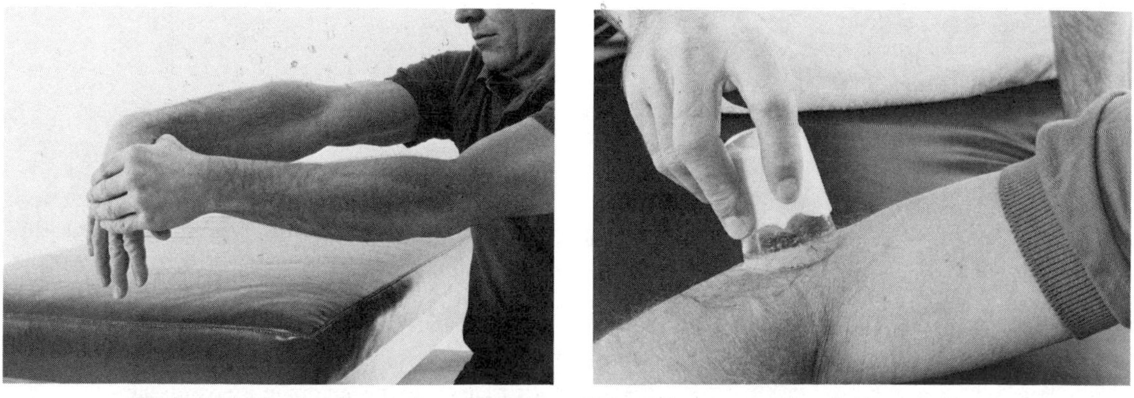

FIGURE 14.10 Gentle passive stretching of the extensor carpi radialis muscles, together with ice-massage, is often useful in treating "tennis elbow."

drocortisone (phonophoresis) may be useful, as may high-voltage galvanic stimulation over the tender area and muscle stimulation to enhance the contractile properties of the extensor carpi radialis muscles.[23]

g. *Medical treatment*: Anti-inflammatory medication can be used in the form of oral aspirin, an ibuprofen-type drug (Motrin), or a short course of phenylbutazone. If necessary, intralesional cortisone injections can be given. The need for these injections is reduced, however, if the previously mentioned suggestions are faithfully followed. Sling immobilization can be used during flare-ups. Cast immobilization is not advised, but is occasionally used. As a last resort, surgery can be undertaken.

TREATMENT: As medial epicondylar symptoms are mainly related to the serving action and occur in advanced and expert players, an expert coach should be acquired to help modify the serving technique. Players should also be sure to warm up slowly and to avoid practicing the serve for too long. They should be aware of the dangers of repetitive all-out serving and should adjust their strategies to include a large number of three-quarter pace serves, using only a moderate

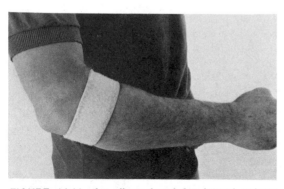

FIGURE 14.11 An elbow band for lateral epicondylitis Elbow band is worn just below the elbow and appears to reduce the tension of the extensor aponeurosis at its attachment to the lateral epicondyle.

amount of spin. Icing and anti-inflammatory medication are very beneficial. Cortisone injections may be used as indicated.

MUSCLE-STRENGTHENING PROGRAM FOR "TENNIS ELBOW"

1. *Shoulder exercises.*

1. *Work on localized muscle weaknesses with elastic tubing and/or isokinetic machines
2. *Military press
3. Pull-ups
4. Dips
5. Pendulum arm stretch—when bent at 90°, swing arm
   a. forward into flexion with weight in hand
   b. sideways into abduction with weight in hand (see Figure 12.38)
6. *Flies, with weight in each hand
   a. to the front (Figure 12.42)
   b. to the side
7. *Ball-squeezing exercise, from external rotation-abduction (Figure 12.35) to internal rotation-abduction (see shoulder rehabilitation exercises, p. 192).

2. *Arm exercises.*

1. *Triceps-elbow extension (Figure 14.12)
2. Bench press
3. Reverse curl

3. *Elbow and forearm exercises.*

1. *"Broom handle exercise"—weight hanging at the end of a string attached to a broom handle, the broom handle held in front of the athlete, who then attempts to curl the string around the handle and so raise up the weight. The

*These are the important exercises; they should be included if only a limited program is performed.

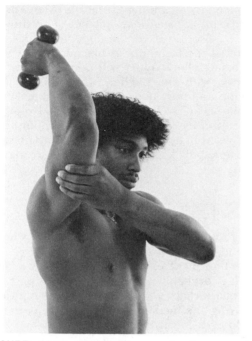

FIGURE 14.12 Triceps-elbow extension exercise The elbow is extended and flexed slowly. Do not allow the elbow to rapidly snap into extension. The nonexercising arm supports the humerus.

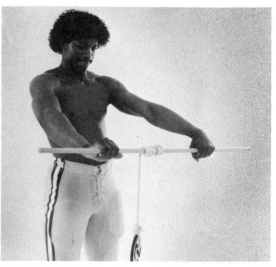

FIGURE 14.13 The broom-handle exercise This helps to develop the wrist extensors.

weight is then lowered in the same manner with a reverse curling action (Figure 14.13).

2. *Wrist extension
3. *Wrist flexion (Figure 14.14). These exercises can be done isometrically, with weights, or with the appropriate iso-

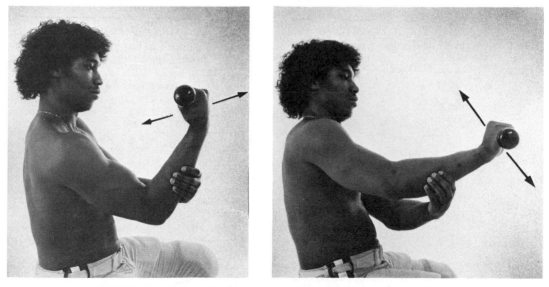

FIGURE 14.14 Wrist flexion and extension exercises using dumbbells

kinetic apparatus, which produces excellent results when used at the faster speeds. Elastic tubing should also be used.

4. Wrist rotation—clockwise and counter-clockwise.
5. Wrist side-to-side motion.
6. *Supination and pronation with the elbow at 90°.

   This can be done isometrically, with weights, with wall pulleys, and, most importantly, with elastic tubing and isokinetically.

4. *Finger exercises.* This involves extension of the fingers at the metacarpophalangeal joint, using elastic bands as resistance. This exercise should be performed relatively rapidly until the muscles of the hand and arm are fatigued (Figure 14.15).

Do not forget to incorporate flexibility exercises into the strength program.

ELBOW INJURIES IN OTHER SPORTS

Javelin Throwing

Throwing a javelin places considerably more stress on the elbow than does pitching a baseball. Some of the factors involved are the heavier javelin and the greater forces produced by a running javelin thrower, compared with the stationary pitcher. The shoulder is also stressed, though to a lesser extent. If the technique is not quite right, an immediate elbow injury will occur. This is in contrast with the pitcher, who will usually develop an injury over a period of time. The technique in javelin throwing is vital to the prevention of injury. The forearm should be kept vertical during the acceleration phase, and the elbow kept from going into a valgus position.

Football

The football quarterback has a limited wind-up and a short acceleration phase. Most of the action involves the wrist flexion or snap, which is probably the most important part of the quarterback's throw. However, injuries involving the medial elbow and triceps muscle do occasionally occur.

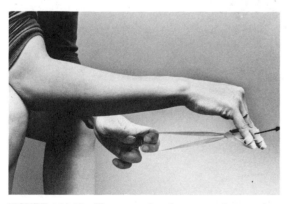

FIGURE 14.15 Finger extension exercise, using rubber bands as resistance The wrist should be kept stationary during this exercise.

REFERENCES

1. Tullos HS, King JW: Lesions of the pitching arm in adolescents. *JAMA* 22:264–271, 1972.
2. Larson RL: Epiphyseal injuries in the adolescent athlete. *Orthop Clin North Am* 4:839–851, 1973.
3. Cahill BR, Tullos HS, Fair RH: Little league shoulder. *J Sports Med* 11:150–153, 1974.
4. Lipscomb AB: Baseball pitching injuries in growing athletes. *J Sports Med* 3:25–34, 1975.
5. Tullos HS, King JW: Throwing mechanisms in sports. *Orthop Clin North Am* 4:709–720, 1973.
6. Jones HH, Priest JD, Hayes WC, et al: Humeral hypertrophy in response to exercise. *J Bone Joint Surg* 59A:204–208, 1977.
7. Woods GW, Tullos HS, King JW: The throwing arm: Elbow joint injuries. *J Sports Med* 1:43–47, 1973.
8. Albright JA, Jokl P, Shaw R, et al: Clinical study of baseball pitchers: Correlation of injury to the throwing arm with method of delivery. *Am J Sports Med* 6:15–21, 1978.
9. Kerlan RK, Jobe FW, Blazina ME, et al: Throwing injuries of the shoulder and elbow in adults. *Curr Pract Orthop Surg* 6:41–58, 1975.
10. Norwood LA, Del Pizzo W, Jobe FW, et al: Anterior shoulder pain in baseball pitchers. *Am J Sports Med* 6:103–105, 1978.

11. Jackson DW: Chronic rotator cuff impingement in the throwing athlete. *Am J Sports Med* 4:231–240, 1976.

12. Lombardo SJ, Jobe FW, Kerlan RK, et al: Posterior shoulder lesions in throwing athletes. *Am J Sports Med* 5:106–110, 1977.

13. Devas M: *Stress Fractures.* London, Churchill Livingstone, 1975.

14. Brown R, Blazina ME, Kerlan RK, et al: Osteochondritis capitellum. *J Sports Med* 2:27–46, 1974.

15. Del Pizzo W, Jobe FW, Norwood L: Ulnar nerve entrapment syndrome in baseball players. *Am J Sports Med* 5:182–185, 1977.

16. Brondy A, Leffert R, Smith R: Technical problems with ulnar nerve transposition at the elbow: Findings and results of reoperation. *J Hand Surg* 3:85–89, 1978.

17. Priest JD, Braden V, Gerberich SG: The elbow and tennis. Part 1. An analysis of players with and without pain. *Phys Sportsmed* 8:81–91, April 1980.

18. Priest JD, Braden V, Gerberich SG: The elbow and tennis. Part 2. A study of players with pain. *Phys Sportsmed* 8:77–85, May 1980.

19. Priest JD: Tennis elbow. The syndrome and a study of average players. *Minn Med* 59:367–371, 1976.

20. Priest JD, Jones HH, Nagel DA: Elbow injuries in highly skilled tennis players. *J Sports Med* 2:137–149, 1974.

21. Nirschl RP: Etiology and treatment of tennis elbow. *J Sports Med* 2:308–323, 1974.

22. Nirschl RP, Pettrone FA: Tennis elbow: The surgical treatment of lateral epicondylitis. *J Bone Joint Surg* 61A:832–839, 1979.

23. Nirschl RP, Sobel J: Conservative treatment of tennis elbow. *Phys Sportsmed* 9:42–54, June 1981.

RECOMMENDED READINGS

Barnes DA, Tullos HS: An analysis of a hundred symptomatic baseball players. *Am J Sports Med* 6:62–67, 1978.

Berhang AM, Dehner W, Fogarty C: Tennis elbow: A biomechanical approach. *J Sports Med* 2:235–259, 1974.

DeHaven KE, Evarts EM: Throwing injuries of the elbow in athletics. *Orthop Clin North Am* 3:801–808, 1973.

Gruchow HW, Pelletier D: An epidemiologic study of tennis elbow. *Am J Sports Med* 7:234–238, 1979.

Gunn CC, Milbrandt WE: Tennis elbow and the cervical spine. *Can Med Assoc J* 114:803–809, 1976.

Indelicato PA, Jobe FW, Kerlan RK, et al: Correctable elbow lesions in professional baseball players: A review of 25 cases. *Am J Sports Med* 7:72–75, 1979.

Ingham B: Transverse friction massage for relief of tennis elbow. *Phys Sportsmed* 9:116, October 1981.

Kulund DN, McCue FC, Rockwell DA, et al: Tennis injuries: Prevention and treatment. A review. *Am J Sports Med* 7:249–253, 1979.

Priest JD, Nagel DA: Tennis shoulder. *Am J Sports Med* 4:28–42, 1976.

Slocum DB: Classification of elbow injuries from baseball pitching. *Tex Med* 64:48–53, 1968.

CHAPTER 15

Wrist and Hand Injuries

FUNCTIONAL ANATOMY

The hand is a very versatile organ, largely due to the wide range of movement possible at the shoulder, the hinge action of the elbow, and the rotation of the forearm. The area between the scapulae is the only region of the body the hand cannot reach. It can open and become completely flat or it can clench into a fist. The fingers can spread wide apart or converge to pick up tiny objects. The thumb has a wide range of movement and works with the fingers to pinch and grasp.

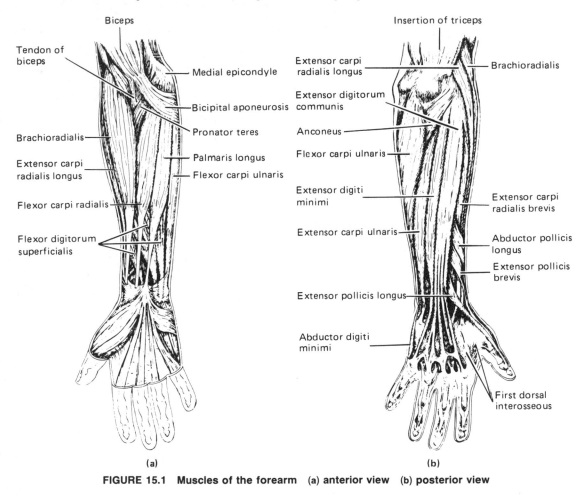

(a)   (b)

FIGURE 15.1 Muscles of the forearm   (a) anterior view   (b) posterior view

Muscles

The muscles supplying the hand are divided into two groups:

1. Those arising from the forearm—the *extrinsic* muscles (these have their muscle bellies in the forearm, but their tendons are in the hand)

2. Those arising from the hand—*intrinsic* muscles

1. *The extrinsic muscles.* The extrinsic muscles play an important part in the following hand movements:

1. Supination of the forearm—mainly controlled by the biceps muscle, assisted by the supinator

2. Pronation of the forearm—pronator teres and pronator quadratus

3. Adduction of the hand at the wrist—produced by the combined action of the flexor carpi ulnaris and extensor carpi ulnaris muscles

4. Abduction of the hand at the wrist—flexor carpi radialis with extensor carpi radialis longus and brevis

5. Flexion of the wrist—effected by the flexor carpi radialis and the flexor carpi ulnaris

6. Extension of the wrist—extensor carpi radialis longus and brevis and extensor carpi ulnaris

7. Flexion of the fingers—due to the action of flexor digitorum sublimis (or superficialis) and the flexor digitorum profundus (assisted by the lumbricals and interosseous muscles)

8. Extension of the fingers—combined action of the extrinsic and intrinsic muscles:

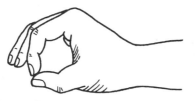

FIGURE 15.2 **Test for ulnar nerve lesion** When the adductor pollicis muscle is inactive, the pinch action of the thumb lacks strength.

a. The extensor digitorum communis extends the proximal phalanges and stabilizes the metacarpophalangeal joints, so that the interossei can extend the middle and distal phalanges and move the fingers laterally. This is the reason why, with a "mallet finger," it is possible to extend the metacarpophalangeal (MP) and proximal interphalangeal (PIP) joints even though the tendon is avulsed from the distal phalanx.

b. The interosseous and lumbrical muscles are intrinsic muscles and will be discussed on p. 230.

9. Movements of the thumb—the most important digit of the hand, capable of many types of movement:

a. Abduction—produced by the abductor pollicis longus and brevis.

b. Adduction—produced by the adductor pollicis (supplied by the ulnar nerve).

c. Opposition—flexor pollicis brevis and opponens pollicis (supplied by the median nerve). In opposition, the opponens pollicis arches the thumb toward the tips of the fingers, while the adductor pollicis slides the thumb across the palm toward the ulnar side of the hand. However, when pinching the tips of the fingers, pressure is exerted by the action of the flexor pollicis longus and adductor pollicis. If the ulnar nerve is damaged and the adductor pollicis inactive, it is difficult to make an *O* with the thumb and index finger (Figure 15.2).

d. Circumduction—of the muscle groups supplying the thumb.

e. Flexion—by the flexor pollicis longus and opponens pollicis, assisted by the flexor pollicis longus.

f. Extension—by the extensor pollicis longus and brevis and the abductor pollicis longus. This muscle not only extends and abducts the first metacarpal, but also stabilizes the first metacarpophalangeal (MP) joint.

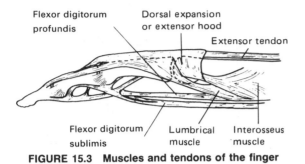

Flexor digitorum profundis

Dorsal expansion or extensor hood

Extensor tendon

Flexor digitorum sublimis

Lumbrical muscle

Interosseus muscle

FIGURE 15.3   Muscles and tendons of the finger

2. *The intrinsic muscles.*   The intrinsic muscles of the hands consist of:

1. Muscles of the hypothenar eminence
2. Muscles of the thenar eminence
3. Interosseous muscles
4. Lumbrical muscles

The seven *interosseous* muscles have three main functions:

1. Abduct and adduct the proximal phalanges, that is, spread and approximate the fingers.

2. Help flex the proximal phalanges (when the extensor tendons are relaxed).

3. Extend the middle and distal phalanges. These latter two movements occur as a result of the attachment of the interosseous and lumbrical muscles into the dorsal expansion or "hood" (Figure 15.3).

In a boutonnière deformity (see p. 237), the central slip to the dorsum of the middle phalanx is damaged, resulting in overactivity of the lateral bands (interosseous and lumbricals). This results in flexion of the PIP joint and extension of the distal interphalangeal (DIP) joint.

The four *lumbrical* muscles arise from the flexor digitorum profundus tendons in the palm of the hand. They are attached to the dorsal expansion (hood) like the interosseous muscles, and they form the lateral bands that insert into the middle and distal phalanges. This enables these muscles to flex the proximal phalanges when the extensor digitorum longus is relaxed and to extend the middle and distal phalanges when the extensor digitorum longus is extending the proximal phalanx. The ulnar nerve supplies the medial lumbricals and the median nerve supplies the lateral two.

Ligaments

Of the many ligaments in the hand, the important ones in athletic injury are:

1. *The ulnar collateral ligament of the thumb.* The collateral ligaments reinforce the capsule on each side of the MP joint of the

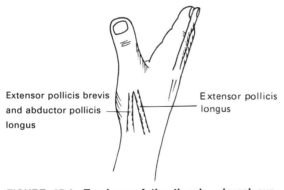

Extensor pollicis brevis and abductor pollicis longus

Extensor pollicis longus

FIGURE 15.4   Tendons of the thumb—dorsal surface

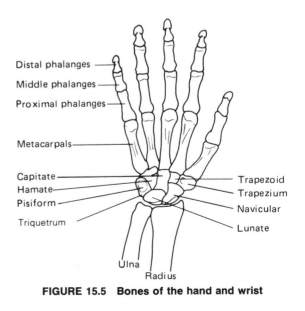

Distal phalanges

Middle phalanges

Proximal phalanges

Metacarpals

Capitate

Hamate

Pisiform

Triquetrum

Trapezoid

Trapezium

Navicular

Lunate

Ulna

Radius

FIGURE 15.5   Bones of the hand and wrist

thumb. They run from the sides of the metacarpal head to the base of the proximal phalanx. There is also an accessory ulnar collateral ligament which links up with the volar plate.

When the thumb is in extension, the accessory ulnar collateral ligament and the volar plate are tight, whereas the ulnar collateral ligament proper becomes tight only when the thumb is flexed (Figure 15.6). Therefore, when one is testing the ulnar collateral ligament for laxity, it is necessary to test with the MP joint in flexion as well as in full extension.

2. *The collateral ligaments and the volar plate of the PIP and the DIP joints of the fingers.* The volar plate and expansion of the joint capsule may be injured if the finger is forced into hyperextension. The collateral ligaments stabilize the interphalangeal joints laterally. If severe lateral stress is placed on the finger, the collateral ligaments tear first, followed by the volar plate.

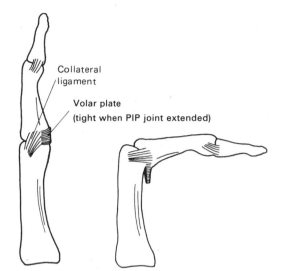

FIGURE 15.7 The collateral ligaments and volar plate of the fingers

Blood Supply

Blood is supplied to the hand by the radial and ulnar arteries. These join to form two arches in the palm: the superficial palmar arterial arch, which is the larger, and the deep palmar arterial arch. The blood supply to the fingers arises from these arches.

Nerve Supply

Dermatomes of the hand. The hand is supplied by three neurological levels: C6, C7, and C8 (see Figure 12.7).

Peripheral nerve supply. The hand is supplied by three nerves: the radial, the median, and the ulnar.

1. *The radial nerve.* The radial nerve supplies sensation to the radial side of the dorsum of the hand. Sensation is best tested between the thumb and the index finger (Figure 15.8). Motor function is tested by extension of the fingers at the MP joints against resistance (Figure 15.9), and by flexion of the elbow against resistance with the forearm in a neutral position (brachioradialis muscle).

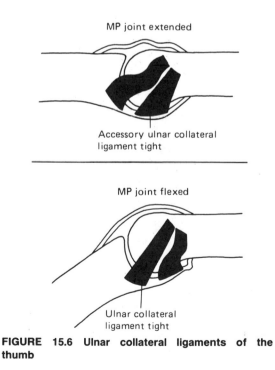

FIGURE 15.6 Ulnar collateral ligaments of the thumb

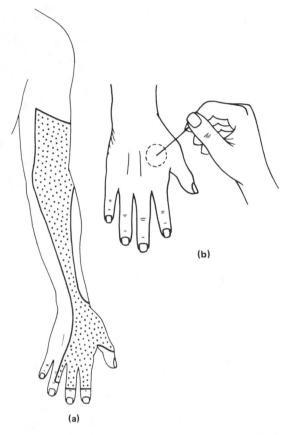

(b)

(a)

FIGURE 15.8 The radial nerve (a) **sensory distribution** (lower forearm dorsally and dorsum of the hand) (b) **sensation test** (dorsum of the hand)

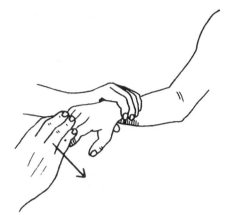

FIGURE 15.9 The radial nerve—motor function test The fingers are extended at the metacarpophalangeal joints against resistance. (Figures 15.9 through 15.14 modified from R. McRae, *Clinical Orthopaedic Examination*, 1976. Printed with permission of Churchill Livingstone, Edinburgh.)

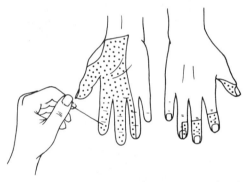

FIGURE 15.10 The median nerve—sensation test

2. *The median nerve.* The median nerve supplies sensation mainly to the radial side of the palm and the fingers, and usually the dorsum of the terminal phalanges of the thumb, the index finger, and the middle finger. Sensation is best tested on the palmar aspect of the index finger (Figure 15.10). To test the motor function of the median nerve, have the athlete resist abduction of the thumb and note the tone of the thenar eminence. This tests the abductor pollicis brevis muscle (Figure 15.11).

3. *The ulnar nerve.* The ulnar nerve supplies sensation to the palmar and dorsal surfaces of the little finger and of the ulnar half of

the ring finger. Sensation is best tested toward the tip of the little finger (Figure 15.12). Muscle tests include adduction (interosseous muscles) and abduction (abductor digiti minimi) of the little finger, adduction of the thumb (adductor pollicis), and abduction of the index finger (first dorsal interosseous) against resistance.

WRIST INJURIES

A diagnosis of a sprained wrist should never be made unless the following conditions have been excluded:

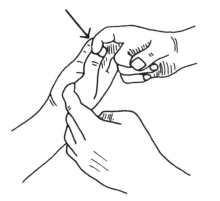

FIGURE 15.11 **The median nerve—motor function test** Test the abductor pollicis brevis by resisting abduction.

1. Fracture of the distal radius (Colles' fracture)
2. Displaced distal radial epiphysis (in an adolescent or pre-adolescent)
3. Fractured navicular (scaphoid)
4. Injury to the distal radio-ulnar joint

Fracture of the Distal Radius (Colles' Fracture)

A Colles' fracture is very common in the general population, but does not occur frequently in athletes. It usually results from a fall on the dorsally flexed hand of an outstretched arm.

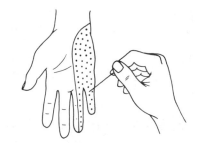

FIGURE 15.12 **The ulnar nerve—sensation test**

SYMPTOMS AND SIGNS: There is usually severe pain, swelling, and deformity in which there is a depression or hollow in the lower third of the forearm, followed by a prominence at the wrist due to the displaced fracture.

TREATMENT:
Initial: Ice, splint, and analgesia.
Definitive: Reduction under anesthesia, followed by immobilization.

Displaced Distal Radial Epiphysis

In the pre-adolescent and the adolescent, the commonest epiphyseal injury involves displacement of the distal radial epiphysis. If this occurs in a child with a fair amount of subcutaneous tissue, the displacement may not be readily visible. For this reason, if a child has tenderness around the wrist after falling, the wrist should be X-rayed.

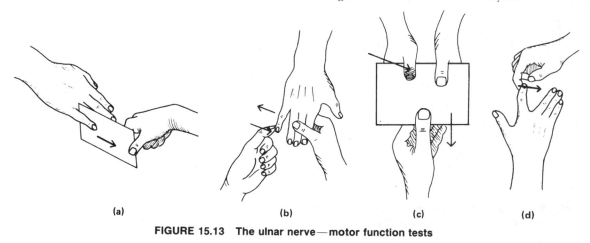

(a)   (b)   (c)   (d)

FIGURE 15.13 **The ulnar nerve—motor function tests**

TREATMENT:

Immediate: Ice, splint, elevation, and analgesia.

Definitive: Reduction if necessary, immobilization for a period of time, depending on the severity of the injury (see Chapter 10).

Fractured Navicular (Scaphoid)

The navicular fracture is notorious for

1. not being readily visible on initial X-rays
2. requiring prolonged immobilization before healing occurs
3. having a high rate of complications, such as nonunion or avascular necrosis

MECHANISM OF INJURY: The fracture is usually due to a fall on the dorsally flexed hand of an outstretched arm.

SYMPTOMS AND SIGNS: Symptoms may be minimal, with little or no swelling. Tenderness is the most important physical finding, being located directly over the navicular ("anatomical snuffbox") (Figure 15.14). A valuable sign is pain in the area of the navicular when the forearm is rotated.

Any athlete who has had a wrist injury and has tenderness in the area of the navicular should be considered to have a fractured navicular until it is proven otherwise. Do not treat this athlete for a sprained wrist. X-rays are mandatory.

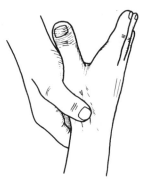

FIGURE 15.14 The "anatomical snuffbox" Tenderness on palpation is highly suggestive of a fractured navicular.

As mentioned, the initial X-rays are frequently negative. In some cases it may be desirable to obtain a tomogram or a bone scan in order to help establish the presence of a fracture. In most cases, tenderness over the navicular dictates that injury be treated as a fractured navicular and the wrist be immobilized. After two weeks the cast is removed and the wrist re-X-rayed.[1]

TREATMENT:

Immediate: Ice, elevation, analgesics, and splinting.

Definitive: A navicular cast is applied, extending from below the elbow to the interphalangeal joint of the thumb, with the wrist in slight radial deviation and dorsiflexion. It is necessary to keep the wrist immobilized until X-rays show the fracture to be healed.

COMPLICATIONS:

1. If the fracture does not mend and the wrist is symptomatic, a bone graft is often necessary.

2. The blood supply to the proximal fragment may be impaired and can result in avascular necrosis (death of the bone due to a lack of blood), which could cause a permanently painful wrist.

Injury to the Distal Radio-Ulnar Joint

MECHANISM OF INJURY: The injury is usually caused by a fall with the wrist hyperextended and the forearm hyperpronated. This results in an injury to the

1. inferior dorsal radio-ulnar ligament
2. ulnar collateral ligament
3. fibrous cartilaginous disc between the ulna and the carpals
4. interosseous membrane

In a mild injury, only the inferior dorsal radio-ulnar ligament is involved, whereas in a severe injury all the structures are damaged.

SYMPTOMS AND SIGNS: Swelling and tenderness are present over the distal radio-ulnar joint, particularly on the dorsal aspect of the wrist. Pain is increased by active and passive pronation. The ulna might be slightly more prominent in some cases, and compressing the distal ulna toward the volar aspect will increase the pain.

X-RAYS: X-rays are frequently interpreted as being normal. However, close inspection may reveal a spread of the distal radio-ulnar joint and possibly some dorsal displacement of the ulna, which can be seen on the lateral view.

TREATMENT: The ulna is reduced by dorsal compression and by supinating the wrist and the forearm. The wrist is held in an above-elbow cast for four weeks or longer.

Rotatory Instability of the Navicular (Scaphoid)

MECHANISM OF INJURY: A fall on the hand of the outstretched arm is the usual cause. The wrist goes into dorsiflexion, and there is damage to the naviculolunate articulation and to the ligaments of the wrist.

SYMPTOMS AND SIGNS: There is pain on dorsiflexion of the wrist, and often a limited range of motion. Tenderness is usually present over the lunate and the naviculolunate joint dorsally. There is frequently a painful click, and occasionally the navicular can be felt to slip as the wrist is moved.

X-RAYS: Special views are usually necessary to confirm the diagnosis. A widening of the space between the lunate and the navicular can be seen on the anteroposterior view.[2]

TREATMENT: Treatment depends on the extent of the instability and on when the diagnosis is made.

Fracture of the Hamate

MECHANISM OF INJURY: Fracture of the hamate is a fairly rare injury that occurs in baseball catchers or tennis players. The fracture is due to repeated trauma to the area, usually of a fairly minor nature (such as holding a tennis racquet or suffering a blow on the hamate from a baseball).[3]

SYMPTOMS AND SIGNS: There is tenderness over the base of the hypothenar eminence, some pain on flexing the fourth and fifth fingers, and possibly a mild ulnar nerve lesion.

X-RAYS: Special X-ray views are often necessary to detect the fracture.

TREATMENT: Surgical treatment is frequently required.

HAND AND FINGER INJURIES

Sprain of the Ulnar Collateral Ligament of the Thumb ("Gamekeeper's Thumb")

An ulnar collateral ligament sprain of the thumb is both a common and an important injury that is often overlooked initially or dismissed as a minor sprain.[4] The ulnar collateral ligament is necessary for the stability of the thumb-index finger pinch. If a tear of the ligament is not diagnosed and adequately treated, the thumb-index finger-pinch ability will be lost and chronic pain will probably

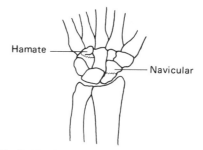

FIGURE 15.15 A diagrammatic representation of fractures of the navicular and hamate

develop at the metacarpophalangeal (MP) joint of the thumb. Instability will be greatest if both the accessory and the ulnar collateral ligament itself are torn. The ligament is most frequently torn at its distal attachment.

MECHANISM OF INJURY: Abduction or hyperextension forces are the usual mechanisms of injury, but damage to the ligament can also occur with a torsion force.

SYMPTOMS AND SIGNS: Pain and swelling are present in the web space at the base of the thumb. There is tenderness over the ulnar collateral ligament and sometimes hemorrhage in the MP joint. Swelling may also be present along the ulnar side of the metacarpal head.

Severe pain is experienced if the examiner attempts to abduct the thumb. Instability will be present if the tear is complete (i.e., a third-degree sprain). It should be remembered that it is necessary to test for instability with the thumb both in extension and in slight flexion, and always to compare the amount of laxity present with that on the opposite side. Very often it will be difficult to assess the degree of laxity because of the pain produced by the stress test, and local anesthesia may have to be administered. The amount of laxity present may be documented by means of X-rays. Arthrography may be useful in confirming the diagnosis in difficult cases.[5,6]

TREATMENT:

Immediate: Ice with some compression, elevation, and splinting of the thumb, usually with tape. Anti-inflammatory medication can be given if necessary.

Definitive: First-degree and mild second-degree sprains are adequately treated with proper taping;[7] the taping can be modified for everyday activity and reinforced for athletic participation (see Figure 5.17). More severe second-degree sprains should be immobilized in a cast for four to six weeks. Third-degree sprains should be treated by early surgery, followed by adequate immo-

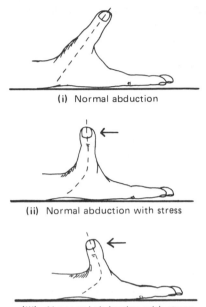

(i) Normal abduction

(ii) Normal abduction with stress

(iii) Abnormal abduction with stress

FIGURE 15.16 Abduction stress test indicating laxity of the ulnar collateral ligament

bilization.[8] When the athlete returns to participation, the thumb should be taped for the first month.

Collateral Ligament Sprain Involving the Proximal Interphalangeal Joint

A proximal interphalangeal joint (PIP) sprain of the collateral ligament is probably the most common athletic injury. It is often mistreated, mainly because of inadequate diagnosis, which may lead to permanent disability with swelling, stiffness, loss of finger movement, and pain.[9]

MECHANISM OF INJURY: The finger is pulled to the side, usually toward ulnar deviation, and any subluxation either reduces spontaneously or is immediately reduced by the athlete.

SYMPTOMS AND SIGNS: Tenderness is present over the collateral ligament involved and over the volar plate. Swelling occurs rapidly.

Stress testing of the PIP joint is usually possible soon after the injury. If the athlete is seen later, however, a local anesthetic should be used at a site proximal to the PIP joint, in order to adequately examine and stress test the ligaments. For complete instability to occur, both the collateral ligament and the volar plate must be torn.[10,11]

DIAGNOSIS:

First-degree sprains do not have any laxity of the collateral ligament, and the X-rays are normal.

Second-degree sprains may have some laxity of the collateral ligament and X-rays are normal.

Third-degree sprains show considerable instability of the joint when stress tested. X-rays reveal an avulsion fracture involving the volar plate.

TREATMENT:

Immediate: Ice and compression should be applied to the involved ligament, and the finger should be splinted. Anti-inflammatory medication should be commenced if necessary.

Definitive: X-rays need to be taken to exclude any fracture or avulsion fracture. The PIP joint is usually immobilized by means of a dorsal splint in 20° to 30° of flexion for three weeks, followed by gentle, active range-of-motion exercises. The finger is then taped to the adjacent finger for the following two to three weeks, and thereafter during all athletic participation for as long as symptoms persist. Surgery is indicated if there is functional instability of the PIP joint or if an avulsion fracture involving 20% or more of the articular surface has occurred.

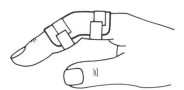

FIGURE 15.17 PIP sprain of the collateral ligaments This may be treated with a dorsal splint. The finger is flexed 20°–30° at the PIP joint, and may be taped to the adjacent finger.

Boutonnière Deformity

The classic boutonnière deformity consists of hyperextension of the metacarpophalangeal (MP) joint, flexion of the proximal interphalangeal (PIP) joint, and hyperextension of the distal interphalangeal (DIP) joint. It results from an injury to the central slip.

MECHANISM OF INJURY: A severe flexion force often causes the injury, though occasionally a direct blow to the PIP joint crushes the central slip.

The PIP joint goes into flexion when the central slip tears, and the lateral bands (hood) then drop anteriorly. This maintains the PIP joint in flexion as the DIP joint is extended.

SYMPTOMS AND SIGNS: There is pain and swelling of the PIP joint. General joint tenderness is present, but specific point tenderness should be looked for over the dorsum of the middle phalanx.

A diagnostic point is that the PIP joint cannot be fully extended. This is often assumed to be due to pain and swelling, so that the diagnosis is missed. A local anesthetic nerve block should be given and the athlete asked to actively extend the PIP joint. If the athlete is unable to fully extend the finger (e.g., there is an extension lag), the diagnosis of a ruptured central slip and a po-

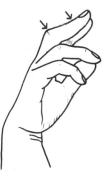

FIGURE 15.18 The Boutonnière deformity The metacarpophalangeal joint is extended, the proximal interphalangeal joint is flexed, and the distal interphalangeal joint is extended.

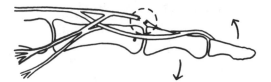

(i) Tearing of the central slip

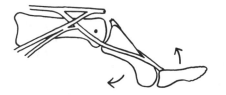

(ii) The extensor hood drops anteriorly, resulting in the PIP joint being held in flexion while the DIP joint is extended.

FIGURE 15.19 The Boutonnière deformity (Modified from R.I. Burton and R.G. Eaton, "Common hand injuries in the athlete," *Orthopedic Clinics of North America* 4:3:812, July, 1973.)

tential boutonnière deformity should be suspected.

Note: Extension of the DIP joint does not usually occur soon after the injury.

TREATMENT:

Immediate: Ice and anti-inflammatory medication should be commenced immediately and the finger splinted.

Definitive: The PIP joint alone is immobilized in full extension for at least eight weeks (Figure 15.20), followed by eight weeks of splinting at night and for athletic participation. The splint should be continued during athletic participation until there is at least 45° of flexion and full extension.

If the diagnosis is missed and the finger is splinted in flexion, the disrupted ends of

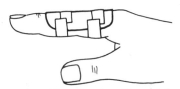

FIGURE 15.20 The Boutonnière deformity The proximal interphalangeal joint is splinted in extension.

the central slip will be held apart. This will only aggravate the condition and establish a deformity. Splinting in as much extension as possible can be tried for awhile to assess the response, but if the extension lag remains, surgical correction should be undertaken.

Pseudo-Boutonnière Deformity

This deformity appears similar to the boutonnière deformity but has a number of differences. It is due to a hyperextension injury (not a flexion injury) to the PIP joint (e.g., a ball striking the end of the finger or a fall on the outstretched finger). The mechanism of injury does not therefore involve the central slip; rather, there is damage to the volar plate. This results in progressive contraction and calcification of the scar tissue that subsequently forms. Radiological evidence of calcification appears three to six months after the injury, usually in the area of the proximal attachment of the volar plate.

TREATMENT: Surgical intervention is often required.

Dislocation of the Metacarpophalangeal Joint

The index finger is most frequently affected. The proximal phalanx is dislocated dorsally on the metacarpal. This is called an "irreducible" dislocation because it often requires open reduction. Immobilization is for three weeks, after which active range of motion is started.

Dislocation of the Metacarpophalangeal Joint of the Thumb

The diagnosis is usually obvious.

TREATMENT:

Immediate: A gentle attempt to reduce the dislocation can be made by a trained physician. If this fails, it should not be repeated. The thumb should be iced, the limb elevated, the athlete transferred for X-rays, and the reduction attempted in a more appropriate setting.

Definitive: After X-raying of the dislocation, a local anesthetic is usually given. Direct traction should not be applied; the
thumb should first be adducted and flexed
across the palm, after which traction usually
reduces the dislocation. The X-rays should
also be taken following the reduction. If attempts at reduction prove unsuccessful, surgery may be necessary. Immobilization is for
three to four weeks, followed by four weeks
of protective taping during athletic participation.

Dislocation of the Proximal Interphalangeal Joint

Dislocation of the PIP joint is usually in a
dorsal direction, that is, the middle phalanx
dislocates dorsally on the proximal phalanx
(rarely in a volar direction). The nature of
this dislocation means there must be either a
tear or an avulsion of the volar plate of the
middle phalanx.

TREATMENT:

Immediate: Reduction is usually relatively
easy. Long-axis traction is applied, together
with gentle hyperextension of the PIP joint.
Following reduction, the joint should be
tested for stability. Ice and a splint should be
applied. The athlete should be sent for X-
rays, to establish whether an avulsion fracture of the volar plate or an articular fracture (which involves the joint) has occurred.

Definitive: Anti-inflammatory medication
should be commenced, and the finger
should be immobilized with the PIP joint in
a position of 20° to 30° of flexion for about
three weeks. This is followed by gentle, active range-of-motion for about three weeks.
The affected finger should be taped to the
adjacent finger for a further two weeks to
keep it immobile. Thereafter, taping should
be continued for athletic participation as
long as there are symptoms.

With a straight dorsal dislocation, the
collateral ligaments are usually intact and so
no collateral instability is present. However,
if a large fracture has occurred which includes the insertion of the collateral ligament, reduction is often unstable and if
functionally unstable, requires surgery.

Dislocation of the Distal Interphalangeal Joint

DIP joint dislocation can be in either a dorsal or a lateral direction or in a combination
of the two. The flexor and the extensor
mechanisms are usually not disrupted.

TREATMENT:

Immediate: Reduction is fairly easily accomplished by gently increasing the deformity while applying traction. Once reduction is
achieved, the joint is usually stable, but it
should be examined both for stability and
for range of motion. If the range of motion
is incomplete, it may indicate that the volar
plate has been entrapped within the joint.
Ice and a splint should be applied and the
athlete referred for X-rays, to exclude any
accompanying fractures.

Definitive: The DIP joint should be
immobilized in a position of function (30° of
flexion) for three weeks, then taped during
athletic participation for at least another
three weeks.

Fractures of the Metacarpals

Fractures of the metacarpals can occur at the

1. base
2. shaft
3. neck

These fractures can be transverse, oblique, or spiral. In addition, there are certain
types (e.g., "boxer's fracture") that can be
impacted.

SYMPTOMS AND SIGNS: The athlete complains of pain and swelling of the hand following the injury. There is tenderness over
the affected metacarpal and crepitation is
elicited in an unstable fracture.

One of the most useful signs for differentiating between a contusion and a fracture is the "percussion" test. In this test the athlete holds the fingers in full extension. The ends of the fingers are firmly percussed, transmitting force down the shaft of the metacarpal and producing pain if a fracture is present (Figure 15.21). The same test can be applied with the fingers flexed while the MP joint is percussed.

Finger alignment should be checked. Most important is nail alignment on flexion of the MP and finger joints. If there is a disturbance in the normal fingernail alignment, a fracture with rotational deformity should be suspected (Figure 15.22). The diagnosis is confirmed by X-ray examination.

TREATMENT:

Immediate: Ice, compression, and elevation of the limb are combined with anti-inflammatory medication if necessary.

Definitive: This varies with the metacarpal involved, the type of fracture, and the amount of displacement or angulation. Generally speaking, the third and fourth metacarpals are usually more stable than the index-finger and the little-finger metacarpals. Immobilization is achieved with the MP joint held in flexion (this allows muscle relaxation because the MP joint is in the position of function). Four or five weeks of immobilization are usually sufficient for healing. Open reduction may be necessary if rotation, shortening, or angulation are detected.

Boxer's fracture is a fracture of the neck of the fifth metacarpal and usually produces

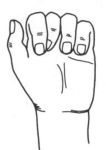

FIGURE 15.22 Rotation of a fractured metacarpal will cause a disturbance in the normal fingernail alignment

a flexion deformity. It usually results from a mistimed punch. Many physicians consider that up to 40° of volar angulation is acceptable for normal functioning, as long as no rotation is present. Some physicians, however, reduce the fracture if less than this. The fracture should be immobilized for four to six weeks.

Fracture-Dislocation of the Base of the First Metacarpal ("Bennett's Fracture")

A fracture-dislocation of the first metacarpal base is really a dislocation in which the small medial fragment of the proximal metacarpal is left in the joint, where it is held by the attachment of the volar ligament. The fracture is very unstable and can usually be diagnosed clinically, and because of this metacarpal instability, maintenance of the reduction may be troublesome. Thus, operative reduction with internal fixation is not uncommon.

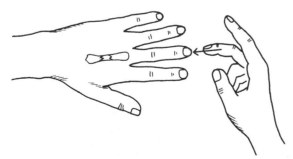

FIGURE 15.21 The percussion test for a suspected fracture of the metacarpal

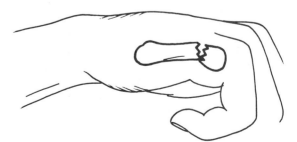

FIGURE 15.23 Fracture of the neck of the fifth metacarpal—the "boxer's fracture"

Fractures of the Proximal Phalanges

The proximal phalanx is fractured more commonly than the other phalanges, usually by a hyperextension force. This fracture is often disabling because of complications.

SYMPTOMS AND SIGNS: The diagnosis may be suspected clinically by the presence of swelling, tenderness, and percussion tenderness. Fingernail alignment should be checked to determine if rotation or angulation has occurred.

TREATMENT:
Immediate: Ice, elevation of the limb, and splinting of the finger are combined with anti-inflammatory medication as required.
Definitive: Since this fracture is frequently unstable, it may have to be surgically immobilized with Kirschner wires (fine wires placed through the bone across the fracture to hold the fragments in place).

COMPLICATIONS: These include rotation, nonunion (if immobilized inadequately), or adherence of adjacent tendons to the healing fracture site. This last complication can limit motion of the finger joints.

Fractures of the Middle Phalanges

Middle phalangeal fractures usually occur in the narrow midshaft and are either transverse or oblique. Diagnosis is based on swelling, local tenderness, possibly crepitus, and percussion tenderness at the end of the extended finger. Rotation should be checked by examining nail alignment. These fractures heal slowly and may require six to eight weeks of immobilization. If unstable, Kirschner wires should be used.

Articular Fractures Involving the Phalangeal Joints

Fractures extending into the joint may require surgery if they involve more than a quarter of the articular surface, if there is displacement of a condylar fracture, or if a volar lip fracture is present.

Fracture-Dislocation of the Volar Lip

A fracture-dislocation usually involves the volar lip of the base of the middle phalanx. There is frequently a history of longitudinal compression force, for example, a ball hitting the fingertip. Some dorsal subluxation of the joint may also occur. If this condition is not adequately diagnosed and treated, permanent stiffness and pain result. Examination usually requires local anesthesia and stress X-rays. If the fracture involves more than approximately 20% of the articular surface, it should be replaced surgically, for it is often found during operation to be considerably larger than expected from the X-rays.[10,11]

Rupture of the Flexor Tendon (Flexor Digitorum Profundus) of the Distal Phalanx

MECHANISM OF INJURY: In a contact sport such as football or rugby, the athlete may grab the opposition's jersey by bringing the fingers into flexion. If the force extending one of the fingers is too great, the attachment of the flexor digitorum profundus may be avulsed from its insertion into the distal phalanx.[12]

SYMPTOMS AND SIGNS: There is pain, swelling, and tenderness of the finger, particularly at the tendon attachment just distal to the DIP joint on the volar surface. Pain and tenderness are felt in the palm if the tendon has retracted, and a small mass can be felt in that area. Ecchymosis can be seen under the skin along the course of the tendon if the athlete is examined a day or two after the injury. The diagnostic feature is an inability to fully flex the DIP joint, particularly when the PIP joint is held in extension (Figure 15.24). An X-ray should be taken to rule out an avulsion fracture.

TREATMENT:
Immediate: Ice, anti-inflammatory medication, and elevation.
Definitive: Surgery as soon after the injury as feasible.

TABLE 15.1 Common Finger Injuries

Mechanism	Injured Structures	Treatment
Injuries to the metacarpophalangeal joint of the thumb Abduction or torsional stress	Ulnar collateral ligaments	First-Degree: Tape Second-Degree: Cast Third-Degree: Surgery
Adduction Direct blow or longitudinal force	Radial collateral ligaments Fracture, proximal phalanx	First- and Second-Degree: Tape Cast
Injuries to the proximal interphalangeal joint Hyperextension	Volar plate Fracture, proximal or middle phalanx	Splint PIP joint in 30° of flexion for 6 weeks
Valgus or varus stress	Collateral ligament with or without the volar plate	Splint PIP joint in 30° flexion, with adjacent fingers as stabilizers, for 6 weeks
Forced flexion or dorsal contusion	Central slip rupture (point tenderness on dorsal surface of middle phalanx—boutonniere deformity)	Splint PIP joint in full extension for 8–16 weeks
Injuries to the distal interphalangeal joint Forced flexion—unable to extend distal phalanx	Attachment of extensor tendon (extensor digitorum—"mallet finger")	Splint DIP joint in extension for 8–16 weeks, occasionally surgery
Forced extension—unable to flex distal phalanx (particularly when PIP joint is held in extension)	Attachment of flexor tendon (flexor digitorum profundus)	Surgery

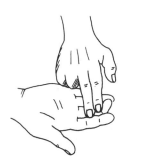

(i) Test for flexor digitorum profundus

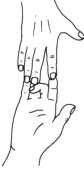

(ii) Test for flexor digitorum sublimis

FIGURE 15.24 Tests for the function of the flexor tendons of the hand (Figures 15.24 and 15.25 modified from R. McRae, *Clinical Orthopaedic Examination*, 1976. Printed with permission of Churchill Livingstone, Edinburgh.)

Acute Mallet Finger

Acute mallet finger (rupture of the extensor tendon of the distal phalanx) can occur in any sport involving catching a ball. The injury is caused by a longitudinal force to the fingertip which occurs when the hand is slightly closed before the ball is caught. The ball therefore strikes the extended finger, forcing it into flexion and avulsing the tendon (extensor digitorum) from the distal phalanx, with or without a piece of bone. The DIP joint thus cannot be fully extended.

SYMPTOMS AND SIGNS: The diagnosis is usually obvious. There is a "dropped finger" and tenderness over the distal phalanx at the attachment of the tendon to the dorsal sur-

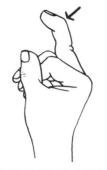

FIGURE 15.25 Mallet finger

face. A secondary reaction can result if the condition is not corrected—the PIP joint may be forced into hyperextension (especially if there are lax ligaments at the PIP joint) as the force of the extensor mechanism is increased due to lack of pull on the distal phalanx. This results in a "swan neck" deformity.

TREATMENT:

Immediate: Treatment is with ice, some compression, splinting of the finger in extension, and anti-inflammatory medication if indicated. An X-ray should be taken to exclude an avulsion fracture.

Definitive: This consists of splinting the DIP joint at 0° of extension. It is not considered necessary to hyperextend the DIP joint, nor to include the PIP joint. Splinting of the DIP joint at 0° should be continued for approximately eight weeks. The splint should not be removed if the joint and distal phalanx are not fully supported, even for a moment. After eight weeks, the splint should be worn only at night and when participating in athletics. This should be continued for at least another six weeks. Surgery should be considered if a large piece of bone is

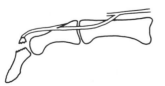

FIGURE 15.26 Mallet finger The extensor tendon itself or the tendon plus a piece of bone may be avulsed.

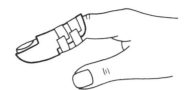

FIGURE 15.27 Mallet finger The distal interphalangeal joint is splinted in extension (0°).

avulsed, particularly if it involves the surface of the joint.

Note: An injury to the PIP joint often co-exists with a mallet finger but is frequently overlooked. When examining a mallet finger, always remember to exclude an injury to the PIP joint.

Tenosynovitis of the Tendons of the Thumb

Inflammation of the tendon sheaths of the extensor pollicis longus, the extensor pollicis brevis, and the abductor pollicis longus (occasionally the extensor digitorum) are particularly common in sports requiring a great deal of wrist action such as in crew or basketball. It occurs especially when the athlete has a deficient technique.

SYMPTOMS AND SIGNS. Pain, swelling, and crepitus along the tendons at the wrist and up the arm are the presenting symptoms. Performance is impaired and there is local tenderness along the tendons. Resistance to abduction and extension of the thumb is frequently painful and weak.

TREATMENT: Ice, immobilization of the wrist and the thumb, and anti-inflammatory medication should be used initially, followed by ultrasound and ice massage. Injection of corticosteriods under the tendon sheath (but not into the tendon) may prove beneficial if a more conservative regime does not work. When the athlete returns to participation, the coach should attempt to correct the faulty technique.

Lacerations

A laceration that involves the hand should not be passed off as a minor injury. It should be taken seriously, and the nerve and tendon function should be carefully checked (see tendon and nerve tests of the hand, p. 231). If there is any doubt as to the integrity of either of these structures, an orthopedic or hand surgeon should be consulted immediately. Standard antiseptic management should be applied before referral.

"Bowler's Thumb"

Bowler's thumb (perineural fibrosis of the ulnar digital nerve) is found in tenpin bowlers, who constantly irritate the ulnar digital nerve of the thumb when placing it within the thumbhole of the ball. Some of these athletes have transient symptoms which subside when bowling is curtailed, but others have permanent damage to the nerve.[13,14] Enlarging the thumbhole and/or padding the thumb are useful for preventing or decreasing symptoms. However, if symptoms do not subside, surgical exploration of the nerve may be indicated.

"Handlebar Palsy"

Handlebar palsy occurs in cyclists, who present with motor weakness involving the ulnar innervated muscles of the hand. There are minimal sensory findings. It results from repeated irritation of the deep branch of the ulnar nerve just distal to the canal of Guyon. Prevention of this condition consists of applying sufficient padding to the handlebars and changing the position of the hand at frequent intervals while cycling.[15,16]

Subungual Hematoma (Bleeding Under the Nail)

A hematoma can develop under the nail of a finger or toe following localized trauma to that area. This is an exceptionally painful condition, due to the sensitivity of the subungual nerve endings to any increased

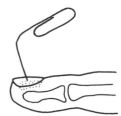

FIGURE 15.28 Releasing a subungual hematoma with a heated paper clip

pressure. As the pressure increases, the pain is accentuated by throbbing that interferes with the athlete's rest.

TREATMENT: Following trauma to a nail, the area should be iced continuously for a number of hours in the hope of preventing the development of a hematoma under the nail.

Once blood is present it should be released. The old technique is to use the straightened end of a paper clip, which is heated until red hot and then immediately placed end-on against the nail. The heat rapidly and painlessly produces a hole in the nail and so releases the entrapped blood.

If a hot paper clip seems objectionable, a wide-bore needle (No. 18) can be used. The needle is rotated like a drill bit, and if done gently, may be an adequate, though time consuming, technique. A number of holes should be made to ensure complete release of all the entrapped blood and serous fluid. The nail should be cleaned with an antiseptic solution, and antibiotic ointment applied for the following few days.

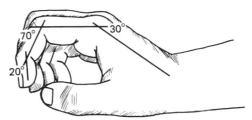

FIGURE 15.29 The so-called "position of function" of the hand

REFERENCES

1. Leslie IJ, Dickson RA: The fractured carpal scaphoid. *J Bone Joint Surg* 63B:225–230, 1981.

2. Mayfield JK, Johnson RP, Kilkoyne RK: Carpal dislocations: Pathomechanics and progressive perilunar instability. *J Hand Surg* 5:226–241, 1980.

3. Stark HH, Jobe FW, Boyes JH, et al: Fracture of the hook of the hamate in athletes. *J Bone Joint Surg* 59A:575–582, 1977.

4. McCue FC, Hakala MW, Andrews JR, et al: Ulnar collateral ligament injuries of the thumb in athletes. *Am J Sports Med* 2:70–80, 1974.

5. Engel J, Ganel A, Ditzian R, et al: Arthrography as a method of diagnosing tear of the ulnar collateral ligament of the metacarpophalangeal joint of the thumb ("Gamekeeper's thumb"). *J Trauma* 19:106–109, 1979.

6. Bowers WH, Hurst LC: Gamekeeper's thumb. Evaluation by arthrography and stress roentgenography. *J Bone Joint Surg* 59A:519–524, 1977.

7. Rovere GD, Gristina AG, Stolzer WA, et al: Treatment of gamekeeper's thumb in hockey players. *J Sports Med* 3:147–151, 1975.

8. Sakellarides HT: Treatment of recent and old injuries of the ulnar collateral ligament of the MP joint of the thumb. *Am J Sports Med* 6:255–262, 1978.

9. McCue FC, Andrews JR, Hakala M: The coach's finger. *J Sports Med* 2:270–275, 1974.

10. Melchionda AM, Linburg RM: Volar plate injuries. *Phys Sportsmed* 10:77–84, January 1982.

11. Bowers WH, Fajgenbaum DM: Closed rupture of the volar plate of the distal interphalangeal joint. *J Bone Joint Surg* 61A:146, 1979.

12. Reef TC: Avulsion of the flexor digitorium profundus. An athletic injury. *Am J Sports Med* 5:281–285, 1977.

13. Howell AE, Leach RE: Bowler's thumb: Perineural fibrosis of the digital nerve. *J Bone Joint Surg* 52A:379–381, 1970.

14. Dobyns JH, O'Brien ET, Linscheid RL, et al: Bowler's thumb: Diagnosis and treatment. Review of seventeen cases. *J Bone Joint Surg* 54A:751–755, 1972.

15. Burke ER: Ulnar neuropathy in bicyclists. *Phys Sportsmed* 9:52–56, April 1981.

16. Smail DF: Handlebar palsy. Letter to editor in *New Eng J Med* 292:322, 1975.

RECOMMENDED READINGS

Burton RI, Eaton RG: Common hand injuries in the athlete. *Orthop Clin North Am* 4:809–839, 1973.

Dobyns JH, Simm FH, Linscheid RL: Sports stress syndromes of the hand and wrist. *Am J Sports Med* 6:236–254, 1978.

MacCollum MS: Protecting upper extremity injuries in sport. *Phys Sportsmed* 8:59–64, July 1980.

McCue FC, Bangher WH, Kulund DN, et al: Hand and wrist injuries in the athlete. *Am J Sports Med* 7:275–286, 1979.

Ruby LK: Common hand injuries in the athlete. Symposium on sports injuries. *Othop Clin North Am* 11:819–839, 1980.

CHAPTER 16

Cervical and Thoracic Spine Injuries

ANATOMY

The *vertebral column* consists of 24 movable vertebrae (7 cervical, 12 thoracic, and 5 lumbar) and numerous fixed vertebrae (5 sacral and a number of coccygeal bones). It is rigid enough to support the body and protect the spinal cord, yet flexible enough to permit a wide variety of movements. This flexibility is largely due to the *intervertebral discs* between all the movable vertebrae (except the first two cervical vertebrae) and to the angle of articulation of the facet joints in the different areas of the vertebral column (see section on functional anatomy of the lumbar spine, p. 267).

Each region of the spine (i.e., the cervical, thoracic and lumbar regions) has its own characteristics. There are also smaller differences within each region.

The *spinal cord* is enclosed within the bony spinal canal. Nerve roots emerge from the spinal cord through the superior portions of the intervertebral foramina which are formed by the pedicles of two adjacent vertebrae (Figure 16.3).

Cervical Vertebrae

Cervical vertebrae are the smallest in the spinal column. They are oblong, and broader from side to side than from front to back. The transverse foramen contains the vertebral artery (Figure 16.4).

The first cervical vertebra is the *atlas*, which articulates with the skull. The atlas has no body, but is pierced by the odontoid process of the second cervical vertebra, the *axis*. This odontoid process allows the head and the atlas to rotate by pivoting on the articular facets of the axis (Figure 16.5).

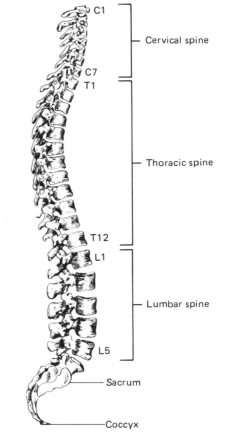

FIGURE 16.1 The spinal column (from the side)

246

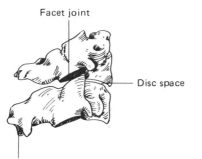

Facet joint

Disc space

Spinous process

FIGURE 16.2 Lateral view of two cervical vertebrae —note angle of facet joints

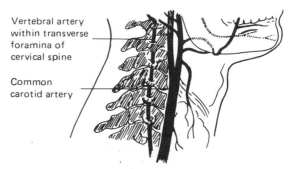

Vertebral artery within transverse foramina of cervical spine

Common carotid artery

FIGURE 16.4 The anatomy of the vertebral artery in the neck

The seven cervical vertebrae normally form a gentle curve which is convex anteriorly. When injured, the paravertebral muscles go into spasm and eliminate the curve. An excessive curve can indicate poor posture of the entire vertebral column and pelvis.

Ligaments

The main ligaments are:

1. *Ligamentum flavum*: Contains much elastin, which gives it its yellowish color. It is able to stretch and contract, unlike most other ligaments. It secures the lamina of the adjacent vertebrae and prevents excessive motion of one vertebra upon another. Another of its important functions is to main-

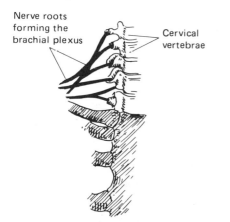

Nerve roots forming the brachial plexus

Cervical vertebrae

FIGURE 16.3 Nerve roots emerging through the intervertebral foramina of the cervical spine

tain the tension on the capsule of the facet joint, thus helping to keep the capsule from becoming trapped within the joint.

2. *Ligamentum nuchae*: Runs from the external occipital protuberance to the posterior spinous processes of the seven cervical vertebrae, after which it becomes the supraspinous and interspinous ligaments. It separates the muscles of the posterior portion of the neck at the midline.

3. *Alar ligaments*: These are strong ligaments that link the skull with the axis. They help to control lateral flexion and rotation, but do not restrain flexion or extension in normal circumstances.

4. *Transverse ligament of the atlas*: This ligament runs horizontally from one side of the atlas to the other. It holds the odontoid process against the anterior arch of the atlas.

5. *Posterior longitudinal ligament*: Attaches to the posterior surface of all the cervical vertabrae and intervertebral discs. It forms the tectorial membrane which helps hold the skull on the atlas and axis.

Cervical Muscles

Because the neck combines extreme mobility with necessary protection of the spinal cord, there is an intricate interdigitation of the muscles that help to support and protect the neck. There is a synergistic use of the muscles so that movement and support can occur at the same time. Some of the important

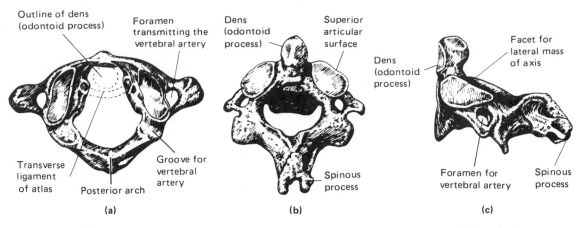

FIGURE 16.5 (a) Looking down on the superior aspect of the atlas (first cervical vertebra) (b) Looking down (and slightly obliquely) on the superior aspect of the axis (second cervical vertebra) (c) Lateral view of the axis

muscles associated with movement of the cervical spine include:

1. *Longissimus cervicis*: From the transverse processes of the fourth and fifth thoracic vertebrae. Inserts at the transverse process of the second through sixth cervical vertebrae. *Function*: Extends the neck.

2. *Longissimus capitis*: From the transverse processes of the fourth and fifth thoracic vertebrae. Inserts at the mastoid process of the temporal bone. *Function*: Extends the neck and rotates the head.

3. *Splenius capitis*: From the lower half of the ligamentum nuchae and the spines of C7 through T8. Inserts into the mastoid process.

4. *Splenius cervicis*: From the spines of T3 to T6. Inserts into the transverse processes of C1 through C3.

Function of the splenii muscles includes extension of the neck when the two sides work together. When one side acts separately, the head is drawn to one side and the face is rotated to the same side.

5. *Iliocostalis cervicis*: From the angles of the first six ribs. Inserts into the transverse processes of the fourth through sixth cervical vertebrae. *Function*: Extends the neck.

6. Other muscles involved in neck movements are:
   a. Trapezius
   b. Levator scapulae
   c. Sternocleidomastoideus

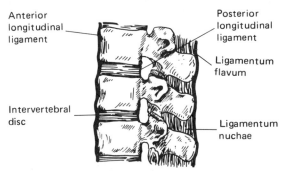

FIGURE 16.6 Schematic representation of the ligaments of the cervical spine

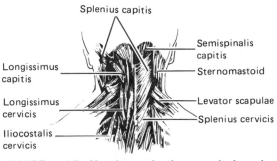

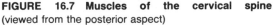

FIGURE   16.7 Muscles of the cervical spine (viewed from the posterior aspect)

Nerve Plexuses of the Cervical Spine

There are two plexuses that arise from the cervical spine. The *cervical plexus* is formed from the anterior rami of C1, C2, C3, and C4 and has three major branches, the *cutaneous*, the *motor*, and the *phrenic*. The *brachial plexus* arises from the anterior rami of C5, C6, C7, C8, and T1, and provides the nerve supply to the upper extremities. The brachial plexus consists of roots that join together to form trunks and then divide to form the cords of the brachial plexus. From these cords arise the *ulnar*, the *radial*, the *median*, and the *musculocutaneous* nerves.

Circulation

The neck contains the vital arteries that supply the brain. Anterior are the external and internal carotid arteries, while the vertebral arteries run posteriorly within the vertebrae.

Thoracic Vertebrae

The thoracic spine is part of the bony cage that encloses the heart, the aorta, the lungs, and other vital structures. Thoracic verte-brae are larger than cervical vertebrae and have a long spinous process which points downward. Each thoracic vertebra (except the eleventh and twelfth) articulates with a rib on each side by means of three articular facets, one of which is located on the transverse process and two on the vertebral body itself. Therefore, each thoracic vertebra that articulates with a rib has six articular facets (Figure 16.9).

Thoracic Muscles

Some of the muscles surrounding the thoracic spine are:

1. *Spinalis thoracis*: Originates from the spinous processes of the upper lumbar and lower thoracic vertebrae and runs to the spines of the upper thoracic vertebrae. *Function*: Extends the thoracic spine.

2. *Longissimus thoracis*: Originates from the transverse processes of the lumbar vertebrae and lumbosacral fascia and inserts into the transverse processes of all the thoracic and upper lumbar vertebrae and the ninth and tenth ribs. *Function*: Extends the thoracic vertebrae.

3. *Iliocostalis thoracis*: Runs from the upper border of the angle of the lower six ribs to the angles of the upper six ribs. *Function*: Helps keep the thoracic spine erect.

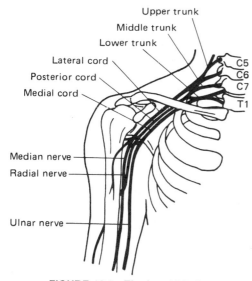

FIGURE 16.8 The brachial plexus

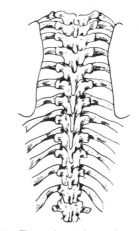

FIGURE 16.9 Thoracic spine—from the back— showing the costovertebral articulations

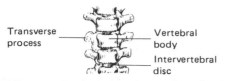

Transverse process — Vertebral body — Intervertebral disc

FIGURE 16.10 Thoracic vertebrae—from the front

4. *Other muscles*: Also involved with the movement of the thoracic spine are the *rhomboid major* and *minor*, the *trapezius*, the *serratus anterior*, and the *latissimus dorsi*.

INJURIES TO THE NECK

The Mechanism of Cervical Injuries

Cervical spine injuries usually result from the neck being forced into hyperflexion, or less commonly, hyperextension, often with rotation.[1] Axial loading is also considered to be a cause in some cases.[2] In football, where the mechanics have been well documented, injuries occur by one of the following mechanisms: the head or face mask is struck by the knee; the face mask is grabbed by an opponent; the athlete receives a karate-type blow; or, most frequently, the athlete lowers his or her head when making contact with an opponent. A number of serious injuries, including quadriplegia and paraplegia, have occurred in recent years from the athlete's using the head as a battering ram, with the crown of the head making contact with the top of the helmet. This action transmits forces axially through the spine.

Most severe injuries from hyperflexion and hyperextension (with or without rotation) result in cord damage from a fracture, a dislocation, or both. Injuries from axial loading usually occur at the level of the third and fourth cervical vertebra. They include acute rupture of the disc between C3 and C4, anterior subluxation of C3 and C4, or unilateral or bilateral dislocation of the joints between the articular processes.[2]

Occasionally a cervical spinal cord injury occurs without a fracture or a dislocation and is thought to be the result of a vascular injury. In the less severe cases, the lesion usually consists of sprained cervical ligaments, with secondary muscle spasm.

Prevention of Neck Injuries

The main *functions* of the cervical portion of the spine are

1. protection of the spinal cord
2. mobility
3. stability

Since mobility is one of the main requirements of the cervical spine, stability suffers. When stability suffers, the spinal cord is placed at increased risk. It is therefore imperative that an athlete engaging in a contact sport use all available methods to strengthen the muscles and ligaments supporting the cervical vertebrae. At the same time, appropriate measures must be taken to decrease the possibility of injury to this area.

The next three topics relate to the prevention of neck injuries.

Neck musculature. Strength, power, and endurance of the neck musculature should be maintained year round, particularly for athletes in contact sports. Too often one sees the big linemen improving their neck musculature while the defensive backs do not consider this necessary. Statistics have shown that it is the thinner, lighter, and speedier defensive back and wide receiver who have the greatest incidence of quadriplegia and paraplegia following neck injuries in football.[3]

Athletes with long necks are theoretically more at risk than those with short thick necks. However, it is not only the length of the neck that is important, but also the ability to fully contract the muscles at the appropriate time (proprioceptive awareness).

Some exercises that should be performed throughout the year by all athletes in contact activities (see section on neck rehabilitation, p. 261) include:

1. Isometric resistance—resistance to flexion, extension, lateral flexion, and rotation

at various angles throughout the range of movement.

2. Manual resistance using a partner—a full range of flexion, extension, lateral flexion, and rotation while the partner applies resistance (Figure 16.11).

3. Isokinetic-type resistance (e.g., Mini-

Gym)—flexion, extension, and lateral flexion exercises.

4. Weighted football helmet, neck harness, or spring resistance—flexion, extension, lateral flexion, and circular motions (see Figure 16.19).

5. Bridging—using the *back of the head*—is

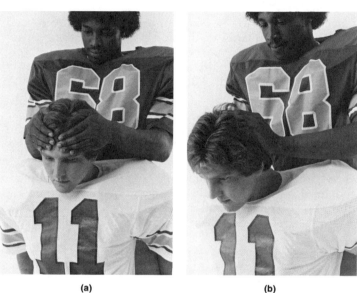

(a)   (b)

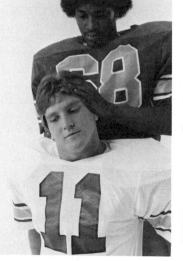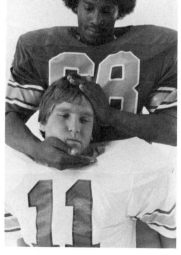

(c)   (d)

FIGURE 16.11 Isometric neck-strengthening exercises (a) Resisting neck flexion (b) Resisting neck extension (c) Resisting lateral flexion (d) Resisting rotation

useful for athletes in wrestling and other contact sports and should be part of the prevention exercise program (see Figure 16.20).

6. Shoulder shrugs—important mainly for the trapezius muscles. They can either be done with free weights or, more easily, using the bench-press bars on the Universal gym (see Figure 16.21).

7. Nautilus equipment—a series of machines using variable isotonic resistance for flexion, extension, lateral flexion, rotation, and shoulder shrugs. These machines are considered to give an excellent neck-muscle workout (Figure 16.12). It is recommended that exercises on these machines be performed slowly, with no more than three workouts per week.

Technique.

1. *Football.* The protection afforded by the helmet has unfortunately allowed the head to be used as a weapon, exposing the neck

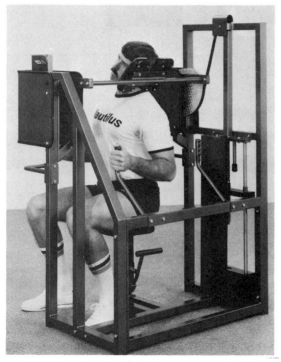

FIGURE 16.12 Nautilus four-way neck machine

to unphysiological forces. This danger should be emphasized to the athlete and the correct techniques of blocking and tackling pointed out. Spearing in any form should not be tolerated.[4] Coaches should emphasize the importance of keeping the paracervical musculature "on guard" (shoulder-shrug position) so an unexpected blow will not catch the neck unprotected.

2. *Rugby.* Neck injuries in rugby are related primarily to the collapse of the scrum, placing the hooker at risk.[5,6,7] If a team purposely collapses the scrum, they should be heavily penalized. The high tackle may also injure the neck.[8]

3. *Wrestling.* Neck injuries in wrestling occur mostly from slamming the opponent onto the mat. The official should disqualify any wrestler who performs this maneuver.[9]

4. *Falling techniques.* Correct falling techniques should be taught so they become automatic and routine for all participants in any sport where a fall from a height might occur.

Equipment.

1. *Football.*

   a. *Helmet*: Experiments are being undertaken to change the helmet to afford adequate head protection yet discourage its use as a weapon. This should save opponents from injuries and save offenders from possible cervical damage.

   b. *Face mask*: "Face-masking" is illegal but occurs with some frequency. Fortunately, very few injuries occur from such a maneuver. Many observers see the face mask as being responsible for the development of an attitude of invulnerability because of the protection it affords. Some authorities feel that removing the face mask would discourage overaggressive use of the head in blocking and tackling and would thereby decrease the chances of serious cervical injury (though the incidence of less serious but potentially disfiguring facial injuries could well increase).

c. *Neck collar*: An appropriately designed and well-fitted neck collar prevents lateral flexion and hyperextension injuries. This is probably as much due to proprioceptive feedback and muscular contraction as to the actual physical limitation of movement by the collar.

d. *Restrictive straps*: Some college teams are utilizing a method of strapping the helmet to the shoulder pads in front, behind, and at the sides, to limit extremes of neck movement.[10] This might help decrease the incidence of recurrent brachial plexus lesions and the chance of serious spinal cord injury.

2. *Gymnastics and wrestling mats.* Mats used in gymnastics and wrestling should give athletes adequate protection for the particular maneuver they are undertaking. It is the coach's responsibility to ensure that the mats give sufficient protection for the purpose for which they are being used. It might mean, for example, that with certain new or difficult maneuvers on the balance beam, the mats should be piled to a height almost parallel to the beam. A foam-filled "pit" should be used for learning new "tricks," so confidence can be developed and mistakes made without the intervention of injury.

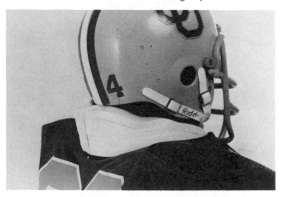

FIGURE 16.13 Football neck-collar

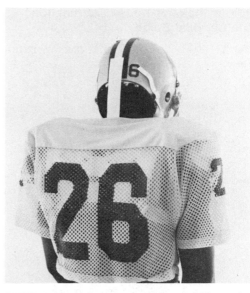

FIGURE 16.14 Helmet-to-shoulder pad strap to restrict excessive neck flexion and extension. These have been used experimentally by some college teams in an attempt to decrease the incidence of neck injuries.

Tragedies from improper use of the trampoline have resulted in the American Academy of Pediatrics issuing a statement urging that the trampoline be banned.[11,12] Suggestions have been made about the safe use of the trampoline,[13] including:

1. The potential for severe injuries on the trampoline should be recognized, and all participants should be well coached before they use the apparatus.

2. All trampolines should be locked when they are not in use.

3. Proper specifications for trampoline equipment should be made including frame, pads, and safety spotting decks.

4. The six basic learning positions should be mastered early.

5. The gymnast should proceed in a systematic progression of twist routines as his or her ability improves.

6. There should be no somersaults in any basic physical education class or tricks requiring inversion of the head. The use of the trampoline should always be elective.

Office or Training-Room Examination of the Cervical Spine

With the athlete sitting on the examination table:

1. Palpate tenderness of the
   a. spinous processes
   b. transverse processes
   c. muscles
   d. brachial plexus—roots and trunks

2. Check active voluntary range of motion (Figure 16.15)
   a. flexion
   b. extension
   c. lateral flexion to both sides
   d. rotation to both sides
   e. circle left and right

3. Check sensation (see Figure 12.7)
   a. occipital area and angle of the jaw (C2, C3)

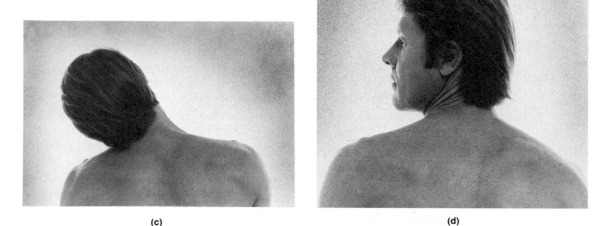

FIGURE 16.15 **Neck range-of-motion**   (a) Flexion   (b) Extension   (c) Lateral flexion   (d) Rotation

b. supraclavicular area (C4)
c. lateral aspect of the shoulder (axillary nerve patch)
d. lateral upper arm (C5)
e. lateral forearm, thumb, and index finger (C6)
f. middle finger—palmar aspect (C7)
g. little finger and ring finger—palmar aspects (C8)
h. medial side of forearm and elbow (T1)
4. Check reflexes
    a. biceps (C5, C6)
    b. supinator (C5, C6)
    c. triceps (C7, C8)
5. Check strength—tested against isometric resistance
    a. neck flexion—chin tuck (C1, C2)
    b. extension (C1–C2)
    c. lateral flexion (C3)
    d. shoulder shrugs (C4)
    e. resistance to elbow flexion, elbow at 90° (C5)
    f. resistance to elbow extension, elbow at 90° (C6)
    g. resistance to wrist extension (C7)
    h. resistance to thumb extension (C8)
    i. resistance to finger opening and closing (T1)

If there is no evidence of neurological deficit and X-rays are normal, test strength of full range of neck movement against resistance.

On-Field Management of a Neck Injury

When dealing with a potential neck injury, the trainer must be aware that the spinal cord may be involved. It is essential that a pre-established plan be developed so the injury can be dealt with in the most satisfactory manner. The following points should be considered by anyone likely to be faced with this situation:

1. Keep an airway and resuscitative equipment on hand during practice and participation in a contact sport.

2. If there is any question as to the seriousness of a cervical injury, always assume that the *most serious* injury has occurred. This approach may result in some relatively minor injuries being dramatized. On the other hand, if a serious injury is neglected, it could cost a life or cause permanent paralysis.

3. Designate a leader to be in charge of evaluation, decision making, and removal of the athlete from the field. Evaluation and removal from the field of play may hold up the event for a period of time. This should not influence the attitude of the examiner, who must be unhurried in the evaluation and beyond reproach in the removal of the athlete from the field.

4. A neck injury that at first seemed to be minor may become complicated later on by some inadvertent movement. It is therefore imperative that any neck injury be thoroughly evaluated and followed. This will help eliminate the tragedies that do occur after the athlete has left the field.

Sideline Evaluation of a "Minor Neck Injury"

These are minor injuries involving the neck, with which the athlete is allowed to walk off the field.

1. Repeat questions about tingling, burning,[14] numbness, or weakness.

2. Ask the athlete to localize the area of discomfort.

3. Check grip strength and leg power.

4. Check sensation along dermatome areas of neck, shoulder, upper arm, forearm, hand, trunk, and legs.

5. Check reflexes of biceps, triceps, supinators, finger flexion, and the patella.

6. If all the above are normal and symmetrical, remove the helmet (if one is worn).[15]

7. Check for tenderness and deformity in the neck area.

8. Ask the athlete to move the neck through a voluntary (active) range of move-

TABLE 16.1   On-Field Evaluation of a Potentially Serious Neck Injury (with particular reference to football)

Athlete Unconscious	Athlete Conscious
1. Assume athlete has *neck injury* in addition to head injury. 2. Check airway. If impaired, cut face mask with bolt cutters or similar tool. Do not remove helmet. Stabilize head and neck. Do not hyperextend neck but bring jaw forward. Insert airway or supply oxygen. 3. Check pulse. If not present, commence CPR with head and neck stabilized. 4. Check blood pressure. 5. Check pupils. 6. Remove from field • on spine board • head and neck stabilized If in any doubt, obtain help from trained EMTs in removing athlete from field.	1. Ask athlete a. Where is the injury? b. Is there any neck pain? c. Is there any tingling, burning, or numbness down the limbs? d. Is there any difficulty with breathing? e. Any problem in moving the limbs? 2. *If any of above are present,* treat as potentially serious neck injury (i.e., take off field on spine board with head and neck stabilized). Do not allow athlete to sit up, stand up, or walk off until thoroughly evaluated. 3. *If neck pain only* (i.e., no limb tingling, burning, numbness, weakness, or difficulty with breathing), check for posterior neck tenderness and deformity (do not remove helmet or move neck). Check for deficiency in grip strength and leg power. 4. *If above are negative,* ask athlete to put neck through voluntary range of movement (flexion, extension, lateral flexion, and rotation). Ask if there is any tingling, burning, or numbness in limbs with any neck movement. 5. *If any are positive,* suspect a neck injury. Remove from field on spine board with head and neck stabilized. 6. *If above are satisfactory,* athlete can walk off the field. Evaluate fully at sideline.

ment (flexion and extension, lateral flexion, and rotation).

9. If the active motion is normal and relatively painless, test these movements against resistance; also test power of shoulder shrugs.

10. Perform the compression test. With the chin directed toward the supraclavicular fossa, apply a compressive force downwards on the head. Any pain in the neck or any radiation of pain down the arm produces a positive test, suggesting a cervical disc protrusion or rupture.

11. If the athlete has normal neck muscle power, a full range of motion, no pain with any maneuver, and no tingling, burning, numbness, or weakness of any limb, a minor neck injury can be assumed. Return to participation can be permitted.

Spinal Cord "Concussion"

A "concussion" of the spinal cord implies a temporary paraplegia or quadriplegia with complete recovery. The mechanisms that can cause spinal cord concussion are the same as those that result in more serious injury with permanent spinal cord damage. Possible causes include:

1. Vertebral impingement of the spinal cord, with or without sprain of the ligaments (see Cervical Stenosis, p. 258)

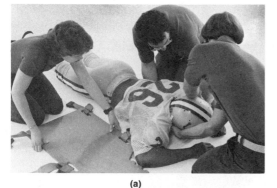

(a)

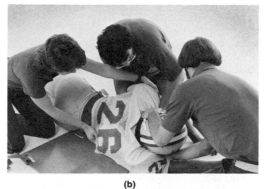

(b)

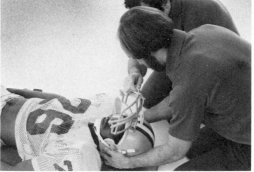

(c)

(d)

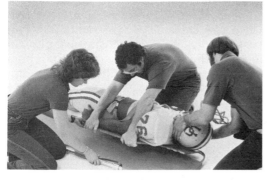

(e)

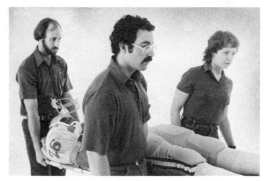

(f)

FIGURE 16.16 Removal of a player with a suspected neck injury from the field

(a) A leader should be designated. He or she should control the position of the head and neck, and apply traction.

(b) The leader directs the other members of the team. The injured player is carefully rolled onto the spine board. The leader continues to apply traction to the neck.

(c) The face mask may need to be removed. The is accomplished either by using a bolt-cutter, or if the face mask is fastened to the helmet by rubber ties, these may be cut by using a sharp penknife.

(d) The face mask is then removed and an airway inserted if necessary.

(e) Secure the player to the spine board, and place on a stretcher. The neck should be controlled, or secured by means of straps.

(f) Place sand-bags on each side of the head to control its position, or secure the head with straps. Under the direction of the leader, the player is lifted and carried off the field for further evaluation or transportation by ambulance.

TABLE 16.2   Criteria for Return to Activity After a Neck Injury

1. Minimal or no neck tenderness
2. Full, voluntary active range of motion
3. Normal and symmetrical neck muscle power when neck movements are tested against resistance—with no pain
4. Normal and symmetrical limb power, sensation, and reflexes
5. No tingling, burning, or numbness in any limb

2. Anterior spinal artery compression or impingement

3. Protruded or ruptured intervertebral disc

Cervical Stenosis

The term *cervical stenosis* implies a narrowing of the spinal canal, usually the mid-cervical area. This narrowing is due to a developmental abnormality and probably predisposes an athlete to a spinal cord injury.[16] Hyperextension force is the usual mechanism of injury when cervical stenosis is present, though some cases may be due to hyperflexion. The athlete presents with paraplegia or quadriplegia which may be temporary or permanent.

The diagnosis is made on examination of the lateral X-ray or by means of computerized axial tomograms (CAT) scan. The width of the spinal canal should not be less than 14.5 mm for vertebrae C3, C4, C5, and C6. If it is less than this, the diagnosis of cervical stenosis should be considered. An athlete who is discovered to have cervical stenosis after recovering from an episode of paraplegia or quadriplegia should be advised to refrain from contact sports, as continued activity might result in permanent quadriplegia or even death.

Contusions to the Posterior Cervical Spine

1. *Involving muscle*: A contusion to the posterior muscle group is usually painful and causes varying degrees of muscle spasm.

Treatment should be with ice, anti-inflammatory medication if indicated, and active range-of-motion exercises when the initial spasm has subsided. Inappropriately or inadequately treated contusions to this area can result in the formation of calcification within the hematoma in the muscle. A blow to this area may also be associated with a sprain or strain, which can further complicate the contusion.

2. *Involving bone*: The posterior spinous process of one or more cervical vertebrae may be fractured from a direct blow to that area or from an avulsion fracture caused by sudden contraction of the neck muscles when, for instance, the head or neck is forceably struck.

Contusions to the Anterior Neck and Throat

A contusion anteriorly to the larynx and/or trachea usually results in severe distress, apprehension, aphonia (inability to talk), and some dyspnea (shortness of breath) lasting for a few seconds. These symptoms should pass rapidly, and relatively normal phonation and breathing should return within a minute or two. If they do not, then a severe injury to the larynx and trachea should be suspected, and the athlete should be immediately referred to a laryngologist.

Pinched-Nerve Syndrome

SYNONYMS: Nerve pinch, burner, stinger, nerve stretch.

ETIOLOGY: A pinched-nerve syndrome can result from one or more of the following causes:

1. Brachial plexus lesions—This is thought to be the most frequent cause. Commonly, the head is forced to one side while the opposite shoulder is depressed. This usually affects the upper trunk of the brachial plexus.[17] However, there are many variations such as stretching, contusing, or, rarely, tearing of

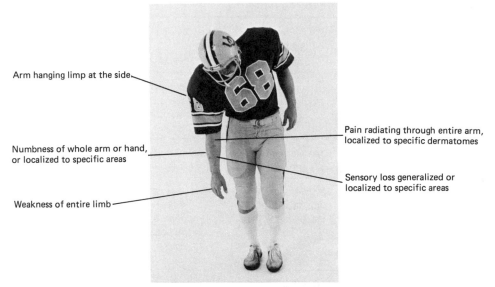

Arm hanging limp at the side

Numbness of whole arm or hand, or localized to specific areas

Weakness of entire limb

Pain radiating through entire arm, localized to specific dermatomes

Sensory loss generalized or localized to specific areas

FIGURE 16.17   Football player with a "pinched-nerve" lesion

the brachial plexus. Occasionally the plexus is compressed between the clavicle and the first rib, particularly when the shoulder is abducted and the neck extended.

2. Entrapment of the nerve root or roots in the spinal column—A hyperextension or hyperflexion injury can cause subluxation of the facets, resulting in entrapment of a nerve root.

3. Protruded or ruptured intervertebral disc—This can result in a combined spinal cord and nerve root lesion, though it is an uncommon mechanism of injury.

4. Combination of nerve root and brachial plexus lesion—The cervical nerves pass almost horizontally through the nerve root canals and are therefore subject to traction injuries.

TABLE 16.3   Differentiation between Brachial Plexus and Nerve Root Lesions

Brachial Plexus Lesions	*Nerve Root Lesions*
1. Numbness and burning of entire arm, hand, and fingers.	1. Numbness and burning confined to one or more definable dermatomes.
2. Sensation loss over two to four dermatomes.	2. Sensation loss confined to a definable dermatome.
3. Complete transient paralysis of arm.	3. Partial transient paralysis of arm.
4. Tenderness over brachial plexus.	4. No tenderness over brachial plexus.
5. No tenderness over neck posteriorly.	5. Tenderness over neck posteriorly.
6. Increase in symptoms with passive movement of head and neck to *opposite side*.	6. Hyperflexion, extension, or lateral flexion of neck to *same side* as the symptoms may cause symptoms.
7. Symptoms do not occur with downward pressure on head with chin in supraclavicular fossa on same side as lesion.	7. Symptoms occur with downward pressure on head with chin in supraclavicular fossa on same side as lesion.

Note: It may not be possible to differentiate these two because the symptoms and signs may be mixed.

TABLE 16.4 Effects of a Brachial Plexus Lesion

Nerve Root	Symptoms: Pain, Numbness, Tingling	Signs: Sensation Impairment	Weakness	Reflexes Absent
C4	Supraclavicular and shoulder area	Supraclavicular and shoulder area	On attempting to resist forced lateral flexion of the neck to the opposite side	
C5	Outer border of upper arm	Outer border of upper arm	Shoulder abduction Elbow flexion	Biceps Supinator
C6	Down radial side of arm to include radial side of hand	Radial side of forearm, thumb, and index fingers	Shoulder abduction Elbow flexion Pronation and supination Wrist flexion and extension	Biceps Supinator
C7	Down arm to hand including middle finger	Middle finger and corresponding area on palmar aspect of hand	Shoulder adduction Elbow extension Wrist flexion and extension Finger flexion and extension	Triceps Flexor finger jerk
C8	Down ulnar side of forearm to include ulnar side of hand	Ulnar side of forearm, ring, and little finger	Elbow extension Finger flexion and extension	Flexor finger jerk
T1	Inner border of mid and upper arm	Inner border upper arm	Finger abduction and adduction	

SYMPTOMS AND SIGNS: The athlete experiences a sudden, severe burning pain that radiates along the shoulder and down the arm, sometimes to the hand, and is usually associated with varying degrees of numbness, weakness, and neck pain. There may be sensation changes and the reflexes may be depressed. The most frequently affected area is the upper trunk of the brachial plexus, involving C5 and C6, leading to weakness of the deltoid, biceps, infraspinatus and supraspinatus. X-rays of the cervical spine should be taken to exclude any bone injury or displacement.

The symptoms and signs are usually transient, but occasionally permanent damage results. Any athlete with a pinched nerve should be watched and checked for at least two weeks, so that objective muscle weakness can be excluded.

GRADING THE SEVERITY OF A PINCHED-NERVE LESION.

Grade I	Full recovery within a few minutes (to a few days)
Grade II	a. Recovery within a few days to two months
	b. Recovery within two to six months
Grade III	Recovery not complete within six months (catastrophic injury)

TREATMENT: There is no specific form of treatment that will "cure" a pinched-nerve lesion. A number of modalities help reduce some of the inflammation around the damaged nerves. Perhaps the most important aspect of treatment is to ensure that the athlete does not return to participation too soon (see criteria for return to play). The treatment of a pinched nerve includes:

1. Cervical collar
2. Ice
3. Anti-inflammatory medication, muscle relaxants and analgesics if necessary
4. Cervical traction and electrical muscle stimulation if necessary
5. Active range-of-motion exercises that are steadily increased within the limitations of discomfort
6. Strength exercises as described under the section on neck rehabilitation when symptoms subside
7. Electromyographic studies if sensation does not recover completely within three to six weeks[18]
8. Investigation for a cervical disc lesion if and when the clinical situation warrants

Other Nerve Lesions

Axillary nerve. An axillary nerve injury may present as an isolated lesion. It is caused by an injury to the anterior aspect of the axilla, either from an anterior shoulder dislocation or from a direct blow. The nerve can also be involved as part of a brachial plexus or cervical nerve root lesion. There is loss of sensation localized to a small patch on the lateral aspect of the shoulder, and often weakness and wasting of the deltoid muscle occurs (see Figure 12.13).

Suprascapular nerve. Injury to the upper root of the brachial plexus may damage the suprascapular nerve, resulting in weakness of the supraspinatus and infraspinatus. No sensation defect will be found, as this nerve is purely a motor nerve.

TABLE 16.5 Criteria for Return to Play Following a Pinched-Nerve Lesion

> 1. *Full range of active neck movement* with minimal pain
> 2. *Full strength of neck movements* as tested against resistance—without pain
> 3. *Full strength, power, and endurance* of shoulder shrugs, abduction, elbow flexion and extension, and grip as compared with the opposite side
> 4. *Normal sensation* over all dermatomes
>
> When a footballer returns to play following a pinched-nerve lesion, use of a cervical collar or straps on the football helmet should be encouraged (see section on prevention, p. 250).

An isolated lesion of the infraspinatus may occur if the nerve is entrapped or damaged in the suprascapular notch. This lesion will present with weakness and atrophy localized to the infraspinatus. Occasionally, pain is a prominent symptom.

Long thoracic nerve. The long thoracic nerve arises from C5, C6, and C7 and can be damaged either at the root level or along its course. It supplies the serratus anterior muscle and, if damaged, results in "winging" of the scapula – see test for winging, p. 167 (see Figure 16.18).

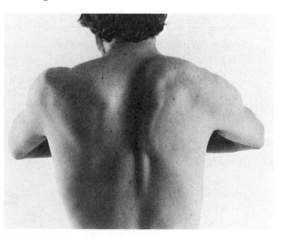

FIGURE 16.18 Winging of the scapula, due to a lesion of the long thoracic nerve

NECK REHABILITATION EXERCISES

The exercises outlined in Table 16.6 can be performed as part of a prevention and conditioning program by athletes who have poor neck musculature but who wish to engage in contact sports such as football, wrestling, and rugby. These sports are the most frequent sources of neck injuries.

Stages of Rehabilitation

The outline presented here is meant purely as a guide. Many variations have been and can be developed on this theme. This program is divided into three stages and each stage should be completed before progressing on to the next, though it is not necessary to perform all the exercises that are mentioned in each stage. The program should always be individualized.

The Roman numerals refer to the stage, and the + indicates in which stage a particular exercise should be performed.

In the neck rehabilitation program, hyperextension exercises should not be attempted until there is painless neck motion. Neck muscle spasm may be helped by one of the many neck traction devices available.

TABLE 16.6   Neck Rehabilitation Exercises

Stage I: There is neck pain and stiffness

No.	Exercise	I	II	III
1.	Traction	+		
2.	Range of movement to point of pain, but no hyperextension	+		
3.	Ice massage and/or heat	+	+	
4.	TENS	+		

Stage II: Almost no pain, though still some limitation of range of movement

No.	Exercise	II	III
1.	Range of movement with isometric contraction at end of movement— flexion, lateral flexion (no hyperextension yet)	+	
2.	Gentle isometric partner resistance exercises—flexion, lateral flexion to left and right, rotation to left and right	+	

Stage III: No pain, full range of movement

No.	Exercise	III
1.	Isometric exercises utilizing athlete's own resistance—flexion, extension, lateral flexion left and right	+
2.	Full isometric resistance using a partner (see Figure 16.11)—flexion, extension, lateral flexion left and right, rotation left and right	+
3.	Shoulder shrugs using free weights	+
4.	Helmet with weights, or weight-loaded head strap (Figure 16.19)—flexion, extension, lateral flexion left and right	+
5.	Bridging—the back of the head or helmet should contact the ground, not the top of the head (variation: athlete face down using forehead or front of helmet as contact point) (Figure 16.20)	+

If machines are available:
1. Universal bench press apparatus for shoulder shrugs (Figure 16.21)
2. Nautilus special neck machines (see Figure 16.12)
   (a) Shoulder shrug machine
   (b) Four-way neck machine
   (c) Rotation neck machine

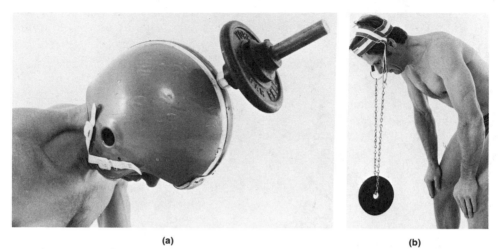

(a)   (b)

FIGURE 16.19 Devices used to strengthen the neck musculature (a) An adapted football helmet   (b) Head attachment, with chain and weights

Bridging is a controversial exercise, as some writers have stated that it may be associated with vertebral artery impingement and potential brain damage. It is the authors' contention, however, that if a wrestler does not strengthen his or her neck and does not practice bridging, limited to the back and foreparts of the head, he or she is in all likelihood at greater risk of a neck injury. Wrestling requires the ability to perform a vigorous bridging maneuver, and if the athlete is going to be engaged in such an activity, then the neck must be strengthened and the correct bridging exercise mastered.

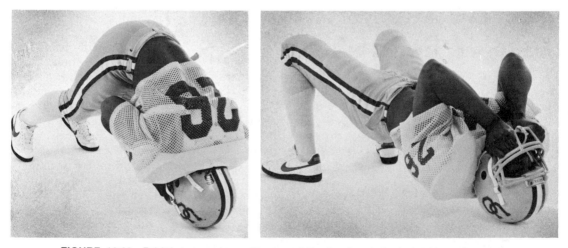

FIGURE 16.20 Bridging exercises The top of the head or helmet should not be used; this avoids hyperflexion or hyperextension of the neck.

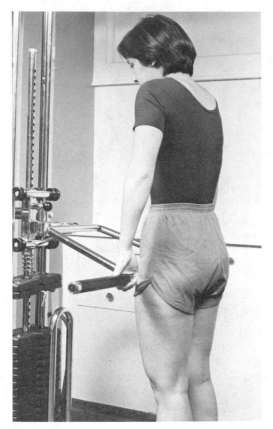

FIGURE 16.21 Shoulder shrugs to build up the tra-pezius muscles

INJURIES TO THE THORACIC SPINE

Examination of the Thoracic Spine

1. *Athlete standing with back to examiner.* Athlete outlines area of pain.

  1. Palpate area of tenderness over
     a. spinous processes
     b. costovertebral joints
     c. muscles
     d. trigger areas (see section on stretch and spray, p. 106)
  2. Note pain and limitation of active, volun- tary range of motion with

  a. flexion—note manner of bend; per- cuss spinous processes, note manner of return
  b. extension
  c. lateral flexion
  d. rotation

2. *Athlete sitting on examination table.*

  1. Note rotation to each side.
  2. Test sensation. Useful landmarks are
     a. medial forearm (T1)
     b. medial side of upper arm (T2)
     c. medial side of upper arm and axilla to the nipple line (T3)
     d. umbilicus area (T10)
  3. Test reflexes.
     a. triceps (C7 and C8)
     b. abdominal (upper—T8 to T10; low- er—T11 and T12).
     c. knee patella (L4)

Injuries to the Thoracic Facet Joint and Costovertebral Articulation

The numerous thoracic facet and costo- vertebral articulations are subject to frequent trauma. Joint dysfunction (called subluxation by some) often results. Many times a joint dysfunction is missed because the pain is re- ferred along the rib, and intercostal muscle spasm is considered the etiology.

The mode of injury is usually from com- pression of the chest, such as when a foot- ball player falls onto a football with another player on top of him. Also, side-to-side com- pression can occur, as in wrestling. A flexion injury to the thoracic spine, as well as land- ing rigidly on the feet, can also cause joint dysfunction involving the thoracic area.

Examination of the thoracic spine and costovertebral articulation should always be carried out in cases of chest and rib com- pression injuries, as well as in cases of inju- ries involving rotation, flexion, and exten- sion.

With rib and thoracic spine fractures ex- cluded by X-rays, joint dysfunction can usually be accurately diagnosed by a combination of localized tenderness, palpation of the position of the posterior spinous processes, skinfold rolling, and sometimes sensory changes. If these are present in the absence of X-ray bone changes, manipulation of the facet joints and costovertebral articulations can safely be undertaken, usually with dramatic improvement of symptoms.

Compression Fracture of the Vertebral Body

A compression fracture of the vertebral body often results from a hyperflexion injury. The anterior aspect of the vertebra is compressed; usually the amount of compression is minimal, but the symptoms may be severe. An extension brace may need to be worn for a few weeks until the symptoms improve.

Occasionally, the force on the spine is directed axially up the spinal column, resulting in a fracture of the hyaline cartilaginous end plate of the intervertebral disc. Nuclear material may be extruded into the body of the vertebra, resulting in a Schmorl's nodule.

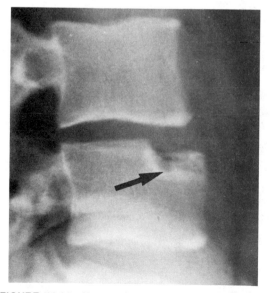

FIGURE 16.22   X-ray—Schmorl's nodule   This end-plate fracture may be seen in the lower thoracic and lumbar vertebrae.

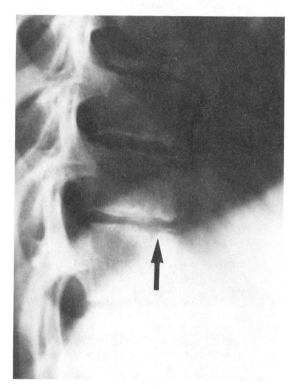

FIGURE 16.23   X-ray—juvenile epiphysitis (Scheuermann's disease)   Note the irregularity of the thoracic vertebrae. The amount of wedging present is minimal.

Dislocation of the Thoracic Spine

A dislocation involving the thoracic vertebrae is a very unusual injury in athletics. When it does occur, the spinal cord is almost always involved. Always test for tingling, numbness, loss of power, reflexes, and sensation of the lower legs in an injury involving the spine. If there is any suggestion of spinal cord damage, the athlete should not be moved except by a highly trained team of emergency medical technicians.

Juvenile Epiphysitis (Spinal Osteochondrosis or Scheuermann's Disease)

The exact etiology of juvenile epiphysitis is unknown. There is a disturbance of the growth plate resulting in a patchy and irregular transition of cartilage to bone. This affects mainly the thoracic vertebrae in the teen-ager and results in wedging of a variable number of dorsal vertebrae. The symptom is usually diffuse thoracic discomfort. If the discomfort is severe, the athlete might need to be placed in a Milwaukee brace. It is possible for this condition to result in kyphosis (forward angulation of the spine) if left untreated.

REFERENCES

1. Schneider RC: *Head and Neck Injuries in Football.* Baltimore, Williams and Wilkins, 1973, p 110.

2. Torg JS, Truex Jr, RC, Marshall J, et al: Spinal injury at the level of the third and fourth cervical vertebrae from football. *J Bone Joint Surg* 59A:1015–1019, 1977.

3. Torg JS, Truex Jr. RC, Quedenfeld TC, et al: The National Football Head and Neck Registry, report and conclusions. *JAMA* 241:1477–1479, 1979.

4. Duff JF: Spearing: Clinical consequences in the adolescent. Sports safety supplement. *J Sports Med* 2:175–177, 1974.

5. Williams JPR, McKibbin B: Cervical spine injuries in Rugby Union football. *Brit Med J* 2:1747, 1978.

6. Scher AT: Vertex impact and cervical dislocation in rugby players. *S Afr Med J* 59:227–228, 1981.

7. Scher AT: Rugby injuries to the cervical spinal cord. *S Afr Med J* 51:473–475, 1977.

8. Scher AT: The high rugby tackle—an avoidable cause of cervical spinal injury? *S Afr Med J* 53:1015–1018, 1978.

9. Roy SP: Intercollegiate wrestling injuries. *Phys Sportsmed* 7:83–94, November 1979.

10. Andrish J, Bergfeld J, Romo L: A method for the management of cervical injuries in football. A preliminary report. *Am J Sports Med* 5:89–92, 1977.

11. Committee on Accident and Poison Prevention: Trampoline. Evanston, Ill., American Academy of Pediatrics, September 1977.

12. Hammer A, Schwartsbach AL, Paulev PE: Trampoline training injuries—one hundred and ninety-five cases. *Br J Sports Med* 15:151–158, 1981.

13. Rapp GF, Nicely PG: Trampoline injuries. *Am J Sports Med* 6:269–271, 1978.

14. Maroon JC: "Burning hands" in football spinal cord injuries. *JAMA* 238:2049–2051, 1977.

15. Long SE, Reid SE, Sweeney HJ, et al: Removing football helmets safely. In Trainer's Corner, *Phys Sportsmed* 8:119, October 1980.

16. Grant T, Puffer J: Cervical stenosis: A developmental anomaly with quadriparesis during football. *Am J Sports Med* 4:219–221, 1976.

17. Robertson WC, Eichman PL, Clancy WG: Upper trunk brachial plexopathy in football players. *JAMA* 241:1480–1482, 1979.

18. Clancy WG, Brank RL, Bergfeld JA: Upper trunk brachial plexus injuries in contact sports. *Am J Sports Med* 5:209–216, 1977.

RECOMMENDED READINGS

Albright JP, Moses JM, Feldick HG, et al: Nonfatal cervical spine injuries in interscholastic football. *JAMA* 236:1243–1245, 1976.

American Academy of Pediatrics; Trampolines II. *Pediatrics* 67:438, 1981.

Hammer A, Schwartzbach A, Paulev PE: Some risk factors in trampolining illustrated by six serious injuries. *Brit J Sports Med* 16:27–32, 1982.

Maroon JC: Catastrophic neck injuries from football in Western Pennsylvania. *Phys Sportsmed* 9:83–86, November 1981.

Maroon JC, Kerin T, Rehkopf P, et al: A system for preventing athletic neck injuries. *Phys Sportsmed* 5:77–79, October 1977.

Mueller FO, Blyth CS: Catastrophic head and neck injuries. *Phys Sportsmed* 7:71–74, October 1979.

Riley D: Strength training for the neck. In Trainer's Corner, *Phys Sportsmed* 9:165, May 1981.

Roback DL: Neck pain, headache, and loss of equilibrium after athletic injury in a 15-year-old boy. *JAMA* 245:963–964, 1981.

Torg JS, editor: *Athletic Injuries to the Head, Neck, and Face.* Philadelphia, Lea and Febiger, 1982.

Torg JS, Quedenfeld TC, Moyer RA, et al: Severe and catastrophic neck injuries resulting from tackle football. *J Am Coll Health Assoc* 25:224–226, 1977.

CHAPTER 17

Lumbar Spine, Pelvis, and Hip Injuries

FUNCTIONAL ANATOMY

Bones

The *lumbar vertebrae* are designed for the attachment of the powerful lumbar muscles and for the support of the body's weight. They are therefore much stronger and larger than the other vertebrae and have short, thick processes (Figure 17.1).

The *pars interarticularis* is subject to severe angular forces from certain athletic activities such as football and gymnastics. This results in a high incidence of spondylolysis and stress fractures of the pars interarticularis (see Figure 17.14).[1,2]

The *sacrum* articulates with the fifth lumbar vertebra above, the coccyx below, and the two iliac bones on either side. The intervertebral disc between the fifth lumbar verte-bra and the sacrum is subjected to severe shear and torsional forces, so that this articulation has the highest incidence of disc protrusion and degeneration.

The *coccyx* articulates with the distal end of the sacrum. It is occasionally contused, leading to annoying discomfort when sitting.

The *pelvis* consists of a ring of bone which articulates with the sacrum posteriorly and with itself at the pubic symphysis anteriorly. The bones of the pelvis consist of the ilium superiorly, the ischium inferiorly, and the pubic bone anteriorly. Landmarks which can be easily palpated are the anterior superior iliac spines, the iliac crests, and the posterior superior iliac spines. All three portions of the pelvic bone meet laterally at the *acetabulum*, a deep socket which, together with the head of the *femur*, forms the hip joint. Below the head of the femur is the neck, which projects at an angle from the main shaft of the femur. At this junction one finds the *greater* and *lesser trochanters*, to which are attached a number of important muscles.

Intervertebral Discs

The intervertebral discs are important structures that are frequently subjected to injury, particularly in the lower lumbar and lumbosacral areas. The disc consists of the *annulus fibrosus*, which is composed mainly of dense fibrous rings surrounding the soft gel-like interior—the *nucleus pulposus*. Connection to the vertebrae above and below is through a hyaline cartilage layer. Most of the resistance

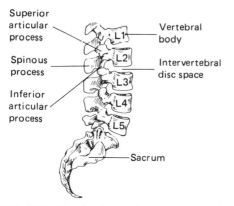

FIGURE 17.1 The lumbar spine—from the lateral aspect

Superior articular process

Spinous process

Inferior articular process

Vertebral body

Intervertebral disc space

L1
L2
L3
L4
L5

Sacrum

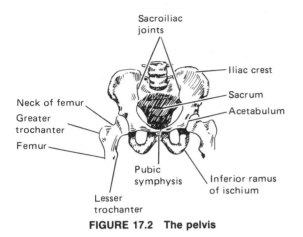

FIGURE 17.2   The pelvis

to rotational or torsional stress appears to be taken by the annulus, the hyaline cartilage, and the facet joints.

The *articular facet* joints are synovial joints with articular cartilage. The capsule surrounding these joints is very sensitive to pressure and motion and is thought to have the same nerve supply as the dura. The synovial lining contains meniscoid-like bodies, which can become entrapped within the joint, causing it to lock and producing pain.

Ligaments

The *anterior longitudinal ligament* is very powerful and helps to limit hyperextension of the spine as well as forward motion of one vertebra upon another, especially of the fifth lumbar onto the sacrum. It is attached to the annulus and the intervertebral discs and prevents forward bulging of the annulus.

The *posterior longitudinal ligament* lies anterior to the spinal cord and has strong attachments to the rim of the vertebral body and to the central portion of the annulus. The posterolateral corner of the annulus is poorly covered and this produces a weak area where disc protrusion frequently occurs.

The *posterior ligamentous system* is well developed in the lumbosacral area. It consists of the lumbar dorsal fascia and the interspinous and supraspinous ligaments. It helps resist shear stress as well as forward bending. However, the interspinous and supraspinous ligaments are frequently found to be weak or ruptured at L4–5, L5–S1, or both in those over thirty years of age.

The most important ligament at the hip joint is the *iliofemoral ligament*, which is usually torn in dislocations of the hip.

Muscles

There are numerous muscles that support the lower back and aid in stabilization of the pelvis and motion of the leg during walking and running. These include:

1. *Longissimus thoracis*: Runs from the transverse processes of the lumbar vertebrae and the lumbosacral fascia to the transverse processes of all the thoracic and upper lumbar vertebrae and the ninth and tenth ribs. *Function*: Extends the vertebral column and maintains posture.

2. *Iliocostalis lumborum*: Runs from the iliac crests to the angles of the sixth and seventh ribs. *Function*: Extends the lumbar spine.

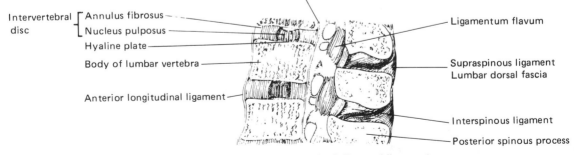

FIGURE 17.3   Lumbar intervertebral disc and ligaments

3. *Quadratus lumborum*: Originates from the iliac crests and iliolumbar ligament and inserts into the last rib and the upper four lumbar vertebrae. *Function*: Flexes the trunk laterally.

4. *Psoas major*: Originates from the transverse processes of the lumbar vertebrae and inserts into the lesser trochanter of the femur. *Function*: Flexes the hip and medially rotates the thigh.

5. *Iliacus*: Runs from the margin of the iliac fossa to the lateral side of the tendon of psoas major. *Function*: Flexes the hip and medially rotates the thigh.

6. *Psoas minor*: Runs from the last thoracic and the first lumbar vertebrae to the iliopectineal eminence. *Function*: Flexes the trunk.

7. *Gluteus maximus*: Runs from the posterior gluteal line of the ilium and the posterior surface of the sacrum and the coccyx to the fasciae latae and gluteal ridge. *Function*: Extends the thigh.

8. *Gluteus medius*: Runs from the lateral surface of the ilium into the lateral surface of the greater trochanter. *Function*: Abducts the hip and medially rotates the thigh.

9. *Gluteus minimus*: Runs from the outer surface of the ilium to the anterior border of the greater trochanter. *Function*: Abducts the hip and medially rotates the thigh.

10. *Piriformis, gemelli, quadratus femoris*, and *obturator* muscles: Run from the sacrum, the posterior portion of the ischium, and the obturator foramen to the greater trochanter of the femur. *Function*: Mainly rotate the thigh laterally.

11. Abdominal muscles

   a. *Rectus abdominis*: Runs from the pubic crest to the xiphoid process, costal cartilages of the fifth, sixth, and seventh ribs. *Function*: Helps flex the lumbar vertebrae, support the abdomen, and control the position of the pelvis.

   b. *Transversus abdominis*: Runs from the costal cartilages of the lower six ribs,

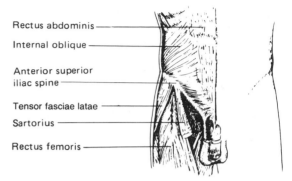

FIGURE 17.4 Superficial abdominal and groin muscles

Labels: Rectus abdominis, Internal oblique, Anterior superior iliac spine, Tensor fasciae latae, Sartorius, Rectus femoris

the thoracolumbar fascia, the iliac crest, and the inguinal ligament to the linea alba through the rectus sheath and the conjoined tendon to the pubis. *Function*: Helps support and control the abdominal viscera.

   c. *Obliquus externus abdominis* (external oblique): Runs from the lower eight costal cartilages to the iliac crest and the linea alba through the rectus sheath. *Function*: Flexes and rotates the vertebral column.

   d. *Obliquus internus abdominis* (internal oblique): Runs from the lumbar aponeurosis, the iliac crest, and the inguinal ligament to the lower three or four costal cartilages, the linea alba, and the conjoined tendon to the pubis. *Function*: Flexes and rotates the vertebral column on the pelvis.

Nerves

The *sciatic nerve* is the longest nerve in the body. It is formed by the sacral plexus of nerves and consists of rami L4 and L5 and S1, S2, and S3. It runs deep to the gluteus maximus after passing under the piriformis muscle. Thereafter, it travels down the posterior aspect of the thigh to supply the lower leg and foot via its main branches, the tibial nerve and the common peroneal nerve.

Nerves forming the sciatic nerve can be compressed by a protruding or herniated lumbar disc, particularly at the L4–L5 and the L5–S1 interspaces. Pain is also produced by irritation or locking of the facet joints. The sciatic nerve can, in addition, be compressed by a spasm of the piriformis muscle, producing radiating pain down the leg. The *femoral* nerve originates from L2, L3, and L4 and supplies mainly the anterior aspect of the thigh. The *femoral artery* and *vein* lie alongside the femoral nerve in the groin.

LOWER-BACK PAIN

Lumbar Backache

Lumbar backache is one of the most common afflictions of the human race, and unfortunately athletes are not exempt from this most annoying and at times incapacitating malady. There are many hypotheses as to the causes of and cures for backache, and, while no unanimous opinion can be reached, two broad schools of thought seem to have the greatest following.

The standard view of lumbar backache suggests that, while backache has many caus-

es, the pain is commonly due to disc degeneration involving the hyaline cartilage, the annulus fibrosus, or both.[3] This subsequently results in subluxation of the posterior articular facet joints.[4] However, disc protrusion or herniation is thought by some to be the main cause, accompanied by symptoms and signs of nerve compression or irritation such as radiating pain.[5]

While not disputing that disc degeneration and disc protrusion are important causes of lower backache, there is a school of thought which contends that most cases of backache without radiating pain are due to joint dysfunction of the facet and sacro-iliac joints. They are of the opinion that normal movement takes place at each sacro-iliac joint independently of each other, and if normal movement cannot take place this joint dysfunction will cause backache.[6,7]

This view is not accepted by many orthopedic surgeons, who generally state that the sacro-iliac joint is of little importance in backache. Some state that pain and tenderness at the sacro-iliac joint area are due to referred pain of disc degeneration (especially from T12–L1 and L5–S1 discs) or from stretching of the supraspinous ligaments.[4]

This division of opinion awaits resolution by further research, but the athletic trainer should be aware of these views, as the controversy surrounding lower back pain is commonly discussed in athletic circles and is a familiar topic to many coaches and athletes.

Prevention of lumbar backache. Many of the lower backaches that occur in the athlete could be prevented by attention to some of the predisposing factors.

1. *Standing posture*: Observe from the side and ask the athlete to hyperextend the knees. Note how this may cause hyperlordosis of the back. Standing in this position for a period of time can aggravate lower backache. A kyphotic position of the thoracic spine can induce both thoracic and lower-back pain as can hyperlordosis of the cervical spine with the head held forward.

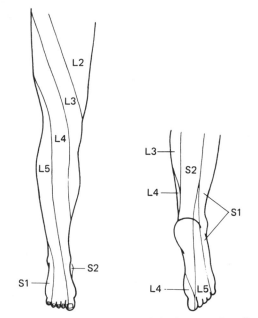

FIGURE 17.5 Dermatomes of the lower extremity

TABLE 17.1 Lower Backache in Athletes

Common causes
1. Mechanical backache (i.e., pain arising from a disorder of one of the structures of the spinal column)
   a. joint
   b. bone
   c. soft tissue (e.g., capsule, ligament, or muscle)
2. Discogenic backache
   a. disc protrusion or rupture which may involve the nerve root
   b. disc degeneration

Rare causes
1. Neurogenic backache—arising from pathology of the nerve root or of the spinal cord.
2. Vascular backache—arising from changes in blood vessels (e.g., an athlete with Marfan's syndrome suffering from a dissecting aneurysm of the aorta may present with back pain).
3. Viscerogenic backache—arising from visceral disorders (e.g., gallbladder or kidney stones may present with backache).
4. Inflammatory disorder—such as ankylosing spondylitis, Reiter's syndrome, etc.

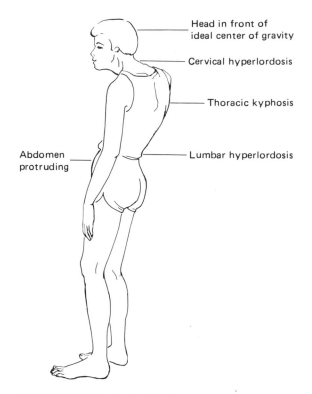

FIGURE 17.6 Postural defects

2. *Sitting posture*: Sitting with the legs extended together and the hips flexed puts a severe strain on the lumbosacral joint. This can produce symptoms in a susceptible athlete. There are some who feel that sitting for a period of time with the back flattened (e.g., with the knees higher than the hips) can induce backache. They contend that a certain amount of lordosis is necessary for normal back functioning.[8]

3. *Lifting posture*: Weight lifting has become an increasingly important part of almost all sports and is commonly performed on a year-round basis by both males and females. The coach and trainer should be aware of the correct technique for each particular type of lift, and should constantly observe athletes while they are lifting, in order to correct deficiencies in their technique. The athlete should keep the back erect and the knees bent, with the weight close to the body at all times. A lumbosacral belt should be used for heavy weight lifting, as this is thought to help stabilize the lumbosacral and

sacro-iliac joints. Rotational movements put a severe strain on the facet joints and can induce acute joint dysfunction or subluxation.

4. *Sit-ups*: Many athletes have surprisingly weak abdominal muscles, which predisposes to hyperlordosis and poor control of the pelvis. This in turn puts a strain on the posterior articular facets, the discs, and the lumbosacral and sacro-iliac joints. To counteract this, an abdominal strengthening program of sit-ups should be used.

There are many variations in technique for performing a sit-up. Some of these may actually be harmful to those with potential back problems. The correct form should be stressed. Incorrectly performed sit-ups tend to increase the strength and tone of the iliopsoas muscle, causing it to be functionally shorter (see Figure 17.17). This in turn can increase hyperlordosis.

5. *Muscle tightness*: Inflexibility of the hamstrings and iliotibial tracts tends to aggravate

lower backache. Stretching exercises for the hamstrings, the iliotibial tracts, and the back muscles help prevent back problems. Tightness of the Achilles tendon can cause a weight distribution problem that affects the articular facets. If inflexibility of the Achilles tendon is noted, heel lifts can be temporarily used while the athlete works on improving the flexibility of both the gastrocnemius and soleus muscles and tendons.

6. *Back exercises*: Using the correct form for back exercises is important in preventing lower-back pain (see section on back rehabilitation, p. 281).

Examination of the Lumbar Spine

1. *Athlete standing with back to examiner.* The athlete outlines area of pain.

1. Note alignment of iliac crests and posterior superior iliac spines.

2. Note range, rhythm, and deviation during voluntary range of motion of
   a. flexion
   b. extension
   c. lateral flexion to both sides
   d. rotation to both sides

3. Note movement and symmetry of posterior superior iliac spines on forward flexion and on return to erect position.

4. Test strength of calf muscles by repeated unilateral heel-raises (this tests for an S1 lesion).

5. Test strength of anterior tibial muscles by heel-walking (L5).

2. *Athlete leaning forward over examining table.*

1. Test tenderness of spinous processes (anterior and lateral pressure) including lower thoracic spines.

3. *Athlete sitting on examining table.*

1. Compare standing and sitting alignments of iliac crests and posterior superior iliac spines.

4. *Athlete lying supine.*

1. Note level of anterior superior iliac spines.

2. Test power of
   a. abdominals (Figure 17.6)
   b. hip flexors (L2)
   c. quadriceps (L3)
   d. anterior tibial (L4)
   e. extensor hallucis longus (L5)
   f. flexor hallucis longus (S1)
   g. hamstrings (S2)

3. Test sensation by dermatome areas
   a. medial mid-thigh (L2)
   b. superior aspect of medial knee (L3)
   c. medial arch (L4)
   d. dorsum of foot (L5)
   e. lateral border and lateral plantar aspect of foot (S1)
   f. popliteal fossa (S2)

4. Test muscle tenderness
   a. quadriceps (L4)
   b. anterior tibial (L5)
   c. calf (S1)

5. Test reflexes
   a. patella (L4)
   b. Achilles tendon (S1)
   c. plantar (Babinski's sign)—pyramidal tract (tensor fasciae latae component of this reflex is lost with S1 lesion)

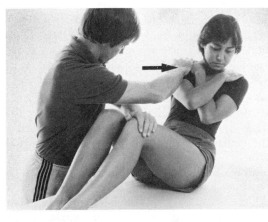

FIGURE 17.7 Abdominal muscle testing Stabilize the thighs. The force is directed obliquely through one shoulder.

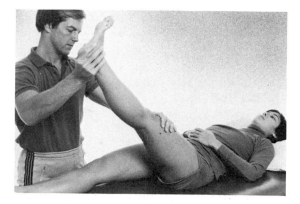

FIGURE 17.8 Contralateral straight-leg-raising test When testing for sciatic nerve irritation, begin by slowly raising the opposite (non-affected) leg with the knee held straight. If pain radiates down the affected leg, this test is strongly suggestive of a disc protrusion or herniation.

6. Test sciatic nerve irritation
   a. straight-leg raising test using the unaffected leg with foot dorsiflexed (contralateral straight-leg raising test)
   b. straight-leg raising test using the affected leg with dorsiflexion of foot and neck flexion—Lasègue's sign (see Figure 17.9)
   c. "bowstring" test (see Figure 17.10).

7. Measure
   a. leg length
   b. muscle bulk of thigh and calf
8. Examine abdomen
9. Examine chest

5. *Athlete lying on side.*

1. Test Gaenslen's sign

6. *Athlete lying prone.*

1. Test tenderness in lower back and buttocks
2. Test stretching of femoral nerve (L4)
3. Test flexibility of Achilles tendon
4. Examine feet (see Chapter 21)

Tests Used to Examine the Lumbar Spine

1. *Straight-leg-raising test* (*Lasègue's sign*): In this test (SLR), the leg is raised with the knee straight until pain is felt. The leg is then lowered by approximately 1″ (2.5 cm) so there is no longer any pain. The foot is then dorsiflexed; if the pain returns, the test is considered positive for sciatic nerve stretch. This test can be made more definitive by flexing the neck at the same time as dorsiflexing the foot (Figure 17.9).

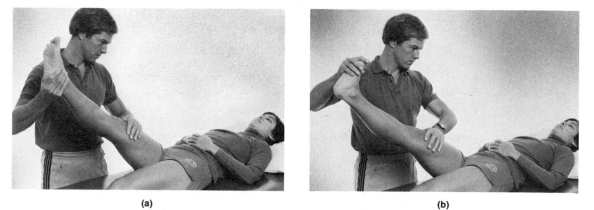

(a)   (b)

FIGURE 17.9 Lasègue's sign This test is performed by (a) raising the straight leg to the point where pain radiating down the leg is experienced. The leg is then lowered slightly so no pain is felt. Then, (b) dorsiflex the foot; if this reproduces radiating pain down the leg, the test is positive for sciatic nerve stretch or irritation.

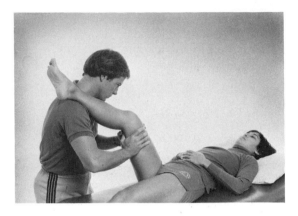

FIGURE 17.10 Bowstring sign Pressure is applied to the sciatic nerve in the popliteal area. If positive, pain is felt locally and frequently radiates up the leg to the back.

2. *Bowstring test*: This test is performed by raising the affected leg until radiating pain is felt. The knee is then bent to relieve the discomfort (Figure 17.10). The lower leg is placed on the examiner's shoulder and firm pressure is applied to and just above the popliteal fossa in the area of the sciatic nerve. If this maneuver produces pain that travels up into the back or down the leg, it suggests the sciatic nerve is under tension, that is, there is likely to be a disc protrusion or rupture.[4]

3. *Babinski's sign*: In the neurologically intact person over the age of two years, stimulation of the plantar aspect of the foot should cause the toes to curl downward; upward fanning of the toes (especially the big toe) is a pathological response. In the context of lower backache, the plantar aspect of the foot is stimulated to elicit a reflex contraction of the tensor fasciae latae. This pertinent feature is lost with an S1 lesion.

4. *Gaenslen's sign*: This tests for pain related to the sacro-iliac joint. It is performed with the patient lying on the unaffected side. The upper leg is retracted by the examiner until the hip is fully extended. At the same time the athlete flexes the opposite hip and knee up against his or her chest. If he or she feels

pain in the sacro-iliac region when the hip is extended, the test suggests a lesion of the sacro-iliac joint.

Presenting History of Lower-Back Discomfort

Mechanical backache

ETIOLOGY:

1. *Sudden onset*: May be due to an unguarded twisting motion such as stepping into a pothole while running or mistiming a particular movement. The athlete will frequently give a history of being "unable to move," or feeling that the "back was locked." He or she may or may not have pain in the buttock, groin, hip, or thigh. Occasionally this pain may go down the leg to the knee or even as far as the ankle.

2. *Slow onset*: The athlete may complain of a dull ache, usually localized to one or the other sacro-iliac joint areas. It is usually relieved by rest, but aggravated by activity. Secondary muscle spasm may follow, further decreasing the range of motion and the effectiveness of running. The legs often feel weak and are felt not to be fully under the athlete's control. There may or may not be referred pain.

TABLE 17.2 Definitions of Radiating Pain and Referred Pain

1. *Radiating pain.* Results from irritation and/or compression of a nerve root. It is localized to the distribution of that particular nerve root, and may travel the entire length of the leg along that particular dermatome. It may present with or without backache.

2. *Referred pain.* Experienced in a site removed from that of the origin—in the back, buttock, groin, or thigh, but usually not beyond the knee. Occasionally a referred pain may mimic nerve root irritation (radiating pain) and present around the ankle and foot.

SIGNS: Tenderness is commonly elicited over the lumbosacral or sacro-iliac joint on one side. The height of the posterior superior iliac spines or the iliac crests may be uneven, indicating either a difference in leg length or pelvic asymmetry. If this finding is present, the athlete should sit on the table and the heights should again be compared. If the crests and spines are not level when standing, but are level when sitting, a discrepancy in length should be suspected of either (a) functional or (b) anatomical origin (see section on backache in the runner, p. 000). If the athlete is asked to bend forward while the posterior superior iliac spines are palpated, an asymmetry of movement, particularly on arising from a flexed position, may be another indication of pelvic asymmetry.

When the athlete lies supine, the reflexes are symmetrical and sensation is unimpaired, but power may sometimes be altered. Ipsilateral straight-leg raising should not cause pain. Contralateral straight-leg raising and the bowstring signs are usually negative.

TREATMENT: Initially, ice in the form of cold towels or ice packs (heat may be used for relaxation if the athlete feels this modality is more helpful than ice). Pain medication when indicated and muscle relaxants can be used, but their effects are variable. Anti-inflammatory medications are often useful. Pelvic traction may provide short-term relief of muscle spasm and pain. A lumbosacral corset is often used if muscle spasm persists.

The athlete should start rehabilitation exercises to ensure improved strength and flexibility, with gentle, active stretching within the limits of discomfort (see section on back rehabilitation, p. 281), and pelvic tilt exercises. Transcutaneous electrical nerve stimulation (TENS) is also useful.

Mobilization and manipulation of the lower back is an everyday form of therapy in training rooms throughout the country, even though these procedures are controversial in some medical circles.[9] Side effects are infrequent or nonexistent provided the guidelines and requirements mentioned next are ad-

hered to (see section on manipulation, p. 110).

1. The diagnosis should be that of joint dysfunction (e.g., mechanical backache).

2. There should be no sign of disc prolapse or rupture or nerve root compression.

3. The therapist should have had adequate training and experience in manipulative techniques.

4. The manipulation should always be gentle and nonforceful.

Relapses, requiring repeated manipulation, are a disadvantage, but these can be minimized by utilizing a full stretching and strengthening program (see section on back rehabilitation, p. 281).

Discogenic backache

ETIOLOGY:

1. *Sudden onset*: Results from a very sudden movement, as, when performing a dead lift with an incorrect technique, the athlete suffers a severe, sharp pain localized to the back with radiation down the leg to the ankle or the foot. Coughing or sneezing aggravates this radiating pain.

2. *Second injury*: Following a fairly severe back injury, a fairly minor incident can initiate back pain with radiating symptoms.

3. *Radiating pain only*: This is the presenting symptom and localizes either in the affected nerve root distribution or in a particular area of the leg (e.g., the lower hamstring area).

The commonest areas for discogenic prolapse or rupture are the L4–L5 disc (L5 nerve root compression) and the L5-S1 disc (S1 nerve root compression).

PATHOMECHANICS OF DISC RUPTURE:

1. The initial injury leads to separation of the hyaline cartilage plate from the adjacent vertebral bodies.

2. Further stress leads to fissuring and weakness of the annulus.

TABLE 17.3   Symptoms and Signs Suggesting Nerve Root Compression and/or Irritation (Radiating Pain)

Decreased sensation Decreased reflexes Decreased power Muscle tenderness (and later wasting) Positive straight-leg raising increased by dorsiflexion (Lasègue's sign) Positive contralateral straight-leg raising Positive bowstring sign	These should all correspond to the same dermatome or nerve root distribution.

3. Subsequent injury leads to the nucleus pulposus protruding or extruding through the torn fibers of the annulus, usually at the posterolateral corner (Figure 17.11).

SIGNS: Tenderness may or may not be present in the back. The posterior superior iliac spines are usually level. Scoliosis, or listing *away* from the site of pain, may be present if the herniation is lateral to the nerve, but listing *to* the side of the pain will happen if the herniation is medial to the nerve (the latter is less common). Forward flexion may produce sciatic nerve radiation down the leg.

Power, sensation, and reflexes may decrease over the affected nerve root distribution, and muscle tenderness may be present in the corresponding muscle group. A sagging of the gluteal fold may be present in an S1 lesion (gluteus maximus weakness). There may be a loss of the iliotibial tract reflex on testing Babinski's sign (S1 lesion). Straight-leg raising tests should then be performed, starting with the contralateral leg (see Figures 17.8 and 17.9). This will indicate tightness of the hamstrings, but, more importantly, if it produces radiating pain down the affected leg, it is very suggestive of a disc protrusion or rupture (this is the contralateral straight-leg raising test mentioned before). Lasègue's sign, using the affected leg, should then be performed, followed by the bowstring test.

The contralateral straight-leg raising test, Lasègue's sign, and the bowstring test are reliable indicators of tension on the sciatic nerve, which in most instances results from a disc protrusion or rupture.

INVESTIGATIONS:

1. *X-rays* include the anteroposterior, lateral, and perhaps oblique views of the lumbosacral spine.

The following investigations are most useful when surgery is contemplated but are not performed routinely.

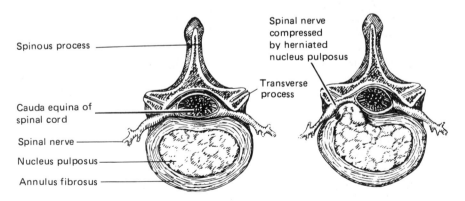

Spinous process

Spinal nerve compressed by herniated nucleus pulposus

Transverse process

Cauda equina of spinal cord

Spinal nerve

Nucleus pulposus

Annulus fibrosus

FIGURE 17.11 A normal and herniated intervertebral disc (Modified from Netter.)

TABLE 17.4   Differentiating Signs of L4–L5 and L5–S1 Disc Lesions

Signs	L4–L5 Lesion (L5 signs)	L5–S1 Lesion (S1 signs)
Power decrease	Extensor hallucis longus (dorsiflexors)	Flexor hallucis longus (plantar flexors)
Sensation decrease	Dorsum of foot and anterior aspect of lower leg	Sole and outer border of leg and foot
Reflexes		Decreased ankle jerk
Plantar stimulation with iliotibial tract response	Iliotibial tract response	No iliotibial tract response
Muscle tenderness	Anterior tibial	Calf muscle
Sciatic nerve stretch tests	Positive	Positive

2. *Epidural phlebography* investigation is particulary useful in the young athlete.[10] Contrast material is injected into the epidural veins; if a disc protrusion is present, an interruption of the dye flow in the veins is usually seen.

3. *Myelography* is used to rule out the possibility of nerve root tumor and to localize the level of a disc herniation.

4. *Nerve root infiltration* is a technique performed with a local anesthetic injected into the root sleeve as the nerve root emerges through the root canal. If the radiating pain disappears following the injection of anesthetic into a specific sleeve, it confirms the particular lesion site.

5. *Electromyography* demonstrates the inability to fully contract a particular group of muscles and thus confirms the diagnosis of nerve compression at a particular level.[11]

6. *Discography*, injection of a disc with dye, is used in some centers.

7. *Computerized axial tomography* (CAT) scan may be very useful.

TREATMENT:

1. Symptomatic therapy (e.g., ice, heat, or both)

2. Pain medication if necessary

3. Anti-inflammatory medication

4. Muscle relaxants

5. Pelvic traction for up to two weeks

6. Lumbosacral corset in conjunction with rehabilitation exercises, continued for at least as long as corset is worn

7. Transcutaneous electrical nerve stimulation (TENS)

8. No manipulation and mobilization if there are signs of nerve irritation, compression, or both

9. Bed rest with or without traction up to three or four weeks (controversial)

10. Epidural cortisone[12]

11. Surgery is indicated when one or more of the following are present:

    a. Bowel and bladder paralysis

    b. Marked muscle weakness, especially if increasing in severity

    c. Worsening of neurological signs in spite of complete bed rest

    d. Unrelieved pain

12. Surgical intervention can be contemplated if an athlete is unable to perform and the diagnosis of a ruptured disc is certain.

OTHER SPECIFIC PROBLEMS

Cauda Equina Syndrome

The cauda equina syndrome results from compression of the cauda equina below L1 (Figure 17.12). This occurs, for instance, with disc protrusion or rupture or from spondylolisthesis. Athletes who develop the cauda equina syndrome usually have lower back pain, sciatica, decreased sensation in the saddle area (most importantly, a lack of the anal wink sign), bilateral weakness of the lower extremities (even frank paraplegia), loss of ankle or knee reflexes, and bowel and bladder incontinence.[13,14] In the early stages, the symptoms and signs may be unilateral and rapidly progressive. The first signs of impending cauda equina compression may be difficulty in voiding and the development of constipation. Signs of loss of sensation, reflexes, and motor function may then become bilateral.

Piriformis Syndrome

Spasm of the piriformis muscle can compress the sciatic nerve, producing sciatica-like symptoms of radiating pain down the leg.[15] Sometimes there is pain in the buttock as well. Localized tenderness may be present in the area of the piriformis muscle. The condition is treated either by applying ice or by ice massaging the piriformis muscle while it

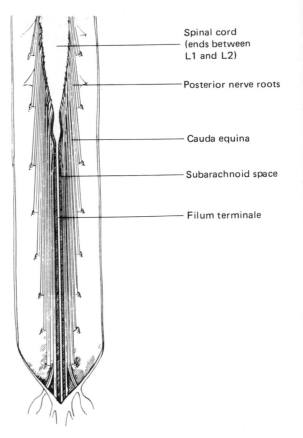

Spinal cord (ends between L1 and L2)

Posterior nerve roots

Cauda equina

Subarachnoid space

Filum terminale

FIGURE 17.12 **The cauda equina** (exposed from behind)

is being stretched. FluoriMethane spray and stretch will usually produce dramatic results (see Figure 7.9).

Contusion to the Lumbar Spine

Contusions to the lumbar spine are common. This area is covered by large muscle groups and so a contusion here should be treated in the same manner as soft-tissue trauma anywhere else (i.e., with ice, anti-inflammatory medication, gentle stretching, and protection from further contusions).

Occasionally the tips of the spinous processes are involved, causing a periosteal hematoma and marked muscle spasm. This may be treated with an injection of cortisone and hyaluronidase into the site of the hematoma, in addition to ice and anti-inflammatory medication. TENS can also be used, and a lumbosacral corset may be useful until adequate muscle relaxation and rehabilitation are achieved.

Fracture of the Transverse Spinous Process of the Lumbar Vertebra

The transverse processes can be fractured by (a) a direct blow or (b) an avulsion due to violent muscular contraction.

Many cases produce relatively little discomfort besides localized tenderness, and the athlete is able to return to activities soon afterward. In severe cases, there is marked iliopsoas spasm, and the athlete is unable to straighten legs and back simultaneously. Treatment includes ice, muscle relaxants, anti-inflammatory medication, analgesics, traction, TENS, and often a lumbosacral corset.

Spondylolysis

Spondylolysis in an athlete is often a stress fracture through the pars interarticularis of one or more of the lumbar vertebrae.[16] If a definite spondylolysis shows on X-rays, it means the condition has been present for weeks or months. Early diagnosis is possible with radioactive isotope scans using technetium, which shows areas of bone stress as "hot spots." If an athlete presents with a backache localized to one of the lumbar vertebrae and ordinary X-rays do not show any lesion, but the scan shows a hot spot, "prespondylolysis" is probably present. If this area continues to be stressed, actual spondylolysis can ultimately develop.[17,18]

Spondylolysis is thought to be a cause of backache, particularly in gymnasts[2] and offensive linemen in football.[1,19] If an athlete has pain at a level other than that of the spondylolysis, it may mean that (a) a prestress fracture is developing at another level, or (b) there is another cause of the pain (e.g., mechanical dysfunction). The X-ray visualization of spondylolysis does not neces-

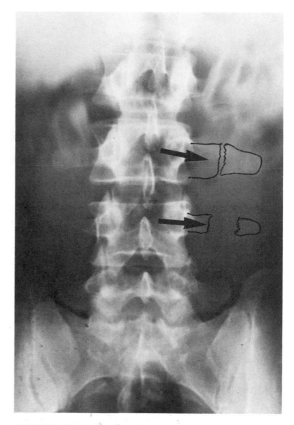

FIGURE 17.13 X-ray—fracture, transverse process lumbar spine

sarily mean the backache is due to the spondylolysis per se. Spondylolysis may, however, predispose the athlete to backache from joint dysfunction, due to the instability it produces.

Spondylolisthesis

Spondylolysis may be the precursor of spondylolisthesis, a group of conditions in which the proximal spinal column moves forward on a distal vertebra. However, spondylolisthesis is often due to hereditary factors. The condition usually occurs in the lower lumbar region. The two commonest types of spondylolisthesis are spondylitic spondylolisthesis and isthmic spondylolisthesis.

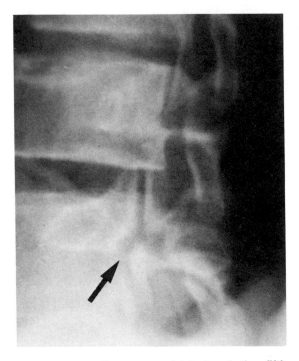

FIGURE 17.14 X-ray—spondylolysis of the fifth lumbar vertebra Note the crack through the neck of the "Scotty dog."

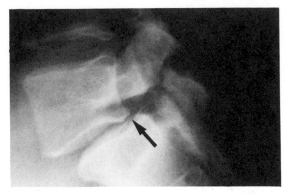

FIGURE 17.15 X-ray—spondylolisthesis—Grade I (out of IV) Note disc-space narrowing between L5 and S1, as well as the spondylolysis of L5.

1. *Spondylitic spondylolisthesis.* The spondylitic spondylolisthesis defect is found in the neural arch in the region of the pars interarticularis, and probably represents a stress fracture. Pain from the spondylolisthesis can develop if the defect is held together by a loose fibrous syndesmosis which separates on flexion or straining, putting additional stress on the supraspinous ligament. However, a forward slip is often associated with degenerative changes of the underlying disc, so the symptoms may be more from the secondary disc changes than the slippage per se. Presenting symptoms are

a. localized back pain

b. referred pain

c. nerve root irritation, or compression, or both (including the cauda equina syndrome)

A clinical sign suggesting spondylitic spondylolisthesis is a step, which can be palpated and often actually seen, usually at the L5 level. There may also be dimples above the posterior superior iliac spines, and the normal lumbar lordosis may be replaced by a very flat lumbar spine.

The diagnosis is made after examining the X-rays. However, the amount of slippage seen on X-rays can be totally out of proportion to the symptoms (e.g., there can be a marked slip on X-rays without any backache or nerve root compression). Again, X-ray visualization of spondylolisthesis does not necessarily mean the backache is due to that condition. It may be due to some other cause, most commonly a mechanical backache (joint dysfunction). Surgery is indicated only if pain becomes progressive, or if nerve root compression or cauda equina symptoms are present. Symptomatic spondylolisthesis in an athlete, such as a gymnast, will probably preclude him or her from further participation.

2. *Isthmic spondylolisthesis.* Isthmic spondylolisthesis usually presents in a young teen-ager. On X-rays the pars interarticularis will appear thinned and elongated, but no actual defect will be seen. This probably represents a number of previous stress fractures, resulting in an elongation of the pars.

This condition behaves differently from the spondylitic spondylolisthesis. The onset can be sudden and dramatic. The athlete presents with a rigid lumbar spine; a functional scoliosis; a pelvis that rotates forward, resulting in a flat sacrum; and hamstring spasm. Walking is possible only with bent knees. In contradistinction to the spondylitic spondylolisthesis, surgery is often required to prevent further slippage as cauda equina symptoms may occur. However, the majority of cases do not have any nerve compression.

Ankylosing Spondylitis

The trainer should be aware of the possibility of this medical inflammatory condition being a cause of backache. Ankylosing spondylitis is a relatively rare condition occurring mostly in males in their late teens or early twenties, and starts as an inflammation of the sacro-iliac joints.

Initially there is vague lower backache with pain around the sacro-iliac joints; some morning stiffness may also be present. Tests such as Gaenslen's sign and pelvic compression may cause pain in the sacro-iliac region. As the disease advances, decreased chest expansion may be noted, together with limitation of back extension. There may also be symptoms related to the iris, the cardiovascular and pulmonary systems, and the pubic area.

The course of this disease is usually slow and variable.

X-RAY: Changes of the sacro-iliac joints include fuzziness, with sclerosis of the iliac and sacral bones developing later. Eventually there is ossification of the vertebral ligaments.

TREATMENT: This consists mainly of anti-inflammatory medication and extension exercises of the spine.

REHABILITATION OF THE BACK

Stages of Rehabilitation

The outline presented in Table 17.5 is meant purely as a guide. Many variations have been and can be developed on this theme. This program is divided into four stages and each stage should be completed before progressing on to the next, though it is not necessary to perform all the exercises that are mentioned in each stage. The program should always be individualized.

The Roman numerals refer to the stage, and the + indicates in which stage a particular exercise should be performed.

The basic concepts in back rehabilitation are to improve the:

a. Abdominal muscle strength and control of the pelvis
b. Flexibility of the lower back, the hamstring muscles, the iliotibial tract, and the Achilles tendons

Once these areas have been strengthened, the athlete can undertake additional exercises to strengthen the back musculature. The first thing the athlete needs to learn is how to perform a pelvic tilt and how to control the position of the pelvis and the amount of lordosis of the lower back. The sit-up (or curl-up) is useful for improving the strength of the abdominal musculature. The athlete bends his or her knees to approximately 90° with the hips at 45°. The legs or feet are not held down. The athlete then performs a pelvic tilt and curls the chin up to the chest. The shoulders and upper back are then slowly curled to approximately 30° off the ground; this position is then held for two seconds. The back is then uncurled, one vertebra at a time, while maintaining the pelvic tilt. The lowering process should take at least two to three seconds. The chin-tuck position is maintained throughout the series of curl-ups. Pelvic tilts are performed before each curl-up. The number of curl-ups is lim-

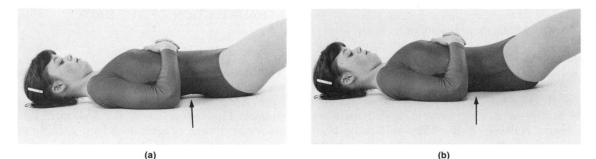

(a)   (b)

FIGURE 17.16   The pelvic tilt   Normally, the lower back has a slight arch (**a**). A pelvic tilt flattens this arch, and holds the lumbar spine against the ground (**b**). This position is maintained for 5 to 10 seconds, and repeated 5 to 10 times. The pelvic tilt forms the basis for many lower back exercises, and is an integral part of the sit-up.

ited by an inability to do a proper pelvic tilt or by loss of form.

Many back injuries are aggravated by improper exercise, such as lowering and raising the legs when held straight out and sit-ups with the legs secured and the back arched into hyperlordosis. These exercises should not be performed, particularly by an athlete prone to back problems.

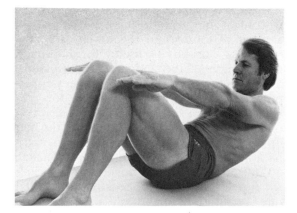

FIGURE 17.17   The sit-up   The knees are bent to 90° and the feet are free. A pelvic tilt is performed and held, and the shoulders are curled forward with the chin tucked in. The movement is slow and held at 30°, and then the trunk is slowly lowered. The chin should be kept tucked in.

INJURIES TO THE GROIN AND THE HIP

Groin Muscle Strain

A strain of one of the groin muscles, be it the sartorius, part of the rectus femoris, one of the adductors, or the iliopsoas,[20] tends to be a slow-healing condition. The athlete complains of discomfort localized to the groin area, particularly when faster speed and a higher knee lift are attempted. Tenderness is usually localized to the muscle involved. Placing the muscle under stress, for instance, isometric resistance or forced hip flexion, reproduces the pain.

TREATMENT: After the initial icing, gentle prolonged stretching of the involved muscle should be instituted, together with a strengthening program for all the groin muscles. These are at first isometric. Once they are performed painlessly, the athlete progresses to high-speed isokinetic workouts.

Taping the upper thigh to hold the hip in slight flexion, which prevents extension, often gives symptomatic relief and may help the athlete to continue participating. Ultrasound and, in particular, TENS are accessory means which might help the athlete return to participation. Corticosteroid injections are sometimes used in resistant cases.

TABLE 17.5 Rehabilitation of the Back

Stage I: Minimal or no muscle spasm present

No.	Exercise	I	II	III	IV
1.	Lying on back—bend knee to chest—one leg at a time.	+			
2.	Lying on back, both legs together—bend knees to chest.	+			
3.	Lying on back—pelvic tilt (Figure 17.16).	+			
4.	Rock backward and forward smoothly (Figure 17.18).	+	+		
5.	Beginning sit-ups—lift to 60° position using elbows and arms, return to table with pelvic-tilt action, arms across chest.	+			
6.	Curl-ups and returns down, arms outstretched in front of body.	+			
7.	Hip-lift—push down with feet and shoulders, raise hips (Figure 17.19).	+	+		
8.	Hanging from overhead bar—do pelvic tilt.	+	+		
9.	Stretching exercises				
	a. Lying on back—rotate legs and lower back slowly to each side, shoulders flat on floor.	+	+	+	+
	b. Iliotibial tract stretch (see Figure 21.30).	+	+	+	+
	c. Hamstring stretch (see Figures 3.1 and 3.2).	+	+	+	+
	d. Achilles tendon stretch (see Figure 3.6)	+	+	+	+

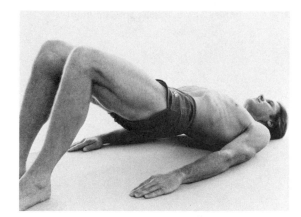

FIGURE 17.19 The hip-lift

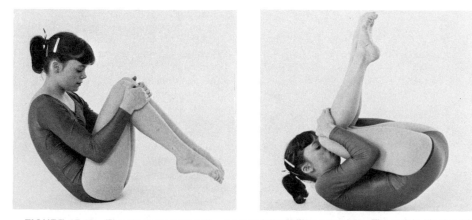

FIGURE 17.18 The rock-up and roll—a useful flexibility exercise The pelvic tilt should be maintained throughout the roll, ensuring a smooth action.

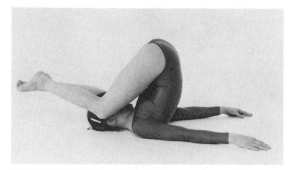

FIGURE 17.20 Back flexibility exercise This is the first stage of the "plow stretch." It should be held for 30 seconds. When this is completed with ease, the second stage may be performed.

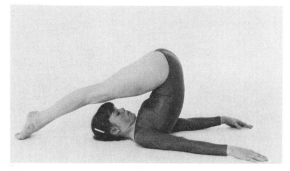

FIGURE 17.21 Back flexibility—the second stage of the "plow stretch" There should be no tension, and the athlete should be able to breathe normally.

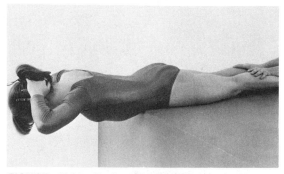

FIGURE 17.22 Back strengthening With the legs held, the athlete should extend to the horizontal only.

TABLE 17.5   Rehabilitation of the Back (*cont.*)

Stage II: No muscle spasm present

No.	Exercise	I	II	III	IV
1.	Lying on back—bring legs over head to a comfortable position, return with knees bent.		+		
2.	Lying on back—bring knees slowly to touch ears (Figure 17.20).		+	+	+
3.	Lying on back—legs straight over head (Figure 17.21).		+	+	+
4.	Isometric pelvic tilts.		+	+	+
5.	Isometric pelvic tilts against a wall.		+	+	+
6.	Curl-ups and return, arms across chest.		+		
7.	Lying prone, legs supported, torso over end of table—extend to 0° only (Figure 17.22).		+	+	
8.	Leg extensions—prone, with legs and pelvis over end of table—raise legs to 0° only, knees bent.		+	+	+

Stage III: More advanced

No.	Exercise	I	II	III	IV
1.	Variations of overhead stretching a. Toes held b. Legs open, toes on ground c. Over end of table				
2.	Shoulder stand (Figure 17.23).			+	+
3.	Hyperextension—in bridging position.			+	+
4.	Curl-ups and return, arms behind head.			+	
5.	Pull-ups from bar.			+	+
6.	Hanging from bar—bring knees up to chest.			+	+
7.	Lying prone, legs supported, torso over end of table—back extensions from 90 to 0° with weight(s).			+	
8.	Psoas stretch—lying on back, bend knee to chest while keeping other leg and thigh flat on table (Figure 17.24).			+	+

TABLE 17.5 Rehabilitation of the Back (*cont.*)

Stage IV: For suitably conditioned, strong and advanced competitive athletes only, with individual prescription and supervision

No.	Exercise	I	II	III	IV
1.	Curl up and touch elbow to opposite knee.				+
2.	Curl up and return, hold weight behind neck.				+
3.	Lying prone, legs supported—hyperextensions without weights, i.e., come up above 0°.				+
4.	Lying prone, legs supported—hyperextensions with weights, i.e., come up above 0° (as long as there is no discomfort).				+
5.	Supine, arms outstretched, holding weight, rotate torso with feet held; or no weight, hands behind head (Figure 17.25).				+
6.	Prone, feet held, torso off end of table—back extensions with rotation.				+
7.	"Good morning" exercise.				+
8.	Dead lifts, cleans, and squats.				+

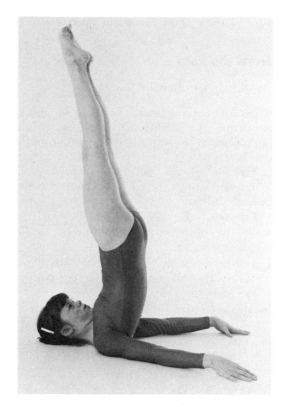

FIGURE 17.23 The shoulder stand The athlete should attempt to bring the ankles, hips, and shoulders into one vertical line, and not allow the buttocks to sag posteriorly.

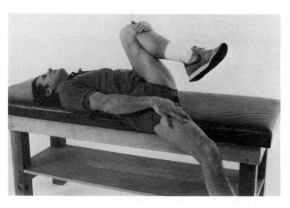

FIGURE 17.24 Psoas stretch To increase the stretch, the leg may be dropped below the level of the table

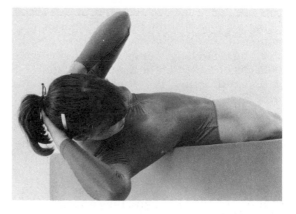

FIGURE 17.25 Trunk strengthening The feet and legs are supported and the buttocks are in contact with the edge of the table. The trunk is held horizontal and slowly rotated. If the athlete is sufficiently strong and well-conditioned, a weight may be grasped while the arms are outstretched.

Lateral Hip Pain

Lateral hip pain may be due to:

1. Strain or weakness of the quadratus lumborum, the abdominal muscles, or the iliotibial tract, presenting with pain along the iliac crest
2. Friction of the iliotibial tract over the greater trochanter, often associated with trochanteric bursitis
3. Strain of the gluteus medius, the piriformis, or both at the attachment to the greater trochanter
4. Lower back dysfunction or discogenic disease, with radiation or referred pain in the hip area
5. Stress fracture of the femur

TREATMENT: Appropriate strengthening and stretching exercises and therapeutic modalities usually relieve the symptoms. A discrepancy in leg length should be sought and corrected. In cases of trochanteric bursitis or iliotibial friction a cortisone injection may be indicated.

"Hip Pointer"

Hip pointer is a term that indicates a *contusion to the iliac crest*, the anterior superior iliac spine, or both. This contusion results in bleeding, swelling, and pain. Sometimes avulsion of a portion of the muscles attached to the crest occurs. Rarely is a fracture of the crest found. The athlete has difficulty walking normally and standing upright, due to the pain and muscle spasm. The area is very tender to the touch. It is important for the trainer to exclude an intra-abdominal injury.

TREATMENT: Ice should be placed on the painful area immediately. Injection of a corticosteroid preparation in conjunction with a long-acting anesthetic agent is often indicated soon after the injury. Following such treatment, symptoms rapidly decrease, though it may take a few days of icing and gentle stretching to enable the athlete to run

normally. Oral anti-inflammatory medication can be used if necessary, and TENS is a useful adjunct. The athlete should wear adequate protective padding upon return to participation.

Injury to the Lateral Cutaneous Nerve of the Thigh

The lateral cutaneous nerve of the thigh supplies the proximal two-thirds of the lateral thigh. It is purely sensory in function. Contusions to this nerve can result in impaired sensation over the thigh laterally. Muscle power is not affected. Recovery depends on the degree of damage the nerve has sustained. No active treatment is usually necessary.

Occasionally the nerve becomes entrapped in scar tissue, producing constant pain in the lateral groin area or along the lateral border of the thigh. This can be treated with a local anesthetic and a cortisone preparation. If this fails to relieve the symptoms, exploratory surgery aimed at releasing the entrapped nerve should be considered.

Dislocation of the Hip

A hip dislocation is a severe injury resulting from a considerable force which usually drives the hip backwards. A fracture may be associated with this posterior dislocation. An anterior dislocation rarely occurs.

The athlete cannot walk after the injury. A large prominence may be felt over the greater trochanteric area with pain localized in the hip. The affected foot will tend to rest on top of the opposite foot. Though the diagnosis may be immediately apparent clinically, no attempt should be made to reduce the dislocation on the field. The athlete should be removed by stretcher and taken to an emergency room for further examination and X-rays.

TREATMENT: Reduction under general anesthesia will most frequently be necessary. It may then take many months before full athletic activity can be resumed.

COMPLICATIONS:

1. Compression of the sciatic nerve can result in an impairment of foot function.

2. Avascular necrosis of the femoral head can occur up to six months after injury. This complication seems to be more common when the femur remains unreduced for a number of hours. It is therefore important to act immediately after the dislocation.

3. Osteoarthritis can occur later in life.

When a dislocation occurs in the adolescent with an unfused capital femoral epiphysis, a *fracture through the epiphysis* can result. This usually presents in a very similar way to dislocation of the hip, and careful X-ray studies may be necessary before deciding on the diagnosis. The condition may require reduction and internal fixation.

Pain around the Pubic Symphysis from Overuse

Pubic symphysis pain can be due to

a. adductor strain

b. stress fracture of the inferior ramus

c. osteitis pubis

Osteitis pubis is an unusual condition that can affect a running athlete, especially a long-distance runner, though it might result from direct local trauma.[21,22,23] Presenting symptoms are pain and tenderness over the symphysis pubis, resulting in spasm of the adductor muscles. In severe cases the athlete may develop a waddling gait. There may be radiation of pain down the inner aspect of the thigh and up into the lower abdomen.

TREATMENT: Anti-inflammatory medication to help alleviate the symptoms is combined with ice, ultrasound, and TENS. If a localized tender spot exists, a local injection of corticosteroid may prove beneficial. In the severely acute case with a markedly inflamed symphysis pubis and high fever, four to six weeks of oral cortisone may be indicated.[24] After the acute symptoms have subsided,

treatment consists of slowly and progressively strengthening any abdominal, groin, adductor, or lower-back muscle weakness.

REFERENCES

1. Ferguson RJ, McMaster JH, Stanitski CL: Low back pain in college football linemen. *J Sports Med* 2:63–69, 1974.

2. Jackson DW, Wiltse LL, Cirincione RJ: Spondylolysis in the female gymnast. *Clin Orthop* 117:68–73, 1976.

3. Levine DB: The painful low back. In *Arthritis and Allied Conditions: A Textbook of Rheumatology* edited by DJ McCarty. Philadelphia, Lea and Febiger, ninth edition, 1979.

4. Macnab I: *Backache.* Baltimore, Williams and Wilkins, 1977.

5. Cyriax J: *Textbook of Orthopaedic Medicine: Diagnosis of Soft Tissue Lesions,* Vol I. New York, Macmillan, seventh edition, 1978.

6. Mennell J McM: *Back Pain.* Boston, Little Brown and Company, 1960.

7. Kirkaldy-Willis WH, Hill RJ: A more precise diagnosis for low-back pain. *Spine* 4:516–523, 1979.

8. McKenzie RA: Prophylaxis in recurrent low back pain. *NZ Med J* 89:22–23, 1979.

9. Schiötz E, Cyriax J: *Manipulation, Past and Present.* London, Heinemann and Son, 1975.

10. Rettig A, Jackson DW, Wiltse LL, et al: The epidural venogram as a diagnostic procedure in the young athlete with symptoms of lumbar disc disease. *Am J Sports Med* 5:158–164, 1977.

11. Leyshon A, Kirwan EOG, Wynn Parry CB: Electrical studies in the diagnosis of compression of the lumbar root. *J Bone Joint Surg* 63B:71–75, 1981.

12. Jackson DW, Rettig A, Wiltse LL: Epidural cortisone injections in the young athletic adult. *Am J Sports Med* 8:239-243, 1980.

13. Gindin RA, Volcan IJ: Rupture of the intervertebral disc producing cauda equina syndrome. *Am Surgeon* 44:585–593, 1978.

14. Floman Y, Wiesel SW, Rothman RH: Cauda equina syndrome presenting as a herniated lumbar disk. *Clin Orthop* 147:234–237, 1980.

15. Pace JB, Nague D: Piriformis syndrome. *West J Med* 124:435, 1976.

16. Wiltse LL, Widell EH, Jackson DW: Fatigue fracture: The basic lesion in isthmic spondylolisthesis. *J Bone Joint Surg* 57A:17–22, 1975.

17. Jackson DW, Wiltse LL, Dingeman RD, et al: Stress reactions involving pars interarticularis in young athletes. *Am J Sports Med* 9:304–312, 1981.

18. Jackson DW: Low back pain in young athletes. Evaluation of stress reaction and discogenic problems. *Am J Sports Med* 7:364–366, 1979.

19. Kotani PT, Ichikawa N, Wakabayashi W, et al: Studies of spondylosis found among weight lifters. *Br J Sports Med* 6:4–8, 1970.

20. Birnbaum DA: Missed avulsion fracture of the lesser trochanter in a tennis professional. *Med Trial Tech Q* 27:121–125, 1980.

21. Koch RA, Jackson DW: Pubic symphisitis in runners. A report of two cases. *Am J Sports Med* 9:62–63, 1981.

22. Cochrane GM: Osteitis pubis in athletes. *Br J Sports Med* 5:233–235, 1971.

23. Williams JGP: Limitation of hip joint movement as a factor in traumatic osteitis pubis. *Br J Sports Med* 12:129–133, 1978.

24. Pyle LA: Osteitis pubis in athletes. *J Am Coll Health Assoc* 23:238–239, 1975.

RECOMMENDED READINGS

Chrisman OD, Mittnacht A, Snook GA: A study of the results following rotatory manipulation in the lumbar intervertebral-disc syndrome. *J Bone Joint Surg* 46A: 517–524, 1964.

Cyriax J, Russell G: *Textbook of Orthopaedic Medicine: Treatment by Manipulation, Massage, and Injection*, Vol II. New York, Macmillan, tenth edition, 1980.

Fahrni WH: Conservative treatment of lumbar disc degeneration: Our primary responsibility. *Orthop Clin North Am* 6:93–103, 1975.

McKenzie RA: Manual correction of sciatic scoliosis. *NZ Med J* 76:194–199, 1972.

Merrifield HH, Cowan RF: Groin strain injuries in ice hockey. Research summaries. *J Sports Med* 1:41–42, 1973.

Micheli L: Low back pain in the adolescent. Differential diagnosis. *Am J Sports Med* 7:362–364, 1979.

Nachemson AL: The load on lumbar discs in different positions of the body. *Clin Orthop* 45:107–122, 1966.

Nachemson AL: The influence of spinal movements on the lumbar intradiscal pressure and on the tensile stresses in the annulus fibrosus. *Acta Orthop Scand* 33:183–207, 1963.

Stanish W: Low back pain in middle-age athletes. *Am J Sports Med* 7:367–369, 1979.

CHAPTER 18

Chest, Abdominal, and Genital Injuries

CHEST INJURIES

Direct blows to the chest can result in one or more of the following injuries:

1. Contusions
2. Rib fractures, which can result in a pneumothorax
3. Costochondral separations
4. Cardiac contusions, which can result in a pericardial effusion with cardiac tamponade (constriction of the heart)

Contusions

A severe contusion to the ribs is often very difficult to distinguish from a fracture. Because of bruising of the intercostal muscles, there may be both pain on inspiration and localized tenderness. These cases should be X-rayed to exclude a fractured rib or other intrathoracic problems such as a pneumothorax.

Having excluded the more serious conditions, the involved area should be iced and anti-inflammatory medication administered if necessary. A rib belt can be used for comfort. If the athlete is participating in a contact sport, sufficient padding should be applied over the contusion for adequate protection.

Rib Fractures

A fractured rib may present with localized tenderness and pain on inspiration, resulting in shallow, rapid breathing. It is sometimes possible to feel crepitus over a fractured rib, but often the symptoms are indistinguishable from those of a contusion. The athlete should always be X-rayed to establish the diagnosis and exclude any complication. Complications include a pneumothorax, which is clinically confirmed by the presence of hyperresonance to percussion and the absence of breath sounds when listening with a stethoscope to the affected site.

Treatment of the uncomplicated case is symptomatic, using a rib belt or tape on the involved side of the chest wall. Healing should be complete before the athlete is allowed to return to participation, mainly because of the danger of a pneumothorax, caused by a fractured rib penetrating the pleura. The healing process in the average case is usually sufficiently completed within three to four weeks, but the athlete should use protective padding over the fracture if participating in a contact sport.

Emergency care of a pneumothorax includes administration of oxygen and rapid removal of the player by stretcher from the area of participation to the nearest emergency room.

Spontaneous Pneumothorax

A spontaneous pneumothorax can occur in a previously healthy athlete. There is sudden shortness of breath and a sharp chest pain, which may be referred to the tip of the shoulder. If a large pneumothorax is present, cyanosis can be seen (blueness of the tongue, mucous membranes, and nails).

Signs include shallow, rapid respiration with poor air entry into the affected lung and hyperresonance to percussion over the affected area. Treatment consists of administration of oxygen and rapid transportation of the athlete to an emergency facility capable of handling this type of problem.

Costochondral Separations

Costochondral separations frequently occur in a sport such as wrestling, when the rib cage is squeezed or when one arm is pulled over to the side, stretching the attachment of the rib at the costochondral junction. Frequently the injured athlete feels a pop.

SYMPTOMS AND SIGNS: Tenderness is localized specifically to the costochondral junction, and often swelling and/or displacement of the rib can be seen and felt. The displaced rib can sometimes be manipulated back into place and held there by means of semicircumferential taping. These cases should be X-rayed to exclude fractured ribs.

TREATMENT: Treatment consists of ice, tape, and analgesics. The judicious use of a corticosteroid injection around the painful area often helps reduce the symptoms and may allow the athlete to return to participation, though many athletes have prolonged discomfort.

Cardiac Contusions

A cardiac contusion can result in a pericardial effusion, which may lead to cardiac tamponade. This is clinically confirmed by muffled heart sounds, engorgement of the neck veins, small pulse pressure when taking the blood pressure, and a pulse that tends to disappear on inspiration.

As cardiac tamponade is a life-threatening condition that needs to be treated immediately, the athlete needs to be taken by ambulance to an emergency room without delay.

ABDOMINAL INJURIES

Injuries to the abdominal viscera are not common in most athletic activities, but they do occur in contact events. Such accidents most frequently cause

1. rupture of the spleen[1]
2. rupture of the liver
3. contusion or rupture of the kidney
4. such uncommon conditions as retroperitoneal hemorrhage and rupture of the bowel

Splenic Rupture

The spleen can rupture at any time but is more likely to do so when it is enlarged and fragile, as it becomes with infectious mononucleosis. Many times the athlete has splenomegaly without being aware of it and can rupture the spleen during a relatively innocent movement or blow. At other times rupture results from a severe impact injury to the left upper quadrant of the abdomen or to the lower left rib cage.

SYMPTOMS AND SIGNS: In most cases the diagnosis is not made initially, though it should be suspected. The athlete may have severe pain immediately after the injury and then recover and be thought to have had either "the wind knocked out" or a contusion to the lower ribs. With continued bleeding into the peritoneal cavity, the athlete will begin to suffer increasing abdominal pain and may have referred shoulder pain from the blood irritating the diaphragm. Because of the blood loss, dizziness or fainting may be the first clue to the diagnosis.[1]

The earliest signs are a pale athlete (from constriction of the blood vessels) and a rapid pulse—this is an important sign. The blood pressure may remain normal for a considerable period of time after the injury. If there is a suspicion of a ruptured spleen, the athlete should be immediately transported to an emergency facility for further investigation and observation. If there is some distance to be traveled to the emergency facility, an intravenous infusion of normal saline or Ringer's lactate solution should be given as a precautionary measure before clinical shock sets in.

TREATMENT: A ruptured spleen almost always needs to be removed surgically, and a blood transfusion is frequently necessary.

Hepatic Rupture

Because the liver is encased in a capsule, it is possible to have a controlled amount of bleeding from a blow to the upper right quadrant. If the liver is severely lacerated and bleeding into the intraperitoneal cavity, symptoms and signs similar to a ruptured spleen rapidly develop.

As with a ruptured spleen, the suspicion of a contused or lacerated liver should be followed by emergency treatment and rapid transfer of the athlete to a facility for further investigation. An athlete with a contused liver is usually kept under observation, as the condition often resolves spontaneously. Lacerations of the liver frequently need to be surgically repaired.

Renal Contusion or Rupture

A renal injury is usually caused by a blow to the flank and presents with a backache, blood in the urine, or both. Any athlete who has a contusion to the flank should be asked to produce a urine specimen which, even though clear, should be tested for microscopic bleeding. If blood is present the athlete should be referred for urological investigation, which frequently includes an intravenous pyelogram (IVP). An athlete with a contusion to or partial rupture of the kidney can be merely placed under observation, as this condition frequently resolves spontaneously. A large laceration of the kidney may need to be surgically repaired.

Contusion to the Solar Plexus ("Getting the Wind Knocked Out")

Solar plexus contusion is a frequent injury resulting from irritation of the solar plexus by a blow to the epigastric area. Spasm of the diaphragm reflexly causes temporary paralysis of respiration. Occasionally, the feeling of having the wind knocked out is due to a forceful expiration of the residual volume of air normally present in the lungs and leads to an inhibition of inspiration for the following few seconds.

The athlete suffering from such a contusion should lie still and wait for spontaneous recovery, then be escorted from the area of participation. The abdomen should be examined to ensure no damage to the spleen, liver, or other abdominal structures and to ensure full recovery, after which return to participation may be permitted.

GENITAL INJURIES

Contusion to the Testes

The intense pain and discomfort associated with contusion to the testes is relieved by a simple procedure. The athlete is given a brief explanation of what is to follow, and is then lifted approximately six inches above the ground. This is accomplished by the trainer placing his or her hands beneath the athlete's axilla. The athlete is then dropped to the ground. The impact appears to break the spasm of the cremasteric muscles, often producing dramatic disappearance of the pain.

If swelling of the scrotum occurs, the area involved should be iced and the scrotum elevated by placing towels between the legs. If a large hematoma develops, the athlete should be examined by a urologist and assessed for possible aspiration.

Contusion to the Vulva

A vulval contusion results from a fall, such as falling astride a balance beam, and a large hematoma rapidly develops. In severe cases, lacerations occur and need to be sutured.

Vaginal Injuries

High-speed water-skiing injuries can result in rupture of the wall of the vagina. Or water may be forced through the fallopian tubes, resulting in localized pelvic peritonitis. If such an injury occurs, the athlete should be referred immediately to a gynecologist. These injuries can be prevented by the athlete's wearing a neoprene wet suit while water-skiing.

REFERENCE

1. Hahn DB: The ruptured spleen: Implications for the athletic trainer. *Athletic Training* 13:190–191, 1978.

CHAPTER 19

Thigh, Knee, and Patella Injuries

FUNCTIONAL ANATOMY

Knee Movements

The knee consists of the *tibiofemoral joint* and the *patellofemoral joint*. The tibiofemoral joint appears to move as a hinge, but actually other movements occur as the knee flexes from the extended position. These movements include[1]

1. a rocking action
2. a gliding action
3. rotational movements

1. In full extension (0°) there is no rotational movement. The tibia is externally rotated on the femur and "locked" in this position.

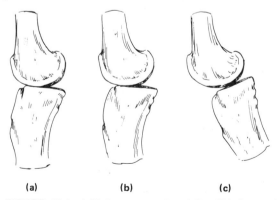

(a) **(b)** **(c)**

FIGURE 19.1 Initial movements of the tibiofemoral joint (a) At 0° the joint is locked (b) With the initiation of flexion, a rocking action occurs (c) From 20° onwards, the tibia glides on the femur. Rotation is now possible.

2. From 0° to 20° of flexion, a rocking action takes place. The tibia begins to internally rotate on the femur (depending on how one looks at it, it is also correct to say that the femur externally rotates relative to the tibia).

3. From 20° on, the tibia starts to glide on the femur. An increasing amount of tibial rotation is now possible—up to 40° when the knee is bent to 90°. More external rotation is usually present than internal rotation.

4. The knee can normally bend until the calf comes into contact with the thigh at approximately 135°.

5. On extension of the knee from the flexed position, the tibia externally rotates relative to the femur during the last 20°.[2] This is the so-called "screw-home" mechanism, which helps to stabilize the knee in full extension.[3]

The *patellofemoral articulation* is a gliding joint. The patella slides along the intercondylar groove between the lateral and medial femoral condyles.

Ligaments

The knee has a complex system of ligaments which enclose it from all directions except over the anterior portion.

Medial stabilizing complex. The medial ligament is divided into two portions:

1. *Medial capsular ligament*: Consists of the meniscofemoral and the meniscotibial bands lying on either side of the joint line and is

attached to the periphery of the medial meniscus. It is divided into anterior, middle, and posterior thirds (Figure 19.2).

The *posterior oblique ligament* is really the posterior third of the medial capsular ligament, but is named as a separate ligament because it is thought to help prevent valgus laxity and medial rotatory instability.

2. *Tibial collateral ligament*: Runs from the medial epicondyle of the femur to the medial side of the tibia and inserts into the tibia underneath the pes anserine group of muscles, about 7 cm below the joint line. It is one of the main stabilizers against valgus stress and medial rotation. The anterior portion of this ligament is taut throughout the range of motion, from full extension to 90° of flexion, which helps prevent valgus opening.[4]

Lateral stabilizing complex.

1. *Lateral capsular ligament*: Similar to the medial capsular ligament in that it consists of both meniscotibial and meniscofemoral bands, and is divided into anterior, middle, and posterior thirds.

2. *Fibular collateral ligament*: Runs from the lateral femur to the head of the fibula and consists of a band of firm tissue that is easily palpated when the knee is held at 90° of flexion and forced into a varus position (such as when the lateral malleolus is placed on the opposite knee while the athlete is sitting). Lateral stability is achieved (Figure 19.4) in conjunction with the

   a. iliotibial band
   b. biceps tendon
   c. popliteus tendon and arcuate ligament complex

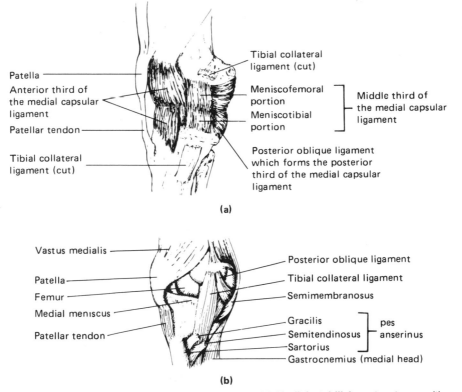

(a)

(b)

FIGURE 19.2   (a) The medial capsular ligament   (b) Medial stabilizing structures   (the capsular ligament is partially removed)

TABLE 19.1 Medial Stabilizing Complex of the Knee

Consists of two parts:
1. *Medial capsular ligament* (deep capsular ligament)
   This is divided into thirds: Anterior third
                                 Middle third
                                 Posterior third (this is the same as
                                            the *posterior oblique
                                            ligament*)
   Each division has a meniscofemoral part and a meniscotibial part
2. *Tibial collateral ligament* (superficial)

Cruciate ligaments.

1. *Anterior cruciate ligament*: Runs from the anterior part of the tibial plateau just medial and posterior to the anterior tibial spine, and goes posteriorly and laterally to attach to the posterior-most portion of the medial aspect of the lateral femoral condyle. This ligament is of vital importance in preventing hyperextension and excessive rotation of the tibia on the femur during running and cutting.[5]

2. *Posterior cruciate ligament*: Lies in the long axis of the leg. It runs from the posterior part of the tibial plateau to the lateral part of the medial femoral condyle. Its main function is to prevent posterior displacement of the tibia on the femur, particularly during the gliding phase of flexion.

Other ligaments.

1. *Popliteal oblique ligament*: On the posterior aspect of the knee, it blends in with the posterior capsule and the fibers from the semimembranosus muscle.

2. *Posterior capsule*: A thick band of tissue situated posteriorly, it appears to be one of the structures preventing hyperextension of the knee. It is taut in extension, but lax in flexion.

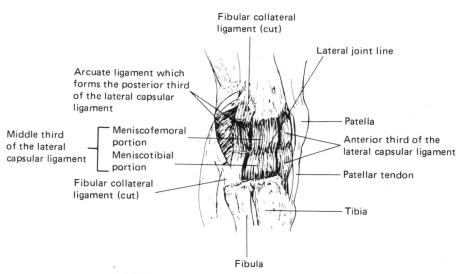

Fibular collateral ligament (cut)

Lateral joint line

Arcuate ligament which forms the posterior third of the lateral capsular ligament

Middle third of the lateral capsular ligament

Meniscofemoral portion
Meniscotibial portion

Fibular collateral ligament (cut)

Patella

Anterior third of the lateral capsular ligament

Patellar tendon

Tibia

Fibula

FIGURE 19.3 The lateral capsular ligament

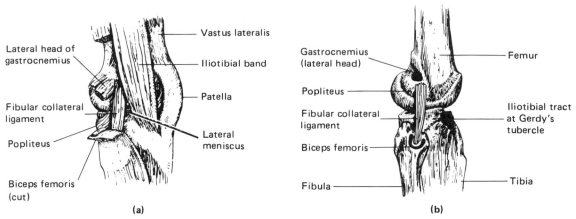

FIGURE 19.4 **(a) Some of the structures comprising the lateral stabilizing complex** (the capsular ligament is not included) **(b) Attachment of the structures comprising the lateral stabilizing complex**

The Menisci

There are two menisci in the knee joint: the *medial meniscus* and the *lateral meniscus*. These fibrocartilaginous disks deepen the joint, thereby permitting a more stable articulation between the femur and the tibia. They also act as shock absorbers (weight transmitters) and help smooth the gliding action of the tibia on the femur (see Table 19.3).

The medial meniscus lies on the medial tibial plateau, which is concave; the lateral meniscus lies on the lateral tibial plateau, which is convex. The menisci move with the tibia during flexion and extension and with the femur during rotation.

The blood supply to the menisci is via peripheral vessels from the synovial and capsular tissues, and is relatively poor, especially that to the central section of the meniscus. Most of the nutritional needs are therefore met by the diffusion of synovial fluid.

The menisci are thicker at their peripheries than at their centers (Figure 19.6) and are circular in shape. Smillie has stated that, "The contour of the lateral meniscus is most accurately described as a large segment . . .

TABLE 19.2   Lateral Stabilizing Complex of the Knee

The following structures support the lateral side of the knee joint:

1. *Lateral capsular ligament*—as on the medial side, this part is divided into thirds: Anterior third
                                                                                  Middle third
                                                                                  Posterior third
   Each of these divisions has a meniscofemoral and a meniscotibial part.

2. *Fibular collateral ligament*—runs between the femur and the fibular head

3. *Biceps tendon*—attaches to the fibular head

4. *Iliotibial band*—attaches to Gerdy's tubercle

5. *Popliteus tendon* and *arcuate ligament complex*—cover the postero-lateral corner of the knee

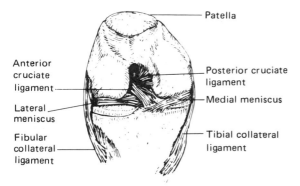

FIGURE 19.5 The ligaments of the knee from the front with the knee bent

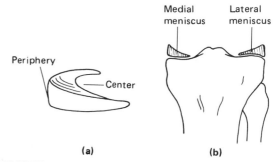

(a) **(b)**

FIGURE 19.6 (a) The meniscus The menisci are thicker at the periphery than at the center **(b) Silhouette of the menisci**

of a small circle. Whereas, by comparison, the medial is a small segment of a large circle."[6]

The *medial meniscus* is C shaped and consists of an anterior portion, or body, and a posterior segment, or horn. There is an important attachment to the deep capsular portion of the medial capsular ligament. A peripheral detachment of the meniscus can result if this medial capsular ligament is torn (Figure 19.7).

The semimembranosus muscle is attached to the posterior aspect of the medial meniscus (via the posteromedial capsule) and tends to pull the meniscus back out of the way during flexion. However, mobility of the medial meniscus is limited, which leaves the posterior horn vulnerable to tearing.

The *lateral meniscus* is more O shaped and is more mobile than the medial meniscus because it does not have any attachment to the deep posterolateral capsule, from which it is

separated by the popliteal tendon sheath. The arcuate ligament is firmly attached to the lateral meniscus, and, as the popliteus muscle is attached to both the arcuate ligament and the lateral meniscus, the posterior segment of the meniscus can be pulled backward during medial rotation of the tibia in flexion.

Muscles

The muscles surrounding the knee joint are of extreme importance in preserving the stability of a basically unstable joint. It has been shown that athletes who condition all the muscles around the knee have a far lower incidence of injury than those who do not. The muscles surrounding the knee are:

The quadriceps muscle group. The quadriceps are the main stabilizers of the knee joint. They lie on the front of the thigh and

TABLE 19.3 Functions of the Menisci

1. Share the load in weight-bearing and increase the joint contact area
2. Absorb shock, thereby protecting the articular cartilage
3. Help stabilize the joint by deepening the articular surfaces of the tibial plateau
4. Help facilitate control of some rotational movements (such as the "screw-home" movement)
5. Aid in joint nutrition and lubrication

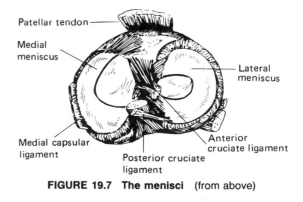

FIGURE 19.7 The menisci (from above)

form the quadriceps tendon, which inserts into the patella. The patellar tendon originates from the inferior pole of the patella and inserts into the tibial tubercle. The main function of the quadriceps muscle group is to extend the flexed knee.

The quadriceps consist of four muscles:

1. *Vastus medialis*—makes up most of the medial bulk of the muscle. It has a separate part, the vastus medialis obliquus (VMO). The vastus medialis is important in stabilizing the patella. It is a very sensitive index of knee derangement, as it is the first muscle to atrophy.

2. *Vastus intermedius*—forms the bulk of the muscle.

3. *Vastus lateralis*—runs on the lateral side. These three vastus muscles originate from the femur and, with the rectus femoris, insert into the quadriceps tendon.

4. *Rectus femoris*—runs from the anterior inferior iliac spine to join the quadriceps tendon above the patella. The rectus femoris is the most superficial of the four muscles. It flexes the hip and extends the knee.

Pes anserine muscle group.   This group is composed of the sartorius, the gracilis, and the semitendinosus muscles, of which the semitendinosus is the strongest. The sartorius runs from the anterior superior iliac spine; the gracilis, from the pubis; the semitendinosus, from the ischial tuberosity. These muscles insert into the tibial crest (as the pes anserine tendon) anteriorly and superficial to the tibial attachment of the tibial collateral ligament, about 7 cm below the medial joint line. They act mainly to flex the knee but can, under certain conditions, internally rotate the tibia (Figure 19.8).

The hamstrings.   The hamstrings are situated on the posterior aspect of the thigh and are nearly as important as the quadriceps in preserving the stability of the knee. The main functions of the hamstrings are to

1. flex the extended knee.

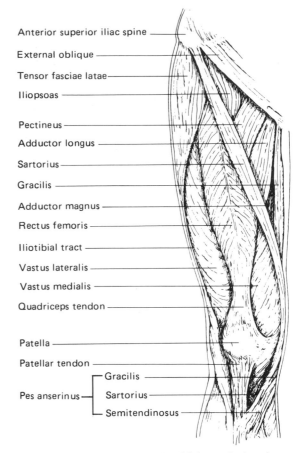

Anterior superior iliac spine
External oblique
Tensor fasciae latae
Iliopsoas
Pectineus
Adductor longus
Sartorius
Gracilis
Adductor magnus
Rectus femoris
Iliotibial tract
Vastus lateralis
Vastus medialis
Quadriceps tendon
Patella
Patellar tendon
Pes anserinus — ⎡ Gracilis
                ⎢ Sartorius
                ⎣ Semitendinosus

FIGURE 19.8   Muscles of the thigh—anterior view

2. work in conjunction with the quadriceps muscle group during knee extension. As the quadriceps extend the knee, the hamstrings act as a brake to slow down the tibia. If the quadriceps are too powerful relative to the hamstrings, a strained (or "pulled") hamstring can result from their being unable to adequately counteract the force of the quadriceps during extension.

3. extend the hip.

The hamstrings consist of three muscle masses which originate from the ischial tuberosity (Figure 19.9).

1. *Semitendinosus*—runs down the medial aspect of the thigh posteriorly and inserts into the tibia with the gracilis and the sartorius as the pes anserine muscle group.

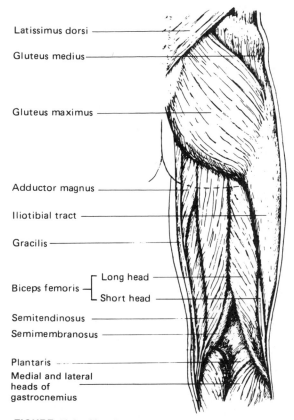

Latissimus dorsi

Gluteus medius

Gluteus maximus

Adductor magnus

Iliotibial tract

Gracilis

Biceps femoris —⌈ Long head
                └ Short head

Semitendinosus

Semimembranosus

Plantaris

Medial and lateral
heads of
gastrocnemius

FIGURE 19.9 Muscles of the thigh—posterior view

from the lateral femur. The biceps runs down the lateral aspect posteriorly and inserts into the head of the fibula. This helps dynamically stabilize the lateral aspect of the knee, particularly in flexion, as contraction of the biceps tightens the fibular collateral ligament and the posterior capsule.

The iliotibial tract. This muscle originates from the anterior superior iliac spine and the iliac crest as the tensor fasciae latae. It becomes the iliotibial tract at the lower third of the thigh and then sweeps across the lateral side of the knee to insert into the tibia at Gerdy's tubercle.

The popliteus. This muscle originates from the femur just above the lateral joint line, where it is covered by the fibular collateral ligament and the biceps femoris tendon. It is intimately connected with the posterior horn of the lateral meniscus, helping to retract it back out of the way. It inserts into the posterior aspect of the upper medial tibia above the soleal line. The popliteus has a number of functions which include:

1. Internal rotation of the tibia relative to the femur or, alternatively, external rotation of the femur if the tibia is fixed

2. Prevention of forward movement of the tibia on the femur when the foot is fixed

3. Tightening of the posterior capsule and the arcuate ligament

4. Retraction of the lateral meniscus

Gastrocnemius. As the gastrocnemius crosses the knee joint, it splits into two heads which insert posteriorly into the medial and lateral aspects of the femur respectively and play a part in stabilizing the knee joint.

THIGH INJURIES

Contusion to the Quadriceps

A contusion to the lateral and, more importantly, the anterior aspect of the thigh is often undertreated. It should be realized that

2. *Semimembranosus*—forms the bulk of the hamstring muscle group. It dynamically tightens the posteromedial corner, helping to prevent excessive rotation of the tibia from medial to lateral. The semimembranosus, on reaching the knee, branches into five divisions which fan out and attach to
   a. the oblique popliteal ligament
   b. the posterior capsule and the medial meniscus, where there is dynamic action retracting the meniscus from the joint
   c. the tibia medially, which helps to increase its internal rotatory action
   d. the posterior tibial tuberosity
   e. the popliteal fascia

3. *The biceps femoris.* This muscle has two heads—the *long head* originating from the ischial tuberosity and the *short head* originating

this can be one of the most disabling injuries to afflict an athlete. Following a severe blow to the thigh, two things occur: (1) Blood vessels are broken and a lesser or greater degree of bleeding occurs and (2) a variable amount of muscle is crushed. The bleeding can be considerable and can increase the damage to the muscle.

SYMPTOMS AND SIGNS: The athlete may attempt to continue participating after the injury. The thigh becomes progressively more stiff while at the same time the quadriceps muscles become more and more unresponsive. If the injury is severe, swelling and tightness of the thigh musculature are observed soon afterwards, together with loss of knee flexion.[7] If the athlete does not receive adequate treatment immediately, there may be increased swelling of the leg, stiffness of the muscles, inability to flex the knee and contract the quadriceps muscles, and severe pain.

TREATMENT: The sooner treatment is commenced the better the prognosis for the athlete.[8] Immediately after the injury, it is usually not possible for either the athlete or the examiner to determine if the injury will result in a major or minor hematoma. It is best to err on the conservative side and treat all contusions to the thigh as potentially serious. The following procedure is recommended:

1. Firmly apply a cold, wet elastic wrap to the thigh at the level of the contusion. After one or two turns of the wrap, apply ice. Further layers of wrap add compression to the contused area; the cold, wet bandage conducts the cold onto the thigh area.

2. While the athlete lies prone, an elastic bandage (or similar device) is tied around the ankle, and the knee flexed until minimal discomfort is felt. The athlete holds the elastic bandage over the shoulder to maintain the desired amount of knee flexion (Figure 19.10). *On no account should any force be applied in flexing the knee.* The idea behind this maneuver is to maintain the flexibility of the knee and the quadriceps muscles; it is *not* designed to increase flexibility. If the leg is kept straight, marked stiffness will be present the next day; with this method, flexibility is usually maintained at or near normal. It should again be emphasized that this procedure does not actually stretch the muscles, rather it holds the leg in a comfortable position.

3. Give analgesics if necessary.

4. Have the athlete use crutches for ambulation.

5. Begin anti-inflammatory medication if necessary.

After a few hours of icing the thigh with the knee held in flexion (the ice should be applied for 45 to 60 minutes at a time, and then taken off for 20 minutes), reassess the injury (Table 19.4). If there appears to be significant damage, continue the ice and the knee-flexed position for at least another twelve to twenty-four hours. If damage is mild, tell the athlete to repeat the icing with the leg in a flexed position two or three times during the night and the following day, each time keeping the ice in place for

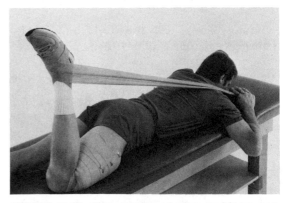

FIGURE 19.10 Early treatment of a quadriceps contusion Ice, together with a cold, wet elastic compression wrap, is applied to the anterior aspect of the thigh. A gentle stretch is then applied to the quadriceps muscle. This stretch should not be forceful, nor should it cause any pain. The stretch should be released and the ice removed for 20 minutes every hour.

about an hour. If the leg continues to swell in spite of these measures, consideration should be given to exploring the hematoma and aspirating the blood.

CONTINUING TREATMENT: Icing in a prone position with the knee flexed for 30 to 60 minutes at a time is continued on a daily or bi-daily basis until full flexibility is achieved, and thereafter, following each workout, until the leg becomes completely asymptomatic.

Quadriceps sets should be started when they can be performed painlessly. Until that time, electrical stimulation of the quadriceps and hamstrings can be used if it causes no pain. When doing isometric setting exercises, the athlete should hold each set for about five to eight seconds, doing ten of these each hour. When full contraction of the quadriceps is achieved, straight-leg raising (as described in the section on knee rehabilitation, p. 346) should begin. The full knee rehabilitation program should then be instituted.

COMPLICATIONS:

Early: As mentioned, a *poorly treated* contusion of the anterior thigh can result in a prolonged recovery, with stiffness, poor

TABLE 19.4 Assessing the Severity of a Thigh Injury

	Mild	Potentially Severe
1. The ability to actively bend the knee through a normal range of motion	Yes	No
2. The ability to actively set the quadriceps and to raise the leg without any discomfort	Yes	No
3. Localized swelling	No	Yes
4. Localized tenderness	+	+ + +

+ = minimal tenderness
+ + + = marked tenderness

TABLE 19.5 Contusion to the Quadriceps

During the recovery phase there should be
NO MASSAGE to the thigh
NO HEAT to the thigh
NO ULTRASOUND
NO CORTISONE INJECTIONS
NO ACTIVE STRETCHING of the quadriceps musculature

quadriceps action, and muscle wasting. A period of four to eight weeks is necessary before the athlete can start to rehabilitate the injured leg. The most important time to start treating this injury is immediately after it happens!

Late: Myositis ossificans (calcification within the muscles at the site of the injury) can develop. Calcification is a feared complication and is particularly apt to occur if (a) the athlete returns to participation too soon, (b) the thigh is re-injured before healing occurs, (c) massage or heat has been applied to the hematoma, (d) the hematoma has been poorly treated, or (e) the bleeding is associated with hemophilia (a rare bleeding disorder).[9]

Myositis ossificans can permanently limit the amount of knee flexion and can also produce a hard, painful lump in the thigh. If this occurs, the athlete should be withdrawn from athletic participation until the calcification has matured (this can be observed on serial X-rays), at which time a decision as to the advisability of surgical removal of the calcified mass can be made. Removal of the mass before it is mature frequently causes a recurrence of the calcification.

PROGNOSIS: If the athlete is adequately treated immediately after the injury, the chance of complications is small. However, if the initial bleeding is severe and the treatment is not started for a few hours, it may be four or five weeks or longer before the athlete can return to participation.

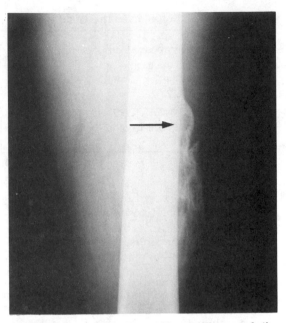

FIGURE 19.11 X-ray—myositis ossificans of the thigh This basketball player suffered a contusion to the thigh six weeks before this X-ray was taken. Note the marked calcification arising from the femur.

Strain of the Quadriceps Musculature

This usually implies a strain of the rectus femoris muscle, but occasionally one or more components of the vastus, the sartorius, or both are involved. A strain may vary from a mild "pull" of the rectus femoris to a

TABLE 19.6   Criteria for Return to Participation after a Contusion to the Quadriceps

1. There should be full flexibility of the thigh musculature when compared with the opposite unaffected leg (Figure 19.13)
2. There should be equal power, strength, and endurance of the quadriceps mechanism compared with the opposite leg
3. There should be minimal or no tenderness present in the thigh
4. The athlete should return to play with substantial protective padding over the affected area (Figure 19.12)

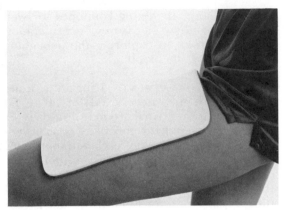

FIGURE 19.12 Anterior thigh pad A heat-molded pad is made from Orthoplast or Plastazote (white material) and a foam inner lining. The pad should be worn to protect the thigh following a contusion. Myositis ossificans is more likely to form if a second contusion occurs to the same area shortly after recovery from the first.

complete rupture of the muscle. When the latter occurs, a large bulge is seen in the upper thigh.

MECHANISM OF INJURY: Most pulls occur in an athlete who is not sufficiently warmed up or stretched out before beginning rapid acceleration during a sprint. Other predisposing factors include (1) tight quadriceps muscles, (2) an imbalance between the quadriceps power of the two legs, and (3) a short leg. The rectus femoris can also be strained when a kick is mistimed in rugby, soccer, or football.

SYMPTOMS AND SIGNS: The athlete is immediately aware that the muscle has been strained. There is pain down the entire length of the rectus femoris, with tenderness localized to the area of the strain. There is inability to contract the rest of the quadriceps mechanism, and knee flexion is usually limited. Swelling, should it occur, may mask a complete rupture of the rectus femoris initially. A complete rupture leaves a permanent bulge high up in the thigh but surprisingly, often produces little functional disability.

TABLE 19.7   Criteria for Return to Participation after a Strain of the Quadriceps Musculature

The athlete should not be allowed to sprint until there is:

1. Equal power, strength, and endurance of both quadriceps muscle groups
2. Equal flexibility of both quadriceps (Figure 19.13)
3. No pain with any of these tests

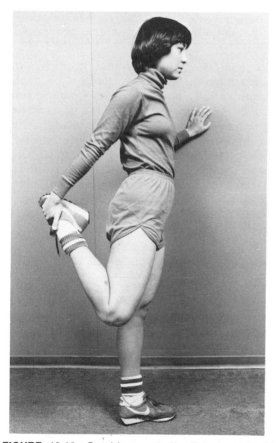

FIGURE 19.13   Quadriceps strain This test should demonstrate equal flexibility of both left and right quadriceps before return to participation is permitted.

TREATMENT:

Initial: Ice on a firmly applied, cold, wet elastic wrap is the treatment of choice. This should be followed by anti-inflammatory medication, analgesics, and crutch ambulation.

Later: Once the initial bleeding has settled down, ice therapy should be combined with TENS, ultrasound, gentle frictional massage, and *gentle, controlled* stretching exercises. At no time should these stretching exercises be painful. As soon as the quadriceps can adequately contract, the athlete should be placed onto an isokinetic machine such as the Cybex or the Orthotron and be put through a limited range of movement at high speed. As healing continues and strength returns, a full quadriceps rehabilitation program should be commenced (see section on knee rehabilitation, p. 346).

Acute Strain of the Hamstring Group

An acute hamstring "pull" is a common and frustrating injury occurring particularly in sprinters. It can be related to some of the following factors:

1. Lack of flexibility of the hamstring group.

2. Imbalance in the ratio of strength and power between the hamstrings and the quadriceps. In sprinters the quadriceps are usually stronger than the hamstrings, while in long-distance runners the quadriceps are usually weaker.

3. Inequality of strength of the left versus the right hamstring group.

4. The fact that the biceps muscle receives two nerve supplies, one to the short head and one to the long head. This theoretically results in an inappropriate contraction of the one head while the other is relaxing.

5. A poor running style, particularly leaning backward when decelerating at the end of a sprint or when attempting to lengthen the stride.

SYMPTOMS AND SIGNS: With an acute strain the athlete is immediately aware of the condition. Occasionally it feels as if something has "popped" in the back of the thigh. In severe cases the athlete will describe an intense tearing sensation, with pain from the ischial tuberosity down to the back of the knee. There is usually generalized pain, but tenderness is localized to the area of the actual disruption. Swelling can occur fairly rapidly and obscure the defect of a severe tear. Passive straight-leg raising is limited, and there is inability to fully contract the hamstrings against resistance. After a few days, considerable ecchymosis might be noted in the back of the thigh, which will gradually descend to behind the knee.

TREATMENT: Immediate treatment is with ice and compression, using a cold, wet elastic wrap. The athlete should gently stretch the hamstrings while icing, to help prevent the loss of flexibililty that would otherwise occur (Figure 19.14). Should spasm of the hamstrings prevent stretching, spraying with Fluori-Methane (see p. 106) and TENS may be useful. An anti-inflammatory drug and analgesics are given as necessary. If the athlete cannot walk normally, crutches should be used.

A few days after the initial bleeding has subsided, ice therapy can be augmented with isometric contractions of the hamstrings, TENS, ultrasound, gentle frictional massage, and gentle, controlled hamstring stretching.

Once hamstring setting exercises are

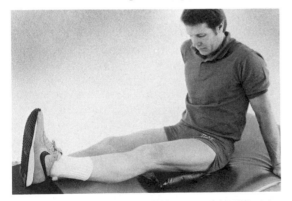

FIGURE 19.14 Acute hamstring strain While icing the injured area, place a gentle stretch on the hamstrings. This may help prevent spasm and loss of flexibility that might otherwise occur. The foot is placed on a stool, the quadriceps are relaxed, and the hamstrings gently stretched. Compression may be added.

TABLE 19.8 Criteria for Return to Participation after an Acute Strain of the Hamstring Group

1. There should be at least equal flexibility of the hamstrings bilaterally (preferably more than was present before the injury)
2. There should be equal bilateral strength, power, and endurance of the hamstring group
3. There should be a satisfactory ratio of quadriceps-to-hamstrings strength, power, and endurance

Hamstring rehabilitation should continue for some time after the athlete has returned to participation.

painless, the athlete should progress onto the isokinetic apparatus (Cybex or Orthotron). Then, both the hamstring and the quadriceps groups should be progressively developed. Stretching should be emphasized. When satisfactory strength, power, and flexibility have been achieved, the athlete may begin to jog. A useful exercise is running backwards. Straight ahead running should be gradually increased, but no sprinting should be allowed until the criteria for return to full participation have been fulfilled.

Slow-Onset Hamstring Strain

With this type of strain, which occurs particularly in the long-distance runner, progressive tightness and discomfort are noted in the uppermost third of the posterior aspect of the leg. Localized tenderness may or may not be present. Hamstring flexibility is limited, weakness is usually apparent, and asymmetry in the heights of the posterior superior iliac spines is sometimes present, suggesting the association of lower-back joint dysfunction or other lumbar spine pathology.[10] Tenderness is sometimes localized to the ischial tuberosity, suggesting either microtrauma of the hamstring attachment or ischial bursitis.

TREATMENT: Progressive stretching of the hamstrings, together with various therapy modalities such as ultrasound, muscle stimulation, TENS, ice massage, cross-frictional massage, and stretching with ice massage, may all effect an improvement. Mobilization of the lower back may be indicated. An intensive muscle-balancing and muscle-strengthening program for the hamstring, gluteal, adductor, and quadriceps muscle groups should then be undertaken. A cortisone injection may be indicated in cases of ischial bursitis.

Complete Rupture of the Quadriceps or Patellar Tendon

A tendon rupture is a major injury which occurs when the athlete lands in an off-balance position from a long jump or from a basketball rebound. There is a sudden giving-in of the knee with severe pain.

SYMPTOMS AND SIGNS: The exact diagnosis might not be immediately apparent and, in fact, it might be possible for the athlete to extend the knee even though the quadriceps mechanism has been completely torn. There is tenderness either at the attachment of the quadriceps tendon into the superior pole of the patella or below the patella in the area of the patellar tendon. In the latter case, the patella is also pulled upward to some extent. A defect in the muscle-tendon at the area of tenderness can be felt.[11]

If the athlete is not seen until some time after the actual injury, a large hemarthrosis of the knee may mislead the examiner into thinking that an intra-articular knee injury has occurred. It is therefore important to consider this condition in the differential diagnosis of a hemarthrosis of the knee.

TREATMENT:

Immediate: Ice, a knee splint (preferably a postoperative knee splint), and crutches or a stretcher should be used. Analgesics will probably be necessary.

Definitive: Surgical repair of the injured tissues frequently needs to be undertaken.

THE KNEE

Prevention of Knee Injuries

Rule changes. Rule changes in contact sports, particularly football, have had a marked effect in reducing certain types of knee injuries. As long as these rules are enforced, many knee injuries will be prevented.

Leg musculature. The development of strength, power, endurance, and proprioception of the muscles surrounding the knee has been shown to be closely related to a decrease in the incidence of knee injuries, particularly in contact sports. However, if the thigh muscles are not in a state of contraction at the time of impact, they cannot contract rapidly enough to effectively protect the ligaments.[12]

The quadriceps are often thought of as the main group of muscles supporting the knee joint; however, it is vital that the other muscles around the knee be given equal attention. These include the hamstrings, the gastrocnemius, the abductors and adductors, the popliteus, and the pes anserine muscles. Not only will development of these muscle groups reduce the rate of acute injuries, but it will also decrease the recurrence of injuries in unstable knees. Surveys have shown that there is up to seventeen times greater chance of suffering a knee ligament injury when the athlete participates with incompletely rehabilitated or atrophied leg muscles.[13] Exercise for developing the muscles around the knee joint are discussed in the section on rehabilitation, p. 346.

Shoe-surface interface. In contact sports such as football, most knee injuries occur when the foot is planted and fixed. A force is applied against the knee, and if the foot cannot move away from its fixed position as contact occurs, knee ligaments are the first to be injured. However, if the athlete is wearing a shoe with a low coefficient of friction, there is a definite chance the foot will move with the blow, thereby eliminating the force on the ligaments. In this way the knee is protected from a potentially serious ligament injury.

Studies have shown that a soccer-style shoe with a relatively large number of cleats (e.g., fourteen) that are low and wide (e.g., ⅜" [9 mm] high and ½" [12 mm] in diameter) is probably the safest type of shoe available. This shoe tends to slip under impact, reducing the incidence of knee injuries, but it holds sufficiently well to enable normal cuts and turns to be performed.[14]

The type of shoe sole in contact with the playing surface is particularly important on artificial turf, where rubber soles have been shown to adhere too firmly, increasing the incidence of knee injuries. For artificial turf, the soccer-style shoe with low, wide cleats and a polyurethane sole is recommended.[15]

Wearing long cleats on grass might be useful for increasing traction, but unfortunately, long cleats have the potential to lock the foot into the surface, increasing the chance of a knee injury. It is suggested that the same soccer-style shoe that is recommended for artificial surfaces also be worn on grass.

The surface. A well-maintained field is always far safer for the athlete than a surface full of potholes and irregularities. This type of surface not only produces a large number of ankle injuries, but is also responsible for many knee injuries.[14]

Controversy exists over whether the artificial surface (AstroTurf) is more dangerous than grass, and over which produces a greater incidence of knee injuries.[16,17] Certain types of injuries tend to predominate on the harder surface of the artificial turf (such as posterior cruciate ligament injuries, which occur when the tibial tubercle comes into contact with the unrelenting surface, forcing the tibia backward).

The History and Evaluation

It has been said that the history in a knee injury is worth 80% of the diagnosis. The following questions should be routinely asked in an *acute injury*:

1. Was it a contact or a noncontact injury? If contact, from what direction was the force applied?
2. Was the foot planted?
3. In which direction did the knee go?
4. Was there a "pop"?
5. Did you feel anything slip out?
6. Where was the pain?
7. Did the knee feel unstable or give way?
8. Did the knee swell immediately?
9. Have you had any previous knee injuries?

The *nonacute* or the *chronic* injury needs to have a number of additional points clarified:

1. Length of time the symptoms have been present
2. Mechanism of injury
3. Primary symptoms
4. Other symptoms
5. Site of the pain
6. Any swelling, locking, or giving in?
7. Is there any pain on going up or down stairs?
8. Are any symptoms related to jumping, running, cutting, or squatting?
9. Are there any abnormal voluntary movements of the knee joint?
10. Has there been any previous knee injury?
11. Has there been any injury to the opposite knee?

Salient points in the history. The examiner should be aware of what the following symptoms might indicate.

1. *Rapid swelling of the knee* within twelve hours of the injury indicates bleeding into the joint and is usually associated with a significant injury.[18,19] In many instances a torn anterior cruciate ligament injury, or possibly a subluxed patella or osteochondral fracture, gives this history.

2. *Swelling of the joint* with relatively gradual onset, occurring more than twelve hours after an injury, is indicative of synovial irritation and a joint effusion. A meniscal tear might be the causative factor.

3. *Giving-in* should be carefully interpreted:

    a. Did the knee give-in while walking straight ahead, which might indicate a meniscal lesion?

    b. Did the knee give-in while rotating, which might indicate a rotatory instability problem?

4. *Locking* is suggestive of a meniscal tear. Locking means that the knee actually locks in one position and is then released by some movement which allows it to become "unlocked." The term "locking" is also used when full extension is blocked, which may be due to a torn meniscus, but may also be caused by spasm of the hamstrings.

5. *The history of a "pop"* in an acute injury is very significant. In most cases it is due to an anterior cruciate ligament tear; in some, it is due to a subluxing patella; and in a few, to a torn meniscus or an osteochondral fracture.

6. *Pain on going up or down stairs,* particularly on walking down, is indicative of retropatellar irritation.

7. *Pain under the patella and along the patellar tendon* after such jumping activities as basketball, is indicative of patellar tendinitis.

8. *Pain behind the patella,* after sitting with the knee flexed at approximately 90° for a period of time, is indicative of retropatellar irritation.

9. *A subluxing patella* can produce vague symptoms, or even symptoms attributable to injuries of other structures; for instance, it can produce a history of giving way, locking, and swelling.

Observation.

1. Note the *bulk and tone* of the quadriceps, the hamstrings, and the calf muscles.

2. Note any *limitation of full flexion or extension or any limp.* Have the athlete stand eight to ten feet away and observe the alignment

TABLE 19.9 **Outline of a Knee Examination**

1. *Observe with athlete standing*
   (1) Stance, leg alignment, attitude of feet
   (2) Swelling, muscle bulk, muscle definition

2. *Functional tests* (if appropriate)
   (1) Hopping (foot externally rotated, then internally rotated)
   (2) Rotational lean-hop (clockwise, then counterclockwise)
   (3) Running-in-place
   (4) Squat
   (5) Duck-waddle
   (6) One-legged squat

3. *Athlete sitting at end of examining table*
   (1) Position of patellae
   (2) Vastus medialis obliquus with legs held at 45° against resistance
   (3) Retropatellar crepitus

4. *Athlete supine on examining table*
   (1) Measure circumference of thighs at 10 cm and at 20 cm above medial joint line
   (2) Check range of motion (note retropatellar crepitus)
   (3) Palpate for swelling
   (4) Palpate for tenderness
   (5) Test muscle strength (quadriceps and hamstrings)
   (6) Lift leg into hyperextension (observe for posterolateral rotatory instability)

5. *Ligament stress tests*
   (1) Valgus and varus stress at 0° and at 30° of flexion
   (2) Lachman test at 10° of flexion
   (3) With the knee at 90° and the hip at 45°, sit on foot and test for anterior and posterior drawer with the foot
       (a) in neutral position
       (b) externally rotated
       (c) internally rotated
   (4) Pivot-shift tests
       (a) MacIntosh test
       (b) Jerk test of Hughston
       (c) Lateral position of Slocum

6. *Meniscus test*
   (1) McMurray's meniscal test

7. *Patella tests*
   (1) Moving the patella laterally with the knee at 0° and at 30° of flexion, test for
       (a) lateral laxity
       (b) pain with movement
       (c) apprehension
   (2) Retropatellar pain on compression

TABLE 19.9 Outline of a Knee Examination
(*cont.*)

8. *Hip movement tests*
   (1) Measure internal and external rotation
9. *Athlete prone*
   (1) Examine the popliteal fossa for tenderness and swelling
   (2) Use Apley's meniscal test
10. *Peripheral circulation tests*
   (1) Always palpate the posterior tibial and the dorsalis pedis pulses after an acute knee injury
   (2) Check peripheral circulation to the toes

of the lower limb, the position of the patellae, the amount of genu varum or genu valgum, the amount of tibia varum, and the position of the feet while standing (particularly with regard to excessive pronation or a high-arched cavus foot). These features can cause knee pain in those undertaking running activities.

3. Apply *functional tests.*

   a. Ask the athlete to hop on the affected leg, first pointing the foot into internal rotation while hopping and then pointing it into external rotation.

   b. Have the athlete hop in a 360° circle while leaning over to the side, first clockwise and then counterclockwise.

   c. Ask the athlete to run in place, first slowly and then with maximum effort, raising the knees as high as possible. Look for any abnormality in the running pattern.

   d. Have the athlete attempt to squat down as far as possible. Note any limitation, crepitus, or pain.

   e. Ask the athlete, while in the squatting position, to walk in a full-squat, duck-waddle fashion. Note any pain or inability to do this maneuver.

   f. Have the athlete lightly hold the examining table with one hand while attempting to squat all the way down on the affected leg. This is a useful test of quadriceps strength. Observe

his or her ability to return to the standing position using the affected leg alone. This test often shows up a latent weakness of the quadriceps.

Measurements. Measurements are sometimes useful, but they are often misleading. Probably a better way to pick out subtle differences in the bulk of the quadriceps musculature is by careful observation. When measurements are taken, a reference point such as the medial joint line or the medial malleolus should be used. Measurements taken from the patella tend to be inaccurate, as the position of the patella varies and the patellae may be asymmetrical.

A useful series of measurements involves the

1. mid-calf area

2. midpatellar area

3. ten centimeters above the medial joint line

4. twenty centimeters above the medial joint line

Palpation. Any swelling in the joint should be noted. One method of determining if the swelling is intra-articular or extra-articular is to perform ballottement on the patella. If the patella is ballotable, then the swelling is intra-articular. Another test for intra-articular swelling involves compressing any fluid to the medial side of the knee. The swelling is then tapped and a fluid wave is felt for on the lateral side (Figure 19.15).

Then palpate for any tender area. Starting on the medial side, palpate along the tibial collateral ligament from the femoral condyle down to the tibia, proceeding down about 7 cm. Tenderness along this area suggests injury to the tibial collateral ligament. Tenderness over the medial joint line is due to injury either to the medial meniscus or to the medial capsular ligament. Continue the palpation posteriorly on the medial side, to include the posteromedial corner. Then palpate the anteromedial joint line. Tenderness here suggests a medial meniscal injury or possibly osteochondral pathology.

Palpate the quadriceps insertion into the

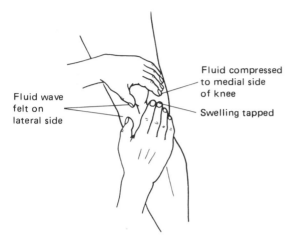

FIGURE 19.15 **Palpating swelling within the knee**

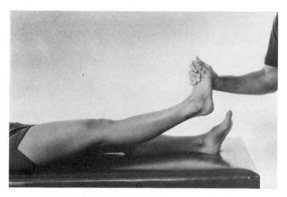

FIGURE 19.16 **Test for hyperextension**

patella, the medial facet of the patella, and the patellar tendon. An important area is the origin of the patellar tendon at the lower pole of the patella. To adequately palpate this area, the patella needs to be stabilized superiorly while the lower pole is palpated firmly with the thumb (see Figure 19.53).

Palpation continues onto the lateral facet of the patella and the anterolateral joint line. Tenderness here can indicate an osteochondral, fat-pad, or lateral meniscal injury. The length of the fibular collateral ligament from the lateral femoral condyle to the fibula should be palpated. Tenderness over the lateral joint line may be associated with a lateral meniscal injury. While palpating the fibular head, do not forget to palpate over the biceps insertion. Palpate the iliotibial tract as it inserts into Gerdy's tubercle. Tenderness over the posterolateral corner suggests an injury to the posterior horn of the lateral meniscus or an involvement of the popliteal tendon and the arcuate ligament complex. Examine the popliteal area for any swelling or tenderness.

Range of movement. Any limitation of flexion or extension should be measured. Compare the two sides. To test for hyperextension, lift both feet off the table simultaneously and note how far the knee drops back (Figure 19.16). Ensure that the thigh muscles are completely relaxed.

Ligament stability tests. There is still controversy as to the exact meaning and interpretation of many of the ligament stress tests. A workable guideline to the interpretation of these tests is presented, but the reader should bear in mind that there may be disagreement on the subject.

1. *Hyperextension test:* The foot is raised so as to let the knee drop back into hyperextension; this is compared with the opposite side (Figure 19.16). If hyperextension is excessive on the affected side, it may indicate rupture or incompetency of the anterior cruciate ligament, with or without a tear of the posterior cruciate ligament. Posterolateral rotatory instability is said to be present if the tibia rotates to the lateral side and drops posteriorly during the hyperextension test.

2. *Valgus and varus stress tests:* The stress tests are designed to demonstrate laxity of the collateral ligaments, but they may also give information on the status of other structures.

    a. Valgus and varus stress at 0°: If there is valgus or varus opening beyond the normal limb, it indicates involvement not only of the stabilizing complex involved, but also of the anterior or posterior cruciate ligaments, and perhaps of other structures as well (Figure 19.17).

    b. Valgus or varus stress at 30°: This localizes the stress to the medial or the lateral stabilizing complex, and

TABLE 19.10   Knee Ligament Instabilities

Instabilities	Tests
One-plane instabilities[a]	
Medial	Valgus stress at 0° and 30° of flexion
Lateral	Varus stress at 0° and 30° of flexion
Anterior	Anterior drawer at 90° of flexion
	Lachman test
Posterior	Posterior drawer at 90° of flexion
Rotatory instabilities[b]	
Anteromedial	Valgus stress at 30° of flexion
	Anterior drawer with foot in external rotation at 90° of flexion
Anterolateral	Anterior drawer with foot in internal rotation at 90° of flexion
	Pivot shift tests
Posterolateral	Hyperextension of leg
	Posterior drawer with foot in internal rotation at 90° of flexion
Posteromedial	Posterior drawer with foot in external rotation at 90° of flexion (rare)
Combined instabilities	
Anteromedial *plus* anterolateral (most common)	
Anterolateral *plus* posterolateral	
Anteromedial *plus* anterolateral and posterolateral	

Note: This classification of instabilities was devised by the Research and Education Committee of the American Orthopaedic Society for Sports Medicine.

[a]*Movement of the tibia in relation to the femur*, that is, medial means the tibia is moving away from the femur on the medial side.

[b]*Movement of the tibia in relation to the femur*, that is, anteromedial rotatory instability means the tibia is rotating anteriorly and moving away from the femur on the medial side.

any excessive opening indicates laxity of that complex of ligaments.

3. *Drawer tests at 90° of knee flexion*: The athlete lies supine, hip flexed to 45° with knee bent to 90°. The examiner sits on the foot to stabilize it and makes sure that the hamstrings are completely relaxed (Figure 19.18).

a. Anterior drawer sign with foot in *neutral* position (Figure 19.19a): Forward movement of the tibia on the femur in this position indicates incompetence of the anterior cruciate ligament. However, it is important to realize that this test may not be positive in a significant percentage of anterior cruciate ligament tears, especially acute injuries.

b. Anterior drawer sign with foot in *external rotation* (15°) (Figure 19.19b): This is the Slocum test for anteromedial rotatory instability.[20] It is positive if the medial tibial plateau advances anteriorly and rotates from the medial to the lateral side. A positive test indicates damage to the anterior cruciate ligament, the posteromedial corner, or both.

c. Anterior drawer sign with foot in *internal rotation* (Figure 19.19c): With anterior stress, the lateral tibial plateau moves anteriorly and rotates medially from the lateral side when there is incompetency of either or both the anterior cruciate ligaments or the lateral collateral ligament and the posterolateral corner.

This test should be repeated with progressive internal rotation of the foot and the tibia. When the tibia is rotated to approximately 20° the test should become negative, as the posterior cruciate ligament holds the tibia from moving forward in this position. If there is forward motion with the foot in maximal internal rotation, suspect the possibility of a posterior cruciate ligament injury.

d. *Posterior drawer sign* with foot in neu-

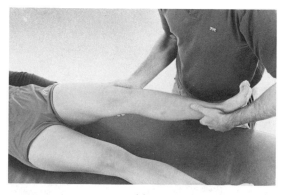

(a)

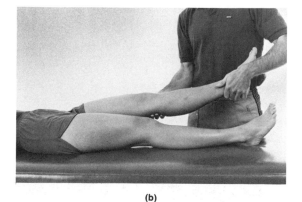

(b)

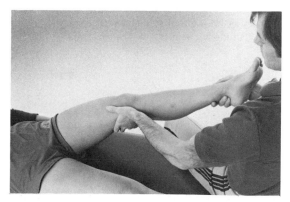

(c)

(d)

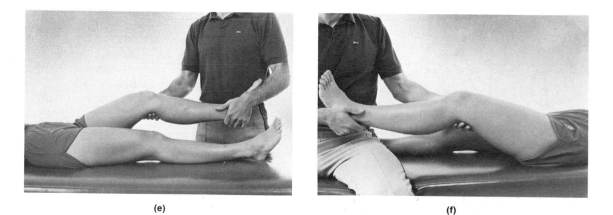

(e)

(f)

FIGURE 19.17 Valgus and varus stress tests (a) Valgus stress test performed at 0°— viewed from above (b) Valgus stress test performed at 0°—viewed from the side (c) Varus stress test performed at 0°—viewed from the lateral side (d) Varus stress test performed at 0°—viewed from above and medially (e) Valgus stress test performed at 30° —viewed from the medial side (f) Varus stress test performed at 30°—viewed from the lateral side

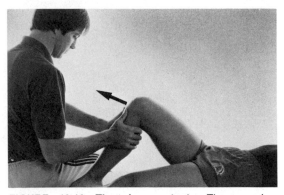

FIGURE 19.18 The drawer tests The examiner should sit on the foot to help stabilize the leg and ensure that the hamstrings are relaxed.

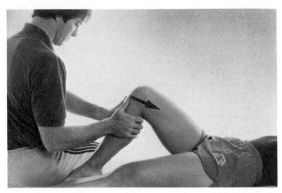

FIGURE 19.20 Posterior drawer test The foot is placed in the neutral position and a posteriorly directed force is applied to the tibia. If the tibia is noted to move posteriorly, then a posterior cruciate ligament injury is probably present.

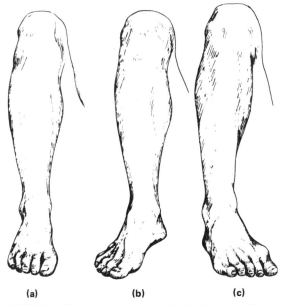

(a)   (b)   (c)

FIGURE 19.19 Anterior drawer test—foot positions (a) The foot is first placed in a neutral position and an anteriorly directed force is applied to the tibia. If anterior motion in excess of the normal opposite limb is produced, an anterior cruciate ligament tear should be strongly suspected. (b) If this motion is also present when the test is performed with the foot in external rotation, and the medial tibial plateau is noted to rotate laterally, anteromedial rotatory instability may be diagnosed. (c) The foot is internally rotated 10° to 15° and the test repeated. If it is noted that the lateral tibial plateau comes forward and medially, then the rotatory instability is anterolateral.

tral position (Figure 19.20): If laxity in a posterior direction is present, it indicates damage to the posterior cruciate ligament.

Sometimes it is difficult to decide if there is an anterior drawer or a posterior drawer sign present, as the neutral position of the knee becomes obscured. A useful way of deciding is to place both knees in the same position of 45° of hip flexion and 90° of knee flexion and note the relative position of the tibial tubercles from the side. If the posterior cruciate ligament is completely torn, the tibial tubercle on the affected side will sag backward in relation to the unaffected leg (Figure 19.21).

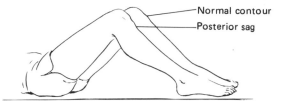

Normal contour
Posterior sag

FIGURE 19.21 Posterior sag When a posterior cruciate ligament tear is present, the tibia may sag posteriorly. The thigh musculature must be relaxed. Line up the legs at 90° of knee flexion and observe the outlines (silhouettes) of the tibiae from the side.

4. *Lachman test*: The Lachman test is one of the most important and sensitive tests for detecting a tear or incompetency of the anterior cruciate ligament.[21] The test will often be positive when all other tests, including the anterior drawer tests, are negative, particularly when performed soon after an injury. It is performed with the knee flexed approximately 5° to 10°. With the thigh supported, the tibia is brought forward on the femur (Figures 19.22 and 19.23). Excessive forward movement of the tibia on the femur suggests a torn anterior cruciate ligament. One can usually observe, as well as feel, any excessive movement but this may be quite subtle.

5. *Pivot-shift tests*: Pivot-shift tests are designed to demonstrate anterolateral rotatory instability and can be used in both acute and chronic situations. Together with the Lachman test, they constitute the most sensitive index for detecting an anterior cruciate ligament injury. In order to appreciate the biomechanics of anterolateral rotatory instability, it is necessary to assume that the tibia is in a subluxed position when the knee is hyperextended. As the knee reaches 20° to 30° of flexion, the tibia relocates on the femur with a sudden shift which is both seen and felt. As the knee returns to extension, the reverse procedure takes place. This is the basis for these tests.

The three tests described all appear to test the same pathological entity. However, in many instances only one or two of the tests will be positive.

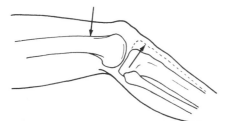

FIGURE 19.22 The Lachman test This test is designed to detect injury to the anterior cruciate ligament. With the knee in 10° to 15° of flexion, the tibia is brought forward on the femur.

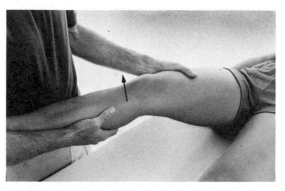

FIGURE 19.23 The Lachman test To detect abnormal motion, observe the tibial tubercle as it moves anteriorly in relation to the inferior pole of the patella.

a. *Pivot-shift test of MacIntosh*:[22] The athlete lies supine and the leg is lifted approximately 30° to 45° at the hip, with the knee fully extended so that it falls backward into hyperextension. The foot and the tibia are internally rotated (sometimes a positive response is elicited when the foot is externally rotated). A valgus force is applied to the knee at the same time as it is flexed. While the valgus force is being applied, pressure is directed against the head of the fibula in an attempt to rotate it forward and around from the lateral to the medial side (Figure 19.24).

b. *Jerk test of Hughston*: This is really the same as the MacIntosh test but is performed in the opposite direction. Start with the knee flexed at about 45° and the foot internally rotated. Apply a valgus force while attempting to rotate the fibula medially as the knee is being straightened. The jerk takes place at approximately 20° of flexion.

c. *Pivot-shift test in the lateral position as described by Slocum*:[23,24] The athlete lies on the unaffected side, the unaffected leg drawn up into flexion and out of the way. The pelvis is positioned

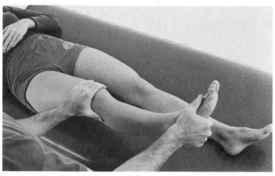

(a)

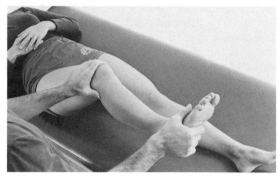

(b)

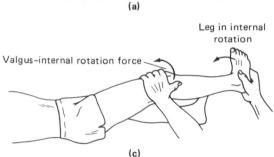

Leg in internal rotation

Valgus–internal rotation force

(c)

FIGURE 19.24 The pivot-shift test of MacIntosh A pivot-shift is produced if anterolateral rotatory instability is present, most commonly as a result of an anterior cruciate ligament injury.

so that the affected leg is internally rotated and the knee fully extended. The thumb of one hand is placed on the fibular head. A valgus force is applied as the knee is flexed. The pivot shift (i.e., reduction of the tibia from its subluxed position) occurs at between 20° and 30° of flexion. As the knee is brought back into full extension, the reverse procedure occurs (Figure 19.25).

Meniscal Tests.

McMurray's meniscal test: The athlete lies supine with the knee fully flexed. The foot is held in one hand while the other hand palpates the joint line on both sides of the knee. Keeping the knee fully flexed, rotate the tibia from external to internal rotation and back again. A click or a grinding probably indicates a tear of the posterior segment of the meniscus (Figure 19.26).

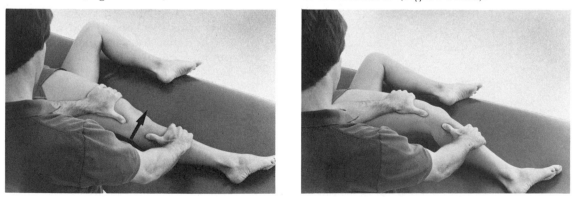

FIGURE 19.25 The pivot-shift test in the lateral position (Slocum test) A valgus force is applied as the knee is flexed. The pivot shift will usually occur at 20° to 30° of flexion.

TABLE 19.11   Clinical Tests for Ligament Instability

Tests	Position of the Knee	Ligaments Involved
Valgus stress	0°	Medial stabilizing complex, ACL,[a] posteromedial corner, and sometimes PCL.[b]
	30°	If stable at 0°, and other tests are negative, then more or less of the medial stabilizing complex is involved, depending on severity.
Varus stress	0°	Lateral stabilizing complex, biceps tendon, posterolateral corner,[c] ACL, and often PCL.
	30°	Same as valgus stress at 30° except the lateral stabilizing complex is involved.
Lachman	5–10°	ACL (with or without other structures).
Anterior drawer	90° 1. neutral position of foot 2. foot externally rotated 3. foot internally rotated	ACL (with or without medial or lateral collateral ligament). ACL and/or medial stabilizing complex and posteromedial corner.[d] ACL (with or without lateral complex and posterolateral corner). If positive at 20° of internal rotation, probably PCL.
Posterior drawer	90°	PCL (with or without structures in the posteromedial and posterolateral corners).
Pivot-shift	Various	ACL (with or without posterolateral corner, and/or lateral stabilizing complex).

[a] anterior cruciate ligament
[b] posterior cruciate ligament
[c] popliteus muscle and arcuate ligament complex
[d] posterior oblique ligament and some attachments of the semimembranosus muscle

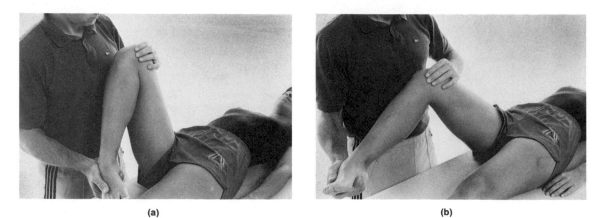

(a)   (b)

FIGURE 19.26 The McMurray test (a) To test for a torn meniscus, the knee is fully flexed, rotated, and extended. The fingers are placed on the joint line and a click or a grinding sensation are palpated for within the joint. (b) By extending the knee while applying a varus force and internal rotation of the tibia, a torn medial meniscus may be compressed and produce a click or pain.

Another method involves extending the leg with the foot internally rotated, at the same time applying a varus force, which will compress the medial compartment. A tear is revealed by a click and by the pain felt in the vicinity of the joint line (Figure 19.27).

The knee is again flexed, the foot externally rotated, and the leg extended while a valgus force is applied to the knee. This compresses the lateral compartment and may reveal a lateral meniscal injury.

Apley's meniscal test: The athlete lies prone and the knee is flexed to 90°. Pressure is then applied to the heel while the foot is rotated. If this produces pain in the knee, it suggests a posterior horn injury. The foot is then pulled upward to distract the joint and remove the pressure from the meniscus. If no pain is felt on rotation of the foot, this adds further weight to the diagnosis.

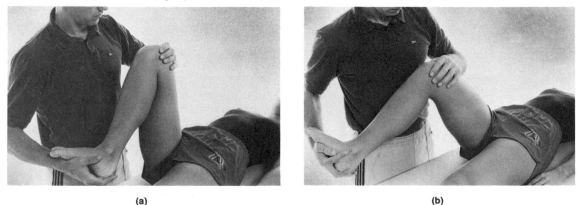

(a)   (b)

FIGURE 19.27 The McMurray test (a) The same procedure is then performed with the foot in external rotation. The knee is hyperflexed and the fibia rotated. (b) The knee is then extended, maintaining the position of external rotation of the foot, and a valgus force is applied to the knee.

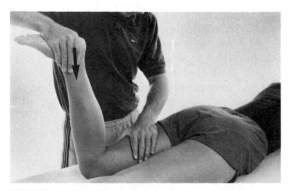

FIGURE 19.28 The Apley test By applying downward pressure and rotating the tibia, a posterior horn tear of the medial meniscus may produce pain. This pain should not be present if the tibia is distracted from the femur and rotated.

Examination of the patella.

1. With the athlete standing, note the alignment, height, and shape of the patella.

2. With the athlete standing, measure the Q angle by taking a line from the anterior superior iliac spine down the thigh to the midpoint of the patella, and from there to the tibial tubercle (Figure 19.29). To be considered normal, it should be under 16° in females and 10° in males; over 20° is probably abnormal.

3. With the athlete sitting at the end of the examining table, legs hanging at 90°, note the position of the patellae, particularly lateral squinting of the patellae or high-riding patellae (Figure 19.30).

Note the tracking of the patella as the knee is extended and flexed. The VMO can be well seen when the knees are held at 45° against resistance (Figure 19.31). Also, note if retropatellar crepitus is present.

4. With the athlete supine and the legs extended, note tenderness of any of the facets of the patella.

5. Then attempt to sublux the patella by moving it laterally. If the patella moves more than half of its width across the lateral femoral condyle, it suggests subluxation, particularly if the so-called "apprehension test" is positive, that is, if the athlete becomes

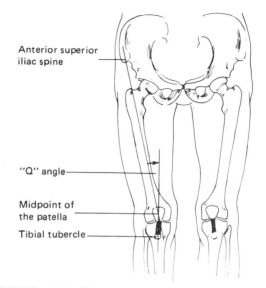

FIGURE 19.29 Measuring the "Q" angle A wide "Q" angle may predispose the athlete to patella problems.

alarmed or grabs the examiner's hand (Figure 19.32). Repeat this maneuver with the knee at 30° of flexion and the quadriceps relaxed and then tightened.

6. To detect the presence of retropatellar crepitus, move the knee through a full range of motion while at the same time palpating the patella. Another test is to move the pa-

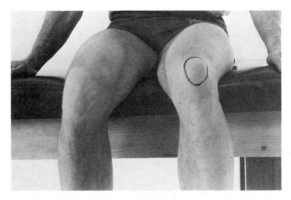

FIGURE 19.30 Patellar position when sitting Note if the patellae are located in the midline or if they squint medially or laterally. Also, note if they point towards the ceiling (patella alta) or are near the tibial tubercle (patella infera).

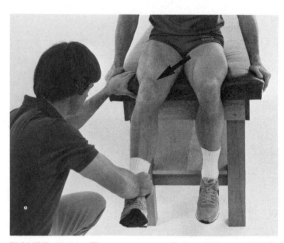

FIGURE 19.31 The vastus medialis obliquus (VMO)
Note the development and insertion of the VMO into the
patella when the knee is held at 45° against resistance.

tella firmly but gently against the underlying
femur with the leg extended and the quadriceps relaxed. Feel for crepitus and inquire if
pain is felt.

Note: The most striking demonstration of
retropatellar crepitus is usually felt when the
athlete squats from a standing position.

Mechanisms of Knee Ligament Injuries

When a knee injury occurs, one or more ligaments may be involved. In addition, the patella, the menisci, or both may be affected.
Most knee ligament injuries result from an

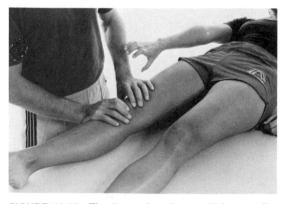

**FIGURE 19.32 The "apprehension test" for patellar
instability** If the athlete becomes alarmed when the
patella is moved laterally, it is suggestive of patellar instability.

external force. However, some knee ligament
injuries occur *without* an external force being
applied to the knee. For instance, a basketball player may stop suddenly, hear or feel a
"pop," and find that the knee gives in (an
anterior cruciate ligament tear). Each major
ligament will now be discussed in turn.

Medial ligament injuries. Medial ligament
injuries are caused by a valgus force, for example:

1. If the foot is planted and fixed, a tackle
or block against the lateral aspect of the
knee will drive the knee medially (Figure
19.33).

2. If one ski becomes entrapped in snow
while momentum carries the skier onward, a
valgus, external rotational movement at the
knee results. In this example the foot is
unweighted (Figure 19.34).

If the force is not severe, only the medial capsular ligament will be involved. This
may also lead to a peripheral detachment of
the medial meniscus. If the force is more severe, there is involvement of the medial capsular ligament, the tibial collateral ligament,
and the posteromedial corner (posterior
oblique ligament). Finally, the cruciate ligaments will tear (the anterior cruciate is more
often involved). A tear through the body of
one of the menisci (usually the medial meniscus) can also occur.

**TABLE 19.12 A "Pop" Associated with an
Acute Knee Injury**

The examiner should always ask if the athlete heard
or felt a "pop" (particularly following a
hyperextension or internal rotation injury).

In most cases, this will indicate an *anterior cruciate
ligament injury*.

In a few cases, it will be due to a *subluxed patella*,
though a tearing sound or sensation is more common with this injury.

In a small number of cases, the "pop" will be due to
a *torn meniscus*.

An *osteochondral fracture* may give more of a
"snap" than a "pop."

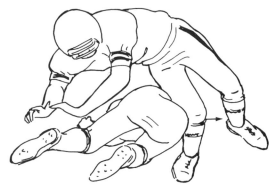

FIGURE 19.33 Valgus knee injury If a valgus force is applied to the knee while the foot is fixed, a tear of the medial ligamentous structures will occur. If the force is sufficiently great, the anterior cruciate ligament may also be torn as well as the medial meniscus.

Lateral ligament injuries. The lateral ligament is injured less than the medial ligament as it is not as vulnerable to injury. This is because the force, or blow, necessary to damage the ligament must be applied to the medial aspect of the knee in order to force it into a varus position.

Usually the lateral capsular ligament and the fibular collateral ligament are the first structures to be torn on the lateral side. With more severe injuries, the biceps tendon and the iliotibial band may come loose from their attachment to the head of the fibula and Gerdy's tubercle respectively, and the

peroneal nerve may be injured. The popliteal tendon and the posterolateral corner of the knee may also be damaged. As with valgus injuries, the cruciate ligaments (particularly the anterior cruciate ligament) may be involved, and one or both of the menisci may be damaged.

Anterior cruciate ligament injuries. The anterior cruciate ligament alone can be torn. This is called an "isolated tear," but it is probably a misnomer because there is usually microscopic damage to other structures around the knee. The anterior cruciate ligament is also injured as part of a more complex injury, which occurs through one of the following mechanisms:

1. Hyperextension.

2. Internal rotation of the leg with external rotation of the body. The leg usually hyperextends as well (Figure 19.35).

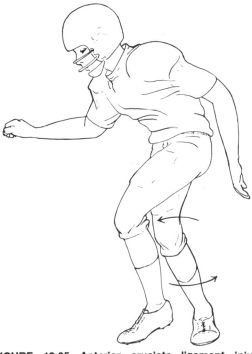

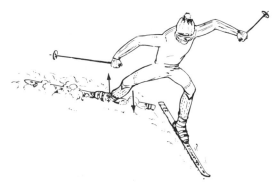

FIGURE 19.34 A valgus, external rotation injury to the right knee, which will result in a medial ligament sprain The anterior cruciate ligament may also be injured.

FIGURE 19.35 Anterior cruciate ligament injury The right tibia is internally rotated, the foot is fixed, the femur and body rotate externally as the athlete cuts to the right.

3. External rotation–valgus cutting action (Figure 19.36).

4. Deceleration, as in basketball.

5. A force which drives the tibia in an anterior direction when the knee is flexed at 90° (Figure 19.37).

6. In conjunction with medial or lateral collateral ligament injuries, as previously described.

Posterior cruciate ligament injuries. The posterior cruciate ligament is also injured in a number of ways:

1. A force applied to the anterior aspect of the tibia while the knee is at 90° will drive the tibia backward and tear the posterior cruciate ligament. Such a force can occur

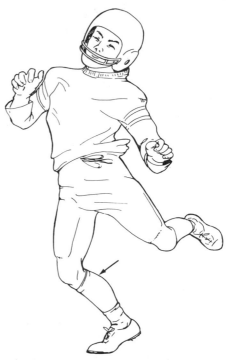

FIGURE 19.37 Anterior cruciate ligament injury If an anteriorly directed force is applied to the tibia when the foot is fixed, the anterior cruciate ligament may be injured.

when a football player lands on the tibial tubercle with his knee flexed, particularly on artificial turf (Figure 19.38).

2. In conjunction with either a lateral or a medial ligament injury, as described.

3. A severe hyperextension injury.

4. Hyperflexion injury.

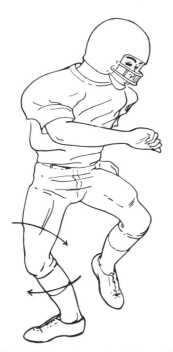

FIGURE 19.36 External rotation injury The tibia is externally rotated, the foot is fixed, the femur rotates internally, and the athlete pushes off and cuts to the left. This mechanism may result in a patellar dislocation, with or without a medial collateral ligament tear. An anterior cruciate ligament tear may also occasionally result from this cutting maneuver.

Classification, Diagnosis, and Treatment of Ligament Injuries:

Medial Stabilizing Complex

A medial stabilizing complex injury may best be described with the example of a football injury. If an athlete's right foot is planted, and the athlete is then blocked or tackled on the lateral side of the right knee, the knee is

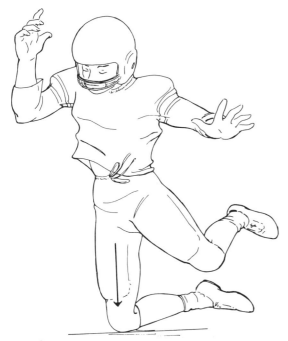

FIGURE 19.38 Posterior cruciate ligament injury A forceful landing on the tibial tubercle may drive the tibia backwards on the femur, rupturing the posterior cruciate ligament.

TABLE 19.13   Forces That Injure Ligaments of the Knee

1. *Valgus force* For example, a block or tackle to the outside of the knee (the foot is fixed) may result in a tear of the: a. medial stabilizing complex ⎫ b. anterior cruciate ligament ⎬ this is the "unhappy triad" or "O'Donaghue's Triad" c. medial meniscus ⎭
2. *Varus force* For example, a force applied to the medial side of the knee, forcing the knee to bend into a varus direction (less common than a valgus force), may tear the: a. lateral stabilizing complex b. anterior cruciate ligament c. lateral meniscus (It should be realized that there are many variations of the above.)
3. *Anteriorly directed force with the knee bent* Results in an "isolated" anterior cruciate tear
4. *Posteriorly directed force with the knee bent* Results in an "isolated" posterior cruciate tear
5. *Hyperextension force* For example, jumping and landing with a straight leg may tear the: a. anterior cruciate ligament b. then the posterior cruciate ligament if the knee is forced posteriorly far enough
6. *Internal rotation force* For example, one ski crossing while the body externally rotates and the leg hyperextends may tear the: a. anterior cruciate ligament b. other structures according to the forces applied

forced into a valgus position. Because of a number of factors (the force involved in the block, the strength of the athlete's leg muscles, and whether the foot remains fixed to the ground, etc.), the injury may vary from a mild, first-degree sprain to a complete rupture of the different structures, perhaps ending as the "unhappy triad" (medial ligament plus anterior cruciate tear plus medial meniscal tear).

First-degree sprain.

SYMPTOMS AND SIGNS: In a first-degree sprain, assume that the integrity of the ligament is undisturbed and that there is almost normal tensile strength (Table 19.14). Visualize the disruption of a few collagen fibers, perhaps in the capsule, sometimes in the superficial portion of the ligament.

The athlete usually complains of some pain on twisting the leg or forcing it into a valgus position. He or she might be aware of the injury, but often continues to play without complaining, only seeking advice afterwards when the leg becomes increasingly stiff.

There is usually minimal or no swelling over the medial side of the knee, and the tenderness is localized to one area, usually

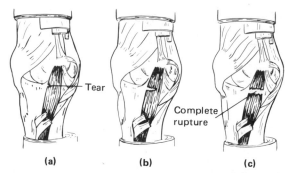

(a)   (b)   (c)

FIGURE 19.39 Degrees of a medial ligamentous injury (a) First degree: only a few collagen fibers are disrupted. There is almost normal tensile strength. Minimal, if any, valgus laxity is present. (b) Second degree: partial tearing of the ligamentous structures occurs. There is a significant decrease in tensile strength. Valgus laxity is present, but an end point can be felt. (c) Third degree: the ligamentous structures are completely torn. No tensile strength remains. There is marked instability on valgus stress.

close to the joint line. There is a full range of movement, with perhaps a minor decrease in flexion due to stiffness. Ligament testing shows normal strength with no abnormal laxity. Functionally, the athlete might run

TABLE 19.14 Criteria for Rapid Rehabilitation of a Second-Degree Grade II Medial Collateral Ligament Sprain

1. No (or minimal) swelling
2. Tenderness localized to one area of the tibial collateral ligament, not diffuse
3. Knee stable when tested at 0° (in full extension)
4. Less than 10° of valgus opening at 30° of flexion
5. A definite end point when valgus stress is applied at 30° (the hamstring muscles should be completely relaxed)
6. No anteromedial rotatory instability with the knee at 90° and the foot externally rotated
7. No other injured ligaments, in particular, no evidence of an anterior cruciate ligament tear

If the injury meets all of these criteria, the athlete may be placed onto a rehabilitation program aimed at returning him or her to participation in the shortest possible time without jeopardizing the knee (see section on knee rehabilitation, p. 360).

with little impairment soon after the injury, or with a slight limp if the leg has become stiff, but is able to perform straight-ahead and backward running. There may be some difficulty in cutting and in running figure-eight patterns.

TREATMENT: Treatment is with ice, compression, perhaps anti-inflammatory medication, and isometric quadriceps and hamstring contractions. This is soon followed by exercise on a stationary bicycle, straight-leg raising, internal rotation at 90°, and knee flexion against resistance (see section on rehabilitation, p. 346). Icing and perhaps protective taping are used until the symptoms subside, probably a few days. The athlete is allowed to return to participation when functionally capable of performing. With this routine, no strength, power, or endurance should be lost. If there is any weakening of the musculature, the athlete should be kept out of contact participation until the leg has developed strength, power, and endurance equal to or greater than the opposite side. Stretching exercises may be undertaken, but they should be performed cautiously immediately after the injury. Rather, the athlete should work gradually toward normal flexibility over a period of days.

Second-degree sprain. A second-degree sprain covers the whole range between a minor ligament injury (first-degree sprain) and a complete rupture of the ligament (third-degree sprain). To make this category meaningful, it is divided into two types:

1. *Second-degree (grade I)*—Sprains that more closely approximate first-degree injuries
2. *Second-degree (grade II)*—Sprains that more closely approximate third-degree sprains

Second-degree sprain (grade I).

SYMPTOMS AND SIGNS: There is some tearing of the medial capsule and the tibial collateral ligament may also be affected. There is usually some decrease in tensile strength of the collagen fibers, but integrity is present. As with first-degree sprains, the athlete might be able to continue playing for a period of time and then afterwards complain of pain and stiffness, but will be more aware that a definite injury has occurred.

Slight swelling may be apparent, though there is no gross hemarthrosis or effusion. Tenderness is more marked but is limited to a small localized area, usually close to the joint line. Full flexion is often difficult to obtain for a while after the injury because of the discomfort, and full extension may be limited by hamstring spasm.

Ligament testing should reveal no laxity on valgus stress at 0° of flexion. There is no, or very minimal (less than 5°), laxity when testing at 30° of flexion. Stressing causes definite pain in the injured area as may testing for anteromedial rotatory instability by means of Slocum's test with the knee at 90° and the foot externally rotated.

TREATMENT: This injury is treated in the same way as the first-degree sprain, except that it is probably wise to keep the athlete in a postoperative knee splint for anywhere from a few days to a few weeks, depending on the severity and amount of ligament damage. Rehabilitation exercises should be started immediately.[25,26]

Second degree sprain (grade II). Grade II implies a more complete tearing of the ligaments, though there is still some tensile strength.

SYMPTOMS AND SIGNS: The athlete usually complains of the knee buckling when attempting to cut, and may feel unhappy or apprehensive about continuing to play (however, some highly motivated athletes will ignore the instability and continue to participate unless restrained by those in charge).

On examination, swelling is usually slight unless there is an additional injury to one of the other ligaments. Tenderness may be localized to one area or may extend along the entire length of the tibial collateral liga-

ment and along the joint line. There is usually a fairly substantial decrease in the range of motion, with flexion being more limited than extension. Ligament stability testing may show the following:

1. At 0° there may be slight laxity, indicating a severe injury.
2. At 30° there may be some laxity (up to approximately 10° of joint opening) but a definite end point can be felt.

The Lachman test should be negative (assuming there is no involvement of the anterior cruciate ligament).

With the knee at 90° and the tibia in the neutral position of rotation, there should be no laxity on testing anterior or posterior drawer signs. Externally rotating the foot with the knee at 90° usually causes severe pain along the posteromedial joint line and the medial ligaments. Testing for anteromedial rotatory instability (Slocum's test) is usually negative or only minimally positive. Rotating the foot into internal rotation at 90° should not cause pain, and the anterior and posterior drawer tests should be stable. Pivot-shift tests should be negative unless there is involvement of the anterior cruciate ligament, but they are often painful and probably should not be performed when there is a damaged tibial collateral ligament.

McMurray's test may be positive for pain if there is peripheral tearing of the meniscus. The test may be negative initially even when there is a meniscal tear, particularly if the knee cannot be fully flexed.

TREATMENT: The grade-II injury does not usually require surgical repair and is treated by immobilization in most instances. The type of immobilization depends on the particular philosophy of the surgeon as well as on the severity of the injury. The choices are usually (a) a long-leg, non-weight-bearing cast with the knee at 15° of flexion, (b) a plaster cylinder from the thigh to the ankle so that the foot is free, or (c) a postoperative knee immobilizer instead of a cast. With the latter, however, the athlete should be reliable, be under responsible and experienced supervision, and be instructed in the dangers of any unauthorized removal of the splint. This splint or cast may have a hinge allowing movement between 30° and 60°.

A modification of the standard treatment of immobilization can be used in certain selected cases. It is aimed at rapid rehabilitation and early return to participation. The athlete must meet strict criteria (Table 19.14), must be in a setting where there is constant supervision, and must be near excellent rehabilitation facilities.[27,28,29,30] (See page 360.)

Third-degree sprain *(grade III)*.

SYMPTOMS AND SIGNS: In a third-degree sprain, there is complete disruption of the ligaments (*no* tensile strength is present). The athlete is fully aware that a serious injury has occurred and usually does not attempt to walk on the leg. There may be severe pain at the time of the injury, which then decreases in intensity and leads into a relatively pain-free period of two or three hours. The athlete should not be allowed to walk on the leg during this time, because of the danger of damaging one of the uninjured ligaments, which are now unsupported and unprotected by the medial stabilizing complex.

On examination, there is usually some swelling (though in some cases there is none). Tenderness is often localized to one end of the tibial collateral ligament and over the joint line. A full range of motion is usually present if the athlete is examined soon after the injury, though this is often followed by severe hamstring spasm which permits only limited movement.

Stress testing of the ligaments demonstrates the following: At 0° there is usually some valgus opening, particularly if the anterior or posterior cruciate ligaments have been torn as well. If complete hamstring relaxation is achieved, testing at 30° will produce marked opening of the joint (greater than 10°) with no definite end point.

The Lachman test is negative unless the anterior cruciate is involved. With the knee bent at 90° and the foot in neutral position, there are negative anterior and posterior drawer signs unless the cruciates are torn. Slocum's test may reveal some anteromedial rotatory instability, especially with a tear of the anterior cruciate ligament. Anterior stress at 90° with the foot internally rotated does not reveal any instability. Pivot-shift tests are usually negative (when there is only a medial ligament injury), but they are very painful and are not advised when a third-degree ligament injury has been demonstrated, as damage to other structures can occur. McMurray's test may or may not be positive (it may not even be possible to perform this test).

TREATMENT: If there is a complete (third-degree) tear of the medial or the lateral stabilizing complex, it should be repaired surgically within the first three to five days following injury.[31] If anteromedial rotatory instability is present as well, a pes anserine transfer procedure may also be performed.[32,33] Rehabilitation can begin soon after the operation.

Lateral Stabilizing Complex

The same findings, classification, and treatment are used for lateral stabilizing complex injuries as for the medial side. There are some differences, however:

1. There is normally some physiological laxity of the lateral stabilizing complex when tested at 30°.

2. Slight instability may be tolerated on the medial side; the lateral side cannot compensate for instability and will collapse into a varus position if stressed.

Anterior and Posterior Cruciate Ligament Tears

Though there may be partial tears of the cruciate ligaments, it is difficult or even impossible to make this diagnosis clinically. If instability of one of the cruciates can be

TABLE 19.15 Medial and Lateral Knee Ligament Injuries

	First-degree Sprain	Second-degree Sprain		Third-degree Sprain
		Grade I	Grade II	Grade III
Tissue Damage	Minimal tissue damage	Partial tearing Some decrease in tensile strength	More complete tearing Serious decrease in tensile strength	Complete disruption Zero tensile strength
Clinical Laxity	Stable	Slight laxity	Moderate laxity	Complete instability
Treatment	Standard immediate care Muscle strengthening exercises Minimal protection	Standard immediate care Muscle strengthening exercises Postoperative splint	Standard immediate care Muscle strengthening exercises Good splinting Cast or cast-brace	Good splinting Early surgery
Prognosis	Normal function No laxity	Good function Minimal or no laxity	Good function if adequate healing occurs	Generally better with primary surgery than reconstructive surgery

demonstrated, a third-degree sprain should be suspected.

The clinical diagnosis of an acute anterior cruciate ligament tear depends on the mechanism of the injury, the history of a pop and the rapid swelling of the knee, together with the findings of a positive Lachman test, possibly a positive MacIntosh test, and occasionally some laxity on the anterior drawer test.[34] An arthroscopic examination of the joint is usually necessary to confirm the diagnosis.[18,19]

On many occasions the cruciates have been found intact at surgery, but instability develops over a period of time. One must envision that a microscopic lesion has occurred with loss of collagen integrity. With continued use, the ligament can stretch and this can lead to functional incompetence even though it is macroscopically intact.

The treatment of *anterior cruciate ligament tears* is exceedingly controversial. Many surgeons, on finding a torn anterior cruciate ligament during arthrotomy, choose not to repair it[35] (see section on the progression of events following an anterior cruciate ligament tear, p. 327). If the ligament is torn in its midportion, the success rate following repair is very low. If a piece of bone is avulsed with the ligament (which is uncommon) and can be replaced, the chances of a full recovery are much increased.

New and experimental procedures aimed at finding a satisfactory answer to acute anterior cruciate tears are constantly being tried. Some surgeons perform a pes anserine transfer to give the knee an extra-articular reinforcement. A combination of intra- and extra-articular procedures is on trial at many centers (e.g., an Ellison[36] or MacIntosh procedure, which reinforces the lateral stabilizing complex, plus transfer of a portion of the patellar tendon through the knee, to act as an anterior cruciate ligament.[37,38] Other structures, such as the semitendinosus tendon[39] or the gracilis tendon,[40,41] can be used instead of the patellar tendon.) Many other methods are also being tried in an effort to find a satisfactory answer to a different problem.

Posterior cruciate ligament partial tears are also difficult or impossible to diagnose. If the history is suggestive of a posteriorly-directed force, and if posterior drawer laxity is present, then the diagnosis of a complete tear of the posterior cruciate ligament should be made.[42,43,44] However, there are some instances in which the clinical tests are negative, and then an arthroscopic examination is needed to make the diagnosis.[45] The hyperextension test may indicate postero-lateral rotatory instability.[46]

Posterior cruciate ligament tears are usually repaired acutely. The success rate is variable.

Rotatory Instabilities

The term *rotatory instability* refers to a *subluxation* of the tibial plateau on the femoral condyles. A number of these rotatory instabilities have been described (see Table 19.10), the commonest ones being:

1. Anteromedial rotatory instability
2. Anterolateral rotatory instability
3. Combined anteromedial and anterolateral rotatory instability

Anteromedial rotatory instability.

SYMPTOMS: The athlete may first become aware of this instability when planting the affected foot in external rotation while attempting to cut to the opposite direction. The tibia rotates and subluxes from the medial side anteriorly, and the knee tends to buckle into a valgus position. Instability varies from mild apprehension to complete giving way of the knee.

PATHOLOGY: The pathology is usually associated with an injury to the posteromedial corner (posterior oblique ligament), the anterior cruciate ligament, or both. However,

the symptoms may only begin after an associated tear of the medial meniscus has occurred. These tears are frequently associated with anteromedial rotatory instability.

EXAMINATION: There may or may not be valgus laxity at 30° of flexion. However, when the anterior drawer test is performed with the knee at 90° and the foot externally rotated 15°, the tibia is seen and felt to move forward and to rotate from the medial side laterally. This condition is also diagnosed with the anterior drawer test with the foot in the neutral position. If the medial tibial plateau comes forward, but the lateral plateau does not, anteromedial rotatory instability is present.

TREATMENT: Conservative treatment is aimed at developing the quadriceps, the adductors, and in particular the hamstrings and internal rotators. A Lenox Hill or similar derotation brace may be worn (see Figure 4.3). If symptoms are severe or athletic performance is compromised, the treatment is surgical and consists of the pes anserine transfer operation. In this operation, the pes anserine group of muscles (consisting, as noted, of the semitendinosus, the gracilis, and the sartorius) is converted from a primary flexor of the knee into an internal rotator of the tibia (Figure 19.40)[47]. In addition, the posteromedial corner of the knee is tightened. An anterior cruciate reconstruction is also performed if necessary. Postsurgical rehabilitation, particularly for developing the pes group, is a vital part of the total treatment.

Anterolateral rotatory instability.

SYMPTOMS: Anterolateral rotatory instability seems to incapacitate the athlete more frequently than does the anteromedial variety. The athlete will state that when cutting to the same side as the planted leg, there is a feeling of instability. This is often described as the tibia subluxing forward and medially while the femur is felt to rotate laterally. Af-

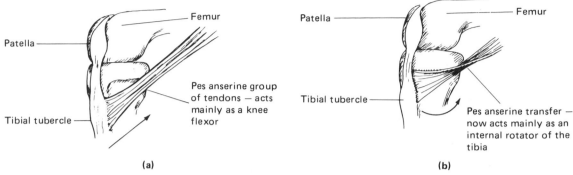

FIGURE 19.40   Pes anserine transfer procedure (a) Normal anatomy   (b) After surgery

ter an episode of this subluxation, pain and swelling are present for a few days. Any sport that uses a pivot-type activity tends to accentuate this instability, particularly basketball and football.

PATHOLOGY: In most cases the basic fault is a rupture or incompetency of the anterior cruciate ligament, together with damage to the posterolateral corner, the lateral stabilizing complex, or both. This injury frequently leads to tears of the medial, and often the lateral, meniscus.

EXAMINATION: The clinical findings associated with this instability usually consist of a positive anterior drawer sign when the foot is in the neutral position and when it is internally rotated to 10°. However, it is possible for these signs to be absent. The main diagnostic criterion is a positive pivot-shift test, obtained by using one or all of the mechanisms presently available:

1. MacIntosh test
2. Jerk test of Hughston
3. Lateral position of Slocum

For the jerk or sudden pivot-shift to occur, the iliotibial band must be intact. If the band has been incised during surgery, the pivot-shift test may be negative, even though anterolateral rotatory instability is present.

TREATMENT: Conservative treatment is aimed at developing the hamstrings, external rotators, and abductors in particular. A Lenox Hill brace or similar derotation device may be useful. Surgical treatment consists of reconstructive operations to control the rotatory instabilities. There are a number of reconstructive procedures for this problem. Such operations include procedures described by Ellison,[36] MacIntosh, Losee[48] and others. This involves transfer of the iliotibial band and the fibular collateral ligament and tightening of the posterolateral corner of the knee. These procedures are aimed at preventing the tibia from subluxing on the femur, and have a fairly high degree of success. Many surgeons augment these extra-articular procedures with an intra-articular substitution of the ACL.[37,38,39]

REHABILITATION EXERCISES: These play an important role in postoperative success. It is necessary to train the relocated muscle groups to perform their new activity, to improve proprioception around the knee, and at the same time to build up full strength in all the muscle groups.[49] It is advisable, however, to avoid pivot-type activities until a very late stage in the rehabilitation process, at which time the status of the knee can be reevaluated (see section on knee rehabilitation, p. 346).

Progression of events following an anterior cruciate ligament tear. Many former athletes give a history of hearing or feeling a "pop" in their knee which resulted from a cutting action or hyperextension. Swelling may have developed rapidly or it may have been completely absent; the initial examination may have been negative for gross ligament instability. A year or two after the injury, the knee will buckle and give way during a cutting maneuver. A torn medial meniscus may be diagnosed and removed.[50]

The athlete then finds that an increasing amount of instability develops and that the knee now gives way both when cutting with the foot externally rotated and when pivoting to the same side as the planted foot. At this stage there might also be pain at the posterolateral corner of the knee. The athlete has now developed anteromedial and anterolateral rotatory instability.[51,52]

The time interval between the initial injury and the subsequent development of instability varies from athlete to athlete and appears to be related to many individual factors. However, the above is a fairly typical sequence of events which belies the often-stated view that a torn anterior cruciate ligament is of no consequence. On the contrary, it is probably the most serious injury that can affect the high-performance athlete, and it has meant the end of many a promising career.[53,54,55,56]

Meniscal Lesions

INCIDENCE: The medial meniscus appears to be injured more frequently than the lateral meniscus. This may be due to the relative lack of freedom of movement of the medial meniscus, since the lateral meniscus can move out of the way of the lateral femoral condyle as it rotates.[57] Also, the medial meniscus is often injured in conjunction with medial ligament injuries. However, in certain sports, for instance, wrestling, there is an increased incidence of lateral meniscal tears. This may be because of the frequently flexed attitude of the knee with the foot in external rotation, and also because lateral ligament injuries occur relatively more often in wrestling.

There appears to be a high percentage of meniscal injuries in such sports as soccer, particularly when compared with football, where ligament injuries predominate. Meniscal tears are rare in pre-adolescents and uncommon in adolescents.

TYPES OF TEARS: Tears of the menisci are divided into

1. Peripheral tears or detachments
2. Tears of the body or substance of the meniscus, which are either longitudinal (vertical) or horizontal cleavage tears

The well-known "bucket-handle" tear is a longitudinal tear through the body of the meniscus (Figure 19.41). In some instances there may in fact be a double bucket-handle tear, in which two separate longitudinal tears are present. This occurs particularly in the midportion and the posterior horn of the medial meniscus.

The type of lesion that occurs differs at different ages, as it appears to be related to the status of the articular cartilage overlying the femur (or tibia), which interacts with the meniscus. A movement in a young athlete can produce the classical longitudinal tear, whereas the same mechanism in an older knee causes a horizontal cleavage tear.

ETIOLOGY: The meniscus is injured in the following ways:

1. In an isolated episode, when the knee is twisted while weight bearing, resulting in a combination of compression and rotational forces being exerted on the meniscus.

The medial meniscus can be injured by a rotational force, in which the tibia rotates externally with respect to the femur. Another

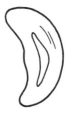

FIGURE 19.41 The "bucket-handle" tear of the medial meniscus

possible mechanism exists when the foot is fixed to the ground by cleats. This prevents the tibia from externally rotating on forced extension of the knee.

The lateral meniscus is protected largely by its mobility. If this mobility is lost due to some aging process, rotational movements may take place within the substance of the meniscus (instead of between the condyle and the meniscus). This results in a horizontal cleavage tear which later causes a "parrot-beak" tear of the meniscus (Figure 19.42).[58] In these cases the ligaments are usually not affected.

2. As part of a ligamentous injury. This is usually, but not always, associated with an external force.

3. When abnormal movements take place in a chronically unstable knee, which occurs particularly with anterolateral rotatory instability. The femur tends to ride over the posterolateral corner of the lateral meniscus, causing a tear to develop with time. Or the abnormal movement can produce an acute medial meniscal tear.

4. When the meniscus is abnormal (e.g., a discoid lateral meniscus).[59]

SYMPTOMS: In the acute injury, there may be a sudden locking of the knee, with inability to move the leg. Occasionally there may also be a "pop" heard as well.

The more common symptoms are joint-line or intra-articular pain localized to one side of the knee. The pain is elicited by squatting or twisting. A feeling of uncertainty may be experienced when the athlete walks on uneven ground, or an actual giving

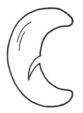

FIGURE 19.42 A "parrot-beak" tear of the lateral meniscus

way of the knee may occur. The athlete may feel that there is a block when attempting to fully extend the knee. Sometimes swelling is the only symptom. If the athlete gives a history of the knee locking near full extension and then suddenly "unlocking" ("snapping back into place"), the diagnosis is fairly certain.

SIGNS: A mild to moderate effusion may be present. There may be some wasting of the quadriceps (particularly the vastus medialis obliquus) if the injury has been present for some time.

Hopping tests may produce a feeling of insecurity, and squatting may cause pain. Duck-waddling is almost always painful. Joint-line tenderness is usually present. If tenderness is experienced over the anterior joint line when the athlete extends the knee from a flexed position, a longitudinal tear of the body of the meniscus should be suspected. Another suspicious finding is tenderness that moves anteriorly with extension and posteriorly with flexion.

There may be limitation to full extension or flexion, and forced flexion may be painful, particularly with posterior horn lesions. Pain on forced extension can indicate an anterior horn tear. Occasionally there will be pain through the midrange of knee movement, with the extremes of flexion and extension being pain-free. This indicates a tear of the midportion of the meniscus and is called the "painful arc sign."

If the knee can be fully flexed, McMurray's test is usually positive if there is a posterior horn tear. This tear causes a palpable or audible click over the torn meniscus (in longitudinal tears) or a grating associated with pain (in horizontal tears). Apley's test is sometimes positive for pain when there is a posterior horn tear.

X-RAYS: X-ray findings are usually normal except in the case of a meniscal tear that has been present for some time and that has produced changes of degeneration within the joint space. This is best appreciated on

TABLE 19.16   Symptoms and Signs of a Meniscal Injury

Symptoms:	Pain
	Pain + swelling
	Pain + giving way
	Locking and unlocking
Signs:	Vastus medialis atrophy
	Effusion
	Joint-line tenderness (important)
	Pain on forced flexion or extension
	Block to complete flexion or extension
	Positive McMurray's test

the standing AP view. Arthrography and arthroscopy are useful procedures for confirming the diagnosis and localizing the tear.

TREATMENT: Small peripheral tears of the attachment of the meniscus to the capsular ligament will heal if the leg is protected for a period of time. These tears can also be sutured.

If the body of the meniscus is torn and is causing joint irritation, surgical removal should be considered. However, it is necessary to bear in mind that a meniscectomy is not a benign procedure. It has been shown that removal of a meniscus increases joint wear, causes the early onset of degeneration, and may cause osteoarthritis in later life.[60,61] On the other hand, if a torn meniscus is left in the joint, it can also cause joint destruction and osteoarthritis.

Another problem that may be associated with a meniscectomy involves the athlete who has subclinical rotatory instability. Following a meniscectomy, this instability may become significant and may render the athlete even more incapacitated than before the meniscus was removed.[50]

The current conservative trend in treating a torn meniscus is shown by the increasing number of partial or incomplete meniscectomies that are being performed, particularly with arthroscopic surgery, as well as by the attempts to repair peripheral tears.[62,63] The

need to remove the meniscus should be carefully weighed against the disadvantages. If there are no symptoms or signs of joint irritation, it is probably advisable to leave the meniscus alone and to observe the athlete at regular intervals.

REGENERATION OF THE MENISCUS: Following a meniscectomy, a new structure which resembles the meniscus in shape and appearance may be found within the joint. This regeneration is variable in amount and can occur between six weeks and two years after the meniscectomy if the peripheral segment left by the surgeon is large enough.[109] The regenerated meniscus consists of fibrous tissue only, no cartilaginous cells being present, and it is thinner and narrower than the original. It does not fulfill the role of a mechanical stabilizer, nor does it seem to affect the development of joint degeneration.

Differential Diagnoses of Meniscal Tears

Osteochondral fractures. An osteochondral fracture (a fracture through the articular cartilage and a portion of the bone) may be associated with a twisting, weight-bearing type of injury, as is a meniscal tear. A dislocating patella can also cause an osteochondral fracture. There may be limitation of extension (as with the meniscal injury) and joint-line tenderness.

Subluxing patella. The athlete with a subluxing patella may also give a history of giving-way and even of "locking." There may be an effusion, vastus medialis wasting, and joint-line tenderness from medial retinacular irritation. There is often pain on forced flexion, though the pain is more anterior than posterior. Tenderness is usually present along the medial facet of the patella, and moving the patella laterally causes pain and sometimes apprehension.

Ligament injury. This injury produces localized joint-line tenderness and pain if the capsular ligament alone is involved. In fact, a capsular ligament tear is often associated with a peripheral tear of the medial meniscus.

Tendinitis—overuse injuries. Pes anserine tendinitis may present with pain and tenderness over and just below the medial joint line. On the lateral side of the knee, symptoms of popliteal and iliotibial tract inflammation, particularly in long-distance runners, can be confused with those of a lateral meniscal injury. Usually the tenderness is just above the joint line, though occasionally it may be over the joint line itself.

Osteochondritis dissecans. Osteochondritis can produce joint-line tenderness, but it is usually anterior and is best felt with the knee at 90° of flexion. It can cause locking if the fragment is detached. Wilson's test may be positive (with the foot internally rotated, the knee is extended from 30° of flexion while a valgus force is applied).[64] Osteochondritis dissecans tends to occur in adolescents (an unusual age for meniscal injuries).

THE PATELLA

Functional Anatomy

The patella is a sesamoid bone situated in the tendon of the quadriceps muscle. The quadriceps muscle group is attached to the superior pole of the patella, while the patella tendon originates from the inferior pole. The main functions of the patella are:

1. To increase the effective power of the quadriceps muscle by
   a. increasing the extensor lever arm of the quadriceps mechanism
   b. increasing the area of the action-force of the quadriceps muscles
   c. decreasing friction associated with quadriceps contraction
2. To protect the femoral condyles from direct blows

The patella glides in the intercondylar groove between the medial and the lateral femoral condyles. This movement is influenced and controlled by a number of factors (Figure 19.43).

1. Quadriceps muscle group, in particular the vastus medialis obliquus (VMO).

2. Medial retinaculum.

3. Medial patellofemoral ligaments (thickening of the deep capsule).

4. Shape of the patella (a patella with a flat undersurface is more likely to move laterally than one with a deep central ridge).

5. Height of the patella. With a patella alta, or high patella, the VMO loses some of its effect in stabilizing the patella.[65]

6. Shape and height of the femoral condyles. A low lateral femoral condyle allows the patella to shift laterally more easily than a high lateral condyle.[66]

7. Vastus lateralis. If there is an imbalance, with the vastus lateralis being more powerful than its medial counterpart, there is a tendency for the patella to be pulled laterally.

8. Lateral retinaculum. If excessively tight, this, too, tends to pull the patella laterally and cause excessive pressure between the patella and the femoral condyles.[67,68]

9. Lateral patellofemoral ligaments (thickening of the deep capsule).

10. Location of the tibial tubercle. A laterally positioned tibial tubercle increases the Q angle.

11. External tibial torsion. This has the same effect as a laterally located tibial tubercle.

12. Q angle (this is the angle formed by a line drawn from the anterior superior iliac spine through the midportion of the patella to the tibial tubercle. This angle is increased by a wide pelvis or external tibial torsion). The normal Q angle is thought to be up to 10° in males and 16° in females.

13. Factors around the hip joint (e.g., anteversion of the femoral neck results in inward squinting of the patella).

14. The position of the foot (e.g., excessive pronation).[69]

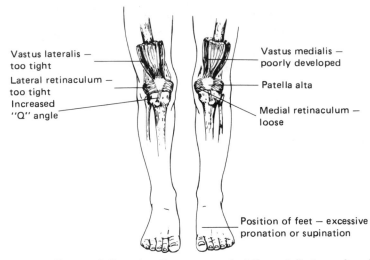

FIGURE 19.43   Factors influencing the movement of the patella towards subluxation (schematic)

The articular surface of the patella is divided into large areas called facets (Figure 19.44). The lateral facet, which is broader and deeper than the medial facet, is divided from the medial facet by the central ridge. This ridge runs vertically and corresponds to the intercondylar groove on the femur. The medial facet has a small area on the most medial aspect termed the "odd facet," which is only in contact with the femur during extremes of knee flexion.

The entire articular surface of the patella is not in contact with the femur at any one time. Various areas of the patella articulate at different angles of the flexing knee. For instance, with the knee in extension, the distal portion of the patella has the highest contact force and the contact area moves proximally as the knee flexes. Between 90° and 135° most of the contact is on the medial facet, and this moves to the odd facet with complete flexion. Any abnormal movement of the patella along its course in the groove results in excessive patellofemoral pressure, pain, and eventually may result in articular cartilage degeneration on the undersurface of the patella or on the femoral condyles.

Patellar shape. The patella has a very individual shape which differs from person to person. This variability may influence congruency and stability of the patella in the patellofemoral joint. A classification by Wiberg[70] and Baumgartl[71] is used to describe the patellar shape (Figure 19.45).

Type I	Medial and lateral facets are equal and slightly concave.
Type II	Medial facet is smaller; both facets are concave.
Type III	Medial facet is smaller and convex; the larger, lateral facet is concave.
Type II–III	Medial facet is small and flat.
Type IV	Medial facet is very small and almost vertical.
Type V	Jagerhut ("hunter's cap") patella is almost flat.

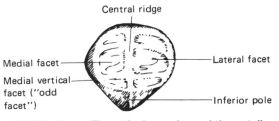

FIGURE 19.44   The articular surface of the patella

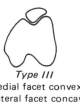
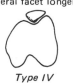
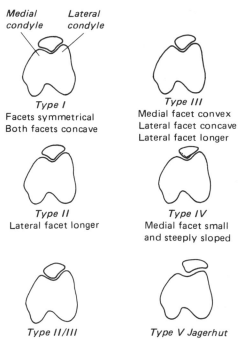

Medial condyle   Lateral condyle

Type I
Facets symmetrical
Both facets concave

Type III
Medial facet convex
Lateral facet concave
Lateral facet longer

Type II
Lateral facet longer

Type IV
Medial facet small
and steeply sloped

Type II/III
Medial facet convex

Type V Jagerhut
No central ridge
No medial facet

FIGURE 19.45 Classification of patellar shapes (by Wiberg and Baumgartl) (Modified from R.L. Larson, "Fractures and dislocations of the knee. Part II, Dislocations and Ligamentous injuries to the knee," in *Fractures,* C.A. Rockwood and D.P. Green [eds.], Vol. 2, p. 1183, published by J.B. Lippincott Co., Philadelphia, 1975.)

Injuries to the Patella

The main injuries affecting the patellofemoral joint are:

1. Patellar fracture

2. Acute dislocation

3. Subluxation and spontaneous reduction of a dislocated patella

Patellar fracture. This is an uncommon injury usually caused by a direct blow. The fracture can be horizontal across the patella, or it can shatter the patella into numerous pieces.

TREATMENT:

Initial: Immobilization with the leg in full extension, plus icing.

Definitive: Surgery is necessary if the fracture is displaced.

Acute dislocation.

1. Commonly, patellar dislocations occur as noncontact injuries and result from the force of contraction of the quadriceps combined with the angle of the leg. For instance, during a cutting maneuver the foot is planted in external rotation and the knee is flexed to about 45° and forced into a valgus position (see Figure 19.36). The quadriceps then forcefully contracts and, because of the angle of pull with the leg in this position, it actively dislocates the patella (Figure 19.46). This type of dislocation occurs in an athlete with a relatively normal lower extremity alignment and without gross abnormality of the quadriceps mechanism, *if* the forces pulling the patella laterally are powerful enough.

2. Dislocation can occur in those with genetic or developmental factors that predispose to lateral displacement of the patella. In these, a very small force may be all that is required to cause a dislocation.

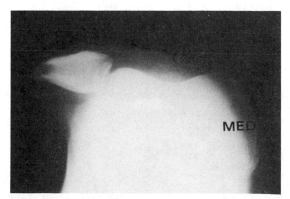

MED

FIGURE 19.46 Patellar dislocation (laterally) With this injury, there is damage to the medial retinaculum, the patellofemoral and patellotibial ligaments, and sometimes the vastus medialis. In addition, articular cartilage fractures frequently occur, particularly of the lateral femoral condyle.

PATHOLOGY: There is usually tearing of the attachments of the following structures from the patella:

1. Medial retinaculum
2. Medial patellofemoral ligaments
3. Vastus medialis obliquus (and perhaps other parts of the quadriceps muscle group)

If these heal in a lengthened position, chronic subluxation or recurrent dislocations can occur. In addition, there is frequently damage to the underlying cartilage or bone, which can result in one of the following (Figure 19.47):

1. Articular cartilage damage—partial thickness: Minimal symptoms.

2. Articular cartilage damage—full thickness: An articular cartilage fracture that can develop significant symptoms.

3. Avulsion fracture—on the medial side of the patella at the attachment of the medial retinaculum and patellofemoral ligaments.

4. Osteochondral fracture—involves the articular cartilage and the underlying bone of either the patella or the lateral femoral condyle. It often occurs during relocation of the patella, as it strikes the lateral femoral condyle.

5. Fracture of the patella—occurs through the entire thickness of bone.

Articular cartilage damage can occur on the patella, the femoral surface, or both, and can lead to permanent patellofemoral joint problems.

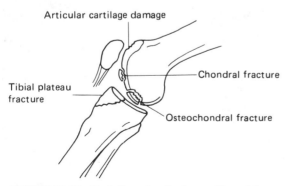

FIGURE 19.47   Varieties of articular cartilage injury

SYMPTOMS: The athlete usually describes feeling the "knee going out of joint." There is intense pain and inability to move the knee.

SIGNS: On observation of the injured knee, the laterally dislocated patella is usually obvious. However, if the athlete is first seen some hours after the dislocation has occurred, gross intra-articular swelling can obscure the position of the patella. There should still be little difficulty in making the diagnosis after palpating the anterior aspect of the knee. While palpating this area, be sure that the quadriceps muscle group and the patellar tendon are intact, because it is possible for one of these structures to rupture, the presenting feature being a large hemarthrosis. In addition, a tibial collateral ligament injury frequently occurs in conjunction with a patellar dislocation, producing medial tenderness and valgus instability.

TREATMENT:

Initial: If the athlete is seen at the site of the injury, the affected leg should be gently straightened. This is sometimes sufficient to produce reduction. If it does not, *gentle* medial pressure should then be applied. When a reduction is achieved, the knee should be packed with ice and splinted with whatever means are available, with the leg fully extended. The athlete is then transported for X-rays and definitive treatment.

If the patella cannot easily be reduced by the simple procedures outlined, no further attempts at reduction should be made. The knee should be iced and splinted with the leg in the position of greatest comfort while the athlete is being transported for X-rays and reduction.

Definitive: Most dislocations reduce easily. A nonsurgical approach to treatment is currently advised, unless the patella cannot be reduced or another indication for surgery exists such as an osteochondral fracture. This is diagnosed by finding fat globules in the hemarthrosis when it is aspirated.

A plaster cylinder is the treatment of choice in most cases. If it is a *first-time dislocation*, the leg should be held in the cast four to six weeks, depending on the assessment of soft-tissue and articular cartilage damage at the time of reduction. The athlete should be kept in bed for the first day or two, with the knee packed in ice, a compression bandage applied, and the limb elevated. During this time, the leg is best immobilized with a plaster cast or postoperative splint. Anti-inflammatory medication is often used and should be started soon after the injury. A full patellar rehabilitation program is then commenced (see section on knee rehabilitation, p. 361).

The athlete should use a knee brace such as a neoprene sleeve with a lateral pad when returning to activity, to protect the patella and prevent lateral displacement (Figure 19.48). In-shoe orthotic devices should also be used if indicated.

Recurrent dislocations.   The athlete who has had previous dislocations need only be kept in a postoperative knee immobilizer until

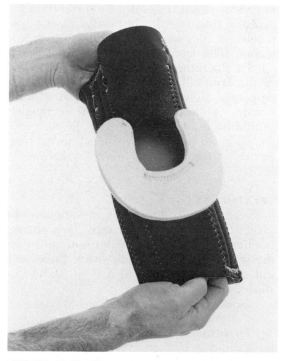

FIGURE 19.48 Neoprene sleeve with a felt patella stabilizing pad

symptoms subside. An assessment should be made as to whether surgical repair is warranted.

Subluxation and spontaneous reduction of a dislocated patella.   The difference between spontaneous reduction of a dislocated patella and subluxation of a patella may be very subtle and difficult to distinguish clinically, though the two are really separate entities. Spontaneous reduction of a dislocated patella is usually a clearly defined event in which the patella is seen or felt to slip over the lateral femoral condyle and then return to the intercondylar groove. With a subluxation, a significant number of athletes are totally unaware that the patella has partially or completely dislocated, only knowing that something serious has occurred in the knee. However, as the two conditions overlap, they will be discussed together.

A subluxation or a dislocation occurs relatively often in athletes.[72,73] The etiology and pathological findings are those described under the section on acute dislocations, p. 333. Many of the symptoms and signs of patellar subluxation are compatible with a meniscal tear, and for this reason the examiner's index of suspicion must be high; otherwise the diagnosis can be missed.

The athlete may state that the knee suddenly buckled and gave way, usually with a tearing sensation and much pain, sometimes with a "pop." Or the history may be much more vague and may include statements to the effect that the knee "went out of joint" or that there was locking, catching, or giving way. It may be stated that when the leg was straightened, something shifted back into place. Occasionally swelling is the only complaint.

If the athlete gives a history of the knee giving way, or of a pop, it is important to try to obtain a description of the mechanism of the injury and the exact position of the affected foot and leg at the time of these symptoms.

SIGNS: In the case of spontaneous reduction of a dislocated patella, there is usually a large hemarthrosis of rapid onset. Any flexion, passive or active, causes intense pain. In less severe or recurrent cases, there may be joint effusion, but this may be absent and the range of movement may be normal.

The athlete should sit at the end of the examining table, legs hanging down at 90° and should be observed for the following:

1. Lateral squinting of the patella. This is a sign which should immediately make the examiner suspect subluxation.

2. Patella alta, or high-riding patella. The patella tends to "look up" at the ceiling (Figure 19.30).

3. Tracking of the patella in the intercondylar notch when the knee is moved through the range of flexion to extension.

The athlete then holds the leg at 45° against resistance, at which time the vastus medialis is inspected and palpated. Then the knee is palpated. Tenderness is often elicited along the medial joint line and over the femoral attachments of the patellofemoral ligaments. The medial retinaculum and the vastus medialis obliquus may also be extremely tender, and the medial facet of the patella is almost always so.

The examiner should then test for lateral hypermobility of the patella, first with the leg fully extended, then at 30° of flexion. The quadriceps muscles should be relaxed. This maneuver can be exceedingly painful to perform in the acute case; if so, further testing for lateral mobility should not be undertaken at this time.

If the medial retinaculum and the patellofemoral ligaments are loose, it may be possible to displace the patella completely without discomfort or apprehension. In most instances, however, as the articular surface of the patella begins to slip over the lateral femoral condyle, the athlete becomes apprehensive and tightens the quadriceps in an attempt to straighten the leg, or grabs the examiner's hand to prevent further lateral displacement. This is termed a "positive apprehension test" and is highly suggestive of patellar instability (see Figure 19.32). Compressing the patella against the underlying

bone should be performed gently, as it may cause exquisite pain.

Testing the medial ligaments produces no laxity, though with valgus stress there is often some discomfort along the medial joint line and the tibial collateral ligament. This might lead the examiner into thinking that a sprain of the tibial collateral ligament has occurred, which indeed may have happened.

Examination of the menisci is usually best deferred in the acute case, as attempts to completely flex the knee will cause severe pain. However, in the chronic case, McMurray's test may also produce tenderness over the medial joint line, again possibly misleading the examiner into thinking that a meniscal injury is present.

X-rays of both knees are most useful in confirming the diagnosis. Sometimes a subluxed patella shows up on an anteroposterior (AP) view. Some osteochondral fractures of the patella or the femur can also be seen on this view (osteochondral fractures of the femur are usually best seen on the tunnel view). Look carefully for osteochondral avulsion fractures off the medial facet of the patella, as they may be difficult to see at first glance. The lateral view will demonstrate a patella alta or an osteochondral defect in one of the femoral condyles. However, it is the tangential view which gives the most information. A number of different techniques should be used to substantiate the diagnosis and to avoid missing any osteochondral fragments[73,74] (see section on knee X-rays, p. 363).

TREATMENT:

Initial: Ice, compression, elevation, and a posterior splint or postoperative immobilizer holding the knee in full extension constitute the initial treatment in the acute case. Anti-inflammatory medication, if used, should be started immediately.

Definitive:

Conservative:

First-time subluxation or dislocation: If no indication for surgery exists, it is best to place the severe case in a cylinder cast from four to six weeks. In the less severe case, or

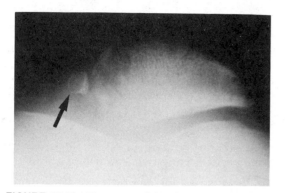

FIGURE 19.49 X-ray—avulsion fracture, medial facet of the patella The attachment of the medial retinaculum and patellotibial ligaments may result in an avulsion fracture if the patella subluxes laterally.

the case of an athlete under close supervision, a postoperative knee immobilizer can be used instead. The main point is to keep the knee straight, in order to avoid any pressure on the articular surfaces of the patellofemoral joint and to allow the soft tissues on the medial side of the patella to heal in the optimal position.

Recurrent subluxation or dislocation: In this case the medial retinaculum and the patellofemoral ligaments have probably elongated, due to previous episodes. There is no value in prolonged immobilization; they are therefore splinted only until asymptomatic, which usually takes from a few days to two weeks. However, they should be assessed for elective surgical repair.

Rehabilitation of both the first-time subluxation or dislocation and the recurrent case should be performed routinely (see section on knee rehabilitation, p. 361).

Surgical: Surgical treatment may be indicated in certain cases.

Patellofemoral Joint Pain

This term covers a number of common conditions associated with the articulation of the patella on the femur. One of these conditions is chondromalacia. The term chondromalacia should be reserved for situations in which there are actual pathological changes of the articular cartilage of the patella, and

should not be used to describe the whole spectrum of patellofemoral joint pain.[75,76,77,78]

As mentioned, there are many causes of patellofemoral joint pain, but *extensor mechanism malalignment* is by far the most common etiological mechanism in athletes. Other causes of pain (many of which are interrelated) include:

1. Direct trauma
2. Recurrent subluxation or dislocation of the patella
3. Knee ligament or meniscal injury
4. Other internal derangements of the knee
5. Insufficiency of the quadriceps muscle group
6. Rotational abnormalities of the transverse plane
7. Patellofemoral joint incongruencies
8. Femoral or tibial torsion
9. Postsurgical or immobilization state
10. Synovial plica

Extensor mechanism malalignment ("the miserable malalignment syndrome") is, as mentioned, the most common cause of patellofemoral joint pain.[69,75] Once an athlete with the typical characteristics of this syndrome is seen, it is not difficult to recognize the more subtle cases (Figure 19.50). The "typical" case has marked bilateral medial squinting of the patellae with "apparent" genu varum when standing. (This is "apparent" because of the genu recurvatum which is usually also present.) There may be patella alta, a prominent fat pad, an increased Q angle, and often external tibial rotation. Tibia varum is often present and usually compensatory pronation of the feet.

Medial patellar squinting is due to anteversion of the femoral neck, or what appears to be anteversion clinically, with greater internal than external rotation, due to an angulation deformity of the femoral neck, or in some cases, to soft-tissue imbalance around the hips. These malaligned angles result in high pressures which localize to particular areas of the patella. This increase in pressure causes pain.

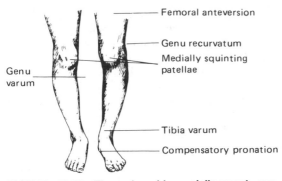

Femoral anteversion

Genu recurvatum

Medially squinting patellae

Genu varum

Tibia varum

Compensatory pronation

FIGURE 19.50 The miserable malalignment syndrome

PATHOMECHANICS: The changes responsible for the development of patellofemoral joint pain have not been clearly defined. The current concept is that the pain is due to irritation of the nerve endings in the subchondral bone (articular cartilage has no nerve supply), and that this irritation occurs because of the loss of the normal energy-absorption function of the intermediate and deep zones of the articular cartilage.[69,79] Other theories state that the pain is secondary to an alteration of the blood supply in the chondral bone, or that it is caused by venous stasis and congestion within the patella.[80] Also, transverse plane rotation malalignments account for abnormal forces on the articular cartilage and subchondral bone in many cases. This is discussed further under the section on the runner's knee, p. 430.

NATURAL HISTORY AND SYMPTOMS: The usual sufferer of malalignment is in his or her teens or early twenties and is usually active and athletically involved at the onset of symptoms. It has been stated that the majority of symptoms resolve spontaneously over a period of time. While some do resolve spontaneously, it is unusual for the person who continues athletic activities to be fortunate enough to have a spontaneous remission of symptoms without receiving treatment or changing the type and/or amount of activity.

Many athletes have pain in only one knee at a time, though some cases are bilateral. The main complaints are:

1. Pain when going up and, particularly, down stairs or hills

2. Aching when sitting with the knees at 90° for a period of time. This is usually accompanied by stiffness which disappears rapidly after walking a short distance

3. Pain during activity, after activity, or both, particularly after squatting and cycling

4. Catching, grating, transient locking, and a feeling of giving way at times

Swelling is an uncommon presenting symptom and if present is usually mild.

SIGNS: When examining an athlete with patellofemoral joint pain, the following sequence should be followed. The athlete should:

1. Stand facing the examiner—observe for signs of malalignment.

2. Stand sideways—examine for genu recurvatum, patella alta, and tight Achilles tendons.

3. Sit with the legs hanging down at 90°—note "squinting" of the patellae and patella alta.

4. Sit with the legs at 45° against resistance—inspect and palpate the vastus medialis obliquus muscles.

5. Lie supine—examine the patellae.

Pertinent physical findings that should be noted are:

1. Tenderness along the medial facet of the patella

2. Pain on compression of the patella against the underlying femur, particularly the lateral facet of the patella (this is the lateral patellar sign and suggests the possibility of the *patellar compression syndrome*, that is, higher-than-normal forces between the patella and the femur)[68,81]

3. Lateral laxity of the patella when tested with the leg in full extension and in 30° of flexion

4. A positive apprehension sign

Crepitus may or may not be demonstrable, but this is not considered an important sign *by itself* in most cases, because there is little association between crepitus and symptoms in the athlete. Crepitus is often present in joints which do not have any patellofemoral pain and vice versa. However, crepitus that becomes more apparent as the severity of the symptoms increases is likely to be related to articular cartilage wear and deterioration.

An examination of hip rotation and feet should be included.

TREATMENT:

Conservative: The mainstay of treatment of patellofemoral joint pain is conservative management, including the following:

1. Improvement of strength and power of the quadriceps muscle group, in particular the vastus medialis obliquus (a schedule of exercises is presented in the section on rehabilitation of the knee, p. 361). Additional help to develop the VMO may be obtained by using an electrical muscle stimulator.

2. In-shoe orthotic devices, particularly useful in malalignment, especially in those cases with excessive compensatory pronation of the feet.[69,82]

3. Increase in flexibility by means of slow, static stretching of the hamstring muscle group and the muscles surrounding the hip joint.

4. TENS can be used at rest, and sometimes worn during activity.

5. Decrease in activities such as cycling, running down hills, jumping, squatting, and sitting with the knees at 90° of flexion, until the condition has become asymptomatic. When asymptomatic, and after increasing the strength and power of the quadriceps muscle group, the athlete may be able to gradually return to these activities. Should the symptoms recur, the activity level must be reduced immediately.

6. Ice after workouts and at other times during the day if symptoms are present.

7. Aspirin or buffered aspirin, taken in a dose of up to 3g or 4g per day.

8. A neoprene patellar sleeve with a supportive ring designed to reduce lateral movement of the patella. The sleeve also helps to keep the knee warm during activity and may give symptomatic relief. Other braces have also been used.[83]

Surgical: Surgery is reserved for the exceptionally unresponsive and difficult case and should not be undertaken until all conservative measures have been tried. Many different surgical procedures have been devised, from a simple lateral retinacular release for patellar compression[84,85] to an operation in which the vastus medialis muscle is advanced, the lateral retinaculum released, and the tibial tubercle moved medially to decrease the Q angle.[86,87] Removal of a localized area of unhealthy articular cartilage is sometimes also performed. The surgical procedure needs to be individualized for each athlete.

Differential Diagnoses

Other causes of anterior knee pain need to be considered.

1. *Recurrent subluxation or dislocation of the patella*. This must be suspected in every case as it is associated with many cases of patellofemoral joint pain due to malalignment.

2. *Patellofemoral compression syndrome*. This may be part of, or independent of, the malalignment syndrome. If the reaction forces between the patella and the femur increase, anterior knee pain may result. The diagnosis is made by finding a tight lateral retinaculum and pain on compression of the lateral facet of the patella (lateral patellar sign), and the pain may be relieved by surgical release of the lateral retinaculum.

3. *Meniscal lesion(s)*. See section on the menisci, p. 328.

4. *Bipartite patella*. The unfused portion of the patella is usually found at the superior lateral pole, and when symptomatic, pain and tenderness are localized to that site. Occurrence is mainly in males and may give rise to symptoms in athletes participating in

sports that require much jumping and squatting.[88] The diagnosis is confirmed by X-rays (best seen on anteroposterior and tangential views of the patella) and often occurs bilaterally.

5. *Infrapatellar fat-pad lesions.* An uncommon finding, these are usually due to direct trauma of the fat pad, which results in swelling and hemorrhage, though the fat pads may become inflamed from general overuse. A differentiating feature is that the pain is often relieved by keeping the knee in slight flexion.

6. *Synovial plica.* The athlete usually complains of pain and swelling, accompanied by a catching or snapping sensation. The articular cartilage can degenerate from recurrent impingement of the plica on the patella and the femoral condyles. This is a relatively rare condition which is becoming more frequently diagnosed with increasing use of the arthroscope.[89]

7. *Quadriceps contracture.* This can occur after a fractured femur or a quadriceps injury, creating pain by increasing the patellofemoral joint reaction forces.

OTHER CONDITIONS IN OR AROUND THE KNEE

Osteochondral Fractures

The term "osteochondral" implies that the fracture is through the articular cartilage as well as a portion of the bone, and that it usually results in a fragment being detached from the underlying bone. While these fractures need to be diagnosed by means of X-rays, they can be suspected clinically.

MECHANISM OF INJURY: There are two basic mechanisms:

1. A direct blow to the knee, for instance, contacting a sharp object like the corner of a table with the knee flexed while moving at speed. The medial femoral condyle is more exposed and therefore more often involved.

2. A noncontact injury. The shearing force of twisting and weight bearing may be enough to cause a fracture through one or the other femoral condyle, for instance, when cutting sharply to the opposite side.

TYPES OF FRACTURES:
Femur. Osteochondral fractures of the medial femoral condyle tend to be smaller than those of the lateral femoral condyle.
Patella: Small or large osteochondral fractures may be produced during a patellar dislocation, when both the lateral femoral condyle and the patella can sustain fractures.

SYMPTOMS: The history is of an acute injury, either contact of the knee against an object or sudden twisting with the knee flexed. This is followed by a "snapping" sensation or sound and the rapid onset of swelling. There is severe pain, particularly if the athlete attempts to walk.

SIGNS: Signs include a large hemarthrosis, joint line tenderness which is usually localized to one specific area, and inability to fully extend the knee.

X-RAYS: X-rays may only show the osteochondral fragment when the special tunnel or tangential views are taken. Arthroscopy is helpful in difficult cases.

TREATMENT: Treatment is by surgery, preferably immediately following the diagnosis. The osteochondral fragment is replaced and pinned into position if this is possible, or else removed. If there is any delay before the diagnosis is made and surgery is undertaken, replacing the fragments may not be possible. Joint degeneration can result.

Osteochondritis Dissecans

Osteochondritis dissecans is a condition in which an area of bone undergoes changes which result in a loose piece of bone (also called a loose body) within the joint. In the knee the area of osteochondritis dissecans is mainly found on the posterolateral aspect of the medial femoral condyle (Figure 19.51)

ETIOLOGY: This is still a matter of debate although a number of factors have been associated with it, such as:

1. Trauma (some think it is a compression fracture)
2. Impairment of the blood supply to the affected area of the femur
3. Heredity in some cases

TYPES: As a generalization, osteochondritis dissecans is divided into two groups. These are distinguished from each other by an age difference.

Under 15 years: In this group, osteochondritis dissecans is generally unrelated to trauma. It presents with nonspecific knee pain that may continue for a period of time (possibly months), and it is often bilateral.

SIGNS: Pre-adolescents and adolescents appear to have external tibial rotation when walking. A slight effusion may be present, and perhaps some quadriceps atrophy. Tenderness to palpation is present over the affected condyle when the knee is flexed beyond 90°.

Wilson's sign for osteochondritis dissecans may be positive.[64] This test is performed by placing the affected knee at 90° of flexion, then internally rotating the tibia and extending the knee. As the knee is extended, a valgus force is applied. Pain at 30° of flexion indicates a positive sign for osteochondritis dissecans, usually of the lateral portion of the medial femoral condyle. However, this test can be negative although osteochondritis dissecans is present.

DIAGNOSIS: The diagnosis is made by means of X-rays, with the lesion commonly seen on the tunnel view.

There is also a growth variant or developmental abnormality affecting the secondary center of ossification, which is seen only on X-rays and does not produce any clinical symptoms and signs. This variant will go on to normal ossification without treatment being necessary.

TREATMENT: Usually the treatment is simple rest from activities that produce pain; sometimes enforced rest in a cast is necessary. The prognosis for this age group is usually excellent.

Over 15 years: These are usually males, and the symptoms are often related to a specific traumatic event. They may present with locking and giving way if the osteochondral fragment becomes detached and slips into the joint, or they may present with the same symptoms and signs as those under 15.

DIAGNOSIS: Diagnosis is made by means of X-rays.

TREATMENT: The over-15 age group, or those with a loose fragment in the under-15 age group, may need surgical pinning or excision of the fragment.

PROGNOSIS: The prognosis for this age group is much poorer than for the under-15 age group, and seems to worsen with increasing age.

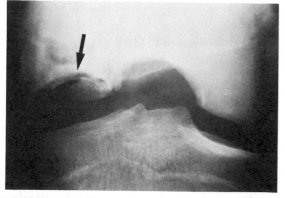

FIGURE 19.51 **X-ray—osteochondritis dissecans of the knee**

Baker's Cyst

Actually a herniation of the synovium, this swelling is usually found on the postero-medial aspect of the knee. The herniation forms a sac and fills with synovial fluid. It is often associated with a tear or a degenerative condition of the medial meniscus.

By itself, the cyst is of little significance, though it can cause discomfort when the athlete is running at full speed. If it causes considerable impairment of athletic performance, or if it is associated with some intra-articular condition, an arthrogram should be ordered to rule out the presence of a meniscal tear. Should a tear be present, it may be an indication for a meniscectomy with or without removal of the cyst. On occasion, the cyst spontaneously ruptures followed by cessation of all symptoms.

Synovial Plica

A normal anatomical variation of the synovium, the plica is a band of tissue that runs from the lateral femoral condyle around the superior and medial aspects of the patella downward to the fat pad anteriorly. It usually does not cause any particular problem, but if it becomes inflexible and taut, it may give rise to symptoms of irritation, usually of the medial facet of the patella, though sometimes the superior or lateral aspects of the knee are involved.[89,90,91]

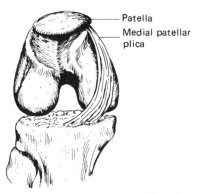

Patella
Medial patellar plica

FIGURE 19.52   Medial patellar plica

SYMPTOMS AND SIGNS: In some cases, direct trauma to the knee (and to the plica) initiates symptoms similar to those of a meniscal injury—pain, pseudolocking, and swelling. Pain referable to the patella, such as retropatellar pain when sitting, with relief on extension of the leg, may also be noticed. A snapping and popping may occur, particularly over the medial femoral condyle, when the knee is moved through about 60° of flexion. Even though a plica may be causing some of the symptoms, there may be other pathology such as a medial meniscal injury or an extensor mechanism malalignment.

TREATMENT: Hamstring and quadriceps stretching exercises relieve symptoms in some cases, though most require surgical removal if symptomatic.

Patellar and Quadriceps Tendinitis ("Jumper's Knee")

Jumper's knee refers to tendinitis involving either the patellar tendon, the quadriceps tendon, or both. This condition is peculiar to athletic activities, particularly those involving constant repetitive jumping and landing such as basketball, the long-and-high jump, and the triple jump.

Patellar tendinitis is the more common of the two and may present with localized pain and tenderness in one of three areas:

1. Attachment of the patellar tendon to the inferior pole of the patella (the most common)
2. Midportion of the patellar tendon
3. Insertion of the patellar tendon into the tibial tubercle

Quadriceps tendinitis usually manifests with pain and tenderness localized to the insertion of the quadriceps group of muscles into the superior pole of the patella.

ETIOLOGY: This appears to be related to microtrauma to the tendon and to the attachment of the tendon to the patella (see section on microtrauma, p. 127). Repetitive jumping with acceleration or deceleration is the primary causative mechanism. It seems that this condition is becoming more common, due to a longer playing season and increasing daily participation. Other factors which may aggravate the condition include squatting with heavy weights and malalignment of the patella.

Patellar tendinitis seldom disappears on its own if the athlete continues to play at the same level and for the same amount of time. A decrease in one of these factors (plus treatment) helps modify the progress of the condition to some extent.

SYMPTOMS: Symptoms are mainly confined to pain in the involved area. Occasionally there may be some catching, giving way, and weakness, which is often due to quadriceps wasting.

SIGNS: Tenderness localized to the involved area is the most prominent sign. In the common variety (i.e., patellar tendinitis localized to the inferior pole of the patella), tenderness is best elicited by stabilizing the patella superiorly with one hand while directing localized pressure against the distal pole of the patella and the most proximal portion of the patellar tendon (Figure 19.53). Occasionally there is swelling localized to the involved area. There is almost never any generalized swelling of the knee. As mentioned, various abnormalities of the extensor mechanism with malalignment of the lower extremity are often present.

X-RAYS: Generally there is little to see on the AP and lateral X-ray views besides radiolucency and sometimes elongation and spurring of the distal pole. Evidence of old Osgood-Schlatter disease may be present. On the tangential view, there may be evidence of patellar instability, that is, lateral patellar tilting. A soft-tissue lateral X-ray may help to identify abnormalities of the tendon.

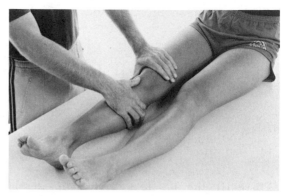

FIGURE 19.53 Patellar tendinitis Stabilize the patella in order to elicit tenderness of the inferior pole of the patella and the proximal portion of the patellar tendon.

DIAGNOSIS: The diagnosis is purely clinical. One can grade the severity of the condition according to the symptoms (as outlined under the section on microtrauma, p. 128):[92]

Phase I: Symptoms only after activity

Phase II: Symptoms during and after activity

Phase III: Symptoms present all the time

TREATMENT: The concept of microtrauma and the progressive nature of patellar tendinitis should be discussed with the athlete. An understanding of this concept by the athlete will facilitate a more successful therapeutic program.

Conservative treatment of Phases I and II:

1. Modification of activity if possible.

2. Removal of any aggravating exercises such as heavy squatting.

3. Icing and ice massage after activity, as well as at various intervals throughout the day.

4. Ice massage or moist heat before activity, depending on which modality is more comfortable to the athlete.

5. Use of a neoprene knee support with a ring to stabilize the patella if patellar instability is present.

6. Use of in-shoe orthotic devices if this is indicated.

7. Quadriceps exercises, particularly isometric contractions, as long as these do not cause any aggravation of the condition. A careful balance needs to be maintained between attempting to prevent quadriceps atrophy and further aggravating the condition.

8. Anti-inflammatory medication (for example, aspirin taken an hour before practice).

Conservative treatment of Phase III: When in Phase III, the athlete will have considerable difficulty maintaining an optimum level of athletic performance. In addition to the treatment program outlined for Phases I and II, the following are suggested:

1. The advantages of modifying activity for a period of time should be discussed with the athlete.

2. More powerful anti-inflammatories such as phenylbutazone (Butazolidin), sulindic (Clinoril), and other similar preparations can be used for short periods of time.

3. It is advised that the athlete *not* receive an injection of a corticosteroid because of the potentially dangerous weakening of an already damaged tendon, and also because of the chronic nature of the condition, which tends to make the athlete desirous of repeated injections in spite of awareness of potential dangers. If a corticosteroid injection is given, it should be placed *around* the tendon and *not into it*. The athlete should understand that this injection is not to be repeated.

4. Ultrasound with 10% hydrocortisone cream is sometimes useful.

5. Occasionally it is necessary to have the athlete walk in a postoperative knee splint, to rest the inflamed area.

6. TENS is sometimes useful in alleviating symptoms but does not appear to halt progression of the condition.

Surgical treatment: Various surgical procedures, from localized excision of the necrotic area in the tendon to major patellar realignment with removal of necrotic material from the inferior pole of the patella, are currently used with relatively good results in selected cases.

ON-FIELD MANAGEMENT OF KNEE INJURIES

Those who are called upon to examine an athlete's knee at the site of injury should be familiar with a definite plan of action so that a quick, yet thorough, evaluation may be made. The on-field examination consists of the initial examination and the sideline examination.

Initial On-Field Examination

This examination is applicable when a decision must be made as to how the athlete will be removed from the field. In essence, the on-field examination is a *screening for ligament stability*. True, a dislocated patella or other serious injury may have occurred, but these are fairly obvious and there is no doubt that the athlete must be removed by means of a stretcher.

A brief history should be obtained as to the mechanism of injury and what the athlete experienced—whether there was a pop, snap, or tearing sensation and where the pain was initially felt. The player should then be asked to lie back and attempt to relax while the knee is being evaluated.

On-field tests for ligament stability.

1. Outline the area of tenderness.
2. Apply valgus stress to the knee at both 0° and 30° of flexion.
3. Apply varus stress at both 0° and 30° of flexion.
4. Perform the Lachman test.
5. Apply anterior and posterior drawer tests with the knee at 90° and the foot fixed.

These tests should enable the examiner to make an accurate assessment as to the stability of the knee. From these findings, a decision should be made as to whether the player can be allowed to walk off the field or whether a stretcher should be used. If there is any doubt, get the stretcher! Do not allow the athlete to be carried off in a sitting position, as this can further disrupt an already damaged knee (Figure 19.54). The athlete should walk off only if the knee joint is completely stable and no other serious injury is found.

The Sideline Examination

When the athlete is at the sideline, both knees should be exposed. The shoe, sock, and tape of the affected limb should also be removed, so that circulation can be monitored. An ice bag should be applied to the knee while the history is reviewed.

The examiner should take great care to record the findings accurately. This is the

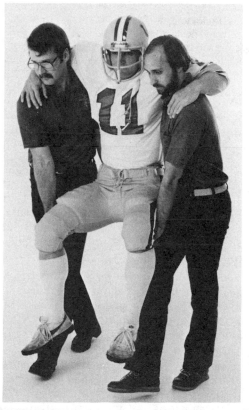

FIGURE 19.54 The incorrect method of removing an athlete with a knee·injury from the field. Use a stretcher!

ideal time to examine the knee, the so-called "golden period," as there is usually very little muscle spasm, swelling, or pain. These will undoubtedly develop later and will then preclude an exact and thorough examination.

Comparison between the healthy and the injured knee should be made at each stage of the examination.

1. Clearly define areas of tenderness.

2. Note any sign of hemarthrosis.

3. Check the range of movement, particularly with regard to hyperextension.

4. Test varus and valgus laxity at 0° and 30° of flexion.

5. Perform the Lachman test.

6. Place the knee at 90° and test the anterior drawer sign:
   a. in the neutral position
   b. with the foot externally rotated 15°
   c. with the foot internally rotated 10°

7. Test the posterior drawer sign at 90° of knee flexion (if positive, carefully monitor the peripheral circulation).

8. Perform pivot-shift tests:
   a. MacIntosh test
   b. jerk test of Hughston
   c. pivot-shift test in the lateral position (Slocum) These pivot-shift tests, if positive, suggest anterolateral rotatory instability. This might be found after an isolated anterior cruciate ligament rupture. Thus, these tests can be very useful in making this diagnosis when other tests are ambiguous.

9. Carefully evaluate the patella for evidence of subluxation. Make sure of the integrity of the quadriceps and the patellar tendons.

10. Attempt McMurray's test of the menisci (not always possible because of pain and limitation of movement; Apley's test is sometimes used).

11. Check the peroneal nerve (sensation on the dorsal aspect of the foot; dorsiflexion of the foot).

12. Check the peripheral pulses.

MANAGEMENT: Apply ice and a postoperative knee splint if there is any evidence of ligament or patellar damage, and start the athlete on pain medication if this is necessary. If there is any suggestion of an unstable knee, the athlete should use crutches when walking and should not bear weight even though in a postoperative splint. The peripheral circulation should also be frequently monitored.

Order of Exclusion of Common Acute Knee Injuries

Table 19.17 presents a line of thinking that a trainer can follow when dealing with an acutely injured knee. Initially, it is important to observe any obvious abnormality, such as a fracture or a dislocated patella. With these conditions excluded, a history of sudden knee pain and disability means that a ligamentous tear is present, until proven otherwise. Once a ligament injury has been excluded (within the limits of clinical evaluation), think of the possibility of patellar subluxation. Then examine for a meniscal tear. Finally, consider the possibility of an osteochondral fracture.

Criteria for Return to Play

The athletic trainer or sideline physician has to decide whether the athlete with a knee injury should return to play. Definite guidelines must be used to avoid further aggravation of an already injured structure.

REHABILITATION OF THE KNEE AND THE PATELLOFEMORAL JOINT

Rehabilitation of the knee is a vital but often neglected part of the treatment program. Even after the best surgery, the athlete's per-

TABLE 19.17 Order of Exclusion in an Acute Knee Injury

1. **LIGAMENT TEAR**
2. PATELLAR SUBLUXATION
3. Meniscal Tear
4. Osteochondral Fracture

TABLE 19.18 Guidelines for Return to Play for an Athlete with a Knee Injury

1. If there is any instability during the examination, no return to play should be allowed.
2. If there is no evidence of any ligament instability or laxity, and the patella and the menisci appear normal, then the athlete should be put through a series of functional tests:
   a. Lean-hopping: the athlete hops on one leg while leaning, rotates 360° clockwise and then counterclockwise
   b. Duck-waddle
   c. Running-and-cutting: the athlete runs fairly rapidly over a 10-yard distance and then cuts to the right and then to the left
   d. Running backwards
   e. Running in figure eights: the athlete starts with fairly large figure eights, then rapidly does progressively smaller ones

If the athlete has no problem with these functional tests, return to play is permitted.

At no time should a local anesthetic or cortisone preparation be injected for the purpose of allowing the athlete to return to competition.

formance will be impaired, and the knee will be placed in jeopardy unless comprehensively and completely rehabilitated. Certain specific points should be noted.

1. *Pre-operative period.* The muscles around the knee should be developed for strength and endurance insofar as the injury permits. This pre-operative therapy also familiarizes the athlete with isometric and other exercises that will be done in the immediate postoperative period.

2. *Immediate postoperative period.* Isometric exercises[93,94] should be started immediately after surgery. Begin with leg lifts, then quadriceps- and hamstring-setting exercises together, so the tibia is stabilized rather than drawn forward by the unopposed action of the quadriceps.[95] Leg lifts should then be performed against resistance, preferably manual.

If the ankle is not incorporated into the cast, range-of-motion and strengthening exercises for the foot and the ankle should be commenced. At the same time, the athlete should start with lower-back and upper extremity exercises, which should be done for both strength and cardiovascular endurance.[96]

TENS has been found to be a useful adjunct to rehabilitation in the early postoperative phase because it decreases the pain and allows the exercises to be performed in relative comfort and with greater intensity. The leads can be applied at the time of surgery or through a window cut in the cast soon afterwards.

Electrical stimulation of the quadriceps and the hamstring musculature has been used with increasing frequency in the past few years.[97] Stimulation can start as early as the first postoperative day via a window cut through the cast. One technique is to stimulate the musculature for one hour per day (five seconds on and five seconds off, increasing up to one minute on and one minute off).

One method of electrode placement puts the negative electrode above the patella and on the quadriceps muscles, with the other lead near the femoral nerve in the groin. The patient monitors the voltage in order to keep it below the pain threshold, but the stimulation should cause a tetanic contraction lasting for the appropriate time. This is followed by an equal period of rest. The pattern is continued for one hour per day, five days per week, for approximately four weeks.

3. *While still immobilized in the cast.* Cardiovascular exercises, for example, one-leg stationary cycling with the unaffected leg, should be done for thirty to forty-five minutes a day.[98] If the cast is made of a material that can be immersed in water, swimming can be used as an alternative to cycling. Care should be taken, however, to dry the leg which is in the cast. The unaffected leg can be put through a vigorous training program, such as one utilizing isokinetic machines. The training program for the upper extremities should continue. Rapid crutch ambulation (i.e., running by means of the crutches)

can be used in selected, highly coordinated athletes.[96]

As the weeks of immobilization progress, motion of the leg within the cast may be permitted, or the cast may have a hinge incorporated to permit a limited range of motion.

4. *When the cast is removed.* The cardiovascular endurance program is continued and swimming is used to help improve the range of motion of the previously immobilized leg. Proprioceptive neuromuscular facilitation techniques can be started as muscle strength returns. Achieving a range of motion early in the program is not necessarily important. In fact, the athlete is often restricted from attempting full extension for a time, particularly after an anterior cruciate repair or reconstruction.[95] The range of motion will develop by itself as a result of the exercises.

5. *Next stage.* As the rehabilitation program develops, all muscle groups around the knee should be exercised—the quadriceps, hamstrings, abductors, adductors, internal and external rotators, and the gastrocnemius. In addition, exercises for hip stabilizers need to be included. Appropriate muscle balance between the quadriceps and the hamstring muscle groups should be achieved.

6. *Later stages.* Exercises specific to the athlete's sport need to be included in the later stages of the rehabilitation program (the SAID principle, sport-specific skills).

7. *Before complete rehabilitation.* The need to wear a *specific brace*, like the Lenox Hill derotation brace, should be assessed for each individual athlete. Many surgeons now prescribe such a brace for a few months postsurgically until the athlete is fully rehabilitated.

Stages of Rehabilitation

The outline presented in Table 19.19 is meant purely as a guide. Many variations have been and can be developed on this theme. This program is divided into five stages. With a mild sprain of, say, the medial collateral ligament, it may be possible to go through all five stages in a few weeks.[25,26] An athlete who has had reconstructive ligament surgery may take three to six months to complete the program.[95] Each stage should be completed before progressing to the next stage, though it is not necessary that all exercises mentioned in each stage be performed. The program should always be individualized.

The Roman numerals refer to the stage, and the + indicates in which stage a particular exercise should be performed. For instance, quadriceps sets (Stage I, No. 1) should be continued throughout the entire program, whereas TENS (Stage I, No. 18) needs to be used only in Stage I. An expla-

nation of some of the exercises accompanies the tables.

Stage I: Leg in a cast or otherwise immobilized.

1. Quadriceps sets consist of tightening the quadriceps muscle group as hard as possible, concentrating particularly on the vastus medialis, and holding the contraction for between five and ten seconds. The athlete is encouraged to do this a minimum of twenty times every hour during the waking day (Figure 19.55).

2. Hamstring sets are performed by pushing the foot backward against resistance and

TABLE 19.19 Knee Rehabilitation after Ligament Injury or Surgery

Stage I: Leg in cast or otherwise immobilized

No.	Exercise	I	II	III	IV	V
1.	Quadriceps sets*	+	+	+	+	+
2.	Hamstring sets	+	+	+	+	+
3.	Quadriceps and hamstring sets together, at 10° and 20° of flexion	+	+	+	+	+
4.	SLR on back, leg neutral*	+	+	+		
5.	SLR on back, leg neutral, against manual-resistance*	+	+			
6.	SLR on side, abduction	+	+	+		
7.	SLR on side, adduction	+	+	+		
8.	SLR on abdomen, hip extension	+	+			
9.	Hip flexion, abduction, adduction, and extension against resistance	+				
10.	Limited motion in cast	+				
11.	Ankle plantar flexion against resistance (or heel raises) and other ankle exercises if ankle not in a cast	+	+			
12.	Cardiovascular endurance—bicycle ergometer with unaffected leg only, swimming, rapid-crutch ambulation	+				
13.	Unaffected leg training program	+	+	+	+	+
14.	Upper extremity training program	+	+	+	+	+
15.	Pelvic tilts, sit-ups, back strengthening, flexibility	+	+	+	+	+
16.	Achilles stretching	+	+	+	+	+
17.	Ice after workouts	+	+	+	+	+
18.	TENS	+				
19.	Electrical muscle stimulation	+	+			

*Should be avoided following ACL surgery.

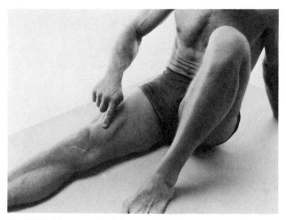

FIGURE 19.55 Quadriceps sets Isometrically tighten the quadriceps. Concentrate particularly on the vastus medialis. Do not allow the knee to hypertextend.

maintaining isometric contraction for five to ten seconds. This is repeated with the same frequency as quadriceps sets (Figure 19.56).

3. It has been suggested that quadriceps sets not be performed for between six and twelve weeks following an anterior cruciate repair or reconstruction procedure for two reasons:
    a. Full extension of the leg should be avoided, as the anterior cruciate ligament or the reconstruction is placed under tension in this position.
    b. Isolated contraction of the quadriceps tends to pull the tibia forward and thus pull on the anterior cruciate ligament or the reconstruction.

What is probably acceptable is to contract *both* the hamstrings and the quadriceps *together* isometrically with the knee bent at 20° of flexion (Figure 19.57).

4 & 5. Straight-leg-raising (SLR) exercises can be performed in a number of ways, but excellent results have been obtained using the following technique: In the initial postsurgical stage, the leg is lifted to approximately 60°, held for three seconds, and slowly lowered under control. Thirty to fifty of these straight-leg raises should be performed each hour that the athlete is awake. When this can be easily performed, manual-resistance should be applied two or three times a day.

The next stage is to modify the leg raises and concentrate on the vastus medialis muscle. Five "stations" of contraction are used. With the leg on the table, the quadriceps muscles are contracted for five seconds. The muscles are then very slightly relaxed and the leg elevated to the next station, approximately 6″ (15 cm) off the table. The muscles are vigorously contracted again and the contraction held for five seconds. Once more the muscles are very slightly relaxed, the leg elevated to about 30° and the muscles contracted. After five seconds the leg muscles are slightly relaxed and the leg elevated to approximately 45°. The same procedure is repeated and the leg elevated to 60°.

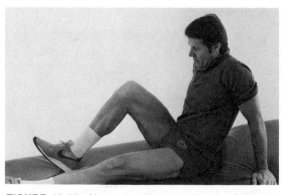

FIGURE 19.56 Hamstring sets performed isometrically The heel is pulled into the table as the hamstrings are contracted.

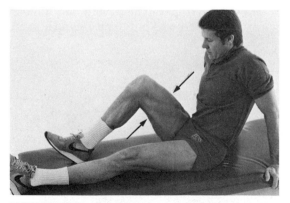

FIGURE 19.57 Quadriceps and hamstring sets— performed together at 30° of flexion This is a particularly useful exercise following surgery of an anterior cruciate ligament injury.

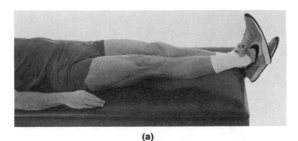

(a)

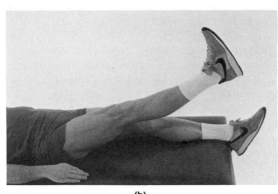

(b)

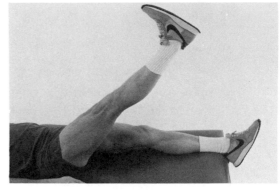

(c)

FIGURE 19.58 Straight-leg-raising Ensure that the vastus medialis is contracted with each change of "station."

The leg is then lowered to 45°, then to 30°, then to six inches (15 cm) above the table, with the muscle contracted and held at each station. This constitutes one repetition. Between five to ten repetitions are used, depending on the capabilities of the athlete. Ankle weights are added when they can be tolerated (Figure 19.58).

6, 7, & 8. The SLR exercise for abduction or adduction is performed with the athlete lying on one side. Three stations are used

(Figures 19.59 and 19.60). Three stations are also used when the athlete lies prone and extends the leg backwards using the gluteal and hamstring muscles (Figure 19.61).

9. Hip flexion, adduction, abduction, and extension exercises are performed with resistance below the knee when a cast is present. Upon removal of the cast, resistance should be placed above the knee, to prevent strain to any of the damaged ligaments.

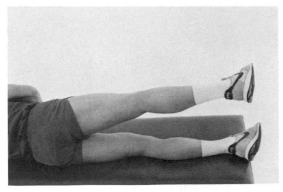

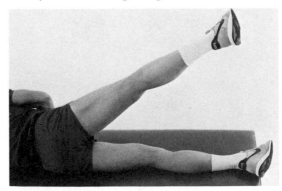

FIGURE 19.59 Straight-leg-raising into abduction

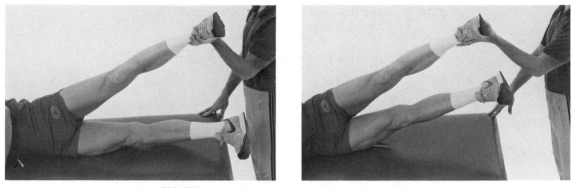

FIGURE 19.60   Straight-leg-raising into adduction

10. Limited isotonic movements or isometric contractions performed at different degrees of flexion can be initiated when the cast becomes loose or if a hinged cast is applied.

11. If the ankle is free, toe-raises, Achilles stretches, toe-curling, and elastic-tubing exercises for inversion, eversion, dorsiflexion, and plantar flexion are used.

12, 13, & 14. These exercises are for cardiovascular conditioning and general improvement of the athlete's feeling of well being, as well as for stimulating a sense of accomplishment at a time when depression and lethargy are common. A crossover effect on the muscles of the affected leg is also possible.

15. The lower-back exercises are described in the section on back rehabilitation, p. 281. These exercises may help decrease the frequency of lower-back problems following surgery or crutch ambulation.

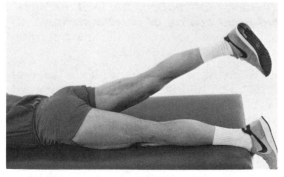

FIGURE 19.61   Straight-leg-raising prone

16. See section on stretching exercises, Chapter 3.

17, 18, & 19. Discussed in Chapter 7.

Stage II: Cast removed, some flexion permitted.

1. SLR exercises aimed at developing the pes anserine group are performed in the same manner as SLR exercise on the back with the leg in neutral position, the difference being that here the leg is externally rotated at the hip while the foot is held in forced inversion.

2. Hip flexion with the knee bent helps to increase knee flexion without actually applying a force to the knee. As the athlete flexes the hip, particularly when a weight or resistance from elastic tubing is applied to the thigh, the knee tends to go into flexion (Figure 19.62). A weighted boot is not used after cruciate ligament injuries as the joint may be distracted apart.

3–6. See Stage I, No. 9.

7. Isotonic hamstring exercises are performed by having the athlete stand facing the wall so that the anterior aspect of the thigh is supported against the wall. The affected leg is then flexed at the knee, with weight bearing on the ankle.

8. Proprioception neuromuscular facilitation (PNF) techniques have been found useful in increasing the range of motion and

TABLE 19.19 Knee Rehabilitation after Ligament Injury or Surgery (*cont.*)

Stage II: Cast removed, some flexion permitted

No.	Exercise	I	II	III	IV	V
1.	SLR—externally rotated (for the pes group)		+	+		
2.	Hip flexion with knee bent, weight on thigh or elastic resistance against thigh		+	+		
3.	Hip flexion, using pulley or elastic resistance*		+	+		
4.	Hip extension, using pulley or elastic resistance*		+	+		
5.	Hip abduction, using pulley or elastic resistance*		+	+		
6.	Hip adduction, using pulley or elastic resistance*		+	+		
7.	Hamstring exercise, knee flexed while standing against wall	+	+			
8.	Proprioceptive neuromuscular facilitation (PNF)	+	+			
9.	Manual-resistance exercises	+	+			
10.	Limited-arc flexion and extension—isokinetic or isotonic	+				
11.	Bicycle ergometer with affected leg	+	+	+		
12.	Walking and/or running in swimming pool	+	+			

*Resistance should be above the knee for movements that may stress the ligament(s); for other movements, resistance may be placed below the knee.

overcoming the neural inhibitions that are frequently present.

9. Manual-resistance exercises can be applied by the therapist with increasing resistance and speed of movement as rehabilitation progresses. Isometric resistance can also be applied, with the duration of the contraction lengthening as the athlete becomes stronger. Examples of manual resistance include knee extension, knee flexion, hip and knee flexion, abduction and adduction, internal and external rotation of the tibia with the knee bent at 90°, and SLR both prone and supine (Figure 19.63).

10. Limited-arc flexion and extension exercises should be done on isotonic or isokinetic machines with light resistance.

11. Unilateral cycling using the affected leg has been found useful, not only for increasing the strength and endurance of the leg, but also for increasing the range of motion.

12. Walking or running in a swimming pool, using a life preserver so the feet do not need to touch the bottom. This technique can be used for cardiovascular fitness as well as exercising the affected leg.

Stage III: Begun when athlete has at least 90° range of motion, no joint irritation, and good control of muscle groups.
After each exercise, stretch the muscle group worked, if this is permitted.

1. Isometric contractions with the knee at 0°, 30°, 60°, and 90° of flexion can be used for both quadriceps and hamstring muscle groups.

2. Isokinetic rehabilitation machines (e.g., the Orthotron and the Cybex) are exceptionally useful in developing strength, power, and endurance. It is suggested that the slow speeds be avoided initially and that the ath-

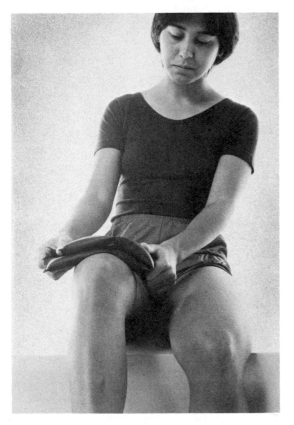

FIGURE 19.62 Hip flexion against resistance
Flexing the hip helps to increase flexion in a stiff knee.

lete commence with a speed of about 120°
per second. A faster speed (e.g., 180° per
second) can be used soon after this and then
progressively moved up to 300° per second.

In the beginning, a limited arc of knee
motion (e.g., from 30° to 60° of flexion)
should be used. Caution should be observed
when dealing with cruciate ligament injuries
and patellar problems, and no pain or feeling of instability should be experienced.
Submaximal intensities should be used during this stage.

3. A knee flexion and extension machine
using isotonic weight resistance is the most
frequently used rehabilitation device. It can
be used in many different ways; for example,
lifting the weight with both legs, lowering
with the affected leg only,[99] and lifting or
lowering with the affected leg only. The

weight is often adjusted to that which can be
lifted at least five times but not more than
ten times, and three sets are performed. If
more then ten repetitions are possible in a
set, the weight is increased by about ten
pounds. The weight can also be increased
with each set, so that fewer repetitions are
possible. The same technique is used for the
hamstring muscle group. However, following
ACL surgery, a light weight should be used
during this stage.[95]

An alternative technique is the daily adjustable progressive resistance exercise
(DAPRE) technique.[100] The quadriceps are
worked in the following way: Each leg is exercised alternately and independently. The
movement is from flexion (90°) to extension
(0°) and back to flexion. This movement is
deliberate, but not slow, with a brief pause
(approximately one-third of a second) at the
extremes of motion. Four sets are used. The
first set of ten repetitions is with a weight
that is 50% of the weight that will be lifted
in set three; the second set of ten repetitions
is with a weight that is 75% of the weight
that will be lifted in set three. Set three
works with the full working weight, with as
many repetitions as possible. The number of
repetitions in set three determines the
weight that will be used in set four. The
weight in set four is adjusted according to
the number of repetitions performed in set
three and as many repetitions as possible are
attempted. This number then determines the
weight that will be used as the working
weight in set three the next day (Table 19.20
and Table 19.21).

4. The ski squat is a useful exercise as long
as no retropatellar pain or crepitus is present.

5. Isometric squats using a power rack are
performed at three or four different angles.
This exercise is useful for developing
strength in the legs and the back. It also has
the advantage of being relatively safe; even if
the athlete finds that the weight is too heavy
after lifting it, the pins under the weight prevent the possibility of injury. The athlete can
also work with a much heavier weight when

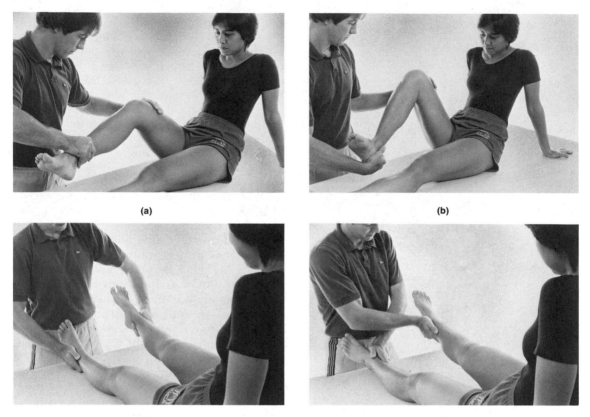

(a) (b)

(c) (d)

FIGURE 19.63 Manual-resistance exercise for the muscles around the knee (a) Resistance to knee extension (b) Resistance to knee flexion (c) Resistance to hip abduction (d) Resistance to hip adduction

using the isometric technique than when using free squats. This is a strenuous exercise and should only be done under supervision.

6. The pes anserine exercise is performed sitting on a chair with the heels placed firmly on the ground about 18″ (45 cm) apart. The feet are slightly internally rotated (adducted) and the medial hamstring group palpated with the hands. The feet are then forced farther into internal rotation, either against resistance or against one another, with the heels firmly fixed on the ground (Figure 19.64). This exercise is particularly indicated after a pes anserine transfer operation in which the pes group has been changed from being primarily a knee flexor to acting as an internal rotator of the tibia.

7. The internal rotation exercise with the knee at 90° achieves the same thing as the pes anserine exercise except that this one uses isotonic resistance, while the pes exercise is isometric. One leg is usually exercised at a time. The resistance may be an elastic band or a pulley on the Universal gym (Figure 19.65).

8. The external rotation exercise with the knee at 90° is the same as no. 7, except that the lower leg and foot move into an externally rotated and abducted position in order to develop the external rotators of the tibia —the iliotibial tract and the biceps femoris.

9. Forward step-ups are useful for increasing endurance and range of motion and can

TABLE 19.19   Knee Rehabilitation after Ligament Injury or Surgery (*cont.*)

Stage III: Begun when the athlete has at least 90° ROM, no joint irritation, and good control of muscle groups

No.	Exercise	Stage I	II	III	IV	V
1.	Isometrics at various angles through limited ROM			+	+	
2.	Isokinetic quadriceps and hamstring exercises (Orthotron) — limited-arc movement			+	+	+
3.	Isotonic quadriceps and hamstring exercises (e.g., DAPRE technique)			+	+	+
4.	Squats held at 90° with back to wall (ski squat)			+	+	+
5.	Isometric squats			+	+	+
6.	Pes anserine exercise			+	+	+
7.	Internal rotation, knee at 90°			+	+	+
8.	External rotation, knee at 90°			+	+	+
9.	Forward step-ups			+		
10.	Lateral step-ups			+	+	
11.	Running in water			+		
12.	Forward stretches			+	+	+
13.	Quadriceps stretches			+	+	+
14.	Bicycle ergometer, one and two legs, high speed with maximum effort			+	+	+
15.	Proprioceptive exercises			+	+	+

TABLE 19.20   DAPRE technique

Set	Weight	Repetitions
1	One-half working weight	10
2	Three-quarters working weight	6
3	Full working weight	Maximum[a]
4	Adjusted working weight	Maximum[b]

[a]The number of repetitions performed during the third set is used to determine the adjusted working weight for the fourth set according to the guidelines in Table 19.21.

[b]The number of repetitions performed during the fourth set is used to determine the working weight for the next session according to the guidelines in Table 19.21.

Reprinted by permission of Kenneth L. Knight Ph.D, A.T.,C., from "Knee rehabilitation by the daily adjustable progressive resistive exercise technique," *American Journal of Sports Medicine* 7:336–337, 1979.

TABLE 19.21   Guidelines for Adjustment of Working Weight

No. of repetitions per set	Fourth set[a]	Next session[b]
0–2	Decrease 5–10 lb[c]	Decrease 5–10 lb
3–4	Decrease 0–5 lb	The same
5–6	The same	Increase 6–10 lb
7–10	Increase 5–10 lb	Increase 5–15 lb
11 to . . .	Increase 10–15 lb	Increase 10–20 lb

[a]The number of repetitions performed during the third set is used to determine the adjusted working weight for the fourth set (Table 19.20).

[b]The number of repetitions performed during the fourth set is used to determine the working weight for the next session (usually the next day)(Table 19.20).

[c]1 kg = 2.2 lb.

Reprinted by permission of Kenneth L. Knight, Ph.D., A.T.,C., from "Knee rehabilitation by the daily adjustable progressive resistive exercise technique," *American Journal of Sports Medicine*, 7:336–337, 1979.

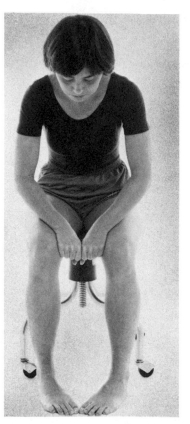

FIGURE 19.64 The "pes anserine exercise" This isometric exercise is particularly useful after pes anserine transfer surgery.

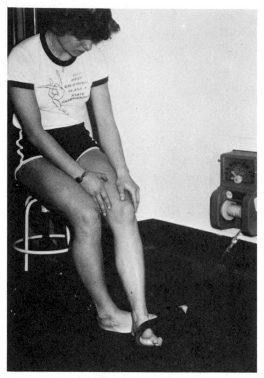

FIGURE 19.65 Tibial rotation exercise for the pes group of muscles

be performed with or without weights. The weights should be dumbbells, as barbells can be hazardous if balance is lost or the knee gives in.

10. Lateral step-ups can be performed in the same way, to develop the gluteal muscles and the hip stabilizers (Figure 19.66).

11. Running in water has been described on p. 352.

12. & 13. See Chapter 3, Figures 3.1—3.4.

14. The athlete should cycle with the affected leg alone, then with both legs. A high speed with maximum effort is maintained for a minimum of twenty minutes.

15. Proprioceptive exercises include mechanisms such as balancing with one leg on a tiltboard or on a rubber ball, both with eyes open and eyes closed.

Stage IV: Begun when the athlete has over 80% of the strength, power, and endurance of the opposite leg.

1. Isokinetic machines are worked from 120° per second to 300° per second. Power and endurance are developed by doing repetitions until the torque falls below 50% of maximum. If the knee is stable in the anteroposterior direction, adequate time for tissue healing has elapsed,[95] and no chondromalacia is present, slower speeds (e.g., 60° per second) can be used.[101,102]

Another technique is to do as many repetitions as possible within a set time period, (for example, 45 seconds with the machine set at the highest speed, Cybex at 300° per second and Orthotron at 10–10). When the

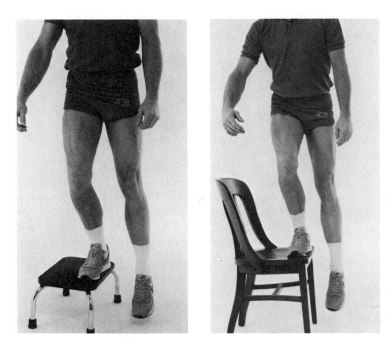

FIGURE 19.66 Lateral step-ups As the rehabilitation program progresses, the height of the step should be increased.

TABLE 19.19   **Knee Rehabilitation after Ligament Injury or Surgery (*cont.*)**

Stage IV: Begun when the athlete has over 80% of the strength, power, and endurance of the opposite leg

No.	Exercise	I	II	III	IV	V
				Stage		
1.	Isokinetic resistance—low and high speeds and endurance				+	+
2.	"Circuit training"				+	+
3.	Rope jumping				+	+
4.	Squat jumps				+	
5.	Side-to-side jumping				+	
6.	Bounding over bench				+	
7.	Running in place				+	
8.	Sprints from start				+	
9.	Sprints 25 to 50 yards, jogging 100 yards (or meters)				+	+
10.	Jogging				+	
11.	Running backward				+	+
12.	Running up stairs				+	+

athlete can do 15 repetitions more than the time (e.g., 60 repetitions in 45 seconds), the time is increased until 110 repetitions can be done in 90 seconds. The speed is then reduced 20% and the process repeated with appropriate modifications of the repetition-to-time ratio.

2. Circuit training. A circuit designed to incorporate power, strength, and endurance[26] with isometric, isotonic, and isokinetic resistance has the athlete starting on a knee flexion and extension machine against a weight of 75% of his or her ten-repetition maximum for 30 seconds. He or she then switches to the Orthotron, which is set at 10–10 (if an Orthotron is not available, a knee flexion and extension machine using a light weight and high speeds can be substituted). High-speed work is then performed on the Orthotron until a burning is felt in the thigh muscles, at which stage the athlete performs an isometric contraction of the quadriceps and the hamstrings, holding it for one minute. The circuit is then repeated as many times as possible without a break.

3. Rope jumping should be performed for at least five minutes at a time.

4. Squat-jumps are performed with the athlete squatting down and then jumping as high as possible. The athlete should have a goal, such as attempting to reach a certain height with each jump.

5. Side-to-side jumping is performed with the legs held together. Two lines are drawn approximately 5 feet (1.5 m) apart and the athlete jumps sideways from one to the other while progressing forward. This is continued for from thirty seconds to three minutes.

6. Bounding over a bench develops dynamic power in the legs. The legs and the feet are kept together; the feet land simultaneously. A low bench is used at first, but this can be raised as the athlete's ability increases. This exercise can be performed with the athlete bounding forward as well as from side-to-side.

7. The running-in-place exercise is an important training mechanism to prevent fur-

ther knee injury. The athlete is told to run as fast as possible in one place while maintaining good posture. The posture includes slight internal rotation of the feet and lower legs; flexion of the knees at about 60° to 80°; and a "ready" position of the back, neck, and upper extremities. The arms pump vigorously during this exercise. When the athlete can maintain the correct posture, the instructor gives orders to turn rapidly to the right or to the left or to shuffle forwards or backwards while continuing to run in place as fast as possible. This exercise, if performed correctly, trains the athlete to respond instantaneously and reflexly while at all times maintaining correct posture of the legs and the knees (Figure 19.67).

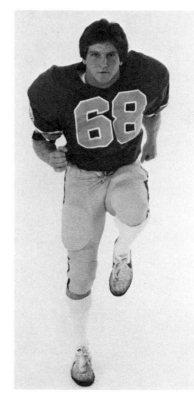

FIGURE 19.67   Running-in-place—rapid   motion
Slight internal rotation of the lower legs, a high knee lift, and a "ready" position of the back, neck, and upper extremities help to develop proprioception and an improved posture.

8–12. The athlete is now ready to begin straight-ahead running, which should begin with sprinting ten yards from a crouched starting position and progressing to wind sprints, long-distance running, and running up stadium steps.

Stage V: The final stage—begun when knee is pain-free, has over 90% of the power, strength, and endurance of the opposite leg, and feels stable both clinically and subjectively. The final stage consists of a functional program which puts the athlete through a number of exercises designed to improve proprioception and co-ordination and to fully test the stability of the knee. Some athletes will not be able to go through this stage without developing problems. Prescription of these exercises should be carefully individualized.

1. Increase the distance and the speed.

2. Figure eights are started in slow, wide circles and then are increased so that rapid, tight figure eights are run.

3. Crossovers or cariocas are used in two different forms. The same leg can cross over in front each time, or the crossover leg can be alternated each time. This exercise should be done in both directions (Figure 19.68).

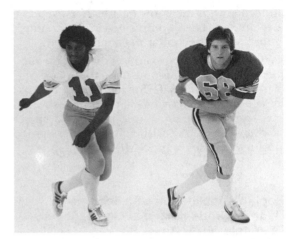

FIGURE 19.68   The cross-over or carioca drill (also called the linebacker's drill) This should be performed slowly initially, and then the speed and intensity gradually increased.

4. Composite circuits consist of running a predetermined course such as a baseball diamond. For example, the athlete runs backwards from home plate to first base, from first to second base, cariocas; from second to third base, half sideways and half backwards; from third base to home plate, cariocas run in the opposite direction. The instructor can alternate the program so that the athlete changes from one movement to

TABLE 19.19   Knee Rehabilitation after Ligament Injury or Surgery (*cont.*)

Stage V: The final stage—begun when knee is pain-free, has over 90% of the power, strength, and endurance of the opposite leg, and feels stable both clinically and subjectively

No.	Exercise	I	II	III	IV	V
1.	Full cross-country running, both up and down hills					+
2.	Figure eights					+
3.	Crossovers (cariocas)					+
4.	Composite circuits					+
5.	Racquetball, basketball, sport-specific exercises (SAID)					+

the other without knowing which movement is coming. This composite-circuit training should be conducted at maximum speed.

5. Other functional exercises can include racquetball and one-on-one basketball, as long as it is considered safe for the athlete to participate in these activities. The athlete should then start on exercises specific to the sport in which he or she wishes to engage (sport-specific exercises—the SAID principle).

Rapid Rehabilitation of a Second-Degree, Grade-II, Medial Ligament Knee Injury[27,28,29,30]

All the criteria must be met before placing the athlete on this program (see section on injuries to the medial stabilizing complex, p. 322). The knee should be immobilized in a postoperative splint immediately after the injury, crutches should be used, and the athlete should be kept non-weight-bearing for the first few days. Non-weight-bearing does not mean, however, that the foot cannot touch the ground. The athlete should always maintain some proprioceptive contact by *touch* weight bearing. Ice and compression are used three to four times a day for a total of about three hours a day. Anti-inflammatory medication, if used, should be started immediately.

Rehabilitation exercises should be started immediately after the injury, commencing with isometric contractions of the quadriceps and the hamstrings and abduction and adduction exercises (resistance at or above the knee). These are done at least fifty times every waking hour, and no pain should be present when doing them.

This is followed by SRL (with weights on the ankles) in three separate positions:

1. Supine
2. On the side (raising the leg into an abducted position)
3. Prone

The athlete can also start with stationary bicycle riding with the seat up high. After a few days, isometric contractions throughout the range of knee movement are commenced. In order for these exercises to be performed, the splint has to be removed, but it should be returned immediately after the icing that follows the rehabilitation session. While the splint is removed, the athlete should be non-weight-bearing, using crutches, and should be under the supervision of a trainer.

It should be emphasized that during the first few weeks after the injury, the postoperative knee splint is worn almost continuously except for periods of rehabilitation. Swimming may be permitted as well as running in the deep end of the swimming pool while wearing a life preserver. The next stage progresses onto internal rotation exercises with the knees flexed at 90°, followed by a full range of isotonic and isokinetic rehabilitation exercises. At no time during the first few weeks should the tibia be permitted to externally rotate.

After three to six weeks, the athlete may begin short periods of jogging if the strength, power, and endurance of the affected quadriceps and hamstrings are equal to or greater than the opposite side. Gradually progress the athlete onto running, sprinting in place, stair running, and finally figure-eight patterns, cutting, and then onto sport-specific exercises.

With high-quality rehabilitation and supervision, there should be a significant functional recovery by this time. It should be fully realized that the ligament is *not* completely healed, but with this type of rehabilitation the muscles have been trained to such a high pitch that the athlete can protect the ligament sufficiently to permit safe return to participation. No pain or swelling should be present during or following tests of strength, power, and endurance or during a full set of functional tests, all of which should indicate that the injured knee is at least as strong as the opposite side. Taping the knee for contact drills is probably advisable, but this is a safety precaution only and should not be relied upon in lieu of full rehabilitation (see Chapter 5).

Post-Meniscectomy Rehabilitation Program

1. *Pre-operative.* Educate the athlete about:
   a. Crutch usage
   b. Quadriceps and hamstring isometric sets
   c. Hamstring stretches
   d. Foot and ankle exercises

2. *Immediately postoperative* until sutures are removed:
   a. TENS and muscle stimulation
   b. Quadriceps and hamstring isometric sets
   c. Hamstring stretches
   d. SRL in all four positions
   e. Hip flexion and extension, abduction and adduction using wall-pulley resistance above the knees
   f. Toe-raises, dorsiflexion exercises
   g. Foot-curls, marble-pickups
   h. Achilles stretching
   i. Stationary cycling with opposite leg
   j. Upper body and abdominal training

3. *After sutures are removed. Add in:*
   a. Stationary cycling—affected leg
   b. Running in swimming pool
   c. Isometric exercises throughout the range of motion
   d. Gait retraining
   e. Then continue on from Stage III through Stage V of knee rehabilitation after ligament injury or surgery.

Rehabilitation Program for Patellofemoral Joint Pain

Patellofemoral joint pain presents with a specific problem. The quadriceps need to be strengthened, and yet a full range of motion against resistance is usually not possible, as it will probably increase pain. The main exercises initially used in rehabilitating an athlete with patellofemoral joint pain are isometric and limited range-of-motion exercises.[103,104] Muscle stimulation (using the technique previously described) is an important means of developing quadriceps muscle action.[105] TENS can also be useful, as it de-creases the pain and allows the quadriceps to contract more effectively.

Initially, quadriceps-setting isometric exercises should be performed with the leg extended (0°). Sometimes, however, especially in those who hyperextend the knee, this exercise causes retropatellar pain. This is overcome by contracting the quadriceps slowly and by placing two or three towels behind the knee so that some flexion is present when quadriceps contraction occurs (Figure 19.69). An alternative is quadriceps sets performed with the knee in minimal flexion (Figure 19.70). If pain is still a problem, TENS should be used during the exercise. The athlete should place a finger on the vastus medialis to ensure that this portion of the muscle is contracting maximally. SRL exercises should also be performed.

Isometric contractions can now be performed at various angles within the pain-free range of motion. This type of isometric exercise strengthens not only the angle exercised, but also the areas above and below this angle to some extent (about 10° in each direction), so that even though the painful angle is not specifically exercised, an increase in strength at this angle is observed.

The DAPRE technique modified for straight-leg static contractions utilizes an isotonic knee flexion and extension machine.[106] The weight is lifted by hand, the leg is ex-

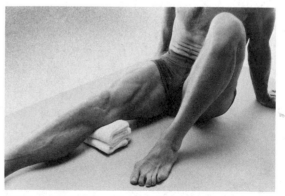

FIGURE 19.69 Quadriceps contraction—submaximal If pain is a problem initially, quadriceps sets may be done with the knee in slight flexion by placing a towel in the popliteal fossa.

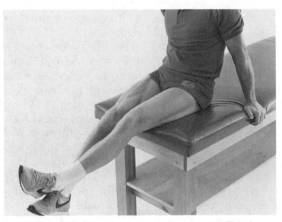

FIGURE 19.70 Eccentric quadriceps set   This is another variation of the quadriceps set should the regular "set" cause retropatellar pain. The affected knee is minimally bent; the opposite leg is placed on top and isometric resistance is applied.

tended, and the weight is applied to the extended leg. It is held for six seconds, followed by a four-second rest, using ten repetitions per set (Figure 19.71). The weights used are outlined in Tables 19.20 and 19.21.

When progressing onto resistance through a range of motion, submaximal isotonics, or isokinetics at 120°/sec., can be attempted on either side of the painful point, if one is present. If general discomfort through the range of motion is present, limited arc (e.g. 30°) isometrics and isotonics should be continued. The motion can be blocked by a stool (Figure 19.72).

Stretching of the hamstrings and the gastrocnemius muscles is important in ensuring that the knee can move through a full range of motion without interference of patellofemoral motion. Very carefully controlled quadriceps stretching can be attempted in individual cases. If the lateral retinaculum is tight, passive medial stretching of this area (for twenty seconds at a time, five times) can be attempted. Ice should be applied for at least twenty to thirty minutes at a time after workouts.

Athletes with patellofemoral joint pain should be educated in the potential dangers

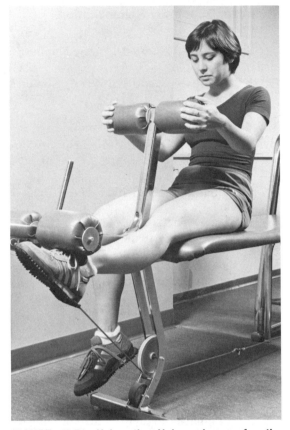

FIGURE 19.71 Using the Universal gym for the DAPRE technique   Lift and control the weight by using the arms.

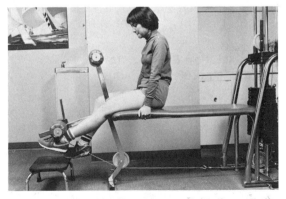

FIGURE 19.72 Blocking range of motion on the Universal machine   The height of the stool may be lowered as the athlete is able to tolerate a wider range of motion.

of squatting (especially full squats), excessive stair climbing, hard uphill cycling, and downhill running, and they should avoid sitting with their knees bent at 90° for a prolonged time.

Relapses and an up-and-down course frequently occur, but if this is discussed with the athlete initially, it is much easier for him or her to accept the problem and work through the setback.

Rehabilitation Program for Patellar Dislocation and Subluxation

Hip flexion, abduction and adduction, isometric hamstring exercises, heel-raising exercises, and Achilles stretching can be started immediately. Contraction of the quadriceps muscle group should be tried only after the first few days, and then only if no pain is experienced. Quadriceps-setting exercises should be increased very judiciously to ensure that there is no pain; if pain is present, then these exercises should not be performed for a few days. Once quadriceps-setting and SLR exercises can be performed painlessly, the patellofemoral joint pain rehabilitation program should be commenced.[107]

X-RAY VIEWS OF THE KNEE

As both students and trainers often wish to obtain more details of X-ray techniques, the following is a brief review of some of the views commonly used in a knee examination.

1. *Anteroposterior view.* The anteroposterior (AP) view is best taken with the athlete standing with both knees on the same plate, so that a comparison of the joint spaces (particularly the medial joint space) can be made.

In acute knee injuries, there should be a careful examination of the lateral aspect of the knee, particularly of the lateral tibial plateau where a lateral capsular sign may be found (Figure 19.73).[108] This sign is an indication that serious ligamentous damage has occurred, and it usually denotes a rupture of the anterior cruciate ligament.

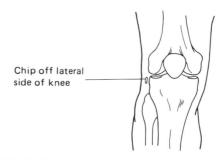

Chip off lateral side of knee

FIGURE 19.73 Lateral capsular sign A chip off the lateral side of the knee following an acute knee injury is suggestive of a major internal derangement, especially an anterior cruciate ligament tear. When seen on X-ray it is called the "lateral capsular sign."

2. *Lateral view.* The lateral view should be taken with the knee bent approximately 30°, in order to standardize measurements of the patellar tendon and the patella. A rule of thumb: If the patellar tendon length exceeds the patellar length by 1 cm or more it is considered a patella alta (Figure 19.74).[65] Patella infera is indicated by a reverse ratio. The femoral condyles should be observed for any osteochondral defect.

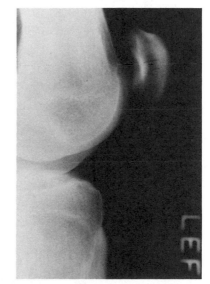

FIGURE 19.74 Patella alta If the distance from the tibial tubercle to the inferior pole of the patella is 1.2 cm greater than the distance from the inferior to the superior pole of the patella, a patella alta should be suspected.

3. *Tunnel view.* The tunnel view is a postero-anterior view taken with the knee bent a varying number of degrees. It is used to visualize the femoral condyles, particularly when looking for osteochondral fractures or osteochondritis dissecans.

4. *Tangential views.* Tangential views are used to obtain information about the patella and the patellofemoral articulation. There are a number of views presently in common use and each has certain limitations. It may therefore be useful to take more than one tangential view when a patellar lesion is suspected (Figure 19.75).

    a. *Sunrise view:* The knee is bent nearly into full flexion, so that views of the inferior surface of the patella can be obtained in cases of a suspected osteochondral fracture.

    b. *Hughston view:* The knee is bent approximately 45°, with the tube angle at 30°. This gives a useful view of

the intercondylar notch as well as the articulation of the patella in the groove. However, the X-ray beam contacts the plate at an angle and thereby distorts the appearance of the joint.

    c. *Merchant view:* The knees are bent approximately 30° with the plate placed on the tibia and held in place by a special piece of equipment. The Merchant view gives an accurate estimation of the intercondylar notch, the congruency angle, and the situation of the patellae.

    d. *Laurin view:* The Laurin view is the same as the Merchant view except that the plate is placed on the thigh and the X-ray tube is held near the feet. Advantages of this technique are: (1) no special piece of apparatus is needed, as the athlete can hold the plate, and (2) the X-ray beam contacts the plate at 90°, giving an

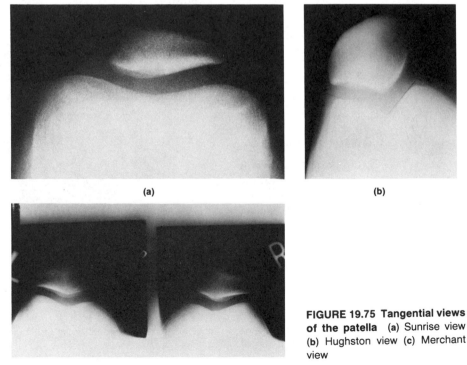

(a)

(b)

(c)

FIGURE 19.75 Tangential views of the patella (a) Sunrise view (b) Hughston view (c) Merchant view

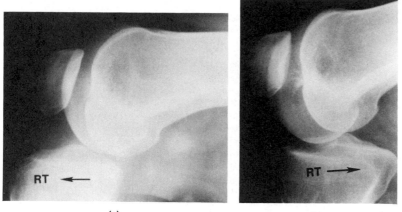

FIGURE 19.76 X-ray—knee, lateral stress view (anterior cruciate ligament laxity) (a) Note the forward movement of the tibia as compared with the "normal" view **(b)**.

(a)

(b)

undistorted picture. It also gives an accurate assessment of the location and articulation of the patella, particularly with regard to subluxation or tilting. The disadvantage is the dose of radiation the patient receives.

5. *Stress views*:

a. *AP stress view*: Used to demonstrate medial or lateral joint opening in collateral ligament rupture or an epiphyseal opening when a fracture through the epiphysis has occurred in the pre-adolescent and the adolescent (see Figure 10.6). Stress is applied in either the valgus or varus direction with the knee at 0° or 30° of flexion.

b. *Lateral stress views*: The knee is flexed to 90°. The anterior and the posterior drawer tests are attempted, in order to demonstrate incompetency of the anterior or posterior cruciate ligaments. Comparison X-rays of the opposite limb are always taken.

REFERENCES

1. Kapandji IA: *The Physiology of the Joints.* London, E & S Livingston, 1970.

2. Lindahl O, Movin A: The mechanics of extension of the knee-joint. *Acta Orthop Scand* 38:226–234, 1967.

3. Hallen LG, Lindahl O: The "screw-home" movement in the knee joint. *Acta Orthop Scand* 37:97–106, 1966.

4. Warren LF, Marshall JL, Girgis F: The prime static stabilizer of the medial side of the knee. *J Bone Joint Surg* 56A:665–674, 1974.

5. Kennedy JC, Weinberg HW, Wilson AS: The anatomy and function of the anterior cruciate ligament. *J Bone Joint Surg* 56A:223–235, 1974.

6. Smillie IS: *Injuries of the Knee Joint.* Edinburgh, Churchill Livingstone, fifth edition, 1978, p 71.

7. Jackson DW, Feagin JA: Quadriceps contusion in the young athlete: Relation of severity of injury to treatment and prognosis. *J Bone Joint Surg* 55A:95–105, 1973.

8. Kalenak A, Medlan CE, Fleagle SB et al: Treating thigh contusions with ice. *Phys Sportsmed* 3:65–67, March 1975.

9. Jokl P, Federico J: Myositis ossificans traumatica. Association with hemophilia (factor X1 deficiency) in a football player. *JAMA* 237:2215–2216, 1977.

10. Muckle DS: Associated factors in recurrent groin and hamstring injuries. *Brit J Sports Med* 16:37–39, 1982.

11. Zernicke R, Garhammer J, Jobe F: Human patellar tendon rupture. *J Bone Joint Surg* 59A:179–183, 1977.

12. Pope MH, Johnson RJ, Brown DW, et al: The role of the musculature in injuries to the medial collateral ligament. *J Bone Joint Surg* 61A:398–402, 1979.

13. Callahan WT, Crowley FJ, Hafner JK: A statewide study designed to determine methods of reducing injury in interscholastic football competition by equipment modification. New York State Public High School Athletic Association, Albany. 1971.

14. Mueller FO, Blyth CS: North Carolina High School Football Injury Study: Equipment and prevention. *J Sports Med* 2:1–10, 1974.

15. Torg JS, Quedenfeld TC, Landau S: The shoe-surface interface and its relationship to football knee injuries. *Am J Sports Med* 2:261–269, 1974.

16. Stanitski CL, McMaster JH, Ferguson RJ: Synthetic turf and grass: A comparison study. *J Sports Med* 2:22–26, 1974.

17. Ryan AJ: Moderator of Round Table on: Artificial Turf: Pros and Cons. *Phys Sportsmed* 3:41–50, February 1975.

18. De Haven KE: Diagnosis of acute knee injuries with hemarthrosis. *Am J Sports Med* 8:9–14, 1980.

19. Noyes FR, Bassett RW, Grood ES, et al: Arthroscopy in acute traumatic hemarthrosis of the knee. Incidence of anterior cruciate tears and other injuries. *J Bone Joint Surg* 62A:687–695, 1980.

20. Slocum DB, Larson RL: Rotatory instability of the knee and its pathogenesis and clinical test to demonstrate its presence. *J Bone Joint Surg* 50A:211–225, 1968.

21. Torg JS, Conrad W, Kalen V: Clinical diagnosis of anterior cruciate ligament instability in the athlete. *Am J Sports Med* 4:84–93, 1976.

22. Galway RD, Beaupré A, MacIntosh DL: Pivot shift: a clinical sign of symptomatic anterior cruciate insufficiency. *J Bone Joint Surg* 54B:763–764, 1972.

23. Cabaud HE, Slocum DB: The diagnosis of chronic anterolateral rotatory instability of the knee. *Am J Sports Med* 5:99–105, 1977.

24. Slocum DB, James SL, Larson RL, et al: Clinical test for anterolateral rotatory instability of the knee. *Clin Orthop* 118:63–69, 1976.

25. Derscheid GL, Garrick JG: Medial collateral ligament injuries in football. Nonoperative management of grade I and grade II sprains. *Am J Sports Med* 9:365–368, 1981.

26. Steadman JR: Rehabilitation of 1st- and 2nd-degree sprains of the medial collateral ligament. *Am J Sports Med* 7:300–302, 1979.

27. O'Connor GA: Functional rehabilitation of isolated medial collateral ligament sprains. Collateral ligament injuries of the joint. *Am J Sports Med* 7:209–210, 1979.

28. Bergfeld J: Functional rehabilitation of isolated medial collateral ligament sprains. First, second, and third-degree sprains. *Am J Sports Med* 7:207–209, 1979.

29. Ellsaser JC, Reynolds FC, Omohundro JR: The non-operative treatment of collateral ligament injuries of the knee in professional football players. An analysis of seventy-four injuries treated non-operatively and twenty-four injuries treated surgically. *J Bone Joint Surg* 56A:1185–1190, 1974.

30. Cox JS: Functional rehabilitation of isolated medial collateral ligament sprains. Injury nomenclature. *Am J Sports Med* 7:211–213, 1979.

31. O'Donoghue DH: *Treatment of Injuries to Athletes.* Philadelphia, WB Saunders, third edition, 1976, p. 575.

32. Slocum DB, Larson RL: Pes anserinus transplantation. A surgical procedure for control of rotatory instability of the knee. *J Bone Joint Surg* 50A:226–242, 1968.

33. Slocum DB, Larson RL, James SL: Late reconstruction of ligamentous injuries of the medial compartment of the knee. *Clin Orthop* 100:23–55, 1974.

34. Marshall JL, Rubin RM, Wang JB, et al: The anterior cruciate ligament: The diagnosis and treatment of its injuries and their serious prognostic implications. *Orthop Rev* 7:35–46, 1978.

35. McDaniel WJ, Dameron TB: Untreated ruptures of the anterior cruciate ligament. A follow up study. *J Bone Joint Surg* 62A:696–705, 1980.

36. Ellison AE: Distal iliotibial band transfer for anterolateral rotatory instability. *J Bone Joint Surg* 61A:330–337, 1979.

37. Jones KG: Reconstruction of the anterior cruciate ligament. *J Bone Joint Surg* 45A:925–932, 1963.

38. Clancy Jr, WG, Nelson DA, Reider B, et al: Anterior cruciate ligament reconstruction using one-third of the patellar ligament, augmented by extra-articular tendon transfers. *J Bone Joint Surg* 64A:352–359, 1982.

39. Puddu G: Method for reconstruction of the anterior cruciate ligament using the semitendinosus tendon. *Am J Sports Med* 8:402–404, 1980.

40. Lindeman K: Uber den plastischen Ersatz der Kreuzbänder durch gestielte Sehnenverpflanzung. *Zsch Orthop* 79:316–334, 1950.

41. Du Toit GT: Knee joint cruciate substitution. *S Afr J Surg* 5:25–30, 1967.

42. Trickey EL: Rupture of the posterior cruciate ligament of the knee. *J Bone Joint Surg* 50B:334–341, 1968.

43. Kennedy JC: Posterior cruciate ligament injuries. *Orthop Digest* 7:19–31, 1979.

44. Loos WC, Fox JM, Blazina ME, et al: Acute posterior cruciate ligament injuries. *Am J Sports Med* 9:86–92, 1981.

45. Lysholm J, Gillquist J, Liljedahl SO: Arthroscopy in the early diagnosis of injuries to the knee joint. *Acta Orthop Scand* 52:111–118, 1981.

46. Flemming Jr, RE, Blatz DJ, McCarroll JR: Posterior problems in the knee. Posterior cruciate insufficiency and posterolateral rotatory insufficiency. *Am J Sports Med* 9:107–113, 1981.

47. Osternig LR, Bates BT, James SL, et al: Rotary mechanics after pes anserinus transplant. *Am J Sports Med* 6:173–179, 1978.

48. Losee RE, Johnson TR, Southwick WD: Anterior subluxation of the lateral tibial plateau. A diagnostic test and operative repair. *J Bone Joint Surg* 60A:1015–1030, 1978.

49. Yamamoto SK, Hartman CW, Feagin JA, et al:

Functional rehabilitation of the knee. A preliminary study. *Am J Sports Med* 3:288–291, 1975.

50. Hughston JC: A simple meniscectomy. *J Sports Med* 3:179–187, 1975.

51. Feagin JA: The syndrome of the torn anterior cruciate ligament. *Orthop Clin North Am* 10:81–90, 1979.

52. Arnold JA, Coker TP, Heaton LM: Natural history of anterior cruciate tears. *Am J Sports Med* 7:305–313, 1979.

53. Feagin JA, Walton CW: Isolated tear of the anterior cruciate ligament. Five year follow-up. *Am J Sports Med* 4:95–100, 1976.

54. Feagin JA, Abbott HG, Rokous JR: The isolated tear of the anterior cruciate ligament. *J Bone Joint Surg* 54A:1340–1341, 1972.

55. Youmans WT: The so-called "isolated" anterior cruciate ligament syndrome: A report of 32 cases with some observations on treatment and its effect on results. *Am J Sports Med* 6:26–30, 1978.

56. Jacobsen K: Osteoarthrosis following insufficiency of the cruciate ligaments in man. *Acta Orthop Scand* 48:520–526, 1977.

57. Yocum LA, Kerlan RK, Jobe FW, et al: Isolated lateral meniscectomy: a study of 26 patients with isolated tears. *J Bone Joint Surg* 61A:338–342, 1979.

58. Smillie IS: *Injuries of the Knee Joint.* Edinburgh, Churchill Livingstone, fifth edition, 1978, p 92.

59. Kaplan EB: Discoid lateral meniscus of the knee joint. *J Bone Joint Surg* 39A:77–87, 1957.

60. Krause WR, Pope MH, Johnson RJ, et al: Mechanical changes in the knee after meniscectomy. *J Bone Joint Surg* 58A:599–604, 1976.

61. Appel H: Late results after meniscectomy in the knee joint. *Acta Orthop Scand Suppl* 133:1–111, 1970.

62. Cargill AO'R, Jackson JP: Bucket-handle tear of the medial meniscus. A case for conservative surgery. *J Bone Joint Surg* 58A:248–251, 1976.

63. Editorial: Partial meniscectomy preferred. *Br Med J* 1:1091–1092, 1978.

64. Wilson JN: A diagnostic sign in osteochondritis dissecans of the knee. *J Bone Joint Surg* 49A:477–480, 1967.

65. Lancourt JE, Cristini JA: Patella alta and patella infera. Their etiological role in patellar dislocation, chondromalacia and apophysitis of the tibial tubercle. *J Bone Joint Surg* 57A:1112–1115, 1975.

66. Brattstrom H: Shape of the intercondylar groove normally and in recurrent dislocation of the patella. *Acta Orthop Scand Suppl* 68:1–148, 1964.

67. Larson RL: Subluxation-dislocation of the patella. In *The Injured Adolescent Knee*, edited by Kennedy JC. Baltimore, Williams and Wilkins, 1979, pp 161–204.

68. Larson RL, Cabaud HE, Slocum DB, et al: The patellar compression syndrome. *Clin Orthop Rel Res* 134:158–167, 1978.

69. James SL: Chondromalacia of the patella in the adolescent. In *The Injured Adolescent Knee*, edited by Kennedy JC. Baltimore, Williams and Wilkins, 1979, pp 205–251.

70. Wiberg G: Roentgenographic and anatomic studies on the femopatellar joint. *Acta Orthop Scand* 12:319–410, 1941.

71. Baumgartl F: *Das Kniegelenk, Berlin,* Springer-Verlag, 1944.

72. Zimbler S, Smith J, Scheller A, et al: Recurrent subluxation and dislocation of the patella in association with athletic injuries. Symposium on sports injuries. *Orthop Clin North Am* 11:755–770, 1980.

73. Hughston JC: Subluxation of the patella. *J Bone Joint Surg* 50A:1003–1026, 1968.

74. Merchant AC, Mercer RL, Jacobsen RH, et al: Roentgenographic analysis of patellofemoral congruence. *J Bone Joint Surg* 56A:1391–1396, 1974.

75. Leach RE: Malalignment syndrome of the patella. *Instructional course lectures.* St Louis, CV Mosby Company, Vol 25, 1976, pp 49–54.

76. Insall J, Falvo KA, Wise DW: Chondromalacia patellae. A prospective study. *J Bone Joint Surg* 58A:1–8, 1976.

77. Goodfellow JW, Hungerford DS, Woods C: Patellofemoral mechanics and pathology. II. Chondromalacia patellae. *J Bone Joint Surg* 58B:291–299, 1976.

78. Insall JN: Current concepts review. Patellar pain. *J Bone Joint Surg* 64A:147–152, 1982.

79. Goodfellow JW, Hungerford DS, Zindel M: Patellofemoral mechanics and pathology. I. Functional anatomy of the patello-femoral joint. *J Bone Joint Surg* 52B:287–290, 1976.

80. Brookes M, Helal B: Primary osteoarthritis, venous engorgement and osteogenesis. *J Bone Joint Surg* 50B:493–504, 1968.

81. Insall J: Chondromalacia patellae: Patellar malalignment syndrome. *Orthop Clin North Am* 10:117–127, 1979.

82. Larson RL: The patella of the female athlete—subluxation, chondromalacia and patellar compression syndrome. *Med Aspects Sport. A.M.A.* 16:12–18, 1974.

83. Levine J: A new brace for chondromalacia patellae and kindred conditions. *Am J Sports Med* 6:137–140, 1978.

84. Merchant AC, Mercer RL: Lateral release of the patella. A preliminary report. *Clin Orthop* 103:40–45, 1974.

85. Micheli LJ, Stanitski CL: Lateral patellar retinacular release. *Am J Sports Med* 9:330–336, 1981.

86. Hughston JC: Reconstruction of the extensor mechanism for subluxating patella. *Am J Sports Med* 1:6–13, 1972.

87. Maquet PGJ: *Biomechanics of the Knee.* New York, Springer-Verlag, 1976, pp 134–143.

88. Weaver JK: Bipartite patellae as a cause of disability in the athlete. *Am J Sports Med* 5:137–143, 1977.

89. Patel D: Arthroscopy of the plicae-synovial folds and their significance. *Am J Sports Med* 6:217–225, 1978.

90. Hughston JC, Andrews JR: The suprapatellar plica and internal derangement. Proceedings of the American Academy of Orthopaedic Surgeons. *J Bone Joint Surg* 55A:1318, 1973.

91. Hardacker Jr WT, Whipple TL, Bassett FH: Diagnosis and treatment of the plica syndrome of the knee. *J Bone Joint Surg* 62A:221–225, 1980.

92. Blazina ME, Kerlan RK, Jobe FW, et al: Jumper's knee. *Orthop Clin North Am* 4:665–678, 1973.

93. Hettinger ERT, Müller EA: Influence of training and of inactivity on muscle strength. *Arch Phys Med* 51:441–462, 1970.

94. Grimby G, Gustafsson E, Peterson L, et al: Quadriceps function and training after knee ligament surgery. *Med Sci Sports Exer* 12:70–75, 1980.

95. Paulos L, Noyes FR, Grood E, et al: Knee rehabilitation after anterior cruciate ligament reconstruction and repair. *Am J Sports Med* 9:140–149, 1981.

96. Steadman JR: Rehabilitation after knee ligament surgery. *Am J Sports Med* 8:294–296, 1980.

97. Eriksson E: Sports injuries of the knee. Their diagnosis, treatment, rehabilitation, and prevention. *Med Sci Sports* 8:133–134, 1976.

98. Costill DL, Fink WJ, Habansky AJ: Muscle rehabilitation after knee surgery. *Phys Sportsmed* 5:71–74, September 1977.

99. Komi PV, Buskirk ER: Effects of eccentric and concentric muscle conditioning on tension and electrical activity of human muscle. *Ergonomics* 15:417–434, 1972.

100. Knight KL: Knee rehabilitation by the daily adjustable progressive resistive exercise technique. *Am J Sports Med* 7:336–337, 1979.

101. Sherman WM, Plyley MJ, Vogelgesang D, et al: Isokinetic strength during rehabilitation following arthrotomy: Specificity of speed. *Athletic Training* 16:138–141, 1981.

102. Wright KE, McNeill A: An Orthotron knee rehabilitation program. *Athletic Training* 14:232–233, 1979.

103. DeHaven KE, Doland WA, Mayer PJ: Chondromalacia patellae in athletes. Clinical presentation and conservative management. *Am J Sports Med* 7:5–11, 1979.

104. Steadman JR: Nonoperative measures for patellofemoral problems. *Am J Sports Med* 7:374–375, 1979.

105. Williams JGP: Vastus medialis re-education in the management of chondromalacia patellae. *Med Aspects Sport* 16:19–24, 1974.

106. Knight KL: Total injury rehabilitation. In Trainer's Corner, *Phys Sportsmed* 7:111, August 1979.

107. Henry JH, Crosland JW: Conservative treatment of patellofemoral subluxation. *Am J Sports Med* 7:12–14, 1979.

108. Woods GW, Stanley RF, Tullos HS: Lateral capsular sign: X-ray clue to a significant knee instability. *Am J Sports Med* 7:27–33, 1979.

109. Smillie IS: *Injuries of the Knee Joint.* Edinburgh, Churchill Livingstone, fifth edition, 1978, p. 108.

RECOMMENDED READINGS

Butler DL, Noyes FR, Grood ES: Ligamentous restraints to anterior-posterior drawer in the human knee. *J Bone Joint Surg* 62A:259–270, 1980.

Detnbeck LC: Function of the cruciate ligaments in knee stability. *J Sports Med* 2:217–221, 1974.

Ellison AE: Skiing injuries. *CIBA Clinical Symposia* 29:3–40, 1977.

Ficat PR, Hungerford DS: *Disorders of the Patellofemoral Joint.* Baltimore, Williams and Wilkins, 1978.

Goldfuss AJ, Morehouse CA, LeVeau BF: Effects of muscular tension on knee stability. *Med Sci Sports* 4:267–271, 1973.

Hughston JC, Andrews JR, Cross MJ, et al: Classification of knee ligament instabilities. Part I. The medial compartment and cruciate ligaments. *J Bone Joint Surg* 58A:159–172, 1976.

Hughston JC, Andrews JR, Cross MJ, et al: Classification of knee ligament instabilities. Part II. The lateral compartment. *J Bone Joint Surg* 58A:173–179, 1976.

Kennedy JC editor: *The Injured Adolescent Knee.* Baltimore, Williams and Wilkins, 1979.

Larson RL: Dislocations and ligamentous injuries of the knee. In *Fractures*, edited by Rockwood Jr, CA, Green DP. Philadelphia, JB Lippincott, Vol 2, 1975, pp 1182–1260.

Outerbridge RE: The etiology of chondromalacia patellae. *J Bone Joint Surg* 43B:752–757, 1961.

Ritter MA, Gosling C: *The Knee: A Guide to the Examination and Diagnosis of Ligament Injuries.* Springfield Ill., Charles C Thomas, 1981.

Staudte HW, Brussatis F: Selective changes in size and distribution of fibre types in vastus muscle from cases of different knee joint affections. *Z Rheumatol* 36:143–160, 1977.

CHAPTER 20

Lower Leg, Ankle, and Foot Injuries

FUNCTIONAL ANATOMY OF THE LOWER LEG, ANKLE, AND FOOT

The Lower Leg

The bones of the lower leg are the tibia and fibula. The tibia is the larger of the two, articulating with the knee superiorly and with the ankle inferiorly. It has an anterior crest and a posteromedial crest, both of which can be palpated subcutaneously. The medial malleolus forms the inner ankle bone.

The fibula articulates with the tibia both superiorly and inferiorly, and bears very little of the body's weight. It does not articulate with the knee; but inferiorly it forms the lateral malleolus, to which are attached the lateral ankle ligaments. At the ankle, the fibula articulates with the tibia and the talus.

The muscles of the lower leg are divided by thick fascial sheaths into four distinct compartments (Figure 20.1). These compartments can give rise to symptoms when the pressure within them rises excessively. The *anterior compartment*, which is the one that most frequently develops symptoms, consists of the anterior tibial, extensor hallucis longus, and extensor digitorum muscles. Within these muscles are the deep peroneal nerve and the anterior tibial artery. The *lateral compartment*, composed of the peroneal muscles, contains the superficial peroneal nerve. The *deep posterior compartment* is made up of the posterior tibial, flexor digitorum longus, and flexor hallucis longus muscles; and the *superficial posterior compartment* is made up of the gastrocnemius, soleus, and plantaris muscles.

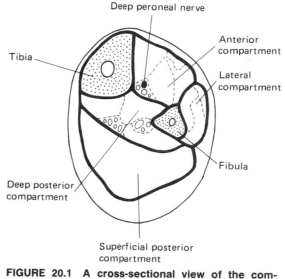

FIGURE 20.1 A cross-sectional view of the compartments of the lower leg

Muscle origin, insertion, and function.

1. *Tibialis anterior*: From the lateral condyle and upper portion of the lateral surface of the tibia to the medial cuneiform and base of the first metatarsal. *Function*: Dorsiflexes and supinates the foot and gently lowers the foot to the ground during the initial contact phase of standing.

2. *Extensor hallucis longus*: From the fibula and interosseous membrane to the dorsal surface of the base of the distal phalanx of the first toe. *Function*: Dorsiflexes the ankle and extends the first toe.

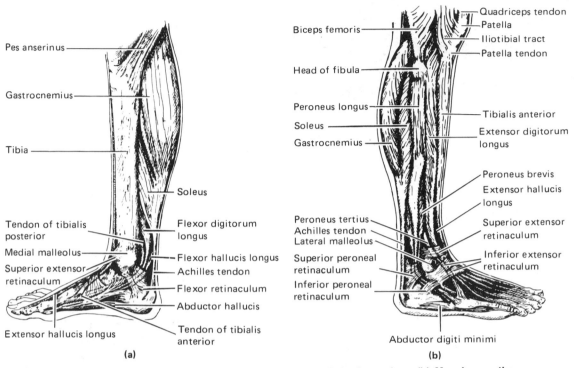

FIGURE 20.2 (a) Muscles on the medial aspect of the lower leg (b) Muscles on the lateral aspect of the lower leg

3. *Extensor digitorum longus*: From the anterior surface of the fibula, the lateral condyle of the tibia, and the interosseous membrane to the common extensor tendon of the lateral four toes. *Function*: Dorsiflexes the foot and extends the toes.

4. *Tibialis posterior*: From the interosseous membrane between the tibia and fibula to the navicular and cuneiforms. *Function*: Plantar flexes and supinates the foot.

5. *Flexor hallucis longus*: From the posterior surface of the fibula to the base of the distal phalanx of the great toe. *Function*: Plantar flexes the ankle and flexes the great toe.

6. *Flexor digitorum longus*: From the posterior surface of the shaft of the tibia to the distal phalanges of the lateral toes. *Function*: Plantar flexes the ankle and flexes the toes.

7. *Peroneus longus*: From the lateral surface of the fibula to the lateral side of the first

metatarsal base and medial cuneiform. *Function*: Everts the foot and plantar flexes the ankle.

8. *Peroneus brevis*: From the lower two-thirds of the lateral surface of the fibula to the base of the fifth metatarsal. *Function*: Everts the foot and plantar flexes the ankle.

9. *Peroneus tertius*: From the lower third of the anterior surface of the fibula to the dorsal surface of the base of the fifth metatarsal. *Function*: Dorsiflexes the ankle and everts the foot.

10. *Gastrocnemius*: Has two heads, one from the lateral and one from the medial condyle of the femur posteriorly to the Achilles tendon. *Function*: Flexes the knee, plantar flexes the ankle, and supinates the foot.

11. *Soleus*: From the posterior aspect of the head of the fibula and the medial border of the tibia to the Achilles tendon. *Function*:

Plantar flexes the ankle and supinates the foot.

12. *Plantaris*: From the lateral condyle of the femur posteriorly to the Achilles or directly into the calcaneus. *Function*: Plantar flexes the foot and slightly flexes the knee.

The Achilles tendon. This is the common tendon of the gastrocnemius and soleus muscles, which unite distally to form it in conjunction with the plantaris muscle that lies between the gastrocnemius and the soleus. The Achilles inserts into the calcaneus.

Two bursae surround the Achilles, one between the skin and the Achilles (subcutaneous bursa) and the other between the Achilles and the calcaneus (retrocalcaneal bursa). The Achilles is surrounded by a peritendon, or, as it is sometimes called, a paratenon (there is no true synovial sheath), which allows it free movement against the surrounding tissue.

The area posterior to the malleoli. Running posteriorly to the medial malleolus are the posterior tibial, flexor digitorum longus, and flexor hallucis longus tendons; the posterior tibial artery; and the posterior tibial nerve (which divides and gives off the medial calcaneal nerve). Behind the lateral malleolus run the tendons of the peroneus longus and brevis. Covering these structures is a thick retinaculum.

The Ankle

Because the bony ankle is shaped like a mortise and tenon, it functions as a hinged joint and allows movement in one plane only—flexion and extension. The mortise is formed by the lateral malleolus of the fibula and by the undersurface and medial malleolus of the tibia. The tenon is the talus, which fits into the mortise. The talus is wider anteriorly, which means it fits more snugly into the mortise when the ankle is in dorsiflexion. Conversely, when the ankle moves into plantar flexion, the narrower part of the talus moves into the mortise, resulting in instability and predisposing the ankle to injury.[1]

The ligaments around the ankle are frequently injured and should be well known to the trainer. On the medial side of the joint is the powerful deltoid ligament, which consists of two parts. The superficial part runs from the medial malleolus to the calcaneus and distally to support the arch of the foot; the deep part runs from the medial malleolus to the talus.

The tibiofibular syndesmosis consists of the anterior and posterior tibiofibular ligaments and the interosseous membrane, allowing very little movement between the tibia and fibula at the ankle joint. The tibiofibular syndesmosis is frequently damaged in rotational-type sprains of the ankle.

The lateral ligaments are much weaker than their medial counterparts and are frequently injured. These ligaments consist of

FIGURE 20.3 The Achilles tendon and the retrocalcaneal bursae (lateral view)

Achilles tendon

Superficial retrocalcaneal bursa

Deep retrocalcaneal bursa

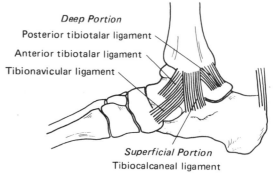

Deep Portion
Posterior tibiotalar ligament
Anterior tibiotalar ligament
Tibionavicular ligament

Superficial Portion
Tibiocalcaneal ligament

FIGURE 20.4 The deep and superficial portions of the deltoid ligament (viewed from the medial side)

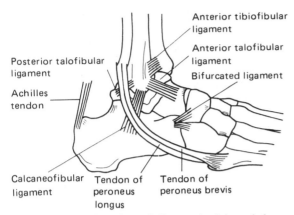

FIGURE 20.5 The lateral ligaments (viewed from the lateral side)

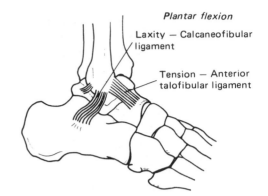

FIGURE 20.7 The position of the foot and ankle, and its influence on the lateral ligaments—plantar flexion

three main parts: (a) the anterior talofibular ligament, (b) the calcaneofibular ligament, and (c) the posterior talofibular ligament. The arrangement of the lateral ligaments is such that at least one of them is tense throughout the range of ankle movement— the calcaneofibular ligament in dorsiflexion, the anterior talofibular ligament in plantar flexion.

The retinaculum securing the peroneus longus and the peroneus brevis behind the lateral malleolus is in close continuity with the calcaneofibular ligament and can be damaged when this ligament is injured.

The Foot

The foot is truly a remarkable organ. It has to absorb shock, adapt to the underlying surface, keep the body balanced, propel the body forward, and change from one of these functions to another—all within a minute period of time. It might be possible to continue to participate with a sore knee or a painful shoulder, but if one or both feet are hurt, the athlete is often incapacitated.

The foot is divided into three areas: (a) rearfoot, consisting of the calcaneous and the talus; (b) midfoot, consisting of the navicular, the cuboid, and the cuneiforms; and (c) forefoot, consisting of the metatarsals and the phalanges.

Two joints often referred to are the *subtalar* and the *midtarsal*. The subtalar joint lies between the calcaneus and the talus. The midtarsal joint is actually two joints: (a) the talonavicular joint and (b) the calcaneocuboid joint.

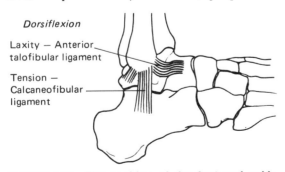

FIGURE 20.6 The position of the foot and ankle, and its influence on the lateral ligaments— dorsiflexion

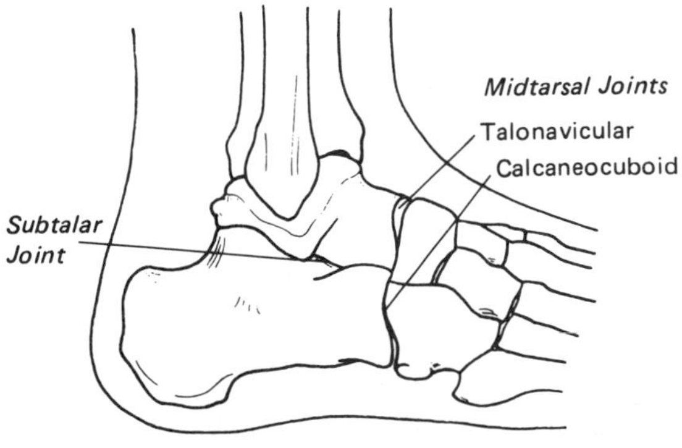

FIGURE 20.8 The subtalar and midtarsal joints

Movements. The subtalar joint imparts a tri-plane movement to the bones that allow motion in a side-to-side direction so pronation and supination can occur. *Pronation* consists of dorsiflexion, abduction, and eversion; *supination* is the opposite, namely, plantar flexion, adduction, and inversion. These movements take place at the subtalar joint.[2] The range of motion of the foot depends on the bony configuration as well as the ligaments and muscles acting on the bones.

When the foot is pronated, it becomes loose and "unlocked," allowing for shock absorbency and adaptation to the underlying surface. Supination of the subtalar joint mechanically aligns the bones of the foot to "lock" the foot. This decreases the range of motion of the midtarsal joint and allows the foot to act as a rigid lever during the take-off and propulsive phase of gait (see biomechanics of running in the section on running injuries, p. 412).

Ligaments and fascia. There are a number of ligaments in the foot. Only a few will be discussed.

"Spring" ligament: The calcaneonavicular or "spring" ligament helps to maintain the medial longitudinal arch. If forces are excessive, injury to this ligament causes discomfort and tenderness localized to the medial arch of the foot in the region of the calcaneonavicular joint.

Bifurcated ligament: A ligament running between the calcaneus, the navicular, and the cuboid, this can be injured with inversion sprains of the foot.

Plantar fascia: A white band of tissue running from the calcaneus to the heads of the metatarsals, the fascia supports the plantar aspect of the foot. It is often subjected to microtrauma, can become inflamed, and can tear under severe stress.

Muscles. Like the hand, the foot is supplied with extrinsic and intrinsic muscles. The extrinsic muscles are discussed on p. 369.

The muscles on the posteromedial aspect of the leg (posterior tibial, flexor digit-

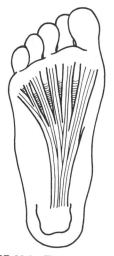

FIGURE 20.9   The plantar fascia

orum longus, and flexor hallucis longus) help to support the arch and promote the rigid lever action of the foot during the propulsive phase of gait.

The anterior muscles (tibialis anterior, extensor digitorum longus, and extensor hallucis longus) prepare the foot for contact with the ground. They also help absorb shock by dorsiflexing the foot before impact and then gently lowering it to the ground.

The lateral muscles (peroneals) act mainly as everters of the foot, helping to stabilize the ankle. They also help plantar flex the foot.

Intrinsic muscles: There are numerous intrinsic muscles in the foot, the main ones being:

1. *Abductor hallucis*: Originates from the medial aspect of the calcaneus and runs to the medial side of the base of the proximal phalanx of the great toe. *Function*: Abducts and flexes the great toe. This muscle is thought to be important in some of the painful conditions around the medial arch.

2. *Abductor digiti minimi pedis*: Arises from the medial and lateral tubercles of the calcaneus in the plantar fascia and inserts into the lateral surface of the base of the proximal phalanx of the fifth toe. *Function*: Abducts the fifth toe.

3. *Flexor hallucis brevis*: Arises from the cuboid and the third cuneiform and inserts into the base of the proximal phalanx of the first toe. *Function*: Flexes the first toe.

4. *Flexor digitorum brevis*: Runs from the medial tuberosity of the calcaneus and the plantar fascia to the middle phalanges of the four lateral toes. *Function*: Flexes the toes.

Nerve supply. The *sciatic nerve* supplies the branches that innervate the lower leg and foot. Thus a lower-back disc herniation or protrusion may present with sensory or motor changes that manifest in the lower leg. The dermatome supplied by L4, L5, and S1 should be noted (see section on the lumbar spine, pp. 269 and 270, and Figure 17.5).

The sciatic nerve gives off a number of branches just proximal to the popliteal fossa. These are the *sural nerve* (supplies the lateral aspect of the foot), the *tibial nerve* (innervates the muscles on the posterior aspect of the leg), and the *common peroneal nerve* which gives off the *deep peroneal nerve*. The deep peroneal nerve then runs within the anterior compartment, where it can become compressed in the anterior compartment compression syndrome. Because it innervates the skin of the first web space of the toes on the dorsal aspect of the foot, this area can lose sensation if the pressure rises sufficiently within the anterior compartment. This nerve also supplies the dorsiflexor muscles. The *superficial peroneal nerve* innervates the evertor muscles that lie within the lateral compartment and the skin of the dorsum of the lateral side of the foot (second, third, and fourth toes).

The *femoral nerve* supplies the saphenous nerve that innervates the medial aspect of the ankle.

Arterial blood supply. Just distal to the popliteal space, the popliteal artery divides into the anterior and posterior tibial arteries. The anterior tibial runs through the anterior compartment and supplies the dorsalis pedis pulse over the dorsum of the foot between the first and second metatarsals (though this pulse may be congenitally absent in some people).

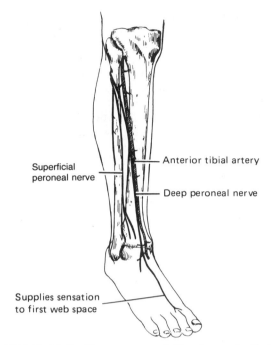

FIGURE 20.10 The nerve and blood supply that passes through the anterior compartment of the lower leg

The posterior tibial artery runs down the posterior aspect of the calf, giving off the peroneal artery to the lateral compartment. The posterior tibial also provides a pulse behind the medial malleolus, where one also finds the flexor tendons and the posterior tibial nerve.

Lymphatic drainage. There is extensive lymphatic drainage from the foot to the lymph nodes in the popliteal area and the groin. Infection of the foot spreads rapidly through the lymphatic drainage system and often presents with a painful swollen lymph node in the groin.

INJURIES TO THE LOWER LEG

Contusions to the Anterior Lower Leg

The results of a contusion to the lower leg may vary from a mild bruise to a serious injury. The increasing popularity of soccer will undoubtedly result in more and more injuries to this area, particularly if the athlete neglects to wear shin guards.

A kick directly on the tibia can cause a *tibial fracture*. When examining an athlete with this injury, gently palpate the tibia. If no fracture is obvious, percuss the tibial shaft and then the heel. If this produces pain over the tender area, a fracture should be suspected. Ice should be applied and the leg splinted. The athlete should not be allowed to bear weight on the leg until X-rays have been taken. Another method of incurring a fracture of the tibia in soccer or football is shown in Figure 20.11.[3]

A blow over the anterior compartment can cause bleeding within the compartment, resulting in increased pressure and development of the anterior compartment compression syndrome (see compartment compression syndrome in the section on running injuries, p. 435). This condition may not develop immediately, and an attempt to prevent it should be made by placing ice over the anterior compartment. Icing and elevation should continue for a number of hours. Anti-inflammatory medication can be given if necessary. Any athlete who has an injury which could develop an anterior compartment compression syndrome should be informed of its symptoms and signs and should be instructed that if they arise, he or she should seek immediate emergency care.

A *hematoma* over the tibia, or elsewhere in the lower leg, can become infected. This should be suspected if, after a few days, the hematoma becomes red, increasingly painful, or swollen. Treatment is drainage of the hematoma and the appropriate antibiotic.

An athlete returning to play after suffering a contusion to the lower leg should ensure that the injured area is adequately protected.

Rupture of the Gastrocnemius Muscle ("Tennis Leg")

"Tennis leg" is a condition formerly attributed to rupture of the tiny plantaris muscle, but it has now been demonstrated by surgi-

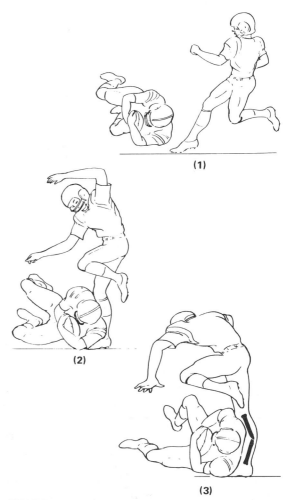

FIGURE 20.11 A mechanism for fracturing the tibia (Modified from S. F. Gunther, "An avoidable soccer injury," *Journal of Sports Medicine* 2:167, 1974.)

cal exploration to be due to a tear of the musculotendinous junction of one of the heads of the gastrocnemius muscle (usually the medial).[4,5]

MECHANISM OF INJURY: The injury occurs when the knee is suddenly extended while the foot is dorsiflexed, or it is caused by a sudden dorsiflexion of the foot while the knee is in extension.

PREDISPOSING FACTORS: Tennis leg tends to occur most in the middle-aged athlete, after some degeneration of the muscle or mus-

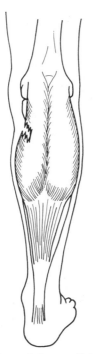

FIGURE 20.12 Tear of the medial head of the gastrocnemius ("tennis leg")

culotendinous junction of the gastrocnemius has occurred.

SYMPTOMS AND SIGNS: A sudden sharp pain is felt in the medial (sometimes the lateral) upper calf. It is often described as feeling like a "shot in the leg." The athlete is unable to bear full weight on the affected leg; swelling is fairly rapid, particularly if a substantial amount of the muscle is torn; and ecchymosis is frequently present.

It is usually very difficult to palpate a defect in the muscle. The affected area can be localized by tenderness to direct pressure. The athlete is often unable to stand on the metatarsal heads of the affected leg, but it is difficult to be certain if this is due to weakness or pain.

Prodromal symptoms (e.g., symptoms appearing before the actual rupture has occurred) have been noticed by some athletes and consist mainly of aching and pain in the musculotendinous junction of the gastrocnemius after activities such as tennis.

TREATMENT:

Immediate: Apply a cold, wet elastic bandage for compression. Apply ice on top of one or two layers of this bandage and hold it firmly in place with further wraps. The leg should be elevated and the foot held in gentle plantar flexion. The athlete should be non-weight-bearing with crutches. Analgesics and anti-inflammatory medication should be commenced if necessary.

Definitive:

1. Mild cases—Limited weight bearing, using a raised heel to reduce pressure on the gastrocnemius, can be recommended when comfortable. Strengthening exercises for the gastrocnemius muscle should be started together with Achilles stretching, ultrasound, and muscle stimulation. Following return from the injury, a heel lift of ¼ " or ½ " (6 or 12 mm) should be placed in both shoes and used for sporting activities.

2. Moderately severe cases—Best treated in a plaster cast, either a below-knee walker or, for more severe cases, a long-leg cast (with the knee held at 60° of flexion and the foot in 10° to 15° of plantar flexion) for three to six weeks. Rehabilitation exercises are important before return to activity and heel lifts should be worn.

3. Severe cases—When there is a substantial tearing of the gastrocnemius muscle together with separation of the affected ends, surgical exploration and repair is considered the best form of treatment by some authorities, but there is controversy on this issue.

PROGNOSIS: If this injury is adequately treated, the prognosis for returning to sports activities is excellent. However, an athlete who has had this condition is likely to suffer the same problem in the opposite leg. For those who have not been treated adequately, or who have not sought attention, return to full sports activity may be delayed for a considerable period of time, and normal function may be impaired.

Total Rupture of the Achilles Tendon

This well-known but relatively uncommon athletic injury occurs particularly in middle age, but can occur in the prime of a young athlete's career.

MECHANISM OF INJURY: The rupture is usually the result of a sudden contraction of the gastrocnemius and soleus complex, such as when pushing off with the knee in extension (as in running) or when the foot is forced into a dorsiflexed position (as in landing from a jump). A direct blow to the Achilles can cause it to rupture, though this is rare. The tendon usually ruptures at its midportion, about 3 cm to 6 cm above the calcaneus, but it may be avulsed from the calcaneus or torn at the musculotendinous junction.

Predisposing factors include nonspecific degeneration of the tendon (possibly due to vascular impairment in the middle third of the tendon) and repeated subclinical tears leading to areas of necrosis. The use of corticosteriods, particularly when given by local injection (but also orally), has been implicated in weakening of the tendon.[6,7]

SYMPTOMS AND SIGNS: The classic case of acute rupture presents with the history of a sudden snap which is clearly audible but often painless. In fact, the athlete may describe a situation in which he or she looked around for the source of the noise. In other cases, the rupture may be associated with the sensation of having been shot or kicked in the leg.

There is subsequent weakness of the foot, particularly when an attempt is made to stand on the metatarsal heads, followed by pain and swelling. However, the swelling may be a very minor symptom, particularly if there is a rupture of an avascular portion of the tendon.

When the athlete stands and is viewed from behind, the affected Achilles tendon appears thicker than the one on the opposite side. Localized swelling may be present over the tendon with possible ecchymosis. There may be tenderness directly over the rupture

site, and sometimes a palpable gap can be felt. Weakness of ankle plantar flexion is demonstrated by inability to stand on the metatarsal heads of the affected limb. There may be some increase of dorsiflexion compared with the other limb, but this is often difficult to determine because of pain.

One of the most important tests is manual compression of the calf (also called the Thompson[8] or Simmonds test[9]). With the athlete prone, the knee bent, and the foot hanging, squeeze the calf. This maneuver normally produces plantar flexion of the foot. If plantar flexion does not occur, a ruptured Achilles tendon should be suspected.

X-RAYS: X-rays are sometimes useful because changes anterior to the Achilles tendon can be seen on the lateral view. Kager's triangle should be carefully examined for any abnormalities (Figure 20.14).[10] Xerography may also help to bring out alterations in the soft tissues. Electromyography is sometimes used to help with the diagnosis in difficult cases.

TREATMENT: *Immediate* treatment consists of applying ice to the affected area, immobilizing the ankle in slight plantar flexion, and having the athlete use crutches. Analgesics and anti-inflammatory medication may be used if desired. Surgical repair is the *defini-*

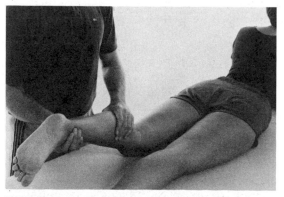

FIGURE 20.13 The Thompson (or Simmonds) test
The foot should plantar flex when the calf muscle is squeezed. If it does not, a rupture of the Achilles tendon should be suspected.

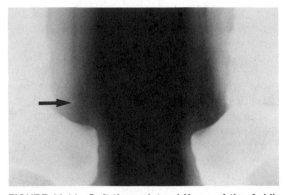

FIGURE 20.14 Soft-tissue lateral X-ray of the Achilles tendons The arrow points to Kager's triangle, which has lost its radiolucency. The Achilles tendon is also noted to be indistinct on that side (compare with opposite Achilles).

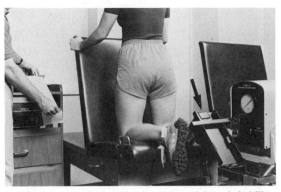

FIGURE 20.15 Rehabilitation of an injured Achilles tendon Isokinetic training has been found to be of value in returning athletes with Achilles injuries to full function. This position exercises the soleus muscle when the foot is plantar flexed. The arrow points to the side being rehabilitated.

tive treatment for an athlete.[11,12] There is some controversy as to whether surgery is indicated in a nonathlete.[13] Cast immobilization is usually from four to eight weeks.

REHABILITATION: A carefully controlled rehabilitation program should be carried out following an adequate period of cast immobilization. The athlete should be started on gentle range-of-motion together with electrical stimulation of the calf muscles. Ice massage can also be used. This should be followed by a graduated exercise program. First use manual resistance, then the Cybex or Orthotron isokinetic machines, which are particularly useful for regaining strength, power, and endurance in the gastrocnemius-soleus complex. Carefully controlled plantar flexion and dorsiflexion stretching exercises should also be started.

Many other rehabilitation exercises, outlined in the section on ankle rehabilitation, p. 392, are applicable to rehabilitating the Achilles tendon.

PROGNOSIS: Following a complete rupture of the Achilles tendon, the prognosis for returning to top-class athletic competition is guarded.[14] It should, however, be possible for the athlete to return to a high level of activity in the majority of cases.

Partial Rupture of the Achilles Tendon

Partial rupture of the Achilles tendon, or tendinosis, is fairly common but infrequently diagnosed. This is due to lack of awareness of the condition, together with the difficulty of making a confident diagnosis.[15] The onset may be dramatic—sudden pain, limited motion, and weakness localized to the Achilles —following an acute dorsiflexion of the ankle, a hard push-off, or even an innocent movement. Or the onset may be more vague, with the athlete presenting with "tendinitis" type symptoms that do not clear with the standard treatment (see section on injuries to the Achilles tendon, p. 439).

SYMPTOMS AND SIGNS: At the one extreme is a picture which may be very similar to that of a complete rupture, only the Thompson test (see p. 377) is negative. At the other extreme is the athlete with the usual symptoms of Achilles tendinitis—swelling, pain with motion, crepitus at times, and inability to perform. Signs include localized tenderness on squeezing the Achilles tendon and pain on either forced passive dorsiflexion or resistance to active plantar flexion. Crepitus may be present. Manual squeezing of the calf muscles does not produce a positive Thompson test, in other words, the foot *will* plantar flex. It is often possible for the athlete to stand on the metatarsal heads without weakness but with much discomfort.

X-RAYS: A lateral X-ray view should be taken and Kager's triangle examined and compared with the opposite side (see total rupture of the Achilles tendon, p. 377). Abnormalities of this triangle are frequently found in a partial rupture.[16]

TREATMENT: Initially, treatment is with ice, immobilization, and anti-inflammatory medication. If the examiner feels strongly enough about the diagnosis and suspects that a substantial portion of the Achilles tendon has been torn, the Achilles should be immobilized in a cast, with the foot in slight plantar flexion, for from four to six weeks. This is followed by a gradual return to normal activities together with a carefully controlled rehabilitation program.

If symptoms do not disappear after an adequate trial of conservative therapy, the question of surgical exploration of the Achilles tendon should be discussed with the athlete.[17] If it is felt on initial examination that a significant portion of the Achilles tendon has been torn, early operative treatment may be considered desirable. It should be remembered that many cases of Achilles "tendinitis" are actually partial tears of the Achilles tendon. This is probably the main reason why injection of a corticosteroid preparation should not be used in or around the Achilles tendon in these cases.

INJURIES TO THE ANKLE

Prevention of Ankle Injuries

Stretching. Recurrent ankle sprains are often associated with tight Achilles tendons. Daily, slow, static stretching of the Achilles tendon can reduce the incidence of recurrent ankle sprains[18] (see technique for Achilles stretching, p. 43, and Figure 3.6).

Exercises. A well-functioning peroneus muscle group helps prevent ankle sprains. The peroneus muscles must contract early enough in the foot's contact cycle to slow down or prevent excessive movement if the foot is forced into inversion.[19] Eversion exercises, as well as other exercises, should be used to train the peroneal muscles to contract maximally when needed[20] (see ankle rehabilitation exercises, p. 392).

Proprioception is also of great importance in preventing ankle sprains. This applies particularly to the athlete who has had previous sprains and who might have injured the proprioception receptor-conduction mechanism. Ankle proprioception is easily tested by having the athlete stand on one foot with eyes closed, to see if balance can be maintained (see Figure 20.26).[21] Athletes with poor proprioception are only able to balance on one foot for a very short time. Proprioception can be improved by various exercises, as outlined in the ankle rehabilitation section, p. 394.

Some athletes are obviously better coordinated than others and have a more highly refined proprioceptive system. This does not mean that the poorly endowed athlete (from the neuromuscular point of view) cannot do anything about his or her genetic plight. By embarking on simple eversion and proprioceptive exercises, the athlete can definitely improve his or her awareness of the body's position in space, and the ability to control previously uncontrolled sudden inversion movements of the foot and ankle.

Shoes.

1. Soccer-style shoes for football: When a field is well maintained, so that ankle sprains from twists in potholes or poorly kept surfaces are eliminated, the type of shoe worn for football can influence the rate of ankle sprains.[22] It appears that the shoe with the lowest incidence of ankle sprains is the same shoe which should be worn to decrease the incidence of knee injuries—a soccer-style shoe with a polyurethane sole and about fourteen relatively flat, wide cleats.[23]

2. Shoe width: Many athletes, particularly football players, are given shoes which are much too narrow for their feet, which tend to bulge over the edges of the soles in a very unstable manner, and may predispose them to ankle sprains. It is therefore important that each athlete be individually fitted with a shoe that is not only adequate for the foot's length but also of correct width.

3. High-top shoes: Though high-top shoes are very uncommon in football these days, they are often used in basketball. A survey of the influence of high-top shoes in preventing ankle sprains in basketball shows that this type of shoe does have some protective value, particularly if used in conjunction with tape.[24] One theory attempting to explain these results suggests that the high top stimulates the proprioceptive receptors, leading to early firing of the peroneal muscles and thereby improving ankle stability.[19] An athlete with a predisposition to ankle sprains should consider wearing high-top shoes as an additional precaution.

Taping. Hundreds of thousands of rolls of tape are used each year in an attempt to reduce the incidence of ankle sprains. Whether tape actually achieves this purpose has never been adequately proven. Most trainers feel that taping a previously sprained ankle or an ankle that is prone to sprains is useful. As mentioned, ankle taping with high-top shoes is effective in preventing ankle sprains in basketball.[24] Whether the athlete who has never sustained an ankle sprain should be taped is controversial and depends on a number of factors, not the least of which is the financial status of the athletic department.

Taping is logical and necessary for those who have recently suffered an ankle sprain and who are still undergoing rehabilitation, as well as for those who are subject to frequent ankle sprains. These individuals should, however, also be maintained on a vigorous rehabilitation program to strengthen the muscles around the ankle, improve their flexibility, and sharpen their proprioception.

Playing surface. An irregular playing surface with potholes in it is an invitation to ankle sprain and negates the positive aspects of the ankle injury prevention program.[22]

Mechanism of Ankle Sprains

Inversion sprains. Over 80% of all ankle sprains are inversion injuries, occurring while the athlete is running straight ahead or cutting. The foot suddenly turns into plantar flexion and inversion, and the athlete feels a sharp pain on the anterolateral aspect of the ankle. With this injury, the talofibular ligament is the first ligament to be affected and it thus is the most commonly injured structure around the ankle. If the sprain is more severe, the calcaneofibular ligament is also involved[25,26] (Figure 20.16).

With the rotational sprain (cutting across the plantar flexed, inverted foot), the tibiofibular ligament and the interosseous membrane may be involved in addition to the lateral ligaments.[27] With this inversion-rotational sprain, it is possible to fracture the neck of the fibula (Maisonneuve fracture).[28]

Occasionally the athlete suffers a pure inversion sprain, for instance when coming down from a rebound in basketball and landing entirely on the side of the foot without any plantar flexion occurring. This is unusual, however.

Eversion sprains. Eversion sprains occur less frequently than inversion sprains, due to the anatomy of the ankle joint and the strength of the deltoid ligament. An eversion sprain may tear the deltoid ligament, or the ligament may be stronger than the bone, in which case the medial malleolus will be avulsed. The pure eversion sprain tears the deltoid ligament only. The milder sprain tears the deeper part of the ligament, whereas more severe forces tear both the deep and the superficial portions.

More often the foot goes into an excessive amount of pronation (this implies abduction, eversion, and dorsiflexion), partic-

TABLE 20.1   Mechanism of Common Ankle Sprains—Ligaments Involved

Mechanism	Stage I	Stage II (more severe)	Stage III (most severe)
Inversion + plantar flexion	Anterior talofibular ligament sprain	Stage I + calcaneofibular ligament sprain	Stage II + posterior talofibular ligament sprain
Inversion + plantar flexion + rotation (most common)	Anterior talofibular ligament sprain + Tibiofibular ligament sprain	Stage I + calcaneofibular ligament sprain	Stage II + posterior talofibular ligament sprain
Pure inversion (rare)	Calcaneofibular ligament sprain	Stage I + anterior talofibular ligament sprain	Stage II + posterior talofibular ligament sprain
Pronation (abduction + eversion + dorsiflexion)	Deltoid ligament sprain or avulsion fracture of medial malleolus	Stage I + tibiofibular ligament and interosseous membrane	Stage II + fibular fracture above mortice line

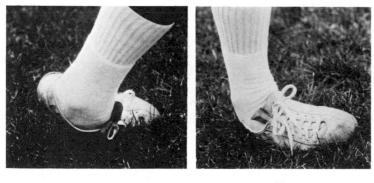

(a)   (b)

FIGURE 20.16   Mechanism of an ankle sprain   (a) An inversion-plantar flexion sprain This motion usually sprains the anterior talofibular ligament, and if severe, the calcaneofibular ligament is also involved. A fracture of the fibula occasionally occurs. **(b) An inversion sprain** This injury may affect only the calcaneofibular ligament, though the anterior talofibular ligament is also frequently sprained.

TABLE 20.2 Anterior Talofibular Ligament Sprain—Symptoms and Signs

Degree	History	Tenderness	Swelling	Pain with Stress	Ligament Laxity	Other Structures
Stable Mild	Plantar flexion-inversion	Anterolateral	Anterolateral	Slight	0	0
Moderate	Plantar flexion-inversion	Anterolateral	Anterolateral	More pain	0	0
Severe	Plantar flexion-inversion + pop	Anterolateral	Anterolateral, more diffuse	Usually very painful; occasionally no pain, especially soon after injury	Slight anterior drawer sign	Calcaneofibular and/or tibiofibular ligaments
Unstable	Plantar flexion-inversion + pop	All over the lateral and anterolateral sides	Anterolateral, more diffuse	Usually very painful; occasionally no pain, especially soon after injury	More definite anterior drawer sign	Calcaneofibular (inversion stress) and/or tibiofibular (side-to-side) stress laxity

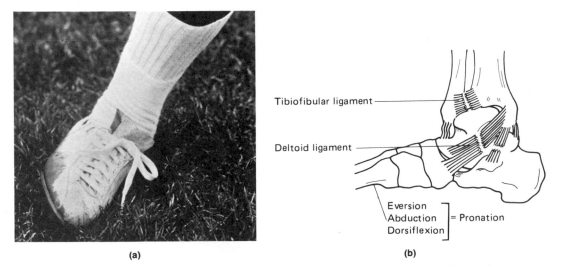

(a)   (b)

FIGURE 20.17 Mechanism of an ankle sprain (a) An eversion sprain This motion may tear the deltoid ligament, or may produce an avulsion fracture off the tip of the medial malleolus. **(b)** An eversion sprain may tear the deltoid ligament and the tibiofibular ligament (viewed from the medial side)

TABLE 20.3 Tibiofibular Ligament Sprain—Symptoms and Signs

Degree	History	Tenderness	Swelling	Pain with Stress	Ligament Laxity	Other Structures that may be involved
Stable Mild	Inversion or eversion rotation	Over tibio-fibular liga-ment	Over anterior aspect in re-gion of syn-desmosis	Slight	0	0
Moderate	Inversion or eversion rotation	Over the tibio-fibular liga-ment and often the me-dial or lateral ligaments	Over anterior aspect in re-gion of syn-desmosis	More pain	0	Lateral or me-dial ligaments and/or interosseous membrane
Severe	Inversion or eversion rotation	Over the tibio-fibular liga-ment and of-ten the me-dial or lateral ligaments	Over anterior aspect in re-gion of syn-desmosis	Usually very painful; occa-sionally no pain, espe-cially soon after injury	Slight laxity on side-to-side test	Lateral or me-dial ligaments and/or interosseous membrane
Unstable	Inversion or eversion rotation	Over the tibio-fibular liga-ment and of-ten the me-dial or lateral ligaments	Over anterior aspect in re-gion of syn-desmosis	Usually very painful; occa-sionally no pain, espe-cially soon after injury	Laxity on side-to-side test	Lateral or me-dial ligaments and/or interosseous membrane

ularly when cutting to the opposite side. The resultant forces may tear not only the del-toid ligament but also the tibiofibular liga-ment and the interosseous membrane, and may even fracture the fibula. Significant in-stability results from this serious injury.

Dorsiflexion sprains. An excessive dorsiflex-ion force jams the talus into the mortise, since the anterior portion of the talus is wid-er than the posterior part. This may separate the syndesmosis and, in addition, cause an osteochondral fracture of the talus. The Achilles may be injured by the stretching forces of dorsiflexion, and the tibia may jam against the talar neck.

Plantar flexion sprains. Pure plantar flexion sprains are rare; there is usually some de-gree of inversion as well. The lateral liga-ments, tibiofibular ligaments, and anterior retinaculum are usually involved. In addi-tion, the os trigonum may be damaged, re-sulting in pain and tenderness over the posterior aspect of the ankle.

Evaluation of the Injured Ankle

The purpose of evaluating an injured ankle is to

1. attempt to exclude the presence of a fracture (relatively uncommon)

TABLE 20.4   Calcaneofibular Ligament Sprain—Symptoms and Signs

Degree	History	Tenderness	Swelling	Pain with Stress	Ligament Laxity	Other Structures
Stable Mild	Inversion	Over ligament	Over lateral side	Slight	0	0
Moderate	Inversion	Over ligament ± anterior talofibular and/or tibiofibular ligaments	Over lateral side	More pain	0	0
Severe	Inversion + pop	Over ligament ± anterior talofibular and/or tibiofibular	Over lateral side with or without anterior swelling	Usually very painful; occasionally no pain, especially soon after injury	Slight inversion laxity	Anterior talofibular and/or tibiofibular ligaments
Unstable	Inversion + pop	Over ligament ± anterior talofibular and/or tibiofibular	Over lateral side with or without anterior swelling	Usually very painful; occasionally no pain, especially soon after injury	Inversion laxity	Anterior talofibular (anterior drawer sign) and/or tibiofibular (side-to-side) laxity

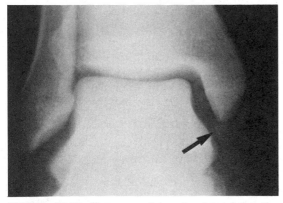

FIGURE 20.18   X-ray—avulsion fracture from the tip of the medial malleolus

2. make an anatomical diagnosis of the structures involved

3. decide on the severity of the injury

4. differentiate the unstable from the stable ankle sprain (probably the most important function of the clinical evaluation)

HISTORY: The following questions should be asked:

1. What was the mechanism of the injury (e.g., inversion with plantar flexion, eversion, rotation, etc.)?

2. Where was the pain initially?

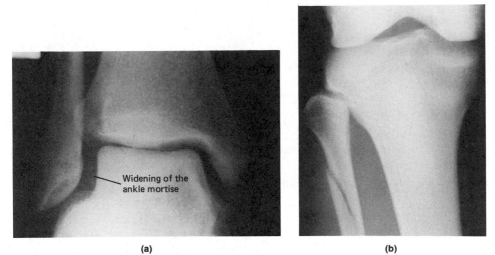

(a)   **(b)**

FIGURE 20.19   X-ray—a tear of the deltoid and tibiofibular ligament, resulting in widening of the mortise (**a**). Part (**b**) shows a fracture of the upper fibula (Maisonneuve fracture) which occurred from the ankle injury shown in part (**a**).

TABLE 20.5   Deltoid Ligament Sprain—Symptoms and Signs

Degree	History	Tenderness	Swelling	Pain with Stress	Ligament Laxity	Other Structures
Stable Mild	Pronation (eversion + abduction + dorsiflexion)	Over deltoid ligament	Over deltoid ligament	Slight	0	0
Moderate	Pronation	Over deltoid ligament + tibiofibular ligament and interosseous membrane	Over deltoid ligament	More pain	0	Anterior tibiofibular sprain
Severe	Pronation	Over deltoid ligament + tibiofibular ligament and interosseous membrane	Over deltoid ligament + anterior ankle	Usually very painful; occasionally no pain; especially soon after injury	Eversion laxity	Anterior tibiofibular sprain ± interosseous membrane
Unstable	Pronation	Over deltoid ligament + tibiofibular ligament and interosseous membrane	Over deltoid ligament + anterior ankle	Usually very painful; occasionally no pain, especially soon after injury	Eversion laxity ± side-to-side laxity	Tibiofibular ligament ± interosseous membrane ± fibular fracture

3. Did you hear a pop, snap, or crack?
4. Were you able to walk immediately after the injury?
5. Did you continue to play?
6. Did the ankle feel unstable?
7. Did the ankle swell up immediately? Later? (Not as important as in knee injuries) (Table 20.6).
8. What treatment was applied immediately? later?
9. Have you hurt either ankle before?

OBSERVATIONS: Note areas of ecchymosis and of localized swelling. Immediate and diffuse swelling is usually, but not always, associated with a severe sprain. If there is bleeding within the joint, suspect a severe sprain. The athlete should then sit with legs hanging over the end of the examining table and the effect of gravity on the position of the ankle should be observed (the leg musculature must be completely relaxed). If there is an obviously noticeable difference in the amount of inversion on the injured side when compared with the unaffected side, there is probably a severe unstable sprain of the lateral ligaments. The same test can be applied to injuries of the medial side involving the deltoid ligament, where a third-degree sprain would result in a position of excessive eversion.

PALPATION: The structures involved can usually be well localized by careful palpation. Start away from the suspected area of injury (leaving the most painful part of palpation to the end) and systematically palpate each important structure in turn. This way, no area will be overlooked. A suggested order for palpating a suspected lateral ligament injury follows (Figure 20.20).

1. Neck of the fibula
2. Squeeze the midshaft of the fibula (pain felt at the ankle during this maneuver may well indicate a fracture)
3. Interosseous membrane and anterior compartment
4. Deltoid ligament
5. Anterior tibiofibular ligament
6. Anterior talofibular ligament
7. Calcaneofibular ligament
8. Posterior talofibular ligament and peroneal tendons
9. Achilles tendon
10. Navicular
11. Bifurcated ligament
12. Base of the fifth metatarsal
13. Any other area indicated

LIGAMENT STABILITY TESTS: After obtaining the history, observing, and palpating, it should be possible to make an anatomical di-

TABLE 20.6   Differences Between Knee and Ankle Injuries

Knee	Ankle
1. Knee joint is anatomically unstable.	1. Ankle joint is basically stable.
2. A third-degree ligament injury requires surgery.	2. Unless very unstable, a third-degree injury can be treated conservatively.
3. With a third-degree injury, an immediate primary repair must be performed.	3. With a third-degree injury, a delayed primary repair can be performed if necessary.
4. Reconstructive procedures are uncertain of success.	4. Reconstructive procedures are usually successful. [29]
5. Taping produces relatively poor support.	5. Taping produces good to excellent support.

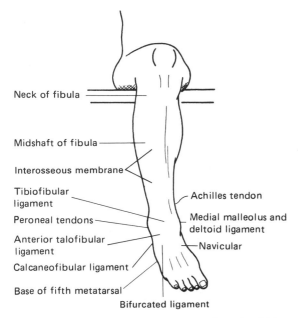

Neck of fibula

Midshaft of fibula

Interosseous membrane

Tibiofibular ligament

Peroneal tendons

Anterior talofibular ligament

Calcaneofibular ligament

Base of fifth metatarsal

Bifurcated ligament

Achilles tendon

Medial malleolus and deltoid ligament

Navicular

FIGURE 20.20 Ankle sprain—areas that should be specifically palpated for tenderness

agnosis as to the structures involved. The ligaments should then be stressed, to determine if the ankle is stable or unstable.

There are four tests used to evaluate stability. Again, start on the unaffected side and move toward the affected side. For example, with a lateral ligament injury, start on the medial side and work across the ankle; with a deltoid ligament injury, start on the lateral side and move medially. Be aware of movement occurring at the subtalar joint when examining the ankle, and differentiate this movement from that of the ankle joint proper. In many athletes with so-called loose ankles, the excessive motion takes place at the subtalar joint and does not necessarily indicate abnormal laxity of the ankle ligaments.[30]

Before testing the affected ankle, remember to check the unaffected ankle and compare the two. Ensure that the athlete is completely relaxed and that no muscles around the ankle are held in involuntary contraction. The four tests (Figure 20.21) are:

1. *Eversion stress.* Stress the deltoid ligament by moving the calcaneus and talus into eversion.

2. *Side-to-side movement of the talus.* The side-to-side motion tests for widening of the mortise, which can occur if the tibiofibular ligament has been stretched.[31] Move the calcaneus and talus to each side as a unit. Do not tilt the ankle into either eversion or inversion. If the mortise (syndesmosis) is widened, the talus will be able to move sideways, producing a definite thud ("clonk") as it hits the fibula, and when moved in the opposite direction, it butts against the tibia.

3. *Anterior drawer test.* The ankle should be held in slight plantar flexion. One hand holds the lower tibia and exerts a slight posterior force while the other grasps the posterior aspect of the calcaneus and attempts to bring the calcaneus and talus forward on the tibia. If there is excessive forward movement, this indicates that at least the anterior talofibular ligament has been completely ruptured.[32] Also test for instability in a posterior direction by moving the tibia forward on a fixed heel.

4. *Inversion stress.* On attempting to tilt the talus into inversion when a severe lateral ligament injury exists, a spongy, indefinite end point will be felt. This test is often very painful and may be difficult to accomplish.

If pain and muscle spasm preclude an adequate evaluation of ligament stability, a local anesthetic can be injected into the joint and around the injured area or around the sural or peroneal nerves. Occasionally it may be necessary to examine the ankle under general anesthesia.

Having completed these tests, you should now be able to

a. make an anatomical diagnosis

b. decide the severity of the injury

c. decide whether the ankle is stable or unstable

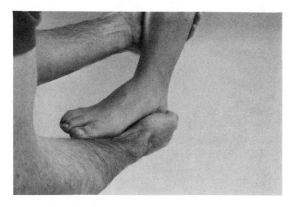

(a) Eversion test The heel is grasped in one hand, the lower tibia in the other, and the ankle moved into eversion.

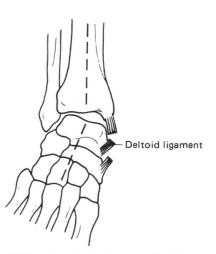

Deltoid ligament

(b) Eversion test A torn deltoid ligament will permit the ankle to open into eversion.

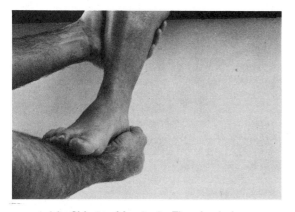

(c) Side-to-side test The heel is moved from side to side, *not* into eversion or inversion. If the tibiofibular ligament is stable, no movement will occur. Attempt to move the calcaneus and talus as one unit.

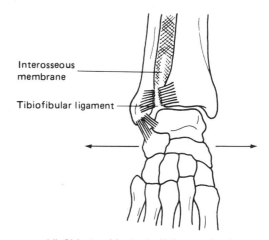

Interosseous membrane

Tibiofibular ligament

(d) Side-to-side test If the mortise is widened, the talus will move from side to side.

FIGURE 20.21 Ankle ligament stability tests

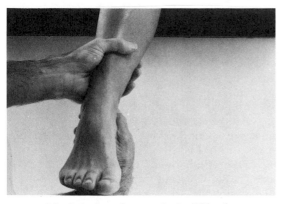

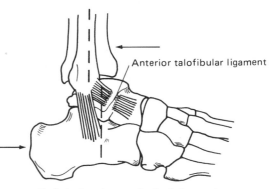

(e) **Anterior drawer test** With the foot in plantar flexion and the tibia stabilized, the heel is brought forward on the tibia. The reverse procedure should also be performed, i.e., moving the heel backwards on the tibia.

(f) **Anterior drawer test** A torn anterior talofibular ligament will permit a positive anterior drawer sign.

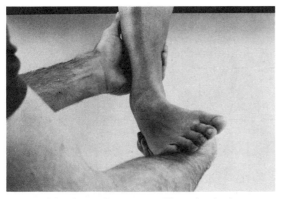

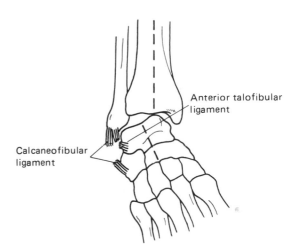

(g) **Inversion test** The heel is brought into inversion while the tibia is stabilized.

(h) **Inversion test** A torn calcaneofibular ligament, usually with a torn anterior talofibular ligament, will permit the ankle to open into inversion.

FIGURE 20.21 (*continued*)

X-RAYS: Most ankle sprains should be referred for routine X-ray examination, to exclude any co-existing fractures. Routine X-rays include AP, lateral, and oblique views. If there is any question about the degree of stability, stress X-rays will further aid the diagnosis.[33,34] However, it should be emphasized that the clinical evaluation is usually sufficient to make the diagnosis; it is not necessary to take stress X-rays routinely. If stress X-rays are considered necessary to define the severity of the injury, they should include both AP and lateral views.[35]

1. *Anteroposterior view (talar tilt):* The stress should be directed either toward inversion or eversion (depending on whether the injury has involved the lateral or deltoid ligament), to demonstrate excessive talar tilt. Always compare with the unaffected side.

2. *Lateral view (anterior drawer test):* Anterior stress is applied to the calcaneus while holding the tibia stable. Again, this is compared with the opposite side.

Arthrography. Ankle arthrography and peroneal sheath arthrography are also used in exceptionally difficult cases. Some reports indicate a high degree of correlation between dye leaking out of the peroneal sheath and a complete rupture of the calcaneofibular ligament.[36] Leakage of dye between the tibia and fibula (after it has been injected into the joint) could indicate a tear of the tibiofibular ligament and interosseous membrane.[37,38]

On-Field Management of the Injured Ankle

Having sustained an ankle injury on the field of play, the athlete should not be allowed to limp around but should be helped off the field, bearing no weight, and should remain non-weight-bearing until the ankle has been evaluated. Immediately on reaching the sideline, the shoe, sock, and tape of the affected leg should be removed. If the athlete is relatively uncooperative because of the amount of discomfort being experienced at that mo-

ment, a cold, wet, elastic wrap (4″ [10 cm] wide) should be applied to support the ankle (eversion support should be given with an inversion sprain). After one or two wrappings have been applied, place an ice bag on the bandage and continue the wrapping. This gives compression and support to the ankle and holds the ice bag in place.

When the athlete has regained composure, usually within three or four minutes, take a history and examine the ankle. The shoe, sock, and tape of the opposite ankle should also be removed, so that the two ankles can be compared. The examination should be as complete as possible for an accurate diagnosis, because examining the ankle soon after the injury is easier than on any subsequent occasion.

If the ankle is completely stable and a fairly minor injury is diagnosed, and if the athlete wishes to return to participation, a series of functional tests should be used before allowing the athlete to return to action (Table 20.7). The ankle should be retaped before these tests are performed.

For the more severe injury, replace the elastic wrap and ice bag and elevate the leg for at least half an hour. If a fracture is suspected, splint the ankle. Do not allow weight bearing until after the X-ray examination.

TABLE 20.7   Criteria for Return to Play Following an Ankle Injury

1. There should be no suggestion from the examination that a fracture might be present.
2. There should be no evidence of ligament instability.

3. The athlete should be able to
   a. run forward
   b. run backward
   c. hop
   d. run-and-cut
   e. run in figure eights at normal speed without any limp

If the above can be accomplished, the athlete is permitted to return to participation. However, protective taping should be applied to support the injured structures. Immediately after the game, the ankle should be re-evaluated and treated as indicated.

Continuing Treatment of the Stable Ankle Sprain

Ice should be applied for at least twenty minutes every hour (longer in more severe cases) during the first twelve to twenty-four hours, while compression and elevation continue. X-rays should have been taken to exclude any fracture. The sprain is diagnosed as a first-, second-, or third-degree sprain.

The stable ankle sprain (first- or moderate second-degree sprain) is treated with tape (Gibney's open basketweave) or an elastic bandage utilizing a left pad for compression over the affected malleolus. This pad is cut into the shape of a horseshoe for compression and can be removed for periodic icing (Figure 20.22). The useful way to achieve elevation is to raise the leg against the wall at 90° to the body while lying down. The elastic bandage holding the pad in place is used mainly for compression and not for stability. Another alternative is to use an air splint (see Figure 4.6).

The athlete should be instructed to elevate the leg and ankle for the rest of that day and night by placing a suitcase or sleeping bag under the end of the mattress. A few pillows beneath the heel are useless.

Over the next twenty-four hours, the athlete should start stretching and eversion exercises. Stretching is performed by placing a band or towel over the end of the foot, which is dorsiflexed and then actively plantar flexed. These movements are performed gently. The ankle should not be forced into either dorsiflexion or plantar flexion. The purpose of this exercise is to inhibit the onset of the all-too-common Achilles-tendon–calf-muscle spasm and tightness. These exercises should not be used with severe ankle injuries.

Eversion exercises should at first be isometric. Elastic resistance can be added later. "Writing the alphabet" with the toes in a slush bucket (ice and water) is also a useful exercise.

The next stage is cryokinetics, in which the ankle is iced for twenty minutes, after which the athlete attempts to walk as normally as possible until the numbing effect of the ice wears off and the ankle again becomes painful. This procedure is repeated a number of times.

Crutches should be used if the athlete is unable to walk normally without pain, and even with crutches the athlete should use partial or touch-weight bearing (see section on crutch usage, p. 91). Use of crutches should continue until the athlete can walk normally without any limp. Touch-weight bearing is used in order to

1. encourage a normal sequence of muscle response to proprioceptive stimuli, which occurs when the foot touches the ground. These responses will be lost if the foot is kept immobilized and away from the ground for a period of time.

2. prevent stiffness of the posterior tissues. Rehabilitation is started immediately in all cases of mild-to-moderate ankle sprains and in some cases of severe, sta-

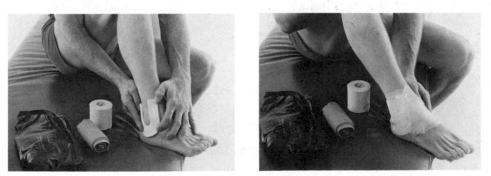

FIGURE 20.22　Ankle sprain　A felt horseshoe pad may be used for compression.

ble sprains (see section on ankle rehabilitation).

Severe second-degree or third-degree sprains.
The severe second-degree or third-degree sprain usually requies a posterior splint or full below-knee cast. With a posterior splint, the athlete can still ice, elevate, apply compression wrap, and do dorsiflexion and plantar-stretching, isometric eversion, and toe-curling exercises.

In very severe cases of ligamentous rupture, surgical repair may need to be undertaken.[39]

ANKLE AND FOOT REHABILITATION

Some differences in the management of ankle and knee injuries are found in Table 20.6. The rehabilitation program is divided into five stages (Table 20.8). Each stage is a relative period of time, varying from perhaps fifteen minutes for a mild ankle sprain to perhaps five to seven days for a more severe injury. The program is designed to literally prevent the athlete from running before he or she can walk. Each stage should be completed before progressing to the next. This means that the athlete should be able to walk before attempting heel-raises; should

do heel-raises before hopping; should hop before jumping rope; should jump rope before jogging; and should jog before running and cutting.[40]

The purpose of ankle rehabilitation is to

1. increase the strength of the muscles around the ankle joint

2. educate the athlete about where the ankle and foot actually are in space, as proprioceptive feedback is frequently impaired following an ankle injury

3. prevent the stiffness that often accompanies a poorly treated ankle sprain

Stage I.   (See sections on on-field management of the injured ankle, p. 390 and continuing treatment, p. 391.)

Stage II.

1. It is often helpful to use a cold whirlpool (4°C to 16°C [39.2°F to 60.8°F]) on the day after an ankle injury. The ankle and foot should be gently but actively moved in the whirlpool.

2. Achilles stretching in the whirlpool is performed with a muslin wrap around the foot (Figure 20.24). This should not be done for more than five minutes at a time, as

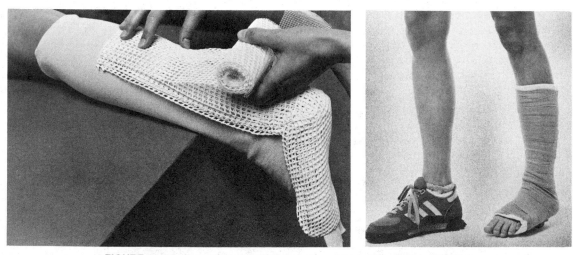

FIGURE 20.23   A posterior splint made from Hexcelite casting material

TABLE 20.8 Outline of an Ankle Rehabilitation Program

Stage I

No.	Exercise	I	II	III	IV	V
1.	Ice, compression, and elevation	+				
2.	Taping—Gibney's open basketweave	+				
	or elastic wrap with horseshoe pad	+				
	or posterior splint					
	(severe or very painful cases)					
	or Airstirrup					
3.	Gentle dorsiflexion and plantar flexion	+				
	(not with severe injuries)					
4.	Crutches with feather-weight bearing	+				

allowing the foot to hang down can increase the swelling. The ankle should be iced and well elevated for about ten minutes.

3. The cycle of pain-immobility-stiffness-pain often hinders rapid return to participation. One way to break this cycle is by means of ice therapy (cryokinetics).[41] Ice or ice massage is applied to the injured area for about ten to fifteen minutes (it is often useful to use ice for about five minutes, followed by ice massage for about five to seven minutes). When the ankle is well numbed, the athlete walks as normally as possible until discomfort is felt. The leg should again be elevated and iced and the walking repeated. It must be stressed that a normal walking motion should be achieved and that there should be no limp. If there is a significant limp, it indicates that the athlete is not yet ready for this exercise.

TABLE 20.8 Outline of an Ankle Rehabilitation Program (*cont.*)

Stage II

No.	Exercise	I	II	III	IV	V
1.	ROM in cold whirlpool		+			
2.	Achilles stretching with muslin wrap		+			
	(can be done in cold whirlpool)					
3.	Alternate icing and walking		+	+		
4.	Contrast application of ice and warmth		+	+		
5.	Isometric peroneal exercises		+			
6.	Partner exercises—eversion, dorsiflexion, and plantar flexion		+	+		
7.	Proprioceptive standing		+	+	+	+
8.	Toe-curls, marble pick-up, alphabet writing		+	+	+	+
9.	Bicycle ergometer—upper body conditioning		+	+	+	+
10.	Swimming and running in swimming pool		+	+	+	+
11.	Ice and elevation after rehabilitation session		+	+	+	+
12.	Supportive taping		+	+	+	+

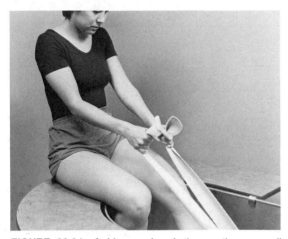

FIGURE 20.24 Ankle sprain Active motion as well as passive Achilles stretching can be performed in a cold whirlpool bath.

4. Some trainers like to use "contrast baths," as they feel this helps remove swelling from around the ankle. If contrast applications are used, they should start and finish with ice.

5. Isometric peroneal exercises are performed by the athlete's keeping the heel fixed against the ground or floor while sitting with the knee bent at 90°. A weighted object, such as a 10 lb (4.5 Kg) sandbag, is placed against the outside of the foot near the toes. The peroneal muscles are isometrically contracted in an attempt to move the foot toward eversion. This contraction is maintained for five seconds or longer.

6. For lateral ligament injuries, the ankle is first moved into eversion against the trainer's light resistance. It is then brought back to the neutral position (but not into inversion). This is repeated about twenty times. The resistance is gradually increased. The same method is used for dorsiflexion and plantar flexion, working eventually toward inversion (see Figure 8.5b).

7. This is a simple way to exercise proprioceptive feedback. The athlete stands on the injured foot, closes his or her eyes, attempts to maintain balance without wobbling or fall-

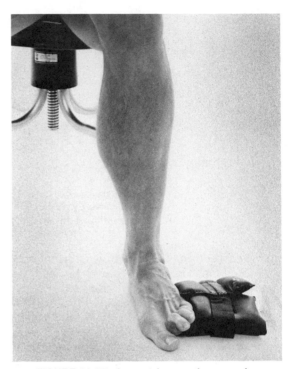

FIGURE 20.25 Isometric eversion exercise

ing over. This exercise should be performed for one or two minutes at a time.[21]

8. Toe-curling exercises can be done with a towel on the floor. The athlete curls up the towel with his or her toes. Other exercises include picking up marbles with the toes or writing the alphabet in a bucket of ice slush.

9. There is no reason for any athlete suffering from an ankle injury to lose cardiovascular fitness. A bicycle ergometer should be used from the first day onward. The ankle can be stabilized by taping the foot or by using a posterior splint. A combination high-resistance, low-speed and low-resistance, high-speed cycling should be used for a minimum of twenty to forty minutes each day. Most fit athletes in their late teens or early twenties should maintain a heart rate of at least 150 beats per minute while working out on the ergometer. Conditioning exercises for the upper body, the unaffected leg, and the

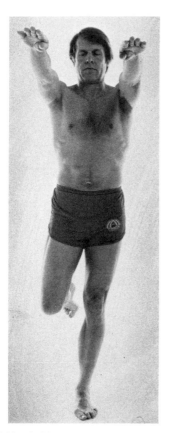

FIGURE 20.26 Ankle proprioception exercise The athlete balances on one leg with eyes closed.

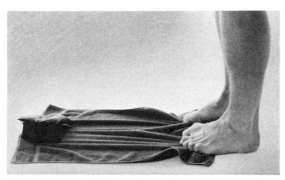

FIGURE 20.27 Toe-curling exercise Using a towel to help develop the smaller muscles of the foot

upper part of the affected leg should be performed.

10. Swimming and running in the swimming pool also maintains cardiovascular fitness. The ankle should be taped, but no vigorous kicking should be permitted.

11. The ankle should be iced and elevated for twenty to thirty minutes at the end of the rehabilitation session. This should continue as long as there is (a) swelling, (b) pain, or (c) tenderness.

12. During the first five to ten days, the ankle should be retaped after each rehabilitation session. The tape should be worn during the day and removed only for whirlpool or icing (see Chapter 5). The ankle should also be taped whenever functional exercises are performed. An alternative to continued taping is the AirStirrup, an air cast which appears to stabilize the ankle relatively satisfactorily (see Figure 4.6).

Stage III.

1. The ice and exercise program is advanced from walking to doing heel-raises. The athlete stands about two feet away from the treatment table and leans forward, hand resting on the table. Both heels are then raised while holding the table. This is repeated a number of times. When the ankle becomes uncomfortable, ice and ice massage are reapplied, followed by repetition of the heel-raises (Figure 20.28).

2. The next stage is to heel-raise without holding onto the table.

3. When the athlete can heel-raise with both legs without any problem, he or she begins heel-raising with the affected leg while holding the table, again using ice before and after.

4. When number 3 is accomplished, the athlete can proceed to heel-raises with the affected leg, holding onto the table only for balance.

5. The same sequence is used for hopping, starting with both legs while holding the ta-

TABLE 20.8   Outline of an Ankle Rehabilitation Program (*cont.*)

Stage III

No.	Exercise	I	II	III	IV	V
1.	Ice, then heel-raises—both legs while holding table			+		
2.	Ice, then heel-raises—both legs without holding table			+		
3.	Ice, then heel-raises—affected legs while holding table			+		
4.	Ice, then heel-raises—affected leg without holding table			+		
5.	Repeat 1–5 while hopping			+		
6.	Isotonic peroneal exercises with elastic band			+	+	+
7.	Achilles stretching—standing			+	+	+
8.	Toe-curls with weighted resistance			+	+	+
9.	Heel-raises with 2″ (5 cm) board			+		
10.	Heel-and-toe walking			+	+	
11.	Isokinetic resistance			+	+	+
12.	Gluteus medius exercise			+	+	

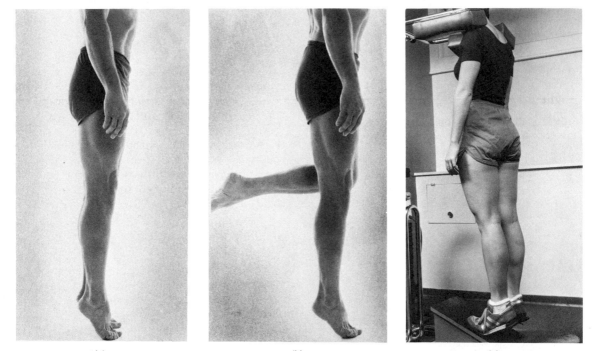

(a)   (b)   (c)

FIGURE 20.28   (a & b) Heel-raising exercise   To progress rapidly, this exercise should initially be performed using both legs and the support of a table. As confidence and strength are gained, the affected leg may be worked independently of support.   **(c) Advanced heel-raising exercise**—weighted resistance plus the use of a slant board.

ble, followed by both legs without support; then the affected leg while holding onto the table, followed by the affected leg without support.

6. The peroneal muscles stabilize and help protect the ankle from inversion sprains. An elastic band (sections of an inner tube) or elastic tubing can be used. The athlete sits with the knee flexed 45° to 90°, the heel resting firmly on the floor. The affected foot is adducted, so the heels are about twelve inches apart and the toes are nearly touching. The band is around the forefoot. The affected foot is then abducted and everted. This maneuver should be repeated ten to thirty times a day and continued for the entire length of the rehabilitation program.

7. Refer to Figure 3.6 for Achilles stretching. One leg is stretched at a time. The athlete leans forward against the wall. The leg is fully extended at the knee and the heel is on the ground. He or she holds for twenty seconds. The knee is then bent and the stretch repeated for twenty seconds. This should be a very gentle stretch without any force or bounce, and though there may be a slight burning, no pain should be felt. It is important that the athlete keep the foot

pointed forward and not abducted, with the weight on the lateral side of the foot, so that the foot does not pronate. A slant board (Figure 20.30) can also be used.[42] Achilles stretching should be done on the affected as well as the unaffected side, and it should become a standard exercise in the athlete's workout schedule.

8. For toe-curls a towel is placed on the floor and a weight added to the far end. The athlete tries to curl up the towel with the toes.[43]

9. When some flexibility returns to the Achilles, heel-raises are performed with the forepart of the foot on a 2″ (5 cm) board. This promotes stretching of the gastrocne-

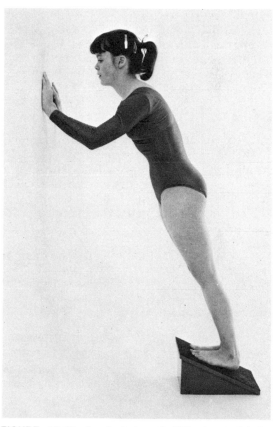

FIGURE 20.30 A slant board This is useful for stretching the gastrocnemius-soleus muscle group and the Achilles tendon.

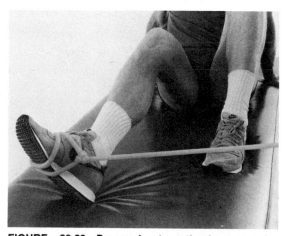

FIGURE 20.29 Peroneal strengthening exercise Elasticized tubing or a rubber band is used as resistance. The heel is kept firmly on the ground as the forefoot is brought into abduction.

mius muscle and strengthening of the Achilles tendon. Resistance is provided by either the bench-press portion of the Universal Gym or a special toe-raising resistance machine. Dumbbells can also be used; barbells are not recommended initially because of the danger of the athlete's losing balance and re-injuring the ankle.

10. Heel- and toe-walking are useful, simple methods of strengthening the lower leg muscles.

11. If isokinetic resistance is available, it should be utilized on a daily basis for strength, power, and endurance. Both inversion-eversion and dorsiflexion-plantar flexion movements should be performed.

12. An interesting phenomenon is the frequent occurrence of gluteus medius weakness following an ankle sprain.[44] To strengthen the gluteus medius, use elastic tubing. The athlete abducts the leg 30°, keeping the knee straight and the body erect (Figure 20.31).

Stage IV.

1. There are various isotonic machines available for strengthening the muscles around the ankle (Figure 20.32). However, if one does not have access to such machinery, a simple sandbag can achieve results. The athlete sits on the end of a treatment table with one or more sandbags attached to the

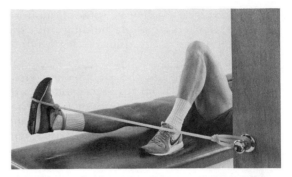

FIGURE 20.31   Strengthening hip abduction (gluteus medius) using elastic tubing The gluteus medius muscle is often found to be weak following an ankle sprain.

foot. Eversion, inversion, dorsiflexion, and rotation are all movements that can be exercised with this method.

2. & 3. Useful proprioceptive exercises are hopping on one foot while bouncing a ball against a wall and balancing on a tiltboard (Figure 20.33). The balance board is a simple device: a croquet ball cut through its top third to produce a flat surface, which is secured to a round board approximately 15″ (37.5 cm) in diameter. The athlete should be careful in the beginning when using this board, and should probably be aided initially, otherwise re-injury might occur.

4. & 5. Running can now be incorporated into the program; at first, straight-ahead jog-

TABLE 20.8   Outline of an Ankle Rehabilitation Program (*cont.*)

Stage IV

No.	Exercise	Stage I	II	III	IV	V
1.	Isotonic ankle machines or sandbags				+	+
2.	Hopping and bouncing a ball simultaneously				+	+
3.	Balance board				+	+
4.	Jogging				+	+
5.	Running rapidly in place				+	+
6.	Jumping rope				+	+
7.	Hopping up stairs and in figure eights				+	+

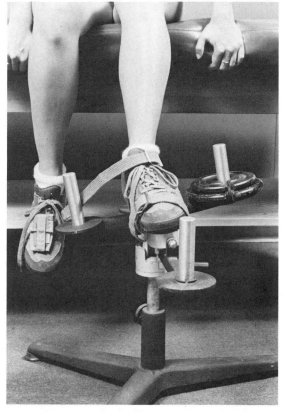

FIGURE 20.32 Ankle-strengthening device

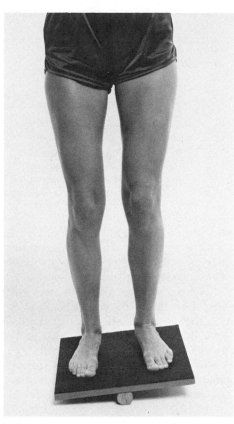

FIGURE 20.33 Balancing on a tilt board This exercise helps improve balance and proprioception. It may be done as a training exercise, but is particularly useful in the later stages of ankle rehabilitation.

ging only. This can be augmented by running rapidly in place with the feet toeing slightly inward and the arms pumping vigorously (see section on knee rehabilitation, p. 346).

6. Rope jumping should begin with low jumps on both feet. One-legged jumping on the affected leg can be started when there is no discomfort or apprehension of instability.

7. Hopping up the stairs and in figure eights develops strength and proprioceptive feedback. Initially, only a few stairs should be attempted, gradually increasing in number.

Stage V. The final functional exercises are designed to put the ankle through its fullest range of movement and to make sure it can withstand the stress of active competition.

1. & 2. Wind sprints alternating with jogging are started, followed by Fartlek-type running.

3. Running backwards is useful for developing proprioception and confidence.

4. Side-to-side jumping is performed with the legs together. Two lines are drawn on the ground approximately five feet apart, and the athlete jumps sideways from one line to another while progressing forward. This can be made more difficult by having the athlete jump sideways as well as forward over a bench.

5. Figure eights, crossovers, sideways running, and sport-specific patterns. Figure

TABLE 20.8   Outline of an Ankle Rehabilitation Program (cont.)

Stage V

No.	Exercise	I	II	III	IV	V
1.	Running sprints					+
2.	Fartlek-type running					+
3.	Running backward					+
4.	Side-to-side jumping					+
5.	Running—figure eights, crossovers, sideways, and in sport-specific patterns					+

eights should be large at first and performed at a slow pace. As increasing confidence is gained, smaller and smaller figure eights are run with increasing speed.

Crossovers are used in two different forms. The same leg can cross over in front each time, or alternate legs can cross over in front. Crossovers should be done in both directions (to the right and to the left).

Sideways running consists of vigorous sprints over a distance of approximately fifteen yards. The athlete runs sideways and touches the ground at the farthest mark, then returns to the starting place. This is repeated nonstop about twenty times.

Sport-specific patterns should also be run where this is applicable.

CONDITIONS ASSOCIATED WITH ANKLE SPRAINS

The following conditions may be associated with an ankle sprain, or they may occur independently but with mechanisms similar to those causing ankle sprains.

Osteochondral Fracture of the Dome of the Talus

These fractures are often missed or may not be detected at all on the initial X-rays.[45] The injury can follow any type of ankle sprain. The commonest area of involvement is the superolateral dome of the talus. Tenderness

over this area should make one suspect this type of fracture (Figure 20.34). These injuries are usually treated conservatively and closely watched—they may need to be treated surgically if they do not heal.[46]

Subluxing Peroneal Tendons

A peroneal tendon subluxation can be confused with an ankle sprain, because it may give the athlete a feeling of instability as well

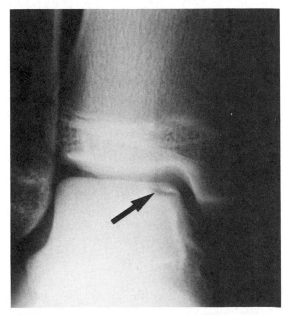

FIGURE 20.34 X-ray—osteochondral fracture of the dome of the talus

as producing tenderness and swelling over the lateral malleolus. The initial injury may follow sudden dorsiflexion and eversion of the ankle, as when correcting an inversion twist.[47] However, it can occur from plantar flexion and eversion. The retinaculum gives way and the tendon slips out over the lateral malleolus and usually spontaneously returns.

The subluxing tendon is best diagnosed with the foot in dorsiflexion and everted against resistance. The tendons may be felt to slip over the lateral malleolus. Treatment, after the inflammation has resolved, is to place a horseshoe-shaped pad around the lateral malleolus, attempting to compress the tendons and keep them in place. If this is unsuccessful, surgery may be necessary if the condition is symptomatic.[48]

Injury to the Os Trigonum

The os trigonum can be fractured or contused during plantar flexion injuries to the ankle. This condition presents with severe discomfort on the posterior aspect of the ankle, particularly with plantar flexion. In certain individuals, like ballet dancers, removal of the os trignonum may be required.

Achilles Tendon Strain

The Achilles tendon and its surrounding soft tissues are sometimes injured during an ankle sprain and, in fact, may require a longer healing period than the ankle itself.

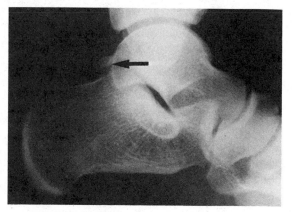

FIGURE 20.35 X-ray—os trigonum

Bifurcated Ligament Sprain

The bifurcated ligament is situated slightly superior to the midpoint of a line running between the lateral malleolus and the base of the fifth metatarsal (Figure 20.36), and it is often involved in sprains of the foot and the ankle. The mechanism is usually in the direction of inversion and may result in either a sprain of the bifurcated ligament or an avulsion fracture of the distal superior pole of the calcaneus.

Diagnosis is made by noting tenderness and swelling directly over the bifurcated ligament. X-rays are normal unless an avulsion fracture of the distal end of the calcaneus is present (Figure 20.37).[49] A bifurcated liga-

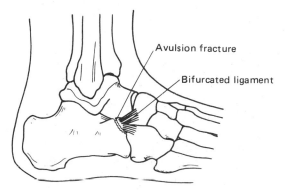

FIGURE 20.36 Avulsion fracture, distal calcaneus

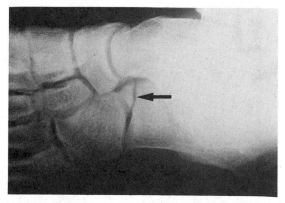

FIGURE 20.37 X-ray—an avulsion fracture off the distal calcaneus at the site of attachment of the bifurcated ligament

ment sprain should be treated like an ankle sprain. Figure eight taping should be used (see Chapter 5). If an avulsion fracture is present, the fragment may need to be excised.[50]

Avulsion Fracture of the Base of the Fifth Metatarsal

An avulsion fracture of the fifth metatarsal base often occurs in conjunction with an inversion sprain. The peroneus brevis or tertius muscle contracts during an inversion, straining the tendon or avulsing a fragment of bone from the base of the fifth metatarsal (Figure 20.38). This condition usually heals if protected as long as the fragment is not avulsed too far off the fifth metatarsal base, in which case surgical correction may be necessary.

OTHER CONDITIONS OF THE ANKLE AND FOOT

Talar Spur (Tibiotalar Impingement)

Repetitive forced dorsiflexion can cause a buildup of spurs over the contact points of the tibia and talus. This can produce pain on dorsiflexion and inability to push off rapidly from a dorsiflexed position. Sometimes the talar spur is palpable. Diagnosis is best made with weight-bearing X-rays and the foot in a maximally dorsiflexed position (Figure 20.39). Treatment consists of surgical removal of the spurs.

Tibiofibular Synostosis

Calcification of the interosseous membrane between tibia and fibula at the inferior

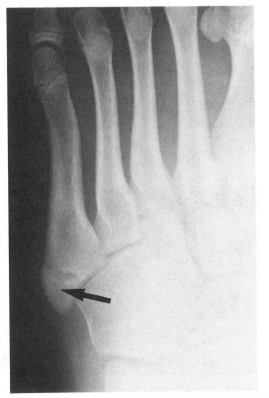

FIGURE 20.38 Avulsion fracture of the base of the fifth metatarsal, due to an inversion injury

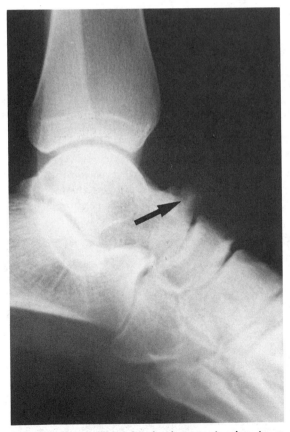

FIGURE 20.39 Tibiotalar impingement—due to a talar spur

tibiofibular syndesmosis can occur after an ankle sprain, particularly after an inversion–internal-rotation sprain, but occasionally after an eversion sprain (Figure 20.40). Some athletes suffer prolonged symptoms, with pain and impaired performance, presumably because of interference with the normal to-and-fro bowing action of the fibula which occurs while running.

Initially, rest followed by rehabilitation exercises may improve the problem in a percentage of these athletes. Some will require surgical treatment, however, which consists of removal of the calcification after it has matured. If surgery is performed too soon, the calcification will recur.[51] Calcification may occur between the tibia and fibula without producing any significant symptoms and does not require any treatment.

Tarsal Tunnel Syndrome

Tarsal tunnel syndrome (entrapment neuropathy of the posterior tibial nerve) generally occurs where the nerve passes through the osseofibrous tunnel between the flexor retinaculum (lacinate ligament) and the medial malleolus. The entrapment is usually the result of abnormal foot function, especially of excessive pronation, which causes tightening of the flexor retinaculum. But it may be caused by a direct injury to the area (i.e., fracture of the medial malleolus or the talus).

SYMPTOMS AND SIGNS: Compression of the medial plantar branch of the posterior tibial nerve results in a burning or tingling sensation or pain in the medial arch region and the ball of the foot. A decrease in sensation may also be present over this area. If the medial calcaneal branch is entrapped, pain may be felt in the heel.

Tenderness is usually elicited over the nerve and just below and above it. Compressing the nerve against the underlying bone may cause pain in the arch or heel area. Tinel's sign (percussion over the nerve) is usually positive for tingling and pain along the course of the nerve.

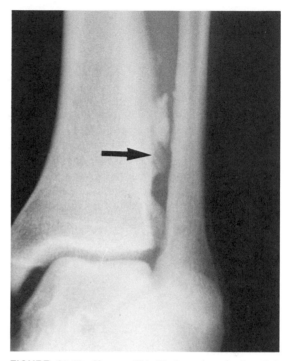

FIGURE 20.40 X-ray—tibiofibular synostosis Calcification of the interosseous membrane between the tibia and fibula

TREATMENT: The tarsal tunnel syndrome may respond to a neutral-position, orthotic device designed to control excessive pronation. Local cortisone injections may be given in an attempt to free the entrapped nerve, but surgical release of the soft tissue causing the entrapment may be necessary.

Fracture of the Diaphysis of the Base of the Fifth Metatarsal

A transverse fracture of the diaphysis of the base of the fifth metatarsal should be differentiated from the more common avulsion fracture (see section on avulsion fractures of the base of the fifth metatarsal, p. 402). The transverse fracture of the diaphysis of the fifth metatarsal frequently begins as a stress fracture (see Figure 20.41). This may become a complete fracture if there is an inversion injury, or it may end in nonunion of the stress fracture as a result of repetitive vertical and mediolateral forces.[52] It can occur in identical places on both feet.

TREATMENT: If a stress fracture occurs, the presently accepted form of treatment is to place the athlete in a non-weight-bearing, below-knee cast (some prefer an above-knee cast with the knee flexed to prevent weight bearing). After four weeks, the stage of healing should be assessed. If it is not healed, a decision must be made about whether to (a) continue with the cast immobilization (this may need to be continued for many weeks, as healing is notoriously slow), (b) remove the cast and see if the athlete can function with a non- or fibrous-union, or (c) proceed with surgery. Surgery is frequently required for running athletes, especially basketball players.

An alternative to the conservative wait-and-see approach is to insert a compression screw across the fracture as soon as it is diagnosed. This approach has led to rapid healing of the fracture and early return to athletic endeavors, especially basketball.

The form of treatment that is most applicable varies from case to case, as it is influenced by many factors, including the type of athlete (whether professional or recreational) and the type of sport in which the athlete participates. For instance, a footballer may be able to participate with a nonunion, whereas a basketball player is unlikely to be able to play unless the fracture is completely united. When healed, in-shoe orthotic devices may help redistribute the forces and prevent a recurrence.

Stress Fracture of the Metatarsal

ETIOLOGY: This appears to be related to excessive hypermobility of the foot, especially of the first ray (navicular, first cuneiform, first metatarsal, big toe). It leads to prolonged pronation during the propulsive phase of gait and places considerable stress on the second, third, and fourth metatarsals.

SYMPTOMS AND SIGNS: Pain and swelling are localized to the metatarsal involved. The pain is particularly noticeable during activity. Percussion of the toes may cause pain in the area of the fracture, as will the tuning-fork test (see section on stress fractures, p. 128).

TREATMENT: Supportive taping and specially formed in-shoe orthotic devices may help the athlete continue with activities. However, the intensity and duration of workouts should be decreased for a time. Ice, elevation, and anti-inflammatory medication may be necessary if swelling is present. If pain with ambulation is a problem, a lower-leg walking cast may need to be applied, but it can be removed for rehabilitation.

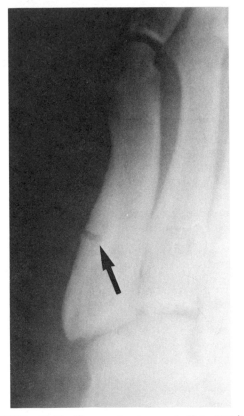

FIGURE 20.41 Stress fracture of the proximal diaphysis of the fifth metatarsal

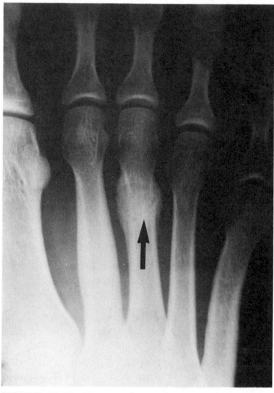

FIGURE 20.42 X-ray—stress fracture of the shaft of the third metatarsal, showing profuse callus formation

Morton's Neuroma (Interdigital Neuroma)

ETIOLOGY: Compression of the bifurcation of the neurovascular bundle between the metatarsal heads can result in the formation of a neuroma (Figure 20.43). This compression is usually due to a shearing force caused by a hypermobile foot with excessive pronation during the propulsive phase of late mid-support and early takeoff.

SYMPTOMS: There are two varieties of presenting symptoms.

Acute—Usually occurring in a sprinter and presenting with an acute electric-shock-like pain radiating from the forefoot down to the toes (usually the third and fourth toes, but it can occur between any two). The ath-

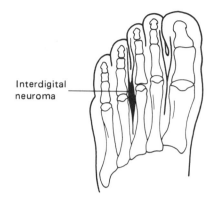

FIGURE 20.43 Morton's neuroma Interdigital neuroma between the third and fourth metatarsal heads

lete rapidly removes the shoe from the foot to obtain relief.

Chronic—Presents with dull discomfort under the foot which, on palpation, is localized to the metatarsal interspace involved. If the condition has been present for some time, changes in sensation along the inside of the toes supplied by that particular nerve can be observed.

TREATMENT: Initially, a metatarsal bar is used to relieve pressure on the nerve, and an in-shoe orthotic device to prevent excessive pronation is prescribed. If these do not produce satisfactory results, a local anesthetic and corticosteroid injection should be used around the neuroma. Surgical excision may be necessary in resistant cases.

Sesamoiditis

A sesamoid bone is one that is found within the substance of a tendon, for example, the patella. In the foot, sesamoids are found within the tendons of the flexor hallucis brevis of the big toe. These sesamoids distribute and disperse the weight of the take-off phase of gait. What is surprising is that so few athletes develop problems related to the sesamoids, as these bones are subjected to considerable force with each strike of the foot.

Usually two sesamoids are present—a medial, or tibial, sesamoid and a lateral, or fibular, sesamoid. The medial sesamoid is not infrequently *bipartite*, that is, the bone shows as two separate pieces on X-rays and this can be confused with a fracture.

Sesamoiditis is an inflammation of the tissues surrounding the sesamoids, which usually affects the medial more than the lateral sesamoid. It occurs most frequently in the cavus type of foot with a rigid, plantar flexed first ray, a high arch, and a tight Achilles tendon, but it can occur in any type of foot.

Tenderness, and sometimes swelling, is localized to the head of the first metatarsal on its plantar aspect. On passive dorsiflexion of the foot and palpation over the head of the first metatarsal, significant discomfort may be felt.

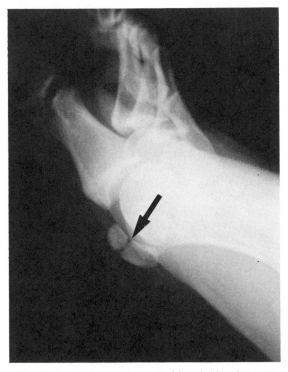

FIGURE 20.44 X-ray—sesamoids A bipartite sesamoid usually has smooth edges, whereas an irregular crack may indicate a fracture or stress fracture.

This condition is best treated with an orthotic device which places the foot near its neutral position and balances the forefoot so that the weight is taken off the painful sesamoid. Ice massage, ultrasound, and other physical therapies, along with anti-inflammatory medication and, occasionally, a cortisone injection may also be used.

The metatarsal sesamoids can also develop stress fractures or, rarely, acute fractures.[53] Conservative treatment, which includes non-weight-bearing on the appropriate part, usually provides adequate results, though surgical removal of the affected sesamoid is sometimes necessary.

Acute Hyperdorsiflexion Injuries to the Metatarsophalangeal Joint of the Big Toe

This type of injury has become more prominent lately, perhaps due to the unyielding surface of artificial turf. Even though the new artificial turf approximates grass in a number of ways, after a few years it becomes much harder. Other predisposing factors include shoes that are very flexible and offer minimal support, and as noted, some athletes' feet are wider than the shoes provided for them, and in an attempt to feel comfortable, they wear longer shoes to obtain more width. These longer shoes have the effect of increasing the forces that act upon the MP joint when hyperdorsiflexed.

Most injuries occur when there is excessive dorsiflexion at the MP joint—the heel is often in the air. If the athlete is then forced toward the ground, the MP joint of the first toe is stressed. Occasionally the second, third, and fourth MP joints are involved, which can cause fractures of the metatarsal shafts, dislocations of the MP joints, or both.

Hyperdorsiflexion of the MP joint results in capsular tears, articular cartilage damage, and possibly a fracture of the medial sesamoid. These injuries may produce major incapacity in terms of discomfort and return to participation.[54]

TREATMENT: Initially, treatment should be with ice, anti-inflammatory medication, and crutches (non-weight-bearing). A posterior plaster splint with a toe extension and walking heel can be used. Walking should be allowed only when performed in a normal fashion without a limp.

In the meantime, the athlete should be cycling, swimming, and doing foot and toe exercises that do not cause any discomfort (see section on ankle rehabilitation, p. 392). As the athlete improves, graduated running activities can be started, but these should only be undertaken when the athlete is pain free, which might take a considerable time. The toe should be taped in plantar flexion, and the shoe should be firm enough to prevent excessive dorsiflexion of the MP joint. A steel spring plate or Orthoplast sole can be incorporated into the shoe. Surgery is usually undertaken only in resistant cases where healing does not occur.

Corns and Calluses

Both corns and calluses are composed of the same type of tissue and are a thickening of the skin in response to friction or trauma. Corns are found on the toes, whereas calluses are lesions on the plantar aspect of the foot.

Corns may be either hard or soft. Hard corns usually occur on top of the toes; soft corns are found between the toes and are kept soft by perspiration. Soft corns result from pressure of one toe against another and are often caused by shoes that are too narrow.

Calluses are generally found beneath the metatarsal heads. They may be divided into shearing or nonshearing types. The nonshearing callus is the most common and is the result of friction between the bottom of the foot and the shoe. It is often not painful but should be controlled with a callus file or a pumice stone. The shearing-type callus is the result of pressure of a metatarsal head against the underlying skin. Like a corn, this callus can be painful and is best treated by

correcting the mechanical problem causing the shearing action of the foot. Customized orthotic devices usually provide relief.

As shoes are the most important causative factor of either corns or calluses, the trainer should examine and evaluate them. In addition to proper length and width, depth of the toe box is of primary consideration in shoe selection. If there is a great deal of deformity in the toes, or there is a plantar displacement of the metatarsal heads, orthotics or protective padding may be necessary. If these measures fail to alleviate the problem, surgical correction provides good results in most cases.

Blisters

Blisters are common in athletes. They result from friction, which causes a separation of skin layers and allows fluid to accumulate between the layers. They may be quite painful and can become infected if not treated properly.

The two primary causes are improperly fitted shoes and abnormal foot function, and they may be prevented by the choice of a proper shoe, orthotic devices if necessary, and/or correct taping techniques. Some athletes use two pair of socks. Vaseline and Spenco SecondSkin may also be helpful.

If the blister is more than one 1 cm in diameter and is painful, it may be desirable to drain it. The skin over and around the blister should be cleansed with alcohol or Betadine, and a sterile needle or blade used to lance the blister. This should be followed by the application of a topical antibiotic to the site, which is then covered with Spenco SecondSkin or with a "sandwich" of Vaseline between two adhesive bandages, the top one being the larger of the two. This allows motion to take place between the bandages without involving the skin.

Ingrown Toenails

Ingrown toenails result from the nail plate becoming imbedded in the surrounding tissue. This occurs for a variety of reasons, in-

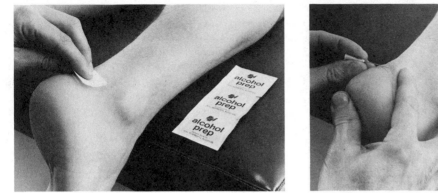

(a)

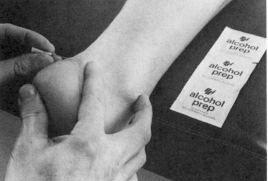

(b)

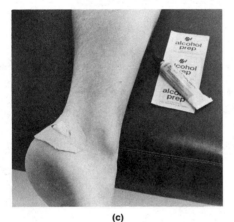

(c)

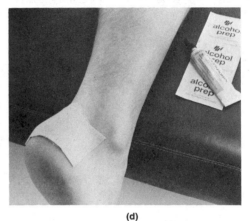

(d)

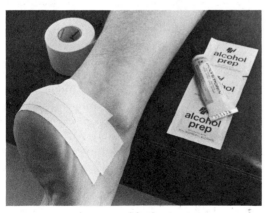

(e)

FIGURE 20.45 Draining a blister (a) The area around the blister is thoroughly cleaned with alcohol or Betadine. (b) The trainer's hands should be surgically clean or sterile gloves should be worn. A sterile needle is used to pierce the blister. (c) The roof of the blister is left on. Antibiotic ointment (such as Polysporin) is applied over the blister. A moleskin "donut" is applied around the blister. (d) A moleskin cover is then applied. (e) If desired, a final layer of tape may be useful in securing the moleskin.

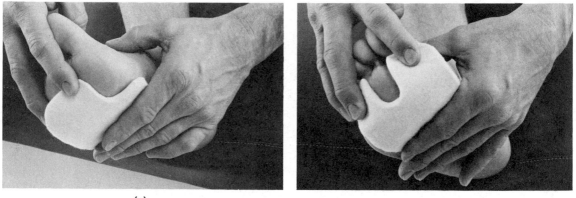

(a) **(b)**

FIGURE 20.46 Felt pad accommodations (a) Pain under the first metatarsal head may result from a callus, blister or sesamoiditis. The felt is cut out to accomodate the painful area, and tapered off towards the second through fifth toes. **(b)** Pain under the head of one of the other metatarsals, from a callus, metatarsalgia, or a neuroma.

cluding direct trauma to the toenail, improperly fitted shoes, and incorrect trimming of the toenails.

The ingrown toenail may require local antibiotic ointment if the area becomes infected, and the offending nail border may need to be surgically removed. If the nail is then kept properly trimmed, and shoes which provide adequate depth, width, and length are worn, permanent relief can result. However, if these measures fail, it may be necessary to remove the offending nail completely. This will usually provide permanent relief from the problem.

Note: Additional injuries of the lower leg and foot are discussed in Chapter 21.

REFERENCES

1. Laurin C, Mathieu J: Sagittal mobility of the normal ankle. *Clin Orthop* 108:99–104, 1975.

2. Root ML, Orien WP, Weed JH: *Normal and Abnormal Function of the Foot.* Los Angeles, Clinical Biomechanics Corporation, 1977.

3. Gunther SF: An avoidable soccer injury. *Am J Sports Med* 2:167–169, 1974.

4. Arner O, Lindholm Å: What is tennis leg? *Acta Chir Scand* 116:73–77, 1958.

5. Miller WA: Rupture of musculotendinous juncture of the medial head of gastrocnemius muscle. *Am J Sports Med* 5:191–193, 1977.

6. Lee HB: Avulsion and rupture of the tendo calcaneus after injection of hydrocortisone. *Brit Med J* 2:395, 1957.

7. Melmed EP: Spontaneous bilateral rupture of the calcaneal tendon during steroid therapy. *J Bone Joint Surg* 47B:104–105, 1965.

8. Thompson TC, Dougherty JH: Spontaneous rupture of tendo achilles. A new clinical diagnostic test. *J Trauma* 2:126–129, 1962.

9. Ranney DA: A good test by any other name. Letter to the editor. *Phys Sportsmed* 8:10, December 1980.

10. Arner O, Lindholm Å, Lindvall N: Subcutaneous rupture of the achilles tendon. *Acta Chir Scand* 119:523–525, 1960.

11. Rubin BD, Wilson HJ: Surgical repair of the interrupted achilles tendon. *J Trauma* 20:248–249, 1980.

12. DiSteffano VJ, Nixon JE: Ruptures of the achilles tendon. *J Sports Med* 1:34–37, 1975.

13. Stein SR, Luekens CA: Methods and rationale for closed treatment of achilles tendon ruptures. *Am J Sports Med* 4:162–169, 1976.

14. Shields CL, Kerlan RK, Jobe FW, et al: The Cybex II evaluation of surgically repaired achilles tendon ruptures. *Am J Sports Med* 6:369–372, 1978.

15. Skeoch DU: Spontaneous partial subcutaneous ruptures of the tendo achilles. Review of the literature and evaluation of 16 involved tendons. *Am J Sports Med* 9:20–22, 1981.

16. Santilli G: Achilles tendinopathies and para-tendinopathies. *J Sports Med* 19:245–259, 1979.

17. Denstad TF, Roaas A: Surgical treatment of partial achilles tendon rupture. *Am J Sports Med* 7:15–17, 1979.

18. McCluskey GM, Blackburn A, Lewis T: Prevention of ankle sprains. *Am J Sports Med* 4:151–157, 1976.

19. Glick JM, Gordon RB, Nishimoto D: The prevention and treatment of ankle injuries. *Am J Sports Med* 4:136–141, 1976.

20. Walsch WM, Blackburn TA: Prevention of ankle sprains. *Am J Sports Med* 5:243–245, 1977.

21. Freeman MAR, Dean MR, Hanham IW: Etiology and prevention of functional instability of the foot. *J Bone Joint Surg* 47B:678–685, 1965.

22. Blyth CS, Mueller FO: *Football Injuries.* Minneapolis, McGraw-Hill Inc., 1974, p 19.

23. Torg JS, Quedenfeld TC, Landau S: The shoe-surface interface and its relationship to football knee injuries. *Am J Sports Med* 2:261–269, 1974.

24. Garrick JG: The frequency of injury, mechanism of injury and epidemiology of ankle sprains. *Am J Sports Med* 5:241–242, 1977.

25. Broström L: Sprained ankles. I. Anatomic lesions in recent sprains. *Acta Chir Scand* 128:483–495, 1964.

26. Almquist GA: The pathomechanics and diagnosis of inversion injuries to the lateral ligaments of the ankle. *J Sports Med* 2:109, 1974.

27. Guise ER: Rotational ligamentous injuries to the ankle in football. *Am J Sports Med* 4:1–6, 1976.

28. Israeli A, Horoszowski H, Chechick A, et al: Beware the "simple" fibular fracture. *Br J Sports Med* 15:269–271, 1981.

29. Broström L: Sprained ankles VI. Surgical treatment of "chronic" ligament ruptures. *Acta Chir Scand* 132:551–565, 1966.

30. Laurin CA, Quellet R, St Jacques R: Talar and subtalar tilt: An experimental investigation *Can J Surg* 11:270–279, 1968.

31. Roy SP: Evaluation and treatment of the stable ankle sprain. *Phys Sportsmed* 5:60–63, August 1977.

32. Frost HM, Hanson CA: Technique for testing the drawer sign in the ankle. *Clin Orthop* 123:49–51, 1977.

33. Cox JS, Hewes TF: "Normal" talar tilt angle. *Clin Orthop* 140:37–41, 1979.

34. Evans GA, Frenyo SD: The stress-tenogram in the diagnosis of ruptures of the lateral ligament of the ankle. *J Bone Joint Surg* 61B:347–351, 1979.

35. Johannsen A: Radiological diagnosis of lateral ligament lesion of the ankle. A comparison between talar tilt and anterior drawer sign. *Acta Chir Scand* 49:295–301, 1978.

36. Black HM, Brand RL, Eichelberger MR: An improved technique for the evaluation of ligamentous injury in severe ankle sprains. *Am J Sports Med* 6:276–282, 1978.

37. Lindstrand A: New aspects in diagnosis of lateral ankle sprains. *Orthop Clin North Am* 7:247–249, 1976.

38. Ala-Ketola L, Puranen J, Koivisto E, et al: Arthrography in the diagnosis of ligament injuries and classification of ankle injuries. *Radiology* 125:63–68, 1977.

39. Broström L: Sprained ankles. V. Treatment and prognosis in recent ligament ruptures. *Acta Chir Scand* 132:537–550, 1966.

40. Garrick JG: When can I . . . . ? A practical approach to rehabilitation illustrated by treatment of an ankle injury. *Am J Sports Med* 9:67–68, 1981.

41. Knight KL: Ankle rehabilitation with cryotherapy. *Phys Sportsmed* 7:133, November, 1979.

42. McCluskey GM, Blackburn A, Lewis T: A treatment for ankle sprains. *Am J Sports Med* 4:158–161, 1976.

43. Grimes DW, Bennion D, Blush K: Functional foot reconditioning exercises. *Am J Sports Med* 6:194–198, 1978.

44. Nicholas JA, Strizak AM, Veras G: A study of thigh muscle weakness in different pathological states of the lower extremity. *Am J Sports Med* 4:241–248, 1976.

45. Smith GR, Winquist RA, Allan NK, et al: Subtle transchondral fractures of the talar dome: a radiological perspective. *Radiology* 124:667–673, 1977.

46. Canale ST, Belding RH: Osteochondral lesions of the talus. *J Bone Joint Surg* 62A:97–102, 1980.

47. Marti R: Dislocations of the peroneal tendons. *Am J Sports Med* 5:19–22, 1977.

48. McLennan JG: Treatment of acute and chronic luxations of the peroneal tendons. *Am J Sports Med* 8:432–436, 1980.

49. Arner O, Lindholm Å: Avulsion fracture of the os calcaneus. *Acta Chir Scand* 117:258–260, 1959.

50. Degan TJ, Morrey BF, Braun DP: Surgical excision for anterior-process fractures of the calcaneus. *J Bone Joint Surg* 64A:519–524, 1982.

51. Levinthal DH, Kaplan L: Post-traumatic ossifying hematoma of the interosseous tibiofibular ligament in the lower leg. *Clin Orthop* 23:171–184, 1962.

52. Dameron Jr, TB: Fractures and anatomical variations of the proximal portion of the fifth metatarsal. *J Bone Joint Surg* 57A:788–792, 1975.

53. Zinman H, Keret D, Reis ND: Fracture of the medial sesamoid bone of the hallux. *J Trauma* 21:581–582, 1981.

54. Coker TP, Arnold J, Weber D: Traumatic lesions of the metatarsophalangeal joint of the great toe in athletes. *Am J Sports Med* 6:326–334, 1978.

RECOMMENDED READINGS

Broström L: Sprained ankles. III. Clinical observations in recent ligament ruptures. *Acta Chir Scand* 130:560–569, 1965.

Broström L: Sprained ankles. IV. Histologic changes in recent and "chronic" ligament ruptures. *Acta Chir Scand* 132:248–253, 1966.

Cetti R: Conservative treatment of injury to the fibular ligaments of the ankle. *Brit J Sports Med* 16:47–52, 1982.

Cleaves G: Orthoplast Splint: Support method for a sprained ankle. *Athletic Training* 15:94–95, 1980.

Freeman MAR: Treatment of ruptures of the lateral ligament of the ankle. *J Bone Joint Surg* 47B:661–668, 1965.

Glasgow M, Jackson A, Jamieson AM: Instability of the ankle after injury to the lateral ligament. *J Bone Joint Surg* 62B:196–200, 1980.

Inman V: *The Joints of the Ankle.* Baltimore, Williams and Wilkins, 1976.

Lindstrand A: Clinical diagnosis of lateral ankle sprains. In *Injuries of the Ligaments and their Repair: Hand — Knee — Foot*, edited by Chapchal G. Littleton MA, PSG Publisher, 1977, pp 178–180.

Symposium: Soft tissue injuries about the ankle. Is there a rational approach to the diagnosis and treatment? *Am J Sports Med* 5:225–257, 1977.

CHAPTER 21

Injuries to the Running Athlete — Particularly the Long-Distance Runner

The Biomechanics of a Normal Running Gait

One of the major differences between walking and running is that during running the body is totally airborne for a period of time. When observing a runner from the side, notice that the stride is divided into two distinct phases:

1. Phase I: The *contact* phase—one foot is in contact with the ground

2. Phase II: The *swing* phase—the leg and foot are swinging through the air[1,2]

Each of these phases may be further broken down as follows:

1. contact phase (Figure 21.1)
   a. foot strike
   b. mid-support
   c. take-off
2. swing phase (Figure 21.2)
   a. follow-through
   b. forward swing
   c. foot descent

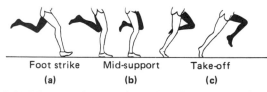

FIGURE 21.1 The running gait—the contact phase
(note the movement of the unshaded leg)

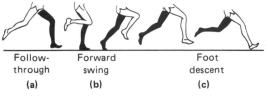

FIGURE 21.2 The running gait—the swing phase

The contact phase. Runners contact the ground in one of three ways[3] (Figure 21.3):

1. With the heel

2. Flat-footed or with the ball of the foot, followed by rocking back onto the heel

3. On the ball of the foot

For purposes of description, this discussion assumes that the contact phase is initiated by heel contact. This phase consists of three parts.

1. *Foot strike*: Initial heel contact is normally on the lateral aspect. This is due to the varus angle formed by the lower leg in relationship to the ground during running, as well as by the supinated position of the foot at the moment of impact. The entire foot then sequentially makes contact with the ground, as the heel moves toward eversion and the midtarsal joint moves toward pronation.

2. *Mid-support*: During foot strike and mid-support, the foot is loose, and is easily able to adapt to the uneven surface and act as a

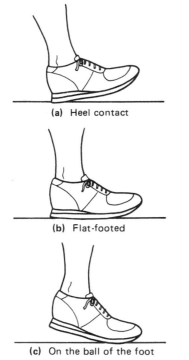

(a) Heel contact

(b) Flat-footed

(c) On the ball of the foot

FIGURE 21.3   Variations in foot contact in runners

shock absorber. This is because of the pronatory action of the subtalar and midtarsal joints, which allows the foot to be a *loose adaptor*. During mid-support, the tarsal joint reaches the limit of pronation. At the same time, the lower leg passes over the foot and the heel starts to rise from the ground. This is a critical time for the foot to change its function—from being a loose "bag of bones" adapting to the surface and absorbing shock to being a powerful and firm lever propelling the body forward.

3. *Take-off*: During this phase the foot is moving toward a supinated position. The muscle action and the angular relationships of the tarsals result in the foot being *locked*. In most athletes the big toe is passively dorsiflexed, and it very seldom actively plantar flexes. In these athletes it does not "flip" the foot off the ground. The value of the big toe being able to actively plantar flex is still an open question.

The Effects of Foot Movements on the Lower Extremities

The lower leg is forced to follow the action of the foot, as can be easily observed by looking at someone who is standing. When the arch of the foot is lowered, the tibia rotates inwardly; when the arch is raised, the tibia rotates externally. This also has an effect on the patella and the femur (Figure 21.4).

When watching an athlete run (particularly with the aid of high-speed movies), notice how the tibia is slightly externally rotated at the beginning of foot strike. As pronation occurs during the mid-support phase, the tibia is forced to follow the subtalar joint movement, and it rotates internally. The tibia again rotates externally when supination occurs during the latter part of the take-off phase.

The angle of the femoral neck influences the angle of the knee and the position of the foot. The femur rotates in the same direction as the tibia (internal rotation during midsupport; external rotation during take-off), but it is not quite so obligated to follow the foot. The patella tends to follow the movement of the femur, by virtue of its position in the intercondylar groove of that bone.

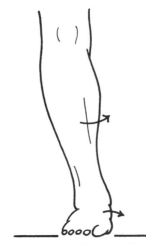

FIGURE 21.4   Foot pronation results in internal rotation of the tibia

The posture of the athlete, particularly that of the lower back, greatly influences the way the legs and feet are able to function. An erect posture allows the legs to work in the most efficient manner and the feet to strike the ground in the optimum position (Figure 21.5). Conversely, foot function also affects the posture of the lumbar spine.

Anatomical Variations

The description just given is of the ideal. There are many variations on this theme, some of which may result in the development of injuries associated with running.

1. Tibia varum and calcaneus varus may require a considerable amount of pronation through the midtarsal joint so that the first metatarsal head is brought down to the ground.

2. A tight Achilles tendon can cause either early heel lift-off or excessive pronation, in order to enable the leg to pass over the foot.

3. A tight Achilles tendon can be associated with a high-arched (cavus) foot, a rigid first ray which is plantar flexed, and a supinated subtalar joint. The cavus foot causes poor shock absorbency and an unstable ankle.

4. Forefoot varus may require excessive pronation to bring the first metatarsal head to the ground.

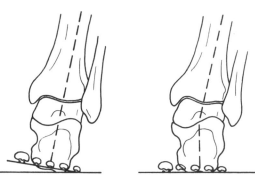

FIGURE 21.6 Tibia varum requiring compensatory pronation

FIGURE 21.7 Compensatory pronation

5. The low-arched (pes planus) foot may have lax ligaments and poor muscle support, resulting in excessive medial movement of the talonavicular joint. This causes many problems from the excessively prolonged pronation and a loose foot (instead of a rigid foot) during the take-off phase.

From this list it is evident that there are two main areas where problems can arise. First, if insufficient pronation occurs (such as with the high-arched, cavus foot), too much shock is transmitted by the foot to the leg;

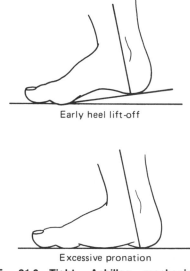

Early heel lift-off

Excessive pronation

FIGURE 21.8 Tight Achilles—mechanisms of compensation

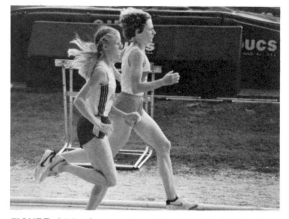

FIGURE 21.5 An erect posture can help the legs drive the body forward.

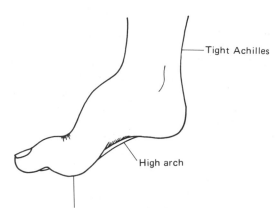

(a) Plantar flexed first ray — forefoot valgus

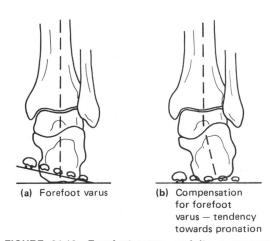

(a) Forefoot varus

(b) Compensation for forefoot varus — tendency towards pronation

FIGURE 21.10 Forefoot varus and its compensation

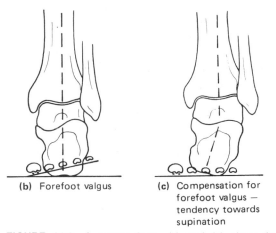

(b) Forefoot valgus

(c) Compensation for forefoot valgus — tendency towards supination

FIGURE 21.9 A cavus foot (a) and (b) show the forefoot valgus. (c) shows the compensatory supination.

second, if excess pronation continues for too long during the mid-support and take-off phases, one of the many "overuse syndromes" can develop.

Causes of Overuse Injuries

It is important for the trainer to understand the mechanism that leads to overuse injuries. With this background, he or she can guide runners in their training routines.

1. Impact shock. Studies have shown that a runner strikes the ground with a force of between three and five times that of walking. It does not take much to imagine what considerable repetitive forces are transmitted to bones, joints, and muscles of the lower extremities of the long-distance runner. This is especially true when an athlete starts distance running for the first time or when he or she starts to move up from, say, three miles a day to seven to ten miles a day. The muscles and bones have to strengthen in order to accept this new challenge. Sometimes they are unable to handle the force, and the athlete is compelled to temporarily back down. Muscle strength usually increases more rapidly than bone strength (in fact, some think the bone actually gets weaker before it gets stronger). This in-between phase, during which the bone is not yet fully ready to accept the force imposed on it, is the time when stress fractures and other "overuse" syndromes are apt to occur.

A very carefully worked out training schedule, avoiding hard surfaces and excessive mileage, is needed to prevent impact-related injuries from developing during this critical time.

2. The varus angle of the leg at foot strike. Most people have a small amount of tibia varum, but this angle is increased during running, particularly in female athletes, who tend to "cross over" during their running gait. An increased varus angle means the foot must compensate in order to bring the first metatarsal head into contact with the ground. This compensation takes the form of an increase in pronation and, if excessive, can result in the foot being unstable rather than rigid during the take-off phase of gait.

3. *Foot function.* Poor foot function results from a poor angular relationship between the bones of the foot or from weak lower extremity muscles and loose foot ligaments. This can, again, result in the development of excessive pronation as well as inability of the foot to move toward a supinated position during the take-off phase. Poor foot function can therefore be the end result of a combination of genetic endowment (a poor bony angular relationship) together with inadequacy of muscles and ligaments to compensate for this defect. How often has one seen a runner with "terrible feet" run long distances without any lower extremity problem at all? If for some reason a weakness in one of the key muscles supporting this foot de-

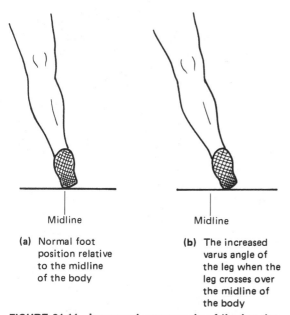

(a) Normal foot position relative to the midline of the body

(b) The increased varus angle of the leg when the leg crosses over the midline of the body

FIGURE 21.11 Increased varus angle of the leg due to "cross-over"

velops, one or other overuse injury occurs and the "terrible foot" takes all the blame.

4. *Muscle tightness.* The more an athlete runs, the greater the likelihood of developing tightness of the gastrocnemius-soleus and hamstring muscle groups. The tighter the gastrocnemius-soleus group becomes, the more it may interfere with optimum foot function. A tight hamstring muscle can alter the movement of the leg, particularly during the swing phase. It can also effect the posture of the lower spine and pelvis and, through this mechanism, influence the biomechanics of foot and leg function.

5. *Muscle weakness.* While the gastrocnemius-soleus and hamstring muscle groups are becoming tighter and stronger with long-distance running, the anterior tibial and quadriceps muscle groups may be getting weaker. A weak quadriceps muscle can cause patellar and peripatellar pain, while a weak anterior tibial muscle is frequently associated with an increase in impact shock and the development of lower leg pain and fatigue.

6. *Overambitious training program.* This is one of the most important, and yet one of the most neglected, reasons why runners develop injuries. Doing "too much too soon," or trying to put in extra miles when the body is not ready to take them, is an almost sure way of developing overuse injuries. Athletes must learn to "listen" to their own bodies. Those who do will learn how to avoid injuries; those who do not may suffer one injury after another.

Prevention of Overuse Injuries

1. *Flexibility.* Flexibility should be maintained or improved by the use of slow, static stretches. The main muscle groups to be stretched are the Achilles tendon (gastrocnemius-soleus group), the hamstring muscles, the lower-back muscles, the groin muscles, and the quadriceps (see Chapter 3).

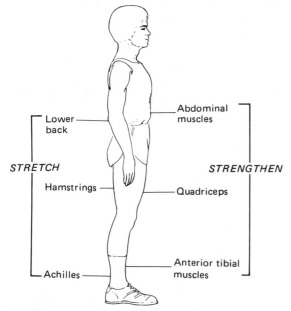

Lower back

STRETCH

Hamstrings

Achilles

Abdominal muscles

STRENGTHEN

Quadriceps

Anterior tibial muscles

FIGURE 21.12 Common muscle imbalances that may develop in the long-distance runner

Stretching exercises should be done *both* before and after a run or workout. The after-workout stretching routine should be emphasized because this is the optimum time to increase flexibility, particularly of those muscle groups that tend to become tighter with long-distance running.

2. Strength, power, and endurance. Developing adequate strength, power, and endurance in all muscle groups, but particularly in those groups which tend to become weak or develop imbalances, should be stressed in a prevention program. In a long-distance runner the muscles to concentrate on are the lower-back and abdominal muscles, the quadriceps, the anterior and posterior tibial muscles, and the intrinsic foot muscles. Simple exercises include

1. Sit-ups: These are best done with knees bent, hands behind the head or arms folded over the chest, and pelvis tilted to flatten out any lumbar lordosis (see section on back rehabilitation, p. 281).

2. Quadriceps exercises: The quadriceps are strengthened with isometric quadriceps sets and SRL's, the muscles being contracted for at least five seconds at a time (see section on knee rehabilitation, p. 348).

Another technique for strengthening the quadriceps group consists of the athlete's sitting on the end of a table with a weight on the foot or ankle and then straightening out the knee. Patellae which are sensitive to this type of isotonic movement can become irritated, so this exercise should be avoided in runners who have peripatellar or retropatellar pain.

To strengthen the anterior tibial muscle group, the athlete sits on the end of a table with legs hanging down and sandbags or similar weights suspended from the feet. He or she then actively dorsiflexes the feet, using the anterior tibial muscles. Variations of this include rotating both feet internally and in circles, to exercise the anterior *and* posterior tibial muscles. The feet can also be rotated externally in a circular motion, which helps strengthen the peroneal muscles.

The intrinsic foot musculature is exercised by the athlete's using his or her toes to curl up a towel placed on a smooth floor. A weight on the towel increases resistance. Picking up marbles with the toes and trying to actively spread the toes apart are other simple forms of exercise designed to strengthen the intrinsic foot musculature.

3. Shoes. Shoes are the runner's only real piece of equipment and should be carefully chosen. They are important in protecting the runner's bones and joints from the hard pavement.[4] During the past few years there has been a revolution in the design and number of brands of shoes used for running, but as yet there is no ideal running shoe, nor is there one shoe that is better than all others for every runner. New models have tended to come on the market before they have been adequately tested, and whole new injury syndromes have been produced by new shoe models. The subject is fraught

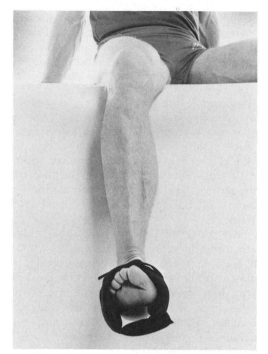

FIGURE 21.13 Anterior tibial muscle strengthening

with numerous difficulties and much confusion.

It is important to realize that though a shoe may obtain a high rating in shoe surveys, these surveys may not relate to a particular athlete's needs. Each shoe has certain qualities of shock absorbency, foot control, and flexibility. Every athlete needs a proportion of each of these qualities which may be totally different from any other athlete's

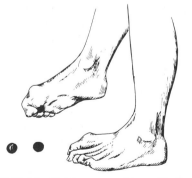

FIGURE 21.14 Picking up marbles with the toes

needs. In the future it may be possible to quantify these unknowns, match them against each other, and choose the ideal shoe for a given foot from the data.

There are certain features to note when examining a running shoe. The heel counter should support the heel and Achilles tendon adequately. The sole at the heel should be built up about ¾″ (1.8 cm). The material used for the heel should not be so soft that it is easily compressed, but it should not be rock-hard either. There should be adequate cushioning for the ball of the foot, because much force is directed through that area. There should be some flexibility of the front sole—otherwise the foot and the lower leg are strained during the push-off phase of gait—but it should not be so flexible that the shoe can easily be bent into a *U* shape.

When trying shoes on, the athlete should wear the actual socks that will be used for running. He or she should try on one shoe at a time, keeping the old running shoe on the opposite foot, lacing it up the same way as the old shoe, and should walk around the store with it on. Then the athlete should try on the other one, wearing the old shoe on the opposite foot. They should both be adequate in length and width. An athlete can certainly accept a little bit of snugness in width, as shoes tend to stretch sideways slightly, but there should be no compromise in length as shoes do not stretch in that direction. The amount of space available in the toe box is also important.

Next, the athlete should try on both shoes at the same time and walk around again, making sure they feel just right. Having done this, and having decided which brand and model to buy, he or she should place these shoes on the counter and view them from the back to see if there is any asymmetry in the way the uppers are placed on the sole. There has, on occasion, been a lack of quality control in the manufacture of athletic shoes and this has led to injuries in a number of runners (Figure 21.15).

An athlete should not run in shoes immediately after purchasing them, but should

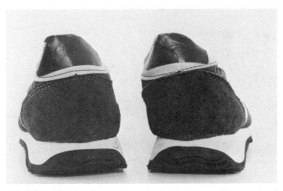

FIGURE 21.15 New shoes—lack of quality control
Note the valgus (or pronated) position of the right heel counter.

walk in them for a day or two, to allow them to adapt to the feet. After a few days of walking around, he or she can go on a short run of about 30% of normal distance, gradually increasing the length of time the shoes are worn so that after about five days the new shoes "fit like a glove."

Most shoes tend to wear down on the outside of the heel, but this should not be allowed to progress too far. The sole in this area should be filled in with either a glue gun made for this purpose or a preparation which is spread on the outside of the sole (e.g., Shoe Goo) to build it up to normal height. When using this type of substance, the athlete should be very careful not to build up the area any higher than the normal height of the rest of the sole. A very thin layer is all that is usually required. If the outside of the sole is built up too high, the foot tends to tilt inward, resulting in increased pronation, which could easily lead to new injuries. Before the shoes wear down completely, it is prudent for the athlete to obtain a new pair, so they can be slowly broken in before the old ones are discarded.

4. *Surface.* As previously mentioned, many injuries are due to impact shock. Though cement might be the only surface available, it should be avoided whenever possible and a more forgiving surface chosen. Conversely, the athlete should be careful not to run on too soft a surface, which can cause excessive pronation or stretching of the Achilles tendon. Uneven ground often causes ankle sprains.

It has been observed that it is not only the surface hardness that is important, but also a change from one type of surface to another. This change, even though to a softer surface, can result in overuse injuries in certain susceptible individuals.

5. *Training schedule.* The sensitivity of some athletes to the body's response to overtraining divides those who suffer from those who continue unscathed. As a rule, it is useful to think of the training schedule as being designed to enable the athlete to reach his or her maximal performance (or peak) when needed. Once over the peak, one has to start at a lower level and build up to the peak once again (Figure 21.16).

General principles of training should include a hard-day, easy-day routine, with enough periods of rest to recover from really hard workouts. Early warning signs of overfatigue include:

1. Faster-than-normal pulse on awakening

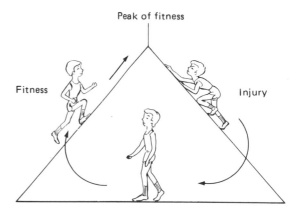

FIGURE 21.16 The pyramid of fitness and injury
As the runner reaches a high level of fitness and nears the peak, the chance of an injury increases. Once over the peak and in the area of injury, the runner cannot immediately return to that same level (as depicted by crawling up the other side of the slope), but must first back down to a lower level and then gradually work up again.

**center for
sports medicine
& running injuries**
of eugene

RUNNER'S HISTORY FORM   DATE:_____

Name _____   Age ____ Sex: M F   Wt:____ Ht:_____

1. When did you first notice symptoms? _____
    Reinjury: ☐ Yes   ☐ No

2. Describe symptoms: (Right, Left, Both) _____
    _____

3. Type of pain: ☐ Dull   ☐ Throbbing   ☐ Intermittant
                  ☐ Sharp   ☐ Constant   ☐ Burning
                  ☐ Sore   ☐ Bruised

4. Onset: ☐ Gradual   ☐ Sudden

5. What was the onset of your symptoms related to?

    ☐ Change in surface   ☐ Running hills: up / down
    ☐ Increase in mileage   ☐ Change in speed: faster / slower / sprints
    ☐ Don't know   ☐ Change in shoes: from_____to_____
    ☐ Other_____

6. When do your symptoms occur?

    ☐ As soon as you start to run   ☐ After you finish the run
    ☐ During the run   ☐ During normal activity (like walking)
    ☐ Always   ☐ _____

7. How long do your symptoms last? _____

8. What helps relieve your symptoms? _____

9. What increases your symptoms? _____

10. Have you been treated for this condition previously? ☐ Yes   ☐ No

    When? _____   By whom? _____

    What treatment? _____

11. Have you had any other running-related problems? ☐ Yes   ☐ No

    What? _____

    When? _____ Treatment _____ By whom? _____

12. What effect do your symptoms have on your workout?

    ☐ Pain during workout but able to run   ☐ Unable to workout
    ☐ Workout compromised by pain   ☐ Self-imposed rest
    ☐ Other _____

FIGURE 21.17 Runner's history form

13. Type of runner:
    - ☐ Fitness
    - ☐ Recreation
    - ☐ Club
    - ☐ Serious

    - ☐ High School
    - ☐ College
    - ☐ Professional
    - ☐ World Class

14. Distance: Daily _____   Speed per mile: Training _____

    Weekly _____   Competition _____

15. How long have you been running? _____

16. How long have you been running at this distance and speed? _____

17. What types of surfaces do you run on ? Check all that apply.

    - ☐ Composition track
    - ☐ Cinder track
    - ☐ Chips

    - ☐ Asphalt
    - ☐ Cross Country
    - ☐ Grass

    - ☐ Beach
    - ☐ Dirt or Gravel
    - ☐ Other _____

18. Where do you do most of your running? Check all that apply.

    - ☐ Hills
    - ☐ Flat

    - ☐ Crowned roads
    - ☐ Trails

19. Brand and model of shoes you wear now? _____

    How long have you been running in these? _____

    Any comments? _____

20. Brands and models of shoes previously worn, plus comments. _____

    _____

21. Do you wear orthotics or other corrective devices now? If yes,...

    What type? _____ How long have you worn them? _____

    Who prescribed them?_____ What effect do they have?_____

22. Have you worn orthotic devices in the past? If yes,...

    What type? _____ How long did you wear them? _____

    Why did you stop wearing them? _____

23. Do you stretch regularly? If yes,...   Before Running   After Running

    How Long?
    - ☐ 5 minutes
    - ☐ 10 minutes
    - ☐ 15 minutes
    - ☐ 20 minutes
    - ☐ More

    - ☐ 5 minutes
    - ☐ 10 minutes
    - ☐ 15 minutes
    - ☐ 20 minutes
    - ☐ More

24. What other sports do you participate in on a fairly regular basis?

    _____

FIGURE 21.17 Runner's history form (*cont.*)

2. Loss of body weight or body fat when in optimum condition

3. Scratchy sore throat

4. Easy fatigability

5. Insomnia

If these signs develop, the athlete should lower the mileage being run and put in a few easy days before returning to the normal schedule of vigorous workouts. He or she should also be aware of undue or unusual stress, such as the changing of time zones.

Probably more athletes have been ruined by overtraining than by any single biomechanical or muscular impairment. The most important injury-prevention advice to give a runner is:

"Listen to your body—work with it, not against it."

Figure 21.17 on pp. 420 and 421 shows a form used to gather information from a runner who has been injured.

BIOMECHANICAL EXAMINATION OF THE RUNNING ATHLETE'S ALIGNMENT

Notice the general alignment of the athlete when he or she is standing. Specifically, notice the heights of the iliac crests, the posterior superior iliac spines, and the greater trochanters; the position of the patellae; the amount of genu varum or valgum, tibia varum; and the angle of the calcaneus. Then, observe the type of arch configuration, the shape and angle of the metatarsals, the shape of the toes in relation to the metatarsals, and the length and general configuration of the toes. Ask the athlete to flex the knees as far forward as possible while keeping the heels firmly fixed to the ground. This indicates the amount of functional Achilles flexibility.

If the iliac crests and posterior superior iliac spines are not level, they should be observed while the athlete is sitting on the examining table. If they then become level, a discrepancy in leg length should be suspect-

TABLE 21.1   Factors Associated with Overuse Injuries in Runners

Impact force	The impact force of running is three to five times that of walking. This can lead to stress fractures or "stress reactions" of bone.
Hard surface	Increases the impact force.
Change of surface	Particularly from soft to hard, but can also be vice versa.
Downhill running	Especially associated with iliotibial tract irritation, popliteus tendinitis, and patellar tendinitis.
Lack of flexibility	Especially the Achilles tendon and the hamstrings.
Muscle weakness	Especially the intrinsic muscles of the foot, the anterior and posterior tibial muscles, and the quadriceps.
Overstriding	Results in hamstring pulls and knee pain.
Poor posture	Especially leaning too far forward and hyperlordosis of the lumbar spine.
Overdistance	There is a relatively high incidence of injuries in runners running over forty miles a week.
Overtraining	Being at the peak of training means being a hair's breadth from an injury.
Anatomical factors	Malalignment of the lower extremity, foot, or the relationship between them. Symptoms are usually associated with muscle weakness.
Shoes	Should provide control and shock absorbency.
Side of road	Running on the same side of a sloped road for a long time can produce knee pain.
Too much too soon!	

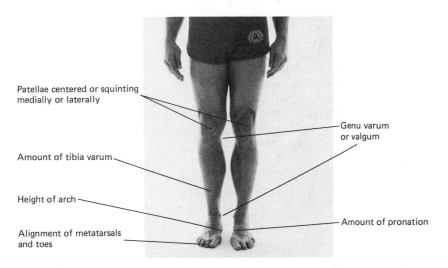

Patellae centered or squinting medially or laterally

Amount of tibia varum

Height of arch

Alignment of metatarsals and toes

Genu varum or valgum

Amount of pronation

FIGURE 21.18 Examination of lower extremity alignment Note the configuration of the feet when observed from the front and from the back.

ed. If they remain unchanged, lower-back joint dysfunction should be suspected.

The amount of tibia varum is determined by having the athlete stand on a firm platform, with the foot in the neutral position. The lowest third of the leg is bisected, and the angle between this line and a line perpendicular to the ground is measured. This should also be measured with the foot in its compensated standing position.

The athlete should then lie prone with feet and ankles hanging over the end of the examining table. Observe the type of calluses present and their positions on the feet. This indicates not only the weight-bearing pressure areas but also what shearing forces are acting on the feet during running.

Grasp the heads of the fourth and fifth metatarsals just proximal to the metatarsophalangeal joint and gently move the relaxed foot through the full range of movement—from full pronation to full supination. This demonstrates whether or not there is limited or excessive range of movement at the subtalar joint, and if the foot is rigid or flexible.

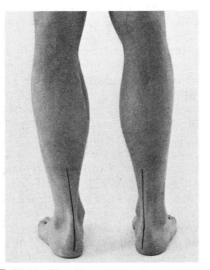

FIGURE 21.19 Bisection of the lower third of the leg (as well as bisection of the heel) assessed while standing

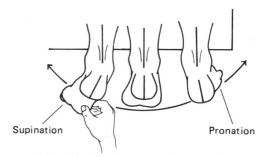

Supination   Pronation

FIGURE 21.20 Testing range of motion of the subtalar joint

The neutral position. To determine the neutral position of the subtalar joint, have the athlete lie prone as previously described. When examining the left foot, use the left hand to move it through the range of movement by grasping the distal heads of the fourth and fifth metatarsals, while the middle finger and thumb of the right hand palpate the talus. The talus is the key to the neutral position and is best felt by placing the thumb just distal to the medial malleolus at the talonavicular joint, with the middle finger distal to the tibiofibular syndesmosis. As the foot is brought into pronation, the talus will be felt by the thumb to bulge on the medial side. As it is brought into full supination, it will be felt by the middle finger to bulge on the lateral side. A point will be reached between full supination and full pronation where the talus will either be felt equally on both sides, or will not be felt at all (Figure 21.21). This has to do with the talus being congruently positioned, so that the subtalar joint is assumed to be in the neutral position. The neutral position can also be felt as a "peak" of movement as the foot is passively moved from pronation to supination and back again.

Having determined the neutral position of the subtalar joint, it is now possible to es-

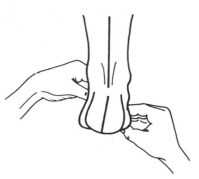

FIGURE 21.22 Determining the neutral position with the athlete lying prone In this example, the rearfoot is in approximately 2° of varus.

timate the relationship of the calcaneus to the lower leg. To do this, bisect the calcaneus and the lowest third of the leg (Figure 21.22) while the subtalar joint is held in the neutral position. In most cases, the calcaneus will be in a slightly varus position (2° to 4°) in relation to the lower leg.

Now determine the angular relationship of the rearfoot to the forefoot, making sure the subtalar joint is in the neutral position and the midtarsal joint is maximally pronated (Figure 21.23). Load the fourth and fifth metatarsal heads in a dorsal direction until resistance is felt. The relationship of the metatarsal heads (the forefoot) to the rearfoot is now estimated by again bisecting the calcaneus and then taking a line from the head of the fifth metatarsal to the first head of the metatarsal. This line is then related to the bisection of the calcaneus. If it is perpendicular (90°), then the forefoot is in a neutral position in relation to the rearfoot. If, however, the first metatarsal head lies on a higher plane than the fifth metatarsal head, the foot is in a forefoot supination or a forefoot varus position. Conversely, if the first metatarsal head is on a lower plane in relation to the fifth metatarsal head, then there is a forefoot valgus (as is commonly found with a cavus, or high-arched, foot).

Estimate the range of movement of the first ray by grasping the heads of the first and second metatarsals and moving the first metatarsal up and down in relation to the

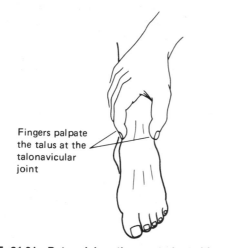

Fingers palpate the talus at the talonavicular joint

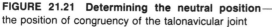

FIGURE 21.21 Determining the neutral position— the position of congruency of the talonavicular joint

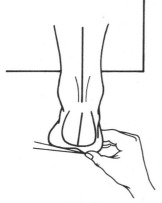

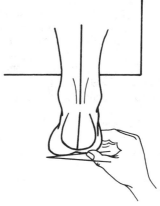

*Subtalar
Neutral position*

Forefoot varus

*Subtalar
Neutral position*

Forefoot valgus

FIGURE 21.23 Determining the position of the forefoot when the subtalar joint is in the neutral position

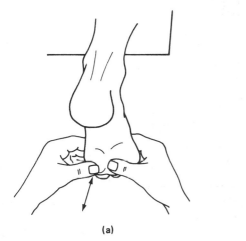

(a)

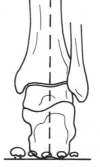

(b) The foot non-
weight-bearing

(c) With weight-bearing,
pronation occurs due to
instability of the first ray

FIGURE 21.24 The influence of first ray motion on pronation (a) Determining the amount of motion of the first ray. (b) and (c) Pronation due to a mobile first ray.

TABLE 21.2   Summary of the Examination of a Running Athlete

1. Athlete standing:
   a. Facing examiner ⎤ View from the hips to
   b. Facing sideways ⎬ the feet (include
   c. Back to examiner ⎦ entire back and
                          shoulders if athlete
                          has back problem)
2. Athlete sitting on examining table:
   a. Level of posterior superior iliac spines and iliac crests
   b. Position of patellae
   c. Lower legs
3. Athlete lying supine on back:
   a. Back
   b. Hip
   c. Knee
4. Athlete lying prone on abdomen:
   a. Hips
   b. Biomechanical examination of feet
      1) Amount of tibia varum of lower third of tibia
      2) Range of motion of subtalar joint and first ray
      3) Heel or subtalar varus with foot in neutral position
      4) Forefoot varus or valgus with foot in neutral position
      5) Position of first ray relative to rest of forefoot
5. Examine area of complaint in detail
6. Observe while walking
7. Observe while running
8. Examine walking and running shoes

second. From this, one can judge whether the first ray is rigid, has some movement, has normal movement, or is hypermobile. A hypermobile first ray allows the foot to pronate more than it may appear to do on the initial examination.[5]

Finally, perform gait analysis to closely study the foot and lower extremity in motion. Ask the athlete to walk back and forth over a distance of about thirty feet, and then to run in the shoes normally worn.

A number of common running-induced injuries will now be discussed according to the anatomical area involved.

COMMON RUNNING-INDUCED INJURIES TO THE LOWER BACK

Foot and Leg as Causes of Lower Backache

Backache in a running athlete is a common complaint. Often the problem arises from faulty mechanics of the foot or leg, the effects being felt in the back. For example, asymmetry of leg length of ⅛″ to ¼″ (3 to 6 mm) is sufficient to produce symptoms in a runner.

Symptoms may be localized to the back, or may be felt in the back buttock, or leg.

EXAMINATION: A full examination of the back and a biomechanical examination of the feet should be undertaken (see section on examination of the back, p. 272). The following points in particular should be noted:

1. Alignment of the lower leg, emphasizing symmetry and amount of pronation or supination of the foot.

2. Heights of the iliac crests and posterior superior iliac spines, with the athlete both standing and sitting.

3. Heights of the greater trochanters.

4. Heights of the anterior superior iliac spines, with the athlete both standing and lying supine.

5. Range of back movement and symmetry of posterior superior iliac spine movement on forward flexion and on return to erect position.

6. Apparent leg lengths, as visualized by the levels of the medial malleoli observed with the athlete lying. Leg lengths are usually measured from the anterior superior iliac spine to the medial malleolus, but this measurement fails to take into account variables of the foot and pelvis.

Having excluded the major causes of backache, discussed in Chapter 17, consider the possibility that back pain in the runner could be due to the following causes:

1. *Functionally short leg.* This means that the actual leg lengths are equal, but that the legs are functionally unequal because of a difference of pronation or supination of one foot relative to the other, or because of some other functional asymmetry. For instance, the right foot may be in its normal position while the left foot is excessively pronated. This causes the left leg to be "shorter" than the right, causing the left posterior superior iliac spine to be lower than the right when the athlete is standing. However, when the back is examined with the athlete sitting on the examining table, the posterior superior iliac spines are horizontally level in height. If the excessively pronated foot is placed in the neutral position, the height of the posterior superior iliac spines should once more be horizontally level when the athlete stands.

2. Anatomically short leg. This means that one leg is actually physically shorter than the other. The posterior superior iliac spine on the shorter side is lower than the opposite side when the athlete is standing, but the spines are level when the athlete is sitting. The body may try to compensate for this leg length difference by, for instance, pronating the foot on the longer side while supinating the foot on the shorter side. This tends to level the pelvis when the athlete is standing.

Both the functionally and the anatomically short leg can cause complications of

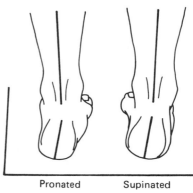

Pronated   Supinated

FIGURE 21.26 If one foot is pronated while the other is supinated, it may lead to a functional leg-length difference. However, if one leg is structurally longer it may result in the foot pronating on that side in order to equalize the leg-lengths and thus balance the pelvis.

joint dysfunction in the lower back. This is detected in an asymmetry of movement of the posterior superior iliac spines on forward flexion and on return from a flexed position, and also by the spines' remaining unequal in height when the athlete is sitting on the examining table.

3. Bilateral excessive pronation of the feet. This results in a forward tilt of the pelvis with excessive lordosis of the back.

4. Muscle imbalances. Weakness of the abdominal, buttock, and lower-back muscles,

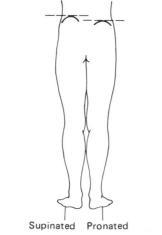

Supinated   Pronated

FIGURE 21.25 Functional short leg

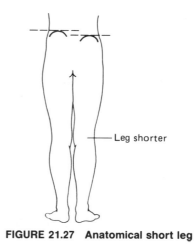

Leg shorter

FIGURE 21.27 Anatomical short leg

with or without excessive tightness of the hamstrings, back, and iliotibial tract, can cause, or predispose to, lower backache.

5. *Muscle spasm.* Spasm of the piriformis or quadratus lumborum muscles occasionally gives rise to lower backache and even to referred pain down the leg to the foot.

TREATMENT:

1. If there is excessive pronation, this should be corrected by an orthotic device and the use of foot and lower leg exercises.

2. Anatomical discrepancy in leg length should be compensated for by building up the height of the heel and the sole of the shoe. For instance, a discrepancy of leg length of ¼ ″ (6 mm) may require ¼ ″ (6 mm) heel lift plus ⅛ ″ (3 mm) continuation of the lift under the forefoot.

3. Any tightness of the Achilles, the hamstrings, or the iliotibial tract should be re-duced by repetitive, slow, stretching exercises.

4. Weakness of the abdominal, back extensor, and buttock muscles should be corrected (see section on rehabilitation, p. 281).

5. If dysfunction of the posterior facets or sacro-iliac joints is a problem, even after implementation of the first four steps listed, manipulative therapy may be performed. Manipulation should be used only if the diagnosis is one of joint dysfunction or posterior facet joint subluxation. If there is evidence of nerve root irritation or compression, manipulation is not advised (see Chapters 7 and 17).

COMMON RUNNING-INDUCED INJURIES TO THE HIP

There are a number of causes of hip pain in a runner, some of which are outlined in Table 21.4 on the next page.

TABLE 21.3   Causes and Treatment of Backache in the Running Athlete

Causes	Complications	Treatment[a]
Functionally short leg (one foot pronates more than the other)	No lumbar complications Lumbar joint dysfunction or subluxation	In-shoe orthotic device In-shoe orthotic device, manipulation if necessary
Anatomically short leg (one leg actually shorter than the other)	Uncompensated for by changes in the feet Compensated for by pronation of longer leg and/or supination of shorter leg Lumbar joint dysfunction or subluxation	Heel-and-sole lift In-shoe orthotic device and a heel-and-sole lift Manipulation and a heel-and-sole lift and/or in-shoe orthotic device
Excessive pronation of both feet	No lumbar complications Lumbar joint dysfunction or subluxation	In-shoe orthotic device In-shoe orthotic device, manipulation if necessary
Dysfunction or subluxation of one of the joints of the lower back—foot alignment or leg length unrelated		Manipulation, stretching and strengthening exercises
Back pathology—other than joint dysfunction (e.g., disc protrusion or rupture)		Orthopedic examination and treatment

[a] *Always stretch*: hamstrings, iliotibial tracts, Achilles tendons, back, and iliopsoas muscles
Always strengthen: abdominals and back extensors

TABLE 21.4   Common Running-Induced Injuries to the Hip

Condition	Symptoms and Signs	Causes	Treatment
Vague hip pain (in one or both hips)	Pain and aching within the hip. No positive findings suggestive of intra-articular hip pathology Normal X-rays Normal bone scan.	Malfunction or malalignment of foot and lower leg. Leg length inequality—anatomical or functional. Lower-back abnormality with referred pain. Muscle imbalance.	Localize and correct cause.
Iliotibial tract irritation	Pain down lateral aspect of thigh, possibly localized to hip. Symptoms worse on downhill running, relieved by uphill running.	Excessive downhill running. Tight iliotibial tract. Shock absorbency problem. Malalignment problem. Leg length discrepancy.	Apply ice. Iliotibial tract stretching. Anti-inflammatory medication and/or ultrasound. Avoid downhill running. Use orthotic devices if indicated. Strengthen any muscle weaknesses. Corticosteroid injection.
Strain of one of the muscles around the hip (iliopsoas, rectus femoris, sartorius, gluteus medius, or piriformis)	Pain localized to one muscle group.	Often due to weakness of other muscles overloading the affected muscle.	Isolate specific muscle weakness and correct. Use physical modalities as indicated.
Trochanteric bursitis	Pain around hip, localized tenderness over trochanteric bursa.	May be associated with irritation of the iliotibial tract and tensor fascia lata. May be associated with leg length difference, malalignment problem, or muscle weakness.	Correct cause. Apply ice. Anti-inflammatory medication and/or ultrasound. Occasionally, inject corticosteroid into the bursa. Rarely, surgery.
Stress fracture of femoral neck	Pain deep within hip. If condition suspected, obtain bone scan (the stress fracture may not show on an X-ray for weeks or even months. This fracture may displace.	Uncertain. May be related to excessive crossover, hard downhill, or mountain running.	Insist on complete rest from all activity, preferably non-weight-bearing using crutches.
Slipped capital femoral epiphysis	Hip pain or only knee pain. X-ray diagnosis.	Often occurs in overweight teenager, usually male.	Usually surgical.
Congenital dysplasia or other abnormality	Vague, constant hip pain after running. X-ray diagnosis.		Requires orthopedic consultation.

RUNNING-RELATED INJURIES TO THE KNEE

Problems related to the knee comprise at least 25% of the injuries incurred by the runner. Many of these conditions have not been clearly defined and are listed according to anatomical area rather than etiology.

Medial Patellar Pain

With a meniscal tear or an internal derangement excluded as the cause of medial patellar pain, pain related to the medial aspect of the patella, the medial joint line, or the medial tibial plateau is usually associated with excessive pronation during the mid-support and take-off phases. One theory about the occurrence of this pain relates to the excessive internal rotation of the tibia which accompanies a prolonged pronatory phase. As the knee starts to extend after reaching its maximal point of flexion, the tibia and femur usually start to rotate externally. As a result of excessively prolonged pronation, the tibia stays in internal rotation. Stress is thus placed on the medial patellar structures because the patella tends to follow the external rotational movement of the femur.

An occasional cause of medial patellar pain is the synovial plica (see p. 342).

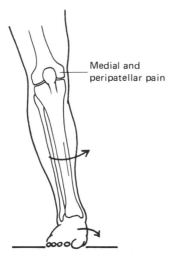

Medial and peripatellar pain

FIGURE 21.28 Excessive pronation may lead to patellar pain in a runner

TREATMENT: Initially, treatment with ice and aspirin four times a day helps. However, it is usually necessary to improve the musculature, particularly of the vastus medialis, the posterior tibial, and the flexor hallucis longus muscles. Orthotic devices are often used as well, and they effect improvement in a high percentage of cases. While the athlete is recovering, it may be necessary to decrease the mileage and perhaps change the running shoe and/or the surface.

Pes Anserine Bursitis

The cause of pes anserine bursitis in a runner is uncertain. Possibly it is related to an attempt by the pes to compensate for excessive tibia varum at heel strike. Frequently a weak vastus medialis muscle is found in association with the condition.

SYMPTOMS AND SIGNS: There is pain and swelling of the pes anserine bursa, which lies in close proximity to the insertion of the pes anserine tendon. This condition needs to be differentiated from a stress fracture of the upper tibia, which can present with the same findings.

TREATMENT: Initially, treat with ice and aspirin or other anti-inflammatory medication, along with exercises to improve the vastus medialis and the pes anserine muscle groups. Orthotic devices are often useful. On occasion, a local injection of corticosteroids helps.

Patellar Tendinitis

Patellar tendinitis can occur in a runner, particularly one who runs hard down hills. (See section on jumper's knee in Chapter 19.)

SYMPTOMS AND SIGNS: Pain and tenderness are localized to the inferior pole of the patella at the origin of the patellar tendon, and sometimes farther down the tendon. An excessive Q angle may be found in association with bowing of the top third of the tibia (not necessarily related to genu varum).

TREATMENT: Of particular relevance to the runner is the use of orthotic devices, ice, and aspirin. Neoprene with a patellar support can be used on those with an excessive Q angle. The quadriceps muscles should be strengthened. Anti-inflammatory medication may also help.

Retropatellar Pain

(See section on patellofemoral joint pain, p. 337.)

SYMPTOMS AND SIGNS: Pain occurs behind the patella when the athlete runs. It may also occur when he or she walks up or down stairs, cycles (or after cycling), or sits for some time with the knee bent at 90°. Frequently there is an extensor mechanism malalignment related to the hips, tibiae, feet, or all three.

TREATMENT: Carefully managed vastus medialis and quadriceps exercises are the mainstays of treatment, along with in-shoe orthotic devices. Gentle quadriceps stretching should be performed as long as this is not painful. High doses of aspirin (perhaps with vitamin C added) may prove helpful. Ice should be used for symptomatic relief of discomfort.

The runner should avoid hills, and he or she may actually have to discontinue running for a period of time, to allow the retropatellar irritation to subside. During this time, treading water or running in place in a swimming pool while wearing a life jacket may prove very beneficial from the cardiovascular and muscular standpoint. Occasionally surgical realignment of the extensor mechanism and/or release of patellar compression has to be performed.

Lateral Patellar Pain

This is thought to be due to an alignment defect involving the patella, but it is sometimes related to the feet as well. There may be a muscle imbalance of the vastus, with the vastus lateralis being more powerful or tighter than the medialis. Rarely is a fat-pad impingement the cause of symptoms.

SYMPTOMS AND SIGNS: There is pain as well as tenderness on the anterolateral aspect of the patella. The lateral patellar structures may be tight, allowing little medial movement of the patella when pressure is applied to the lateral facet.

TREATMENT: Ice and aspirin may be used initially. Quadriceps exercises need to be carefully controlled, emphasizing the vastus medialis. It is important to attempt to gently stretch the quadriceps over a period of time. In-shoe orthotic devices and the occasional cortisone injection may be helpful. A lateral retinacular release procedure is sometimes used.

Lateral Knee Pain

Frequently, lateral knee pain is due to a soft-tissue problem, which is due to tendinitis or friction of the iliotibial tract as it runs over the lateral femoral condyle.[6,7,8,9] Occasionally the popliteal tendon or the lateral ligament become inflamed.[10] Irritation of these tissues appears to be related to increased mileage beyond normal and to poor shock absorbency either through the shoes or through the

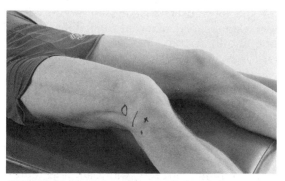

FIGURE 21.29 Lateral knee pain in a runner Most commonly this is due to iliotibial tract friction over the lateral femoral epicondyle. The illustration shows the area of frequent tenderness (0) as well as other areas that might be tender (X). The line marks the lateral joint line.

body alignment, and it therefore shows up quite frequently in runners with rigid feet.

SYMPTOMS AND SIGNS: Pain occurs during running and may be localized to the lateral epicondyle or run diffusely along the iliotibial tract. It is usually initiated by hard downhill running and may disappear when the athlete runs uphill. Often pain is felt as the leg is brought forwards through the swing phase.[11]

There is tenderness over the lateral epicondyle (occasionally over the lateral joint line), at the origin of the popliteal tendon, or at Gerdy's tubercle. There is inflammation where the iliotibial tract crosses the lateral epicondyle, and occasionally crepitus can be palpated. The iliotibial tract is frequently noted to be tight in these runners. Pain is usually elicited by full weight bearing with the knee at 30° of flexion. Compressing the iliotibial tract against the lateral epicondyle while moving the knee through 30° of flexion may reproduce the symptoms.

TREATMENT: Athletes with this problem need to wear shoes with good shock absorbency and should attempt to run on a softer surface. They should also avoid hills. Carefully designed orthotic devices may help. Ice, aspirin, or other anti-inflammatory medication may be necessary. Iliotibial tract stretching has been found useful.[11] Strengthening of specific muscle weaknesses should be undertaken. Corticosteroid injections around the iliotibial tract and/or popliteal tendon are beneficial. In very resistant cases, surgical exploration and partial release of the iliotibial tract may be necessary.[12,13]

Biceps Femoris Tendinitis

SYMPTOMS AND SIGNS: Biceps femoris tendinitis may present with pain and tenderness at, or just proximal to, the insertion of the tendon into the head of the fibula. Swelling occasionally localizes at the tendon insertion.

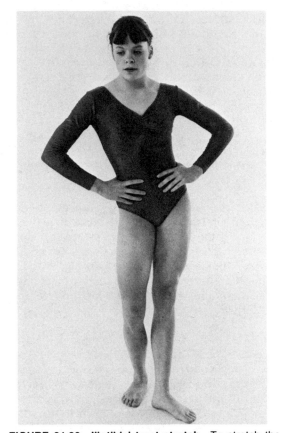

FIGURE 21.30 Iliotibial tract stretch To stretch the left side, place the left leg slightly forward with the body's weight on that leg. Drop the pelvis down on the right side. This will result in a stretching of the tensor fasciae latae and iliotibial tract on the left. Placing the hands on the iliac crests may help reinforce the sensation of when the correct position is obtained.

TREATMENT: Ice, decreased running activities, anti-inflammatory medication; occasionally a corticosteroid injection.

It should be clearly understood that there are many conditions within the knee joint that may be unrelated to running (such as a torn medial meniscus), but that can be brought out by running. These are not discussed here, but should *always* be included in the differential diagnosis and excluded by means of a thorough knee examination.

COMMON RUNNING-INDUCED INJURIES TO THE LOWER LEG

The term "shin splints" is a lay term that refers to any lower leg pain in a runner or in any athlete engaged in a running activity.[14] It is a nonspecific term—avoid using it. Make a specific diagnosis—this is the only way that the appropriate treatment can be instituted. The anatomical classification of lower leg pain in the runner is based on knowledge of the anatomical compartments (see Figure 20.1).

Tibial Stress Reaction and Stress Fracture

The name *tibial stress reaction* applies to a condition in which the tibia is attempting to adapt to the stress placed on it. The main components of a stress fracture are microfractures, which will heal if circumstances permit. This condition could be called a *prestress fracture* or micro-fracture. However, if the stress continues or increases, a proper stress fracture can occur.[15]

The tibial stress reaction therefore encompasses a spectrum of conditions. At the one end is the athlete with slight tibial pain, no X-ray changes, and no increase in uptake on bone scan (there may be X-ray evidence of bone adaptation over a period of time if the stress continues). With a slight decrease in intensity of training, or perhaps an alteration of footwear, the pain may subside and not return when the previous level of activity is again reached.

At the other end of the spectrum is the athlete who suddenly develops severe pain, usually at the junction of the mid- and lower third of the tibia. The symptoms are severe enough to prevent the athlete from continuing training. A bone scan at this time demonstrates a dense localized area of uptake. After two weeks, ordinary X-rays reveal a definite fracture line extending at least part of the way, if not completely, through the cortex of the tibia. Callus is minimal or nonexistent. This represents a definite stress fracture.

TABLE 21.5 Anatomical Classification of Lower Leg Pain in the Running Athlete ("Shin Splints")

1. *Posteromedial pain* (pain and tenderness along the posteromedial aspect of the tibia—the commonest area)
   a. Tibial stress reaction, which can develop into a stress fracture
   b. Muscle strains, inflammation, tendinitis, and periosteal irritation of the posterior tibial muscle and tendon and other soft tissues attached to the posteromedial border of the tibia ("medial tibial stress syndrome")
   c. Combination of the above
   d. Deep posterior compartment compression syndrome

2. *Tibial pain* (pain and tenderness directly on the tibia)
   a. Tibial stress reaction, which may develop into a stress fracture
   b. Pes anserine tendinitis and/or bursitis

3. *Anterior tibial compartment pain* (pain and tenderness within the anterior compartment)
   a. Muscle strains, inflammation, and tendinitis
   b. Anterior compartment compression syndrome

4. *Lateral compartment pain* (pain in the lateral compartment of the leg)
   a. Muscle strains, inflammation, and tendinitis
   b. Lateral compartment compression syndrome

5. *Fibular pain* (pain and tenderness directly on the fibula)
   a. Fibular stress reaction, which may develop into a stress fracture
   b. Biceps tendinitis at the head of the fibula

6. *Posterior pain* (pain on the posterior aspect of the lower leg)
   a. Muscle strains, inflammation, and tendinitis
   b. Posterior compartment compression syndrome of either the superficial or deep posterior compartment
   c. Thrombophlebitis

7. *Miscellaneous*
   a. Fascial herniae
   b. Popliteal artery entrapment syndrome
   c. Interosseous membrane calcification
   d. Varicose veins
   e. Pain referred from the lower back

Between these two extremes are many variations. One common variation is chronic recurrence of pain whenever an athlete exercises beyond a certain point. X-rays will be normal initially, but may change if the athlete is followed over a period of many months or years, providing activity is continued at the same level. The cortex becomes thick and the actual width of the bone increases. Bone scans demonstrate a diffusely increased uptake, which is usually vertical, localized to the posterior aspect of the tibia, and less intense than the acute stress fracture. This area of increased uptake indicates the area of bony change that will be visualized much later on regular X-rays.

Another frequent occurrence is pain in the tibia—not severe enough to prevent the athlete from performing, but constantly present with activity. Bony adaptation is much more rapid and is visualized on X-rays within a month or two as new periosteal bone and tibial molding. An actual stress fracture line is not visualized. Bone scans usually show a more diffuse uptake than that seen in the acute stress fracture, but of a similar horizontal pattern.

It should be understood that bone is an ever-adapting structure, but it adapts less rapidly than muscles and soft tissues. During running activities, certain muscles may increase in strength, adding to the forces generated across the bone, particularly if one set of muscles is considerably stronger than another. This muscle imbalance is thought to be the main etiologic mechanism of both stress reactions and stress fractures.[16,17] Impact is undoubtedly important in the case of the tibia, as are biomechanical factors, foot and leg alignment, flexibility, and other variables; but the one constant feature of stress reactions and stress fractures is related to muscle action (see section on stress fractures, Chapter 9).

It is important to try to differentiate the tibial stress reaction from inflammation of the soft tissues of the lower leg (posterior tibial, flexor digitorum, and hallucis muscles and tendons). Differential points are shown in Table 21.6.

TABLE 21.6   Differentiation Between Tibial Stress Fractures and Lower Leg Soft-tissue Inflammatory Conditions

Tibial Stress	Posterior Tibial Muscle-Tendon Inflammation
Tenderness may be at an area devoid of muscles (lowest third of the tibia) or it may be on the tibial shaft itself.	Tenderness mainly over the soft tissues.
Percussion of the tibia increases intensity of the pain.	Percussion on the tibia does not increase intensity of the pain.
Tuning fork vibration test may or may not be positive.	Tuning fork vibration test is negative.
Swelling is present over the bone and possibly in the soft tissues.	Swelling is usually present over the soft tissues.
Stressing the muscles does not increase pain.	Stressing involved muscles may cause increased pain.

Medial Tibial Stress Syndrome

This stress syndrome includes tendinitis and periosteal irritation involving the posterior tibial muscle and tendon, the flexor muscles and tendons, and other soft tissues attached to the posteromedial border of the tibia. It is a very common condition and is frequently confused with the tibial stress reaction.

ETIOLOGY: The usual cause is abnormal foot pronation, with the posterior tibial, flexor hallucis, and digitorum longus muscles attempting to stabilize the foot. If the forces are severe, microtearing of the soft-tissue attachment to the periosteum can cause inflammation of the musculotendinous attachment to the bone.

An excessive number of foot strikes or the impact force of each foot strike, combined with an attempt at stabilization by the muscles mentioned, can cause the same result ("excessive" is relative and depends on the level of training of a particular athlete and the degree of adaptation of the tibia and the tissues connected to it; excessive may be 150 miles (240 Km) per week for one athlete, but only 5 miles (8 Km) per week for another).

SYMPTOMS AND SIGNS: There is pain and some swelling over the muscles on the posteromedial crest of the tibia, particularly in the middle third. The pain may be localized, or it may extend down the leg along the course of the posterior tibial muscle and tendon and around the medial malleolus to the attachment of the tendon to the navicular and first cuneiform.

In the early stages of the condition, the symptoms can occur after running only, but as it becomes more severe the pain also occurs at other times. Tenderness is present over the muscles and over the muscular attachment to the tibia (see Table 21.6). Small lumps of hematoma are often felt on the posteromedial aspect of the lower leg, usually in the middle third.

There is seldom tenderness over the tibia itself, and percussion and vibration tests are negative.[18] Testing the posterior tibial and the flexor hallucis longus muscles often produces pain and weakness of the muscle being tested.

TREATMENT: The painful area should be iced and ice massaged. Anti-inflammatory medication may be given if necessary. In-shoe orthotic devices are usually successful in controlling the pronation and relieving the excessive forces on the muscles. The posterior tibial, the flexor digitorum longus, and the flexor hallucis longus muscles should be strengthened, as should the intrinsic muscles of the foot.[17,19]

Good, shock-absorbent shoes that do not allow excessive pronation should be worn, and a softer training surface should be used for a time. Occasionally, taping the arch and lower leg helps. If necessary, decreased frequency and duration of weight-bearing workouts, with swimming as a substitute, should be suggested.

Compartment Compression Syndromes of the Lower Leg

There are four osseofascial compartments in the lower leg (see Figure 20.1):

1. Anterior
2. Lateral
3. Superficial posterior
4. Deep posterior

Any of these can develop a compartment compression syndrome. This syndrome is defined as a condition in which the circulation and function of the tissues within the compartment become compromised by an increase in pressure within that compartment.

ETIOLOGY: The anterior compartment will be used as an example to explain the development of the syndrome, as it is an almost closed compartment and the one most commonly affected. In the case of the anterior compartment, the interosseous membrane lies posteriorly, the tibia on one side and the fibula on the other. Anteriorly there is a relatively nonexpansile fascia covering the compartment. If pressure within the compartment rises, there is no space for the compartment to expand and accommodate it. Therefore symptoms and possibly changes in the muscles develop.[20,21,22]

The exact initiating mechanism of compartment compression in a runner is unknown in most cases. Sometimes mild trauma with bleeding into the compartment is the cause. (Severe bleeding into the compartment, for instance after a fracture, is probably the most common etiologic mechanism of the syndrome, but this does not apply to the runner.) In the case of runners, it is thought that muscle swelling produces the initial increase in pressure. This increased pressure leads in turn to impairment of venous outflow, resulting in a further rise in intracompartmental pressure. If the pressure becomes great enough, arterial circulation is then impeded, leading to ischemia (lack of blood supply) of the muscles and then necrosis[23] (see Figure 21.31).

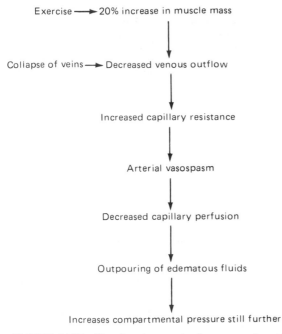

Exercise ⟶ 20% increase in muscle mass

↓

Collapse of veins ⟶ Decreased venous outflow

↓

Increased capillary resistance

↓

Arterial vasospasm

↓

Decreased capillary perfusion

↓

Outpouring of edematous fluids

↓

Increases compartmental pressure still further

FIGURE 21.31 The development of a compartment compression syndrome

VARIETIES: The compartment compression syndrome manifests in one of three ways:

1. Acute
2. Recurrent (less severe than the acute)
3. Acute-on-recurrent

1. _Acute._ An acute compartment compression syndrome is a surgical emergency. Those involved with athletes should always be aware of the possibility of this condition suddenly presenting in the guise of "shin splints." The commonly affected compartment is the anterior. The lateral is less often affected, and acute compression of the posterior is rare.

SYMPTOMS AND SIGNS: The symptom is intense pain developing during a run but not subsiding afterward. Palpation reveals a "woody-hard" tender muscle mass. Passive plantar flexion stretching of the foot may evoke pain. The dorsalis pedis and the anterior tibial pulses are usually present. However, decreased sensation may be noted in an area localized to the web of the first and second toes. If this is found, it suggests that the condition is quite advanced and is a definite indication for emergency surgical evaluation. Other signs of advanced tissue change include spreading numbness over the dorsum of the foot and weakness of the anterior tibial muscle, the extensor hallucis longus muscle, the extensor digitorum longus muscle, and the ankle evertors (Figure 21.32). When other compartments are involved, signs relative to their anatomy are found.[24,25,26,27]

DIAGNOSIS AND TREATMENT: The diagnosis should be made on clinical grounds. It may be confirmed by using a wick catheter or similar device to measure the intracompartmental pressure.[28,29,30] If the pressure is only slightly raised, the athlete may be treated conservatively with ice and observed carefully. If, however, the pressure reaches dangerous levels for more than a short while, surgical incision of the entire length of the fascia covering the affected compartment (fasciotomy) is indicated.[31]

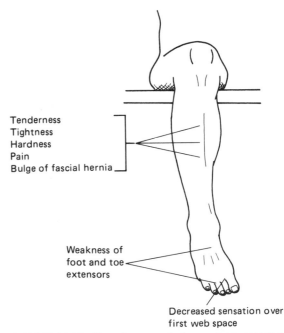

Tenderness
Tightness
Hardness
Pain
Bulge of fascial hernia

Weakness of foot and toe extensors

Decreased sensation over first web space

FIGURE 21.32 Symptoms and signs of an anterior compartment compression syndrome

2. Recurrent. This is more common in athletes than the acute variety. The etiology is unclear. It is also unclear what regulates the pressure so that dangerous levels are not reached.

SYMPTOMS AND SIGNS: The athlete complains of pain localized to the affected compartment whenever a particular level of activity is reached. Symptoms are much less severe than in the acute variety, but performance can be affected by pain and weakness of the muscles in the affected compartment. There is pain during or after a workout, but there is never "woody hardness" or extreme pain. The symptoms disappear fairly rapidly after activity ceases, especially if ice is applied. There is usually no evidence of any change in sensation over the dorsum of the foot.

TREATMENT: Ice applied after activity is the most valuable form of therapy. Some athletes find it useful to apply ice before exercising as well. Other suggestions for helping decrease symptoms include: stretching the anterior tibial muscles, balancing the strength of the muscles of the lower leg, changing the surface, wearing shoes with beveled heels, and using in-shoe orthotic devices.[32]

If the condition persists, the diagnosis should be confirmed by obtaining intracompartmental pressure readings before and after exercise, to help in the decision about whether a fascial release should be performed.[33]

A recurrent compartment syndrome involving the deep posterior compartment has been described. Athletes with this condition have medial tibial pain with tenderness over the middle or lower portion of the postero-medial crest.[34,35,36]

Tightness of the deep posterior compartment is difficult to evaluate clinically, but is sometimes mentioned by the athlete. There may be a feeling of numbness deep within the plantar aspect of the foot, and weakness of toe-off which coincides with the onset of pain. There is usually no pain or weakness on testing the posterior tibial, the flexor hallucis longus or the flexor digitorum longus muscles when in a resting state, though these muscles may demonstrate weakness at the time that symptoms are present.

This condition is usually treated with ice, exercises, anti-inflammatory medication and stretches, but if the symptoms do not rapidly improve, surgical release of the fascia frequently gives good results in spite of difficulty in documenting compartmental pressure increase.[37]

3. Acute-on-recurrent. Any athlete with symptoms of recurrent compartment syndrome should be informed that it is possible for those with long-standing symptoms to suddenly develop the acute variety, necessitating urgent fascial surgery.

The athlete with recurrent compartment syndrome should be warned that if the symptoms are more intense than usual, and do not subside within a short period of time, urgent medical help should be sought.

Fascial Hernia

ETIOLOGY: Occasionally defects occur in the fascia overlying the compartments, particularly over the anterior and lateral compartments. These defects allow the underlying muscle to bulge through when increased compartment pressure occurs during exercise. When the muscle herniates through the fascia, it may be caught in this defect and cause pain. This condition is often associated with the compartment compression syndrome.[38]

SYMPTOMS AND SIGNS: Pain and a bulge are the usual symptoms. It is often possible to palpate a hole in the fascia when the limb is in a nonexercised state. A definite bulge can be felt protruding through the defect during or immediately after exercise.

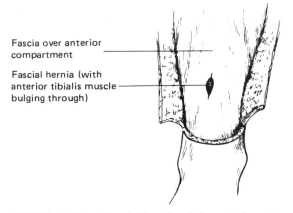

Fascia over anterior
compartment

Fascial hernia (with
anterior tibialis muscle
bulging through)

FIGURE 21.33   A fascial hernia of the anterior compartment of the leg

TREATMENT: Initial treatment is to tape a felt pad firmly over the defect, in an attempt to prevent the muscle from bulging through the fascia. This leads to resolution of the symptoms in some cases. If it does not produce the desired results, a fascial release (incision of the fascia) should be considered, particularly if there are also symptoms of a compartment compression syndrome.

Inflammation of the Anterior Tibial Tendon and Muscle

Inflammation of the anterior tibial tendon and muscle should be differentiated from the anterior compartment compression syndrome.

Inflammation of the muscles and tendons in the anterior compartment appears to be due to microtrauma, which is related to the inability of these muscles to adequately absorb the forces of foot deceleration at or after foot strike. These muscles place the foot in a dorsiflexed position just before impact and then control the speed of pronation during the initial contact and early mid-support phases. Factors frequently precipitating inflammation of these muscles are sudden increase in mileage or hard downhill running.

SYMPTOMS AND SIGNS: There are pain, tenderness, and sometimes swelling over the anterior muscle group. Occasionally, crepitation along the anterior tibial tendon can be felt. There is usually no increase in pressure over the anterior compartment. The tibialis anterior muscle is often weak and/or painful when tested. In addition, other muscles of the lower leg may also be weak, including the tibialis posterior, the extensor hallucis longus, and the extensor digitorum longus muscles.

It is important to feel the tone or firmness of the anterior compartment and to compare this with the opposite side. This tone should also be felt before, during, and after exercise, particularly when symptoms are present, to rule out the possibility of an anterior compartment compression syndrome in which a "woody hardness" is felt.

TREATMENT: Initially, icing and ice massage are performed while gently stretching the anterior muscles in a plantar flexed direction. Good, shock-absorbent shoes with beveled heels may take some of the strain off the anterior tibial tendon. If a biomechanical abnormality is present and is considered to be related to the symptoms, an in-shoe orthotic device may be indicated. Training should be done on a softer surface, and the duration and length of training should be decreased until symptoms have subsided. If symptoms are severe, anti-inflammatory medication and physical therapy, such as ultrasound and hydrocortisone, may be useful.

Once symptoms have improved, the anterior and posterior muscle groups should be strengthened and the anterior muscle group regularly stretched.

Fibular Stress Reaction and Stress Fracture

ETIOLOGY: The exact etiology is uncertain, but it occurs particularly in the undertrained, rather than the more advanced, runner. Sometimes it occurs when a well-conditioned athlete suddenly steps up the number of miles run per week. It may be related to the forward movement and torsional forces of the fibula during pronation.

SYMPTOMS AND SIGNS: Pain is commonly localized to the lower end of the fibula, about 7 cm to 10 cm above (or proximal to) the lateral malleolus, but is sometimes in the mid or upper portion of the fibula (Figure 21.34). Swelling may or may not be present. The tuning fork vibration test may be positive if a stress fracture is imminent.

TREATMENT: The athlete should be encouraged to decrease mileage and to run on a softer surface. Good, shock-absorbent shoes as well as soft orthotic devices may help the symptoms. Ice and aspirin may also be indicated.

If symptoms persist or increase, or swelling develops, it may be advisable to the athlete to stop running for a time. During this time, the athlete should run in place in a swimming pool while wearing a life jacket, to help maintain cardiovascular endurance. Stationary cycling is also useful. If symptoms are severe, it may occasionally be necessary to immobilize the lower leg with a posterior splint.

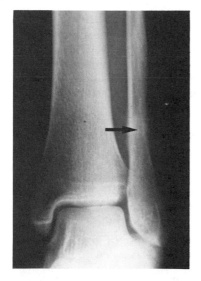

FIGURE 21.34   Stress fracture of the fibula

Popliteal Artery Entrapment Syndrome

The entrapment is an uncommon condition which usually occurs unilaterally in young men who are nonatherosclerotic, but may occur bilaterally. It can also occur in women.

ETIOLOGY: The cause of this syndrome is intermittent compression or entrapment of the popliteal artery by one of the heads of the gastrocnemius muscle, usually the medial.[39]

SYMPTOMS AND SIGNS: The athlete complains of paresthesia and/or pain in the foot and/or calf after running a specific distance. Walking may relieve the discomfort, after which a return to running may be possible. In some cases, symptoms are only produced while walking, and the athlete is able to run without pain.

There may be a decrease in the dorsalis pedis and posterior tibial artery pulses on active continuous plantar flexion of the foot or after passive dorsiflexion. A Doppler apparatus can be used to define the blood flow more clearly. Angiographic investigation shows entrapment of the popliteal artery.

COMPLICATIONS: Repetitive compression can result in chronic trauma to the popliteal artery, which can lead to an aneurysm or a thrombosis within the artery and subsequent loss of the limb. It is therefore vital to make the diagnosis before complications develop.

TREATMENT: Treatment of the entrapment is surgical. The offending head of the gastrocnemius muscle is completely divided to remove the pressure from the popliteal artery, which may need to be grafted with a saphenous vein graft.

Overuse Injuries to the Achilles Tendon

Though Achilles tendon overuse injuries are common problems, the nomenclature of these injuries is sometimes confusing. As mentioned earlier, the Achilles tendon does not have an actual sheath but rather a peritendinous tissue (the paratenon), and the classification is based on whether this tissue or the tendon itself is involved.[40]

1. Achilles peritendinitis—inflammation of the peritendinous tissue surrounding the tendon.

2. Achilles peritendinitis with tendinosis— the Achilles tendon itself shows areas of degeneration, in addition to inflammation of the paratenon. Partial tears—either microscopic or macroscopic—may be present. Bone spurs at the attachment of the Achilles to the posterior aspect of the calcaneus can also occur.[41]

3. Partial tears or tendinosis (see section on lower leg injuries, p. 378).

4. Total rupture (see section on lower leg injuries, p. 377).

ETIOLOGY: It is thought that overtraining, biomechanical malalignments, lack of adequate heel height, or unaccustomed use may lead to an inflammatory response to microtrauma of the peritendinous tissue or to microscopic tears within the tendon. If the tendon is involved, areas of necrosis can develop. In some cases, peritendinous inflammation develops as a response to tears within the tendon. Achilles tendinitis is often associated with a cavus foot configuration in conjunction with a tight Achilles, or with compensatory pronation due to a varus position of the lower leg, rearfoot, or forefoot.

SYMPTOMS AND SIGNS: The athlete presents with pain and swelling over the Achilles tendon and inability to perform. There is local tenderness on squeezing the Achilles tendon, and pain is present on forced passive dorsiflexion, resistance to active plantar flexion, or both. Crepitus may occur. If there is a nodular or fusiform swelling of the tendon, it suggests that microtrauma has led to an area of degeneration within the tendon.

X-RAYS: Soft-tissue lateral views may show changes in the outline of the Achilles tendon or within Kager's triangle.[42] (See Figure 20.14.)

TREATMENT: Initially, treatment is with ice and ice massage, heel lifts in the shoes, anti-inflammatory medication, and ultrasound. Running should be limited if symptoms persist.

If symptoms do not improve within a few days, any biomechanical abnormality should be corrected with in-shoe orthotic devices. If symptoms do not improve within a week to ten days with this treatment, it may be necessary to place the foot and ankle into a posterior splint, which rests the tendon but allows physical therapy to continue. If the symptoms are severe, it may be necessary to place the foot and lower leg in a cast, though this should be avoided if possible.

On occasion, surgical exploration may need to be undertaken. The paratenon is opened and stripped, the tendon incised to reveal any areas of degeneration, and bone spurs on the calcaneus removed.[41,43]

Rehabilitation includes gentle Achilles stretching done with the knee bent as well as straight (see section on stretching, p. 43). The whole lower extremity should be thoroughly rehabilitated, isokinetic machines being the most suitable form of resistance. If isokinetic machines are not available, exercises include toe-raises while standing on a 2″ (5 cm) board or on the edge of a stair, so the heel can drop below the level of the foot. These should be carefully done, and the number and excursion of dorsiflexion should be progressively increased. Exercises should also be prescribed for the anterior tibial and posterior tibial muscles, the quadriceps, and the hamstrings.

Retrocalcaneal Bursitis

This condition may be divided into two categories:

1. Inflammation of the deep, or retrocalcaneal, bursa lying between the Achilles tendon and the calcaneus

2. Inflammation of the superficial or subcutaneous bursa lying between the skin and the Achilles tendon (see Figure 20.3)

ETIOLOGY: Excessive compensatory pronation from whatever cause is the usual etiology of irritation of one of the bursa, particulary the deep bursa. However, retrocalcaneal bursitis is frequently found in those with cavus feet, particularly if a bone spur on the posterosuperior aspect of the calcaneus is also present.

SYMPTOMS AND SIGNS: Tenderness, pain, swelling, and redness involving the posterosuperior aspect of the heel and calcaneus, particularly on the lateral side, results in an inability to wear certain types of shoes, and thus performance is often impaired.

TREATMENT: Initially, ice and anti-inflammatory medication should be prescribed. It is important to protect the heel. In the case of the inflamed superficial bursa, the heel counter of the shoe may need to be incised and separated or have a hole cut in it (this will not help the deep retrocalcaneal bursa).

Control of excessive pronation with in-shoe orthotic devices helps control heel eversion and thus reduce inflammation of the deep retrocalcaneal bursa. Cortisone injected into or around the inflamed area might help in resistant cases. Occasionally it is necessary for surgery to be performed to remove any irritating soft tissue and bone spurs.

COMMON RUNNING-INDUCED INJURIES TO THE FOOT

Medial Arch Pain

ETIOLOGY: There are a number of conditions which may present with medial arch pain in the runner. The most common cause of "arch collapse" is associated with stretching of the *spring ligament*, which is caused by inadequate functioning of the supporting tibialis posterior muscle and leads to excessive pronation. This mechanism may also give rise to *entrapment of the medial calcaneal nerve*, with further aggravation of the problem. *Abductor hallucis spasm* may add to medial arch discomfort, and *medial plantar bursitis* is also often present.

SYMPTOMS AND SIGNS: Commonly there is pain and tenderness around the medial prominence of the navicular and the talonavicular joints. Swelling is occasionally present. There is often an accessory navicular as well as poor intrinsic foot musculature and insufficient functioning of the tibialis posterior muscle.

TREATMENT: Ice, anti-inflammatory medication, and LowDye taping should be commenced initially (see Chapter 5). Excessive pronation should be controlled with in-shoe orthotic devices and with exercises that develop the intrinsic musculature and the tibialis posterior and flexor hallucis longus muscles. Sometimes it is necessary to inject a corticosteroid into the plantar bursa or around an entrapped nerve. Surgery is occasionally necessary to relieve entrapment of the medial calcaneal nerve.

Plantar Fasciitis

Plantar fasciitis can be caused by an acute injury (strain) from sudden excessive loading of the foot. More often it is due to chronic irritation from excessive pronation, resulting in microtears of the plantar fascia. A high-arched, cavus foot is also at risk, as a tight plantar fascia is usually present in this type of foot (see Figure 21.9).

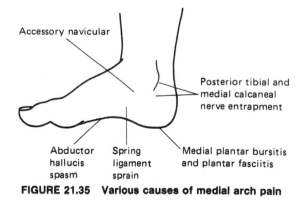

FIGURE 21.35 **Various causes of medial arch pain**

SYMPTOMS AND SIGNS: Pain and tenderness are localized to the plantar aspect of the foot, and they usually radiate from the heel forward, particularly when the athlete takes his or her first steps in the morning. Swelling may be seen near the heel. Localized tenderness is present at the plantar fascial attachment into the calcaneus, just distal to this attachment, in the area of the medial arch, over the medial band of the plantar fascia, and in the abductor hallucis muscle. There may be pain on actively and passively dorsiflexing the foot, especially if the big toe is also dorsiflexed. A tight plantar fascial band can be palpated (see Figure 20.9).

TREATMENT: Ice-massage and anti-inflammatory medication should be used initially. Excessive pronation should be limited by means of LowDye taping, in-shoe orthotic devices, or both. In the case of a high-arched foot, a carefully selected in-shoe orthotic device with good shock absorbency can be used. Local corticosteroid injections should be used judiciously. Surgery is rarely necessary.

Cuboid Dysfunction (Sometimes Called Subluxation)

ETIOLOGY: The etiology is uncertain but may be related in some cases to dysfunction of the calcaneocuboid joint or to passage of the peroneus longus tendon through a groove on the inferior aspect of the cuboid.[44] It occurs particularly in middle- and long-distance runners.

SYMPTOMS AND SIGNS: Presentation is fairly acute, with severe pain, tenderness, and sometimes swelling localized to the calcaneocuboid joint. There is localized tenderness to palpation on the plantar aspect of the foot and laterally over the joint.

TREATMENT: After X-rays of the foot have been taken to exclude bony pathology, the cuboid may be manipulated by one of a num-

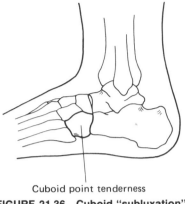

Cuboid point tenderness

FIGURE 21.36   Cuboid "subluxation"

ber of methods. This should be followed by LowDye taping. If the athlete is seen some time after the onset of the condition, swelling and inflammation may be present, necessitating the use of ice, elevation, and anti-inflammatory medication. In long-standing cases resistant to other forms of therapy, surgical exploration of the cuboid and peroneus longus tendon has been undertaken.

Black Toenails

Black toenails are notorious among runners, but are becoming less frequent with the increased room in the toe box of the newer shoes. A shoe that allows the foot to slide forward also predisposes the athlete to this condition.

Black discoloration of a toenail results from pressure which damages the small blood vessels beneath the nail, forming a blood blister. The nail is usually elevated from the nail bed. If this occurs on the big toe, it may be necessary to release the pressure beneath the nail. This is accomplished by heating a straightened paper clip until red hot and melting a number of small holes through the nail with it, thus allowing the fluid to drain. Often the injured toenail falls off within two to four weeks. The new nail may be somewhat thicker and deformed compared with the original, however.

IN-SHOE ORTHOTIC DEVICES

In-Shoe Orthotic Devices for Overuse Running Injuries

In-shoe orthotic devices in athletics, particularly for runners, have gained acceptance and popularity in recent years. Orthotic devices (or *orthotics* as they are commonly called) are not a panacea for all running-related problems, though they are certainly useful in particular conditions (to be discussed). They may cause new problems if they are not made accurately or are used for conditions for which they are not indicated.

In order to judge whether a particular foot type or lower extremity alignment will respond to orthotics, it is necessary to examine the foot and to note the angular measurements. The athlete should then be observed running, as there may be marked pronation when standing, but excellent function when running, as the muscles are able to control the position of the feet. Conversion from the flexible adaptor to a rigid lever should take place in the latter half of the mid-support phase. If the foot is still flexible and loose during take-off, it is quite likely that the athlete will benefit from an in-shoe orthotic device.[45,46]

The purpose of such a device is to place the foot in a position of improved mechanical advantage or efficiency, so the joints and muscles will be more favorably positioned to deal with the repetitive forces applied to them. Some symptom complexes that have been responsive include:

1. Medial longitudinal arch pain and plantar fasciitis

2. Generalized foot pain—the foot is placed in a neutral position and the orthotics suitably posted

3. Morton's neuroma—a metatarsal bar is added to the orthotic

4. Sesamoid pain—controlled by posting behind the metatarsal head with a cutout made for the sesamoid

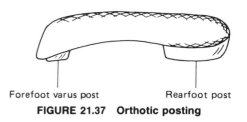

Forefoot varus post   Rearfoot post

FIGURE 21.37   Orthotic posting

5. Heel bruises—cushioned by a donut which surrounds the tender area

6. Medial tibial pain from the medial tibial stress syndrome

7. Medial and peripatellar pain due to malalignment, in particular the malalignment syndrome of anteversion, medially squinting patellae, tibia varum, and pronated feet

8. Patellar tendinitis associated with a wide Q angle and excessive pronation

9. Hip pain or backache due to a short leg from either an anatomical or functional cause

Be careful with more rigid feet that need precise control. Often, additional shock absorbency is needed, especially with the rigid cavus foot, as incorrect posting of the orthotic may produce new symptoms!

With experience in using orthotics, the indications for their use in a particular condition will become clearer and better defined.

Types of Orthotics

The numerous types of available orthotics can be grouped into three categories:

1. Soft, temporary orthotic devices such as felt placed on podiatry mold or cork, and Spenco, etc.

2. Semirigid devices such as Sporthotics and combinations of Plastazote with Aliplast.

3. Rigid orthotic devices such as one of the many types of Rohadur acrylic.

Temporary soft orthotics are often initially useful for evaluating the athlete's re-

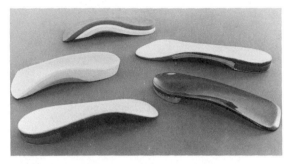

FIGURE 21.38 **Various types of orthotics** Starting at the top and moving clockwise: Regalite with Plastazote (very soft); Sporthotic for the long-distance runner (slightly flexible plastic with cushioned undersurface); Rohadur (hard plastic); Sporthotic (slightly flexible plastic); Plastazote with Aliplast (soft but firm).

sponse. After that, the more permanent semirigid or rigid devices can be prescribed if the response is favorable. Semirigid devices are commonly used for runners and laterally moving sports. A few athletes, mainly long-distance runners, need more precise control of their biomechanical foot function, and they do best with rigid (or acrylic) supports.

The soft devices are usually made from an outline of the foot and posted with felt according to the type of foot encountered. Adjustments are made by clinical experience, attempting to balance the foot toward a neutral position (Figure 21.39). Devices such as Plastazote and Aliplast are heat-molded to the foot, with the subtalar joint placed in or near its neutral position, as it is currently assumed that the foot functions best at, or nearly at, its neutral position (Figure 21.40). Rigid, and some semirigid, devices need to be made from a cast of the foot, usually taken when the foot is non-weight-bearing and in the neutral position (other methods of obtaining casts include: fully weight-bearing, semi-weight-bearing, non-weight-bearing with the subtalar joint in neutral position but the forefoot brought down perpendicular to the rearfoot). These casts are then sent to a podiatric orthotic laboratory, where a positive mold of the negative cast is made.

Taking the Cast Impression

The technique describes a *non-weight-bearing* cast impression with the subtalar joint in the neutral position.

1. The athlete should have been examined and all necessary measurements recorded (see examination of a running athlete, p. 422).

2. The athlete lies supine with the lower third of the leg unsupported over the end of the examining table. The pelvis should be adjusted so the feet are perpendicular to the ground and neither abducted nor adducted. This is accomplished by placing a pillow under one or both hips, to bring the feet to the perpendicular position.

3. Strips of plaster of Paris 4″ (10 cm) (or sometimes 5″ (12 cm)) wide are used. The length of each strip is determined by measuring the distance from the head of the fifth metatarsal, around the heel, to the head of the first metatarsal around the toes. Four strips of this length are cut to size. Two strips are used together to provide adequate strength for the cast. The first double layer is dipped into warm water for a few seconds (a teaspoon (5 ml) of alum is added to facilitate hardening of the cast). Most of the water is then squeezed out and the plaster placed along the side of the foot, from the head of the fifth metatarsal around the heel to the head of the first metatarsal, and smoothed down to eliminate creases. The excess plaster is then brought up behind the heel.

4. The second double layer of plaster of Paris is applied from the head of the first metatarsal around the toes to the lateral side of the foot, with the excess folded beneath the toes (Figure 21.40).

5. The foot is then brought into the neutral position by grasping the heads of the fourth and fifth metatarsals just proximal to the metatarsophalangeal joint while palpating the relationship of the head of the talus to the navicular, as previously described. The foot is then dorsiflexed in this position until

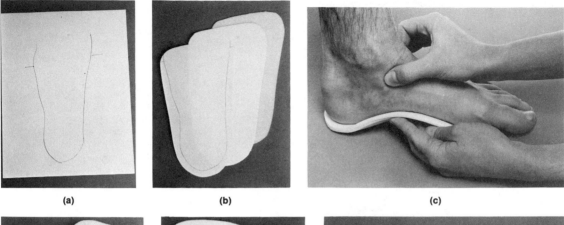

(a)   (b)   (c)

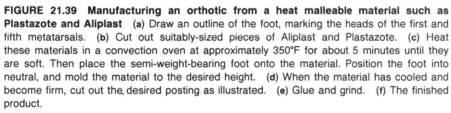

(d)   (e)   (f)

FIGURE 21.39 Manufacturing an orthotic from a heat malleable material such as Plastazote and Aliplast (a) Draw an outline of the foot, marking the heads of the first and fifth metatarsals. (b) Cut out suitably-sized pieces of Aliplast and Plastazote. (c) Heat these materials in a convection oven at approximately 350°F for about 5 minutes until they are soft. Then place the semi-weight-bearing foot onto the material. Position the foot into neutral, and mold the material to the desired height. (d) When the material has cooled and become firm, cut out the desired posting as illustrated. (e) Glue and grind. (f) The finished product.

resistance is felt (which indicates that the midtarsal joint is "locked"). This position is then held until the plaster of Paris has dried.

6. It is important to ensure that the athlete is completely relaxed and does not contract any of the muscles of the lower leg or foot. In particular, the anterior tibial tendon should not be able to be palpated during the casting procedure. If any of the lower leg muscles are tense, a false impression of the rearfoot-to-forefoot relationship will be obtained.

7. The other foot is then put into a cast in the same manner.

8. When the casts are dried they are easily removed from the feet. However, care should be taken to ensure that the casts are not distorted as they are removed.

PREVENTION OF HEAT INJURIES DURING LONG-DISTANCE RUNNING

With more and more recreational athletes participating in an increasing number of distance running events, prevention of heat in-

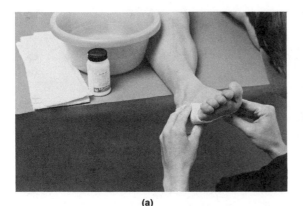

(a)

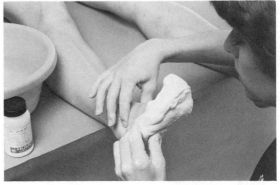

(b)

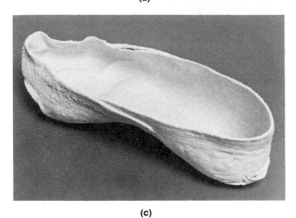

(c)

FIGURE 21.40   **Obtaining a neutral cast of the foot, non-weight-bearing, for the manufacture of an orthotic device**   (a) Strips of plaster of Paris are applied to the heel and sole. (b) Strips of plaster are then applied to the forefoot and the foot positioned into neutral. The fourth and fifth metatarsal heads are then loaded until resistance is felt. The foot is held in this position until dry. (c) The finished cast.

juries has assumed an important place in the organization of these races. If a runner loses 3% of body weight from sweat and fluid loss during a race, the body fatigues more easily. When 5% to 10% of body weight is lost the runner is in danger. Dehydration of this magnitude severely limits subsequent sweating, places a dangerous demand on the circulation, reduces exercise capacity, and exposes the runner to possible serious heat injury[47,48] (see Chapter 25). It is thought that middle-aged and aging men and women possess significantly less heat tolerance than their younger counterparts and so are at increased risk.

The American College of Sports Medicine has published a position statement[49] with guidelines for preventing heat injuries in runners. These suggestions include the following:

1. No long-distance race should be run when the wet-bulb globe thermometer (WBGT) is higher than 28°C (82.4°F).

2. Races should be held early in the morning or late in the evening in areas where the daylight dry bulb temperature exceeds 27°C (80°F).[50]

3. Race organizers should provide adequate quantities of fluids at the start of a race and at water stations. These should be available every 3 Km to 4 Km (2 to 2½ miles).

4. There should be adequate medical and paramedical coverage of the race including medical personnel at each station.

5. Organizational personnel should reserve the right to stop runners who exhibit clear signs of heat stroke or heat exhaustion.

6. Runners should be educated by means of a printed pre-race instruction sheet con-

taining recommendations on training, suggestions on pre-race nutrition and fluid intake, and guidelines for consumption of fluids and recognition of heat symptoms during a race.

7. Immediately before the race, the existing as well as the predicted temperature and relative humidity should be announced to the runners, and an interpretation of these values made. If the temperature exceeds 24°C (75°F), novice runners should be advised to decrease their planned running pace by about forty-five to sixty seconds per mile.

8. Organizers should remind runners of fluid requirements and the symptoms of heat injury, and should suggest that if a runner notices these symptoms in another, he or she should offer or summon aid.

9. Sprinkling down the runners with a garden hose or similar apparatus along the course of the race is a useful way of preventing excessive temperature buildup.

The best protection against development of heat injury is adequate consumption of fluid in the form of water. The athlete should prepare by consuming

1. One liter or more of fluid 2 hours before the race

2. Five hundred milliliters 15 minutes before the race (one tall glass).

3. At least 300 to 500 milliliters of fluid every 15 minutes during the race

Adequate rehydration must be achieved over the 24 hours following the race. Waiting until thirsty is *too late*.

REFERENCES

1. Slocum DB, James SL: Biomechanics of running. *JAMA* 205:97–104, 1968.
2. James SL, Brubaker CE: Biomechanics of running. *Orthop Clin North Am* 4:609–615, 1973.
3. Mann RA, Hagy J: Biomechanics of walking, running, and sprinting. *Am J Sports Med* 5:345–350, 1980.
4. Drez Jr, D: Running footwear. Examination of the training shoe, the foot, and functional orthotic devices. Symposium. *Am J Sports Med* 8:140–141, 1980.
5. Subotnick SI: The flat foot. *Phys Sportsmed* 9:85–91, August 1981.
6. Renne J: The iliotibial band friction syndrome. *J Bone Joint Surg* 57A:1110–1111, 1975.
7. Orava S: The iliotibial tract friction syndrome in athletes—an uncommon exertion syndrome on the lateral side of the knee. *Br J Sports Med* 12:69–73, 1978.
8. McNicol K, Tauton JE, Clement DB: Iliotibial tract friction syndrome in athletes. *Can J Appl Sports Sci* 6:77–80, 1981.
9. Sutker AN, Jackson DW, Pagliano JW: Iliotibial band syndrome in distance runners. *Phys Sportsmed* 9:69–73, October 1981.
10. Mayfield GW: Popliteus tendon tenosynovitis. *Am J Sports Med* 5:31–36, 1977.
11. Noble HB, Hajek MR, Porter M: Diagnosis and treatment of iliotibial band tightness in runners. *Phys Sportsmed* 10:67–74, April 1982.
12. Noble CA: The treatment of iliotibial band friction syndrome. *Br J Sports Med* 13:51–54, 1979.
13. Noble CA: The iliotibial band friction syndrome in runners. *Am J Sports Med* 8:232–234, 1980.
14. Slocum DB: The shin splint syndrome: Medical aspects and differential diagnosis. *Proceedings of 8th National Conference on the Medical Aspects of Sports*, AMA November 1966.
15. Stanitski CL, McMaster JH, Scranton PE: On the nature of stress fractures. *Am J Sports Med* 6:391–396, 1978.
16. Devas MB: Stress fractures in athletes. *J Sports Med* 1:49–51, 1973.
17. Clement DB: Tibial stress syndrome in athletes. *J Sports Med* 2:81–85, 1974.
18. Jackson DW: Shin splints: common, painful, and confusing. *Consultant* 16:75–79, February 1976.
19. Rasmussen W: Shin splints: Definition and treatment. Sports safety supplement. *J Sports Med* 2:111–117, 1974.
20. Leach RE, Zohn DA, Stryker WS: Anterior tibial compartment syndrome. Clinical and electromyographic aspects. *Arch Surg* 88:187–192, 1964.
21. Leach RE, Hammond G, Stryker WS: Anterior tibial compartment syndrome. Acute and chronic. *J Bone Joint Surg* 49A:451–462, 1967.
22. Leach RE, Corbett M: Anterior tibial compartment syndrome in soccer players. *Am J Sports Med* 7:258–259, 1979.
23. Reneman RS: The anterior and lateral compartmental syndrome of the leg due to intensive use of muscles. *Clin Orthop* 113:69–80, 1975.
24. Lunceford Jr, EM: The peroneal compartment syndrome. *Southern Med J* 58:621–623, 1965.
25. Lipscomb AB, Ibrahim AA: Acute peroneal compartment syndrome in a well conditioned athlete:

A report of a case. *Am J Sports Med* 5:154–157, 1977.

26. Goodman MJ: Isolated lateral-compartment syndrome. Report of a case. *J Bone Joint Surg* 62A:834, 1980.

27. Mubarak SJ, Owens CA, Garfin S, et al: Acute exertional superficial posterior compartment syndrome. *Am J Sports Med* 6:287–294, 1978.

28. Mubarak SJ, Hargens AR, Owen CA, et al: The wick catheter technique for measurement of intramuscular pressure. A new research and clinical tool. *J Bone Joint Surg* 58A:1016–1020, 1976.

29. Mubarak SJ, Owen CA, Hargens AR et al: Acute compartment syndromes: Diagnosis and treatment with the aid of the wick catheter. *J Bone Joint Surg* 60A:1091–1095, 1978.

30. Matsen FA, Winquist RA, Krugmire RB: Diagnosis and management of compartmental syndromes. *J Bone Joint Surg* 62A:286–291, 1980.

31. Whitesides Jr, TE, Haney TC, Morimoto K, et al: Tissue pressure measurements as a determinant for the need of fasciotomy. *Clin Orthop* 113:43–51, 1975.

32. Veith RG, Matsen FA III, Newell SG: Recurrent anterior compartmental syndromes. *Phys Sportsmed* 8:80–88, November 1980.

33. Puranen J, Alavaikko A: Intracompartmental pressure increase on exertion in patients with chronic compartment syndrome in the leg. *J Bone Joint Surg* 63A:1304–1309, 1981.

34. Orava S, Puranen J: Athletes' leg pains. *Br J Sports Med* 13:92–97, 1979.

35. Puranen J: The medial tibial syndrome. Exercise ischemia in the medial fascial compartment of the leg. *J Bone Joint Surg* 56B:712–715, 1974.

36. Matsen FA III, Clawson DK: The deep posterior compartmental syndrome of the leg. *J Bone Joint Surg* 57A:34–39, 1975.

37. D'Ambrosia RD, Zelis RF, Chuinard RG: Interstitial pressure measurements in the anterior and posterior compartments in athletes with shin splints. *Am J Sports Med* 5:127–131, 1977.

38. Garfin S, Mubarak SJ, Owen CA: Exertional anterolateral-compartment syndrome. Case report with fascial defect, muscle herniation, and superficial peroneal nerve entrapment. *J Bone Joint Surg* 59A:404–405, 1977.

39. Darling RC, Buckley CJ, Abbott WM, et al: Intermittent claudication in young athletes: Popliteal artery entrapment syndrome. *Trauma* 14:543–552, 1974.

40. Santilli G: Achilles tendinopathies and paratendinopathies. *J Sports Med* 19:245–259, 1979.

41. Leach RE, James SL, Wasilewski S: Achilles tendinitis. *Am J Sports Med* 9:93–98, 1981.

42. Pudu G, Ippolito E, Postacchini F: A classification of achilles tendon disease. *Am J Sports Med* 4:145–150, 1976.

43. Clancy WG, Neidhart D, Brand RL: Achilles tendinitis in runners. A report of five cases. *Am J Sports Med* 4:46–57, 1976.

44. Newell SG, Woodle A: Cuboid syndrome. *Phys Sportmed* 9:71–76, April 1981.

45. Bates BT, Osternig LR, Mason MS, et al: Foot orthotic devices to modify selected aspects of lower extremity mechanics. *Am J Sports Med* 7:338–342, 1979.

46. Scranton Jr, PE, Pedegana LR, Whitesel JP: Gait analysis. Alterations in support phase forces using supportive devices. *Am J Sports Med* 10:6–11, 1982.

47. Wyndham CH, Strydom NB: The danger of an inadequate water intake during marathon running. *S Afr Med J* 43:893–896, 1969.

48. Wyndham CH: Heat stroke and hyperthermia in marathon runners. *Ann NY Acad Sci* 301:128–138, 1977.

49. American College of Sports Medicine Position Statement on prevention of heat injuries during distance running. *Med Sci Sports* 7:VII–IX, 1975.

50. Smith WB: Environmental factors in running. Symposium. *Am J Sports Med* 8:138–140, 1980.

RECOMMENDED READINGS

Bates BT, Osternig LR, Mason BR, et al: Functional variability of the lower extremity during the support phase of running. *Med Sci Sports* 11:328–331, 1979.

Blatz DJ: Bilateral femoral and tibial shaft stress fractures in a runner. *Am J Sports Med* 9:322–325, 1981.

Brody DM: Running injuries. *CIBA Clinical Symposia* 32:2–36, 1980.

Brubaker CE, James SL: Injuries to runners. *J Sports Med* 2:189–197, 1974.

Clancy WG: Lower extremity injuries in the jogger and distance runner. *Phys Sportsmed* 2:46–50, June 1974.

Clancy WG: Runners' injuries. Part One. Symposium. *Am J Sports Med* 8:137–138, 1980.

Clancy WG: Runners' injuries. Part Two. Evaluation and treatment of specific injuries. Symposium. *Am J Sports Med* 8:287–289, 1980.

Clement DB, Taunton JE: A guide to the prevention of running injuries. *Austr Fam Phys* 10:156–164, 1981.

Clement DB, Taunton JE, Smart GW, et al: A survey of overuse running injuries. *Phys Sportsmed* 9:47–58, May 1981.

Corrigan AD, Fitch KD: Complications of jogging. *Med J Aust* 2:363–368, 1972.

Costill DL, Branam G, Eddy D, et al: Determinants of marathon running success. *Int Z Angew Physiol* 29:249–254, 1971.

Costill DL, Kammer WF, Fisher A: Fluid ingestion during distance running. *Arch Environ Health* 21:520–525, 1970.

Costill DL, Saltin B: Factors limiting gastric empyting during rest and exercise. *J Appl Physiol* 37:679–683, 1974.

Detmer DE: Chronic leg pain. Symposium. *Am J Sports Med* 8:141–144, 1980.

Drez Jr, D, Young JC, Johnston RD, et al: Metatarsal stress fractures. *Am J Sports Med* 8:123–125, 1980.

Goergen TG, Venn-Watson EA, Rossman DJ, et al: Tarsal navicular stress fractures in runners. *Am J Roentg* 136:201–203, 1981.

Hanson PG: Heat injury in runners. *Phys Sportsmed* 7:91–96, June 1979.

James SL, Bates BT, Osternig LR: Injuries to runners. *Am J Sports Med* 6:40–50, 1978.

James SL, Brubaker CE: Running mechanics. *JAMA* 221:1014–1016, 1972.

Krissoff WB, Ferris WD: Runners' injuries. *Phys Sportsmed* 7:54–64, December 1979.

Noble HB, Bachman D: Medical aspects of distance race planning. *Phys Sportsmed* 7:78–96, June 1979.

Raether PM, Lutter LD: Recurrent compartment syndrome in the posterior thigh. Report of a case. *Am J Sports Med* 10:40–43, 1982.

Root ML, Orien WP, Weed JH, Hughes RJ: *Biomechanical Examination of the Foot.* Los Angeles, Clinical Biomechanics Corporation, 1971.

Root ML, Orien WP, Weed JH: *Normal and Abnormal Function of the Foot.* Los Angeles Clinical Biomechanics Corporation, 1977.

Ryan AJ: Moderator Round Table Discussion on: Leg pains in runners. *Phys Sportsmed* 5:42–53, September 1977.

Slocum DB, Bowerman W: Biomechanics of running. *Clin Orthop* 23:39–45, 1962.

Smart GW, Taunton JE, Clement DB: Achilles tendon disorders in runners—a review. *Med Sci Sports Exerc* 12:231–243, 1980.

Stewart PJ, Posen GA: Case report: Acute renal failure following a marathon. *Phys Sportsmed* 8:61–64, 1980.

CHAPTER 22

Swimming Injuries

Overuse injuries resulting from the long and grueling workouts that competitive (and recreational) swimmers undergo have only recently been explored and documented. Most of these injuries affect the shoulder, the knee, and the anterior aspect of the ankle and are related to a particular stroke. Each stroke is liable to provide its own peculiar injury complex, but freestyle is the most commonly used stroke, no matter what stroke the swimmer uses in competition.

"Swimmer's Shoulder"

The shoulder is the most commonly injured anatomical area in swimmers. Most cases of swimmer's shoulder are due to *impingement of the supraspinatus and biceps tendons* (and other rotator-cuff tendons) under the acromial process and coraco-acromial ligament (the coraco-acromial arch).[1,2,3] The shoulder of the average competitive swimmer is put through the cycle of abduction–forward flexion–internal rotation many thousands of times each day, leading to an inflammatory response to microtrauma that takes place under the coraco-acromial arch. It has been shown that the part of the rotator cuff that impinges against the coraco-acromial arch is poorly vascularized, which further exaggerates the pathology.

PREVENTION: Gentle, slow static stretching exercises should be performed both before and after workouts. A period of easy swimming before any vigorous workout should be routine. A change to different strokes, especially the backstroke, should be made every now and then during a workout. The use of handpaddles should be limited, as a correlation has been found between their use and shoulder symptoms. If any discomfort is felt, ice should be applied after the workout. While the ice is being applied, the shoulder should be put through a full range of movement and gently stretched.

Evidence is being collected on the importance of adequate muscle function in preventing the development of impingement. Muscle tests, especially of the posterior deltoid and the internal and external rotators, should be conducted on swimmers at regular intervals in an attempt to elicit weaknesses before shoulder symptoms and pathological changes arise. Any imperfections of technique which could produce an impingement should also be looked for and corrected.

SYMPTOMS: Pain and inability to perform are the usual symptoms. The pain may be anterior or anterolateral but is usually diffuse. Most symptoms are produced during the recovery or pull-through phases of the swimming motion, especially at or just after hand entry, at which the shoulder is fully abducted.

SIGNS:

1. Tenderness over the greater tuberosity and acromial process, the biceps tendon, or both
2. A positive "impingement sign" (see section on shoulder injuries, p. 167)
3. Weakness of the posterior deltoid and other individual muscles

TREATMENT: Treatment depends on the phase of the condition.

Phase I: Symptoms are present only after the workout. Ice is applied to the shoulder before and particularly after workouts. During this time a full range of movement and stretching of the shoulder girdle should be performed. Any muscle weakness or dysfunction should be corrected. Anti-inflammatory medications, starting with aspirin, ibuprofen (Motrin), or a similar drug, can be commenced. TENS and ultrasound may be useful. Changing strokes during the workout is important, as is a change in workout schedule. Examination of the swimmer's technique may bring to light an underlying problem. Swimming with hand paddles should be discontinued.

Phase II: Symptoms are present during and after workouts. More powerful anti-inflammatory medication, in the form of phenylbutazone, may be useful for a short period of time (from four to eight days). Icing of the shoulder should continue before and after workouts, possibly during workouts if the shoulder begins to be uncomfortable. TENS can be used before and after workouts, as can ultrasound. There should be a decrease in the total yardage swum.

Phase III: Pain is present at all times. At this stage of the condition, the swimmer should cease swimming and continue with the treatment outlined in Phase II. Cardiovascular endurance should be maintained by kicking, though a kickboard should not be used, as this can put a strain on the arm and possibly produce some impingement. Other cardiovascular conditioning exercises include running in place in the swimming pool while wearing a life preserver and dry-land exercises such as cycling, running, and jumping rope.

Corticosteroid injections should not be used except in the most resistant cases, and they should be followed by a layoff of six weeks. The shoulder musculature should be completely rehabilitated before return to the pool. In resistant cases, a decision may need to be made as to whether surgical release of the coraco-acromial arch is indicated. Though the surgery is frequently successful in selected cases, it does not always result in completely pain-free swimming.

Anterior Subluxation of the Glenohumeral Joint

Anterior subluxation of the glenohumeral joint can be produced by repeated use of the backstroke, particularly on entering the flip-turn, when the shoulder is in full external rotation and abduction.

SIGNS: The standard apprehension test for anterior subluxation can be used to clinically confirm the diagnosis. The swimmer should also be examined in the position of a backstroke turn, with pressure applied to the posterior aspect of the humeral head, thereby forcing it into an anterior direction.[4] X-ray views of the shoulder, particularly the West Point view, may be useful in showing a bony defect of the anterior glenoid.

TREATMENT: Specific muscle testing may expose weaknesses which can often be strengthened. If the rehabilitation does not succeed, the swimmer will have to decide whether to live with it, stop swimming the backstroke, or undergo surgery for anterior subluxation.

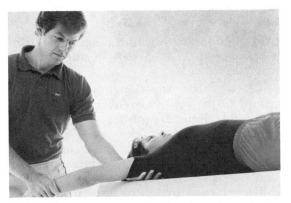

FIGURE 22.1 The apprehension test for anterior subluxation in a swimmer

"Breaststroker's Knee"

Breaststroker's knee has long been associated with the whip kick, but the exact pathology and the anatomical area involved appear to be a matter of controversy. Evidence seems to favor an injury of the tibial collateral ligament, but chondromalacia patellae, medial synovitis, or irritation of the medial retinaculum may be involved in certain individuals.[5,6,7] The area involved may depend on the type of technical fault in a particular swimmer's whip kick,[8] especially in the less-than-top-level swimmer, while the stress of 15,000 to 20,000 whip kicks per week may play a role in the elite swimmer.

MECHANISM OF INJURY: Studies with underwater photography have shown that during the whip kick a valgus stress is applied to the knee when the hip is in an abducted and internally rotated position and as the knee rapidly moves from flexion to extension in an externally rotated position. This movement may put a considerable strain on the medial aspects of the knee and patella, particularly when external rotation, abduction, or both accompany full extension.

PREVENTION:

1. Adjustment of technique, possibly with the aid of an underwater camera, to help prevent an incorrectly performed whip kick from producing symptoms.

2. Isolation and correction of any muscle weakness.

3. General strengthening program for the lower extremity as a part of the training schedule.

4. Slow, static stretching of the muscle groups of the lower extremity. For instance, the swimmer stands with legs apart and feet in external rotation. The knees go slowly into a valgus position, thus placing gentle tension on the medial stabilizing complex. This may allow the tibial collateral ligament and the medial joint structures to adapt to the position that seems to produce the most stress on the knee.

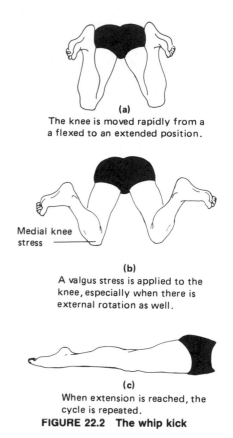

(a)
The knee is moved rapidly from a a flexed to an extended position.

Medial knee stress

(b)
A valgus stress is applied to the knee, especially when there is external rotation as well.

(c)
When extension is reached, the cycle is repeated.
FIGURE 22.2   The whip kick

5. Avoidance of the breaststroke for two months each year by the breaststroke swimmer, with frequent variations in the stroke used.

SYMPTOMS AND SIGNS: Initially, pain is present only when the athlete performs the whip kick, but if participation is continued in spite of pain, symptoms may occur with other strokes and even with walking. Clinically there is usually no swelling, but tenderness may be localized to the course of the tibial collateral ligament, to its attachment to the tibia, or to the medial aspect of the patella. Applying a valgus stress with the tibia in external rotation and the knee in 20° to 30° of flexion may cause pain, as may passively moving the patella laterally.

TREATMENT: As soon as any symptoms arise, the swimmer should be told to ice the affected limb before and after workouts and should be evaluated for any muscle weaknesses. Aspirin or some other anti-inflammatory agent and ultrasound can be started. Consulting the coach about possible technique changes is important because correcting the technical fault can prevent further injury. Should the symptoms persist, the whip kick should not be used for a few weeks.

Irritation of the Extensor Retinaculum of the Ankle

The "flutter kick" is used extensively in freestyle and backstroke swimming. This motion tends to produce a position of excessive plantar flexion of both the foot and the ankle, placing pressure on the structures running under the extensor retinaculum. Tendinitis can develop, with pain, swelling, and crepitation of the anterior tibial, the extensor digitorum longus, and the extensor hallucis longus tendons. The extensor retinaculum itself can become inflamed.

TREATMENT: Changes of technique have been suggested to prevent the problem, that is, using the arms more than the legs and training on a two-beat instead of a six-beat crossover leg kick. Ice, ultrasound, a local corticosteroid injection around the extensor retinaculum, and walking and sleeping in a posterior splint with the ankle at 90° may help reduce symptoms.

REFERENCES

1. Kennedy JC, Hawkins RJ: Swimmer's shoulder. *Phys Sportsmed* 2:34–38, April 1974.
2. Richardson AB, Jobe FW, Collins HR: The shoulder in competitive swimming. *Am J Sports Med* 8:159–163, 1980.
3. Dominguez RH: Shoulder pain in swimmers. *Phys Sportsmed* 8:37–42, July 1980.
4. Kennedy JC, Hawkins RJ, Kristoff WB: Orthopedic manifestations of swimming. *Am J Sports Med* 6:309–322, 1978.
5. Stulberg SD, Shulman K, Stuart S, et al: Breaststroker's knee: pathology, etiology, and treatment. *Am J Sports Med* 8:164–171, 1980.
6. Keskinen K, Eriksson E, Komi P: Breaststroke swimmer's knee: A biomechanical and arthroscopic study. *Am J Sports Med* 8:228–231, 1980.
7. Kennedy JC, Hawkins RJ: Breaststroker's knee. *Phys Sportsmed* 2:33–38, January 1974.
8. Counsilman JE: *The Science of Swimming.* Englewood Cliffs NJ, Prentice-Hall Inc, 1968, pp 117–123.

RECOMMENDED READING

Penny JN, Smith C: Prevention and treatment of swimmer's shoulder. *Can J Appl Sport Sci* 5:195–202, 1980.

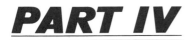

PART IV

Other Areas
for Consideration

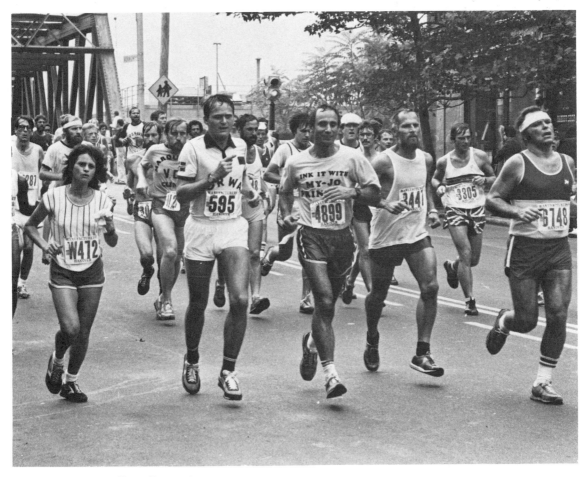

Photo by Yan Lucas, Photo Researchers

CHAPTER 23

The Female Athlete

INTRODUCTION

Over the past decade there has been a dramatic increase in participation by women in both organized and unorganized athletic activities. The passage of Title IX of the United States Education Amendment of 1972, part of which was related to the establishment of equal athletic facilities for males and females in schools receiving federal funds, facilitated the means by which women could better participate in organized athletics. The resulting unprecedented swing by women towards competitive athletics not only demanded a change in social attitudes, but also raised numerous questions that needed to be answered, such as the following:

Are women really genetically inferior to males in their physical makeup, or is this concept a product of society's attitudes and women's previous activity level?

Are women more likely to suffer injuries than males, and are these injuries likely to be different?

Do women have the ability to increase their strength and, if so, will they develop male-type physiques as a result of weight training?

Will women be harmed by participating in endurance events?

Even though the past few years have seen the accumulation of more and more research data, the volume is still relatively small. Many of the questions are just beginning to be answered. A review of some of the research information is presented in this chapter.

THE PREPUBERTAL PERIOD

Many attitudes toward female physical inferiority are initiated at the prepubertal level. For instance, even though the six-year-old male is only slightly taller and heavier than the female, their gym classes have traditionally been separated. This separation of the sexes may imply to the young male that the female is not able to perform as adequately as he can, even though in many school situations the fastest runners in the class are girls. This may also sow the seeds of an inflated male ego, and with it difficulty in adjusting to situations of competing with, and possibly being beaten by, a girl of the boy's own age, height, and weight.

At the present time, the prepubertal male can throw farther, more accurately, and with a better action than his female counterpart. Does this imply that the male is genetically stronger and more coordinated and therefore better able to accomplish this task? Or is the reason that the prepubertal female does not throw as much as the male due to society's orientation to throwing as a "male activity"? Espenschade tested the motor performance of boys and girls between the ages of five and seventeen in sprint running, jump-and-reach, standing long jump, softball throw for distance, and the Brace test of motor ability. For ages five through eleven-to-thirteen, the sexes were identical except for the softball throw.[1] However, Wilmore then conducted a study where he tested the same age groups for the softball throw, but this time used the nondominant arm, thereby removing the factors of practice and experience. He found that the distances thrown were identical for the sexes up to the ages of ten to twelve.[2] The influence of culture and social orientation is strongly implied in these results.

Do organized sporting activities that allow males and females to participate together pose a danger to the female? From the data collected, there does not seem to be any reason to restrict any organized sporting activity at the prepubertal age level so long as contact events are based on equal weight, size, and maturity.

Does intense competitive training of prepubertal girls have adverse effects? While this practice does not appear to result in any physical harm, some questions might be raised regarding the psychological health and development of either a male or female eight-year-old when subjected to three, four, or more hours of strenuous training per day, as might occur in gymnastics or swimming.

THE ADOLESCENT PERIOD

Puberty occurs, on the whole, approximately two years earlier in the female than in the male. By eleven, the female is taller and heavier. At twelve to fifteen years she may be more mature and physically stronger than the male. At this stage it is necessary to make sure that the participants in contact sports are divided into groups of approximately equal maturity and size. However, this is the time when the female has traditionally felt the pressure to confine herself to "ladylike" activities. She might not cut down on running and walking, but her use of the upper extremities has, in the past, largely decreased. Not only can the male teen-ager throw a softball twice as far with his dominant arm, but Wilmore found that at this stage of development the nondominant arm also showed a difference in favor of the male.[2]

During adolescence, the female starts to

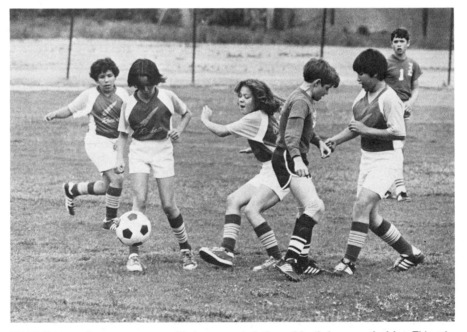

FIGURE 23.1 A soccer game with teams consisting of both boys and girls This mixing of the sexes is becoming more frequent in the prepubertal age group. (Photo by Mimi Forsyth, Monkmeyer)

deposit subcutaneous fat and develops the adult female physique. Whether some of this subcutaneus fat is due to inactivity is discussed in a later section.

THE POST-ADOLESCENT PERIOD

The adult male is generally heavier, taller, and stronger than the average female. Most world records are held by males with at least a 10% superiority over females (though this gap is narrowing in some events). Whether this is a genetically determined phenomenon or the result of social and cultural influences remains to be answered. Some factors related to muscular strength, body type, and endurance will now be discussed.

Muscular Strength

It is commonly assumed that the male is inherently stronger than the female, but what is the female's real potential for muscular strength development in the light of changing attitudes and increasing athletic participation? This is as yet an unanswered question.

At the present, there is a vast difference between the strength of the female and the male when the upper limbs are compared (43% to 63% weaker in the female). However, this difference in strength is much smaller when the lower limbs are compared (27% weaker). There does not appear to be any reason to assume that the upper limbs are inherently weaker. In fact, recent research suggests that with adequate weight training, the relative differences between the female's upper and lower limbs can be equaled out. As the result of a ten-week training course, untrained college females improved their strength between 30% and 100% and were able to increase their strength levels beyond those of normal untrained males of similar ages. In Brown and Wilmore's group of nationally ranked female field athletes on a progressive resistance weight-training program, some of the women were able to bench press several hundred pounds.[3] However, on an average, the women were still well below the level of males who had been weight training.

In studies by the armed forces' academies, 96% of the young women tested between 1973 and 1975 could not do a single pull-up. For these reasons the Naval and Air Force academies modified their entrance tests, requiring three-second, flexed-arm hangs instead of pull-ups. In 1977, however, 41% of the entering class could do one or more pull-ups, and, after being there for six months, 70% could perform at least one pull-up. As a result of these findings, regular pull-ups have been instituted at the Air Force Academy since July of 1978. From these and other findings, it begins to appear that weakness of the upper extremities in the female is socially and not genetically determined.[4,5,6,7]

If recent research is correct, the muscular strength of the female, when adjusted to body weight (strength per body weight), is very similar to the male's. The female's lower body strength is 27% lower than the male's, but if adjusted to strength per body weight, only a 7.6% difference in favor of the male is found. If these results are then expressed relative to lean body weight (lean body weight equals total weight minus fat weight), the female is at least as strong as, if not stronger than, the male. It will be interesting to see in the future whether these results apply to the upper limbs as well.[8]

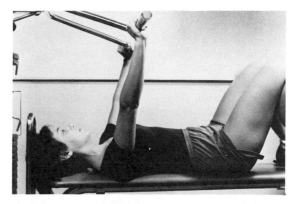

FIGURE 23.2 At one time women were seldom seen in the weight-room.

The present difference in *actual* strength between male and female (as opposed to lean body weight strength or theoretical potential for strength) is the main reason for separating males and females in contact sports. Injury is a real factor, not because the female is more susceptible to injury, but because of the difference in actual strength. An open mind is necessary, however, as continued exposure of the female to athletics may decrease her percentage of adipose tissue and result in her actual strength approximating that of the male.

A point that needs to be studied is the ability of an individual to fully utilize the strength he or she has. Is strength output only a matter of muscle fibers, or is it possibly also derived from a neurological ability to direct energy to the chosen muscle group? If so, would a woman's change in attitude from being ''ladylike'' to giving her body full freedom to perform change her ability to utilize her muscles to their fullest potential? And is this potential equal to or perhaps greater than that of the male? What about the 99-lb mother who, when she saw her son trapped under an automobile, managed to lift it off him? Such questions as these are open to considerable speculation.

Muscle Bulk

It does not appear that muscle bulk is necessarily related directly to strength. This point has to be clarified with further research. What is clear is that the female does not put on bulk with weight training in the same way as the male, *even though she may increase her strength manyfold.* There may be improved muscle definition and some decrease in subcutaneous adipose tissue, but even with intensive weight training, her muscle bulk does not approximate that of the male. Women with a higher level of endogenous androgenic steroids tend to develop more bulk than women with a lower level.

Body Fat

It seems that most people have just accepted the idea that women have a predisposition to a thicker layer of subcutaneous fat and a higher percentage of body fat than males. However, some female long-distance runners approach very low values, and can approach the relative values for fat and lean weight which are found in the male distance runners.

Cardiovascular Endurance

In 1970 Astrand[9] published data which showed that females had a smaller stroke volume and less lung capacity. Average college females were found to have an average maximum oxygen uptake (VO_2 max) of between 30 and 45 ml/kg-min, whereas their male counterparts ranged between 45 and 53 ml/kg-min. In 1977 the U.S. Air Force Academy tested some of its female cadets.[4] This group of select women had a VO_2 max of close to 50 ml O_2/kg-min, which is higher than many top-class male marathon runners. The question once more needs to be asked: Does the VO_2 max relate to genetic limitations of women, or are the lower values culturally related and destined to change with increased athletic participation?

There is no doubt that women are quite capable of participating in endurance events. For some reason, the concept that such events are suitable for males only held sway for many years. Some researchers now feel that, because of the subcutaneous adipose tissue of most women, they may have an advantage in their ability to metabolize free fatty acids after their glycogen supplies have been exhausted. Whether women are more efficient in their ability to metabolize lipids is an open question, but it is certain that they are just as efficient in this as males, and more than able to compete in prolonged endurance events.

INJURIES

Genitals

One of the strongest arguments that has been stated against the female's participation in contact sports is related to the possibility of injury to the reproductive organs. Statistics have, however, shown that the genital areas have the lowest incidence of injuries. The breasts occasionally suffer contusions, though these are usually minor. Some sports, such as soccer, have modified rules for women so that they may cross their arms in front of their chests. Protective brassieres do not seem to be necessary in most cases. However, the large-breasted female may be inconvenienced by excessive breast movement while running. A properly designed and fitted brassiere certainly helps limit movement that is counter to the direction of the chest wall. Those with small breasts are usually unaffected by running activities and, in fact, often find it more comfortable to run braless—the only problem occasionally being friction of the nipples against the overlying clothes.

Another theory is that there is danger of developing breast cancer secondary to trauma, though no statistics or evidence have been accumulated linking trauma of the breast with the development of cancer.

Probably the most serious injury encountered is vaginal wall rupture and peritoneal irritation from water skiing accidents in which the skier, after falling, is dragged through the water. Women participating in this sport are advised to wear neoprene wet suits.

A vulval hematoma may occur occasionally in gymnastics.

Injuries Related to Skiing

In the 1960s, studies were performed on the frequency of fractures in downhill skiers. From these results it was concluded that the female is more susceptible to fractures. It was suggested that this higher rate is due to a combination of

1. less bone density
2. less strength
3. a lower level of skill

First it should be pointed out that in downhill skiing, gravity assists the momentum and so increases the magnitude of any

physical deficiency. Are these deficiencies inherent or will they be modified by the female's increased athletic participation? These studies need to be reviewed in terms of the information available today.

1. *Bone density.* Whether bone density is an endocrine-determined factor or whether it is related to activity and usage is unanswered in the case of females. However, in male baseball pitchers and tennis players it has been shown that increased density in bone diameter occurs in the dominant arm. This appears to be related to the constant repetitive action. Whether the female of the 1980s will have a bone density equal to that of the male remains to be seen.

2. *Strength.* From what has been discussed previously, it seems reasonable to assume that the female does not necessarily have to be less strong relative to her body weight, and this risk factor should rapidly decline with improved and intensified training techniques. By improving her strength, the female athlete will improve her potential in the sport in which she is engaged, no matter what it is. She will also be adding the important element of protection from injury.

3. *Skill.* The question of skill is almost certainly related to the female's upbringing, and it should rapidly disappear as an injury-related factor as females start to ski earlier and continue at a higher level of intensity through adolescence and beyond.

In summary, therefore, the three factors implicated in the higher rate of skiing fractures are all likely to change with the female's increased participation in sports. It will be interesting to see if the statistics on skiing injuries in the 1980s reflect this.

High School and College Injuries

Statistics show that between 1973 and 1975 a 59% increase in female participation in high school athletics occurred, while between 1975 and 1977 almost a twofold increase took place. During this time it was found that the frequency of injury for men was greater than for women, mainly because of the contact sports of football and wrestling. If these sports are excluded from the statistics, the injury rate for males and females is almost identical. There is about one injury for every five participants per season for noncontact sports, while adding in male contact sports doubles the rate.[10]

Many injuries that occur today are the result of the fact that the female has to (a) learn to be an athlete and (b) learn the sport. A substantial number of females participating in high school sports are relative novices because the sports were not offered to them previously. They are, therefore, open to injuries related to adaptation to exercise. This is likely to change as girls start to participate at a younger age and continue to participate throughout high school (it should also be pointed out that in 1978 only about 15% of females in the high schools studied were participating in an athletic program).

As mentioned, most injuries were a result of adaptative problems, which are divided into two broad categories:

a. Overuse syndrome—e.g., stress fractures and tendinitis
b. Strength problems—manifested by peripatellar pain

Overuse injuries.

1. *Stress fractures.* As noted before, cardiovascular fitness is achieved relatively quickly, but the muscles, muscle-tendon junctions, and particularly the bones take a considerable time to adapt to the stress of increasing exercise. This is why tibial stress reaction or actual stress fractures appear to be more common in the female athlete, due to her lower level of previous athletic activity and lack of adequate conditioning.[11,12]

The West Point survey showed that 10% of the females developed stress fractures, compared with only 1% of the males. Stress fractures of the lower third of the fibula tend to be prevalent in the beginning jogger or in an athlete from another sport who starts jogging for conditioning.[13] The junction of the lower and middle thirds of the tibia is particularly likely to develop a stress fracture when a conditioned or skilled athlete is put into a tougher training program. If the conditioning program is gradually increased in intensity, these injuries appear to be no more frequent than in the male athlete.

2. *Tendinitis.* A slow, progressive conditioning program accommodating the adaptive process also helps reduce the incidence of this type of injury. The frequency of tendinitis is also reduced when strengthening and flexibility are emphasized. Once girls are provided with the same chance for musculoskeletal development that boys have had since they entered school, the rate of overuse injuries and tendinitis may decrease, at least until the elite levels of competitive athletics and training are reached, at which time they may again become more frequent.

Patellar problems.

This is one area where the female may be more at risk, but again statistics are uncertain. These problems include patellofemoral joint pain, peripatellar pain, and subluxation of the patella. It is thought that these injuries occur more frequently in females than in males, but that they are related to muscle tone and development rather than to anatomical differences (particularly lack of tone of the vastus medialis muscle). However, they may be related to a combination of malalignment, femoral anteversion, and medial squinting of the patella. The impression is that this type of malalignment is more common in the female, but if functionally corrected, and if the vastus medialis is strengthened, then the predisposition to peripatellar pain does not seem to be any different from that of the male. The wide female pelvis may not influence the occurrence rate of injuries per se, once the malalignment is corrected.

At-Risk Sports

Studies by Garrick and Requa of high school girls show that the sports with the highest rates of injuries are softball, gymnastics, and track and field/cross-country.[10] Activities in which the risk is particularly high are gymnastic practices and softball games (Figures 23.3 and 23.4).

HEAT STRESS: THE FEMALE'S RESPONSE

As has been noted, the body's response to physical exercise includes, among many things, a rise in the heart rate, an increase in the core temperature, and the production of sweat. It has been observed, however, that these changes are magnified by an increase in the environmental temperature and that this response to heat and exercise differs in men and women. For instance, women tend to begin sweating at a higher body temperature and sweat less than men. Conversely, heart rates and rectal temperatures increase more rapidly in women, particularly in humid conditions.

Thermoregulation is, however, adequately achieved by women at a lower sweat rate than men. "The male athlete is a prolific, wasteful sweater, whereas the female adjusts her sweat rate better to the required heat loss and thus maintains a better control of the body's temperature."[14] The reason for the difference is not as yet clearly under-

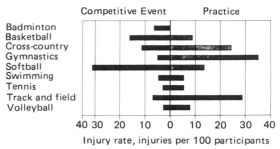

FIGURE 23.4 **Rates for injuries sustained during competitive events and during practices** (Tables 23.3 and 23.4 from J.G. Garrick and R.K. Requa, "Girls' sports injuries in high school athletics," *Journal of the American Medical Association* 239:21:2245–2248, 1978)

stood, but postulates include the female's sex hormones,[15] the influx of fluid from the intestine to the plasma compartment in the female, and the female's greater cardiovascular component in thermoregulation.[16]

It seems that each sex has particular mechanisms for coping with the stresses of exercising in the heat and that each does so to a similar extent, though the female may be more efficient at regulating her body temperature.

GYNECOLOGICAL PROBLEMS OF WOMEN ATHLETES

Menstruation

The menstrual cycle does not seem to have an adverse affect on world-class athletes, as world records have been broken and Olympic gold medals won during menstruation as well as during all other phases of the menstrual cycle. Whether these elite athletes were not bothered by their menstruation, or whether they did not let themselves be affected by menstrually related discomfort is uncertain, as is the influence of their upbringing and the role of their society in forming their attitudes toward menstruation.

On the other hand, there is no doubt that some women are disturbed by premenstrual tension and dysmenorrhea (painful menstruation). It seems possible that these

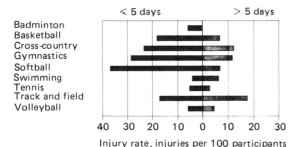

FIGURE 23.3 **Rates for those injuries resulting in ≤5 and >5 days missed from practice and competition**

women eliminate themselves from first-class athletic participation because of their inability to train fully during menstruation.

The relationship between exercise and menstruation needs to be studied more fully. For instance, exercise has often been cited as a therapy for dysmenorrhea. The West Point study tended to add weight to this argument by reporting that dysmenorrhea decreased in 55% of the women cadets after they had undergone a year of intense physical training.[17] There are many more questions like this related to menstruation and physical exercise that need definitive answers. For instance, secondary amenorrhea, e.g., cessation of periods unrelated to pregnancy, is frequently reported by athletes undergoing heavy training (such as running 100 miles per week in a track program) or a combination of physical and mental stress (as in the U.S. military academies' programs). The study from West Point revealed the following figures:

In their first year (1976) 86% of the women cadets had regular menstruation before camp started. One month later, 73% had amenorrhea. Twenty percent still reported amenorrhea after a year, while after fifteen months the figure was down to 7%, but 23% still had irregular periods.

Experience with track athletes suggests that most resume menstruation when training and intensity are reduced, but they may still have less flow then before, infrequent or irregular periods, or both.

Another side effect of physical activity is delay in the onset of menstruation in some young females who have trained intensively for some years.[18] What long-term effects this might have are as yet unknown.[19,20]

Iron loss associated with menstruation. Because the menstruating female loses blood, and therefore iron which is incorporated in the hemoglobin, the iron needs to be replaced. Only about 10% of the iron found in food appears to be absorbed and retained. This means that females need almost twice as much iron as males to maintain adequate stores. If the iron store becomes depleted,

anemia follows. The female athlete is often on the brink of anemia; if the hematocrit drops below 40% in a woman, she should certainly consider taking iron orally. Tests such as those measuring the level of iron circulating in the blood, and others, are even more sensitive means of establishing the need for iron supplements.

Pregnancy adds to the drain on the stores of iron, and during pregnancy a woman requires three to four times the normal daily iron intake. Women who have heavy periods, either spontaneously or because of an intrauterine device (IUD), also need additional iron.

Exercise During Pregnancy

Normal, and even strenuous, amounts of exercise do not seem to be related to spontaneous abortion. Exercise, if suitably adapted, can be continued throughout pregnancy (with the proviso that no complications are present). Many expectant mothers have experienced a feeling of well-being with continued exercise. Nor is there a need for women to abandon athletics after pregnancy. On the contrary, certain females have attained their best athletic performances after having had children.[21]

Contraceptive Steroids

The contraceptive pill may help with some of the discomfort of primary dysmenorrhea by preventing ovulation. However, it can also lead to some side effects, depending upon the athlete's physiology and the type and ratio of hormones used. The effect of these agents on athletic performance is not yet clear. However, in nonathletes, up to 40% of users develop mild to moderate depression. Also, weight gain is a relatively common side effect and may be incompatible with athletic activity in certain individuals.

Anabolic Steroids

The American College of Sports Medicine has stated its position on the use of anabolic steroids by females.[22]

The use of anabolic steroids by females, particularly by those who are either prepubertal or have not attained full growth, is especially dangerous. The undesired side effects include masculinization, disruption of the normal growth patterns, voice changes, acne, abnormal hair growth, and enlargement of the clitoris. . . . For these reasons, all concerned with advising, training, coaching, and providing medical care for female athletes should exercise all persuasion available to prevent the use of anabolic steroids by female athletes.

PSYCHOLOGICAL ASPECTS OF WOMEN'S PARTICIPATION IN SPORTS

Society's attitudes will need to undergo considerable revision to allow the female to enjoy equal participating opportunities. There is no doubt that the values of participating in athletics are not sex linked, and many of the differences in performance and skill level associated with being female have been shown to be more related to sociological than to genetic influences.

Often after menarche (the beginning of menstruation) the female is greatly influenced by other's attitudes toward what constitutes appropriate behavior. These attitudes also affect her choice of and level of intensity in athletic participation. Studies have shown that the male is encouraged to become independent, while the female is encouraged to become dependent. This can obviously stunt self-confidence. However, there is evidence that females who are involved in competitive sports are more likely to be independent and autonomous.[23] They are also more achievement orientated than nonathletic females, even though achievement orientation appears to be strongly influenced by society's attitudes and is certainly not sex related. Because of these attitudes, the female becomes a threat to the male's ego and image; the woman may therefore take a psychological risk if she competes with, or beats, a male. Many females may wish to avoid this by not participating in athletics. One way of changletics. One way of changing this attitude is by encouraging coeducational athletic activities from an early age.

At present, women athletes are often deprecated both by themselves and by their peers of both sexes. They feel they are inferior to males, even though, as has been discussed, the female is not necessarily weaker per pound of lean body weight, nor does she necessarily have less cardiovascular endurance. Also, for a female to participate she has to be able to take the risk of involvement without being threatened. In order not to feel threatened, she must be secure about being a female. If she is insecure about her femininity, she will not take risks that threaten her and will tend to avoid engaging in vigorous activities and competition, considering these to be "unladylike" (on the other hand, the male uses his participation in sports to reinforce his masculinity).[24]

Another problem the female athlete faces is the dissonance she feels between how she perceives herself as an athlete and how society expects her to be. In addition, society's attitude can lead to development of an image of success that is different for the female and the male. Culturally, the rewards and reinforcements the male receives from athletic participation are not yet a reality for the female.

Dorothy Harris feels that we should stress human behavior rather than break it down into sexual roles.[23] She found that when male and female athletes were scored on the same scales and compared with the same norms, they were more alike than different.

Are females more vulnerable to other areas of psychological stress when competing in athletics? Studies on high-quality male and female athletes have shown remarkable similarities in motivation, psychological strategies for coping with athletic performance, and handling of their own special problems such as lack of time for dating and social participation.

From what has been explored regarding the psychological aspects of women's increased athletic participation, it appears that the male will have to adapt as much as the female to the changes that will occur. It is always amusing to observe the expression of a male during a fun run, when on a steep hill he is passed by "a little old lady." Male egos may have to be shaken, but it will inevitably result in a better and healthier relationship between the sexes and allow the female to explore the physical limits of which she is capable.

REFERENCES

1. Espenschade A: Motor development. In *Science and Medicine of Exercise in Sport*, edited by Johnson WR. New York, Harper and Row, 1960.
2. Wilmore JH: Body composition, strength, and development. *J Health Phys Ed Rec* 46:38, 1975.
3. Brown CH, Wilmore JH: The effect of maximal resistance training on the strength and body composition of women athletes. *Med Sci Sports* 6:174–177, 1974.
4. Thomas JC: Women's sports and fitness program at the US Air Force Academy. *Phys Sportsmed* 7:59–68, April 1979.
5. Lenz HW: Women's sports and fitness programs at the US Naval Academy. *Phys Sportsmed* 7:42–50, April 1979.
6. Cox JS, Lenz HW: Women in sports. The Naval Academy experience. *Am J Sports Med* 7:355–357, 1979.
7. Anderson JL: Women's sports and fitness programs at the US Military Academy. *Phys Sportsmed* 7:72–80, April 1979.
8. Wilmore JH: The application of science to sport: Physiological profiles of male and female athletes. *Can J Appl Sport Sci* 4:103–115, 1979.
9. Astrand P-O, Rodahl K: *Textbook of Work Physiology.* New York, McGraw-Hill Book Company, 1970, p 175.
10. Garrick JG, Requa RR: Girls' sports injuries in high school athletics. *JAMA* 239:2245–2248, 1978.
11. Orava S, Hulkko A, Jormakka E: Exertion injuries in female athletes. *Br J Sports Med* 15:229–233, 1981.
12. Kowal DM: Nature and causes of injuries in women resulting from an endurance training program. *Am J Sports Med* 8:265–269, 1980.
13. Franklin BA, Lussier L, Buskirk ER, et al: Injury rates in women joggers. *Phys Sportsmed* 7:105–111, March 1979.
14. Wyndham CH, Morrison JF, Williams CG: Heat reactions of male and female caucasians. *J Appl Phys* 20:257–364, 1965.
15. Kawahata A: Sex differences in sweating. In *Essential Problems in Climatic Physiology*. Kyoto, Japan, Nankada Publishing Company, 1960, pp 169–184.
16. Weinman KP, Slabochova Z, Bernauer EM, et al: Reactions of men and women to repeated exposure to humid heat. *J Appl Physiol* 22:533–538, 1967.
17. Anderson JL: Women's sports and fitness programs at the US Military Academy. *Phys Sportsmed* 7:72–80, April 1979.
18. Frisch RE, McArthur JW: Menstrual cycles: fatness as a determinant of minimum weight for height necessary for their maintenance or onset. *Science* 185:949–951, 1974.
19. Drinkwater BL: Moderator Round Table on: Menstrual changes in athletes. *Phys Sportsmed* 9:99–112, November 1981.
20. Speroff L, Redwine DB: Exercise and menstrual function. *Phys Sportsmed* 8:42–52, May 1980.
21. Zaharieva E: Olympic participation by women: Effects on pregnancy and childbirth. *JAMA* 221:992–995, 1972.
22. American College of Sports Medicine. Position statement on the use and abuse of anabolic-androgenic steroids in sports. *Med Sci Sports* 9:xi–xii, 1977.
23. Harris DV: Psychological considerations of the female athlete. *J Health Phys Ed Rec* 46:32–36, 1975.
24. Kingsley JL, Foster LB, Siebert ME: Social acceptance of female athletes by college women. *Res Q* 48:727–733, 1977.

RECOMMENDED READINGS

Albohm M: How injuries occur in girls' sports. *Phys Sportsmed* 4:46–49, February 1976.

Bodnar LM: Women, sports and the law. *Am J Sports Med* 8:291–293, 1980.

Campbell CJ, Bonen A, Kirby RL, et al: Muscle fibre composition and performance capacities of women. *Med Sci Sports* 11:260–265, 1979.

Christensen CL, Ruhling RO: Thermoregulatory responses during a marathon—a case study of a woman runner. *Br J Sports Med* 14:131–132, 1980.

Corbitt RW, Cooper DL, Erickson DJ, et al: Female athletics. *JAMA* 228:1266–1267, 1974.

Drinkwater BL: Aerobic power in females. *J Health Phys Ed Rec* 46:36–38, 1975.

Drinkwater BL: Physiological responses of women to exercise. In *Exercise and Sports Sciences Reviews*, Vol I, edited by Wilmore JH. New York, Academic Press, 1973.

Gerber EW, Felshin J, Berlin P, Wyrick W: *The American Woman in Sport.* Reading MA, Addison-Wesley, 1974.

Harris DV: The female athlete—strength, endurance, and performance. In *Toward an Understanding of Human Performance*, edited by Burke EJ. New York, Mouvement Publications, 1977.

Haycock CE: Editorial in *Phys Sportsmed* 7:36, April 1979.

Haycock CE, Gillette JV: Susceptibility of women athletes to injury. Myths vs reality. *JAMA* 236:163–165, 1976.

Heyward V, McCreany L: Analysis of the static strength and relative endurance of women athletes. *Res Q* 48:703–710, 1977.

Kabayashi Y, Ando Y, Okuda N, et al: Effects of endurance training on thermoregulation in females. *Med Sci Sport Exerc* 12:361–364, 1980.

Oglesby CA, editor: *Women and Sports: From Myth to Reality*. Philadelphia, Lea & Febiger, 1978.

Protzman RR: Can women be overextended in physical conditioning programs? *Am J Sports Med* 7:145–146, 1979.

Ryan AJ: Moderator Round Table on: Women in sports, are the "problems" real? *Phys Sportsmed* 3:49–56, May 1975.

Snyder EE, Spreitzer E: *Social Aspects of Sport*. Englewood Cliffs NJ, Prentice-Hall Inc, 1978.

Trussell J: Menarche and fatness: re-examination of the critical body composition hypothesis. *Science* 200:1506–1513, 1978.

Wells CL: Sexual differences in heat stress response. *Phys Sportsmed* 5:79–90, September 1977.

Wilmore JH: Inferiority of female athletes: Myth or reality? *J Sports Med* 3:1–6, 1975.

CHAPTER 24

Nutrition and the Athlete

History tells us that athletes have often attempted to use various foods to improve their athletic capabilities. Primitive people attached meaning to many of the foods they ate; for example, eating the meat of a strong or aggressive animal was supposed to confer courage and strength. Today, psychologists believe that many people subconsciously associate the eating of meat, especially steaks, with being masculine.

NUTRITIONAL QUACKERY

The sports world is replete with nutritional faddism and misinformation propagated by coaches, athletes, and the media. Why is this so? There seem to be a number of factors involved.

First, food appears to have an emotional rather than an intellectual value to many athletes, and as a result, food faddists can successfully appeal to their emotional drives.

Second, there is the phenomenon of collective food faddism, that is, the patterning of food habits after successful individuals or teams. Whether the athlete becomes successful because of these practices or in spite of them does not really seem to matter.

Third, there is the impact of direct advertisements that extol the virtues of a given product relative to increased performance capacity.

And last, many athletes and their coaches have a blind craving for "the winning edge." They still believe that there is a special diet or special nutritional ingredient that is essential to success.

At the present time it is generally agreed that no type of dietary supplementation will improve the performance of a normal person who is on a well-balanced diet. No special diet changes a moderately endowed athlete into a champion, but a sound dietary regimen is necessary to produce maximal fitness. Also, there is no evidence that special foods or vitamin supplements are necessary *as long as* the athlete eats a sufficient amount in his or her diet. If the athlete needs an increased amount of an essential nutrient, he or she should consume larger quantities of well-selected foods, not nutritional supplements. Perhaps the most important supplements were summarized by the late Bob Kiphuth of Yale, who issued this menu to his swimmers:

> Breakfast of Champions—Long workouts for stamina
>
> Lunch of Champions—Grueling sessions for strength
>
> Supper of Champions—Exhausting practice for speed

THE WELL-BALANCED DIET

A well-balanced diet should provide all the nutritional and caloric* needs of an individual. Since an athlete is constantly burning up calories and breaking down tissue, the food that he or she needs is food that supplies all the nutrients necessary for repair, growth, and energy.

*See glossary.

The foods in a well-balanced diet fall into four major groups:

1. *The meat group*: Includes meat, fish, cheese, beans, dried peas, eggs, nuts, and poultry. These foods are high in protein, vitamins, and minerals; the red meats are often high in fats as well.

2. *The milk group*: Includes whole and skim milk, buttermilk, yogurt, cottage cheese, ice cream, and cheese. Protein, fat, and calcium are found in these products.

3. *The fruit and vegetable group*: Includes both yellow and green fruits and vegetables, which are excellent sources of carbohydrates, vitamins, and minerals.

4. *The bread and cereal group*: Whole-grain breads and cereals make up the bulk of this group, which primarily provides carbohydrates but also contains some protein, vitamins, and minerals.

This diet, as outlined in Table 24.1, provides almost all essential nutrients for the athlete, except perhaps iron for some women athletes. However, it only supplies about 1,500 kilocalories (Kcal), which is insufficient for most athletes unless they are on special low-calorie diets. Most competing athletes require somewhere in the region of 3,000 to 6,000 Kcal per day, which should be supplied by additional servings and selected foods. The athlete should keep in mind which foods are basic to the nutritional program (Tables 24.1 and 24.2) and which are eaten in addition to increase caloric intake.

TABLE 24.1 Recommended Daily Food Pattern

Food Group	Servings for Teenagers	Servings for Adults
Milk: 1 cup milk, yogurt, or calcium equivalent: 1½ slices (1½ oz) cheddar cheese[a] 2 cups cottage cheese	4	2
Meat: 2 ounces cooked, lean meat, fish, poultry, or protein equivalent: 2 eggs 2 slices (2 oz) cheddar cheese ½ cup cottage cheese 1 cup dried beans or peas 4 tbsp peanut butter	2	2
Fruit-Vegetable ½ cup cooked or juice 1 cup raw Portion commonly served such as medium apple or banana	4	4
Grain: whole grain, fortified, enriched 1 slice bread 1 cup ready-to-eat cereal ½ cup cooked cereal, pasta, or grits	4	4

[a]Count cheese as a serving of milk or meat, not both simultaneously.

Adapted from the National Dairy Council *Guide to Good Eating*. Reprinted with permission.

TABLE 24.2   Important Nutrient Sources

Nutrient	Major Food Source	
Protein	Meat, poultry, fish Eggs Milk	Dried beans, peas Cheeses
Carbohydrate	Cereal Dried beans Bread	Potatoes Corn Sugar
Fat	Shortening, oil Butter, margarine	Salad dressing Sausages
Vitamin A (Retinol)	Liver Sweet potatoes Butter, margarine	Carrots Greens
Vitamin C (Ascorbic Acid)	Broccoli Grapefruit Mango	Orange Papaya Strawberries
Thiamin (B_1)	Lean pork Fortified cereals	Nuts
Riboflavin (B_2)	Liver Yogurt	Milk Cottage cheese
Niacin	Liver Meat, poultry, fish	Peanuts Fortified cereals

Calcium	Milk, yogurt
	Sardines,
	  salmon
	  w/bones
		Cheese
		Collard, kale,
		  mustard and
		  turnip greens

Iron	Enriched farina Liver Dried beans, peas	Prune juice Red meat

Adapted from the National Dairy Council *Guide to Good Eating*. Reprinted with permission.

The proportion of the different food groups in the diet depends to some extent on the type of event for which the athlete is training. The basic caloric requirement for a sedentary person is around 1,500 calories; the caloric intake needed in excess of this amount depends on the quantity of exercise performed by the athlete each day. For instance, an endurance athlete training 70 to 100 miles per week may require up to 6,000 calories per day, whereas a gymnast performing a two-hour workout may not require more than 3,000 calories per day.

On the average, the diet should consist of approximately 10% to 20% protein, 20% to 30% fat, and 50% to 70% carbohydrate. These percentages are based on the body's needs.

Protein is needed to restore the tissue broken down in the body and is only used for energy when the stores of carbohydrate and fat have been depleted. Seldom is more than 0.8 g of protein per kilogram of body weight needed each day. This equates to a 10 oz steak (70 g protein) for a 90 kg (plus or minus 200 lb) athlete. This is the total protein needed by that athlete per day. In exceptional cases, if repeated trauma results in major tissue breakdown, the quantity of protein may be raised to 1 g per kilogram of body weight per day. This often brings the fat value up to 30% because of the red meat eaten, though with a properly worked out diet, this need not be the case.

Carbohydrate is the principal source of energy in endurance events and is actually the only source of energy in explosive or anaerobic activities. It is necessary to replace the carbohydrate stores in the muscles on a daily basis or else the athlete will become fatigued. This replacement is in addition to the four basic food groups. The type of carbohydrate eaten is important—it should almost always be a complex carbohydrate rather than the simple sugars, which are not stored as efficiently. In addition, the simple sugars lead to an outpouring of insulin and a resultant drop in the level of blood sugar.

When compiling a diet, the trainer should consider the following questions:

1. What is the ideal proportion of carbohydrate, fat, and protein for the particular athlete and for the particular event in which he or she is engaged?

2. What is the total caloric intake necessary, considering the athlete's energy expenditure?

3. What is the ideal meal pattern for that athlete, considering the timing of practices and workouts?

4. What types of food are most acceptable to the athlete?

5. What effect will this diet have on the athlete's current and future health?

For instance, the footballer who is force-fed, particularly with meat and cholesterol-containing foods, may, if maintained on this diet, become a prime candidate for coronary artery disease later in life. Or, as another instance, an athlete might habitually oversalt food without realizing the effect this can have on the blood pressure.

Some athletes, because of improper education, a poor diet in the past, or lack of sufficient funds, may eat irregularly or inadequately and may underperform as a result. In this situation, it is important to obtain a "food diary" of exactly what food has been eaten. Daily energy expenditures should also be calculated. In this way, nutritional needs and status can be estimated.

PRE-EVENT NUTRITION

The pre-event meal needs to be carefully planned by the athlete, the trainer, or the coach, because it definitely influences the athlete's performance. Some important guidelines to consider include the following:

1. No food substance gives an athlete special energy, strength, or endurance.

2. Poor nutritional practices can adversely affect an athlete's performance.

3. Every athlete is an individual and each will react differently to different foods before an athletic event. Those involved with the athlete should recognize this individual variability and take it into account.

The athlete should be allowed to select pre-event foods based upon his or her individual preference, so long as they fall within the confines of sound scientific principles and present-day knowledge. This means that the type of food eaten should be able to pass through the stomach and the upper intestine by the time of the scheduled event, although because of many factors, this passage may be slower than normal. Food should be eaten far enough in advance of the scheduled event to allow for at least a three-to-four-hour digestion period.

The length of time necessary for food to leave the stomach depends on many factors. For instance, the emotional state of the athlete prior to the event can severely delay the emptying time. In a study of gastrointestinal motility before a football game, it was found that a meal eaten five hours before the game was still present in the upper small intestine and stomach at the beginning of the game. The type of food also influences gastrointestinal motility. Fats take as long as five hours (without anxiety) to leave the stomach, whereas carbohydrates average two hours and protein three hours. When the athlete is nervous and excited, these times may be considerably longer. Thus bland, nongreasy, easily digestible foods containing higher-than-normal amounts of complex carbohydrates should be consumed in the pre-event meal.

An example of the wrong kind of precontest feeding is the traditional meal composed of a 12-to-16-ounce steak, scrambled eggs, baked potato, coffee, and sugar. Some of the disadvantages of this meal include:

1. This food leaves the stomach slowly because of its high fat content.

2. This type of meal does not contribute anything to the performance of the athlete.

3. The large protein intake may increase urination, inducing some degree of dehydration, and may contribute to early fatigue, due to the buildup of uric and ammonia acids that are not eliminated by the kidney during exercise stress.

4. After such a large meal, the intestinal tract will be loaded.

5. This meal may leave players feeling hungry three or four hours later, which is just the time when they will be competing.

Foods that tend to irritate the intestine, produce stool bulk, or cause excessive gas should be avoided, as should foods that cause abdominal cramps or slow stomach emptying. When planning the pregame meal, foods such as cabbage, cucumbers, nuts, beans, salads with lettuce, oils, spices, and vegetables which may produce gas should not be included. Whole milk should also be avoided because of its high fat content. The pre-event meal should be limited to 500 calories or less. Large amounts of food eaten before competition are useless and may impair the athlete's ability to perform. A liquid meal may be ideal for some athletes.

The athlete should become familiar with the foods that seem to agree with his or her metabolism and personal idiosyncrasies. For instance, there are many athletes who cannot tolerate dairy products because they lack the enzyme lactase. If they do not realize this, drinking milk an hour or two before an event can cause nausea, flatulence, or diarrhea. Black and Asian athletes tend to be more prone to this condition than Caucasians.

INCREASING WEIGHT

An athlete who wishes to increase his or her body weight should consider the following:

1. Any weight increase should consist of muscle tissue and bone only, and should *not* be made up of fat.

2. An increase of muscle tissue and bone is accomplished by specific training programs (e.g., weight training) and an increase in caloric intake.

3. The increased caloric intake should be for a limited time only. It is important for the athlete to realize that this diet should not be continued for a lifetime.

4. Continuous monitoring of the lean body mass and the percentage of body fat (by means of a skinfold-thickness test or underwater weighing technique) should be performed every two weeks to ensure that the weight being gained is not in the form of fat. If the percentage of body fat rises, there should be a reduction in caloric intake and an increase in energy expenditure. Only by strenuous and vigorous muscle work is muscle mass increased.

5. Supplemental protein, anabolic steroids, and antihistamines are all potentially dangerous and/or have not been proven effective.

DECREASING WEIGHT— PARTICULARLY IN WRESTLERS

In such sports as wrestling or light-weight crew, there is a stringent weight limitation. Even in sports without definite weight categories (e.g., gymnastics and long-distance running) low body fat is desirable. Many long-distance runners have achieved levels of 5% and 6% body fat. It is undesirable for any athlete, including a wrestler, to decrease body fat below this level.

The maximum amount of weight an athlete should lose is 1 kg to 1.5 kg (2 to 3 lb) per week (if more than this is lost, it will be lost in the form of muscle mass). To achieve this weight loss, the athlete needs to increase training by about an hour a day, while subtracting at least 1,000 Kcal from the diet. However, the intake should not be less than 1,500 to 2,000 Kcal per day.

The most important points when attempting to lose weight include:

1. Even though the athlete is on a weight-reducing diet, the diet should still be well-balanced and contain selected foods from all four groups discussed earlier. Smaller portions should be eaten. Only carefully selected desserts (fruits) or between-meal snacks (e.g., carrots) are allowed.

2. Normal fluid intake should be maintained at all times. This means at least eight large glasses of water a day.

3. Other methods of losing weight (e.g., rubber suits, saunas, and dehydration) should be banned.[1,2,3]

4. In order to establish the amount of weight an athlete can safely lose, the percentage of body fat will have to be determined. This can be done by means of the formula given in Table 24.3.

TABLE 24.3   Weight-loss Formula

A useful formula for determining the amount of weight that can be safely lost is:

(1) $\dfrac{\text{percentage body fat}}{100} \times \dfrac{\text{weight in kg}}{1} = \text{total kg fat}$

(2) $\dfrac{\text{percentage body fat to lose}}{\text{actual percentage body fat}} \times \text{kg fat} = \text{kg to lose}$

(3) actual weight − kilograms to lose = goal weight

Example: A 70 kg male wrestler with 15% body fat wishes to achieve an optimum of 5% body fat.

$\dfrac{15}{100} \times 70 = 10.5$ kg of body fat (total)

$\dfrac{10}{15} \times 10.5 = 7$ kg to lose to achieve 5% body fat

70 − 7 = 63 kg—the lowest weight that this wrestler should drop to in order to achieve 5% body fat without becoming dehydrated

Not more than 1 to 1.5 kg (2 to 3 lb) should be lost per week. As 1 kg equals 7,700 Kcal, 1.5 kg per week equals 11,500 Kcal, which equals 1,650 Kcal per day. If this wrestler decreases his caloric intake by 1,000 Kcal per day, and increases the amount of training so that another 700 Kcal per day are lost, the goal weight will be met in 4½ weeks.

Effects of Dehydration

Studies have shown that when food and fluids are restricted, the weight loss comes from the body's supply of water, fats, and proteins. Even when five hours are allowed for rehydration after a weigh-in, there is insufficient time for fluid and electrolyte homeostasis to be reestablished.[1,2,3,4,5,6,7,8] Results of this fluid restriction include:

1. Reduced muscular strength
2. Decreased work performance time
3. Lower blood and plasma volumes
4. Reduced cardiac function during submaximal work
5. Higher resting heart rate
6. Smaller stroke volume
7. Reduced cardiac output
8. Lower oxygen consumption
9. Impairment of thermal regulatory processes
10. Decreased renal flow
11. Decreased volume of fluid filtered by kidneys
12. Depletion of liver glycogen stores
13. Increased amount of electrolytes lost from the body

If water and fluid restrictions are repeatedly practiced during the growing phase, these changes can impede normal growth and development.

It needs to be emphasized that the minimal caloric requirements of adolescent wrestlers range from 1,200 to 2,400 Kcal per day, depending on the size of the wrestler. The minimum fluid requirement is four to eight glasses of water a day. No athlete should voluntarily go below these limits.

Fluid-Retaining Foods

It is essential that those involved in weight-controlled sports be aware of foods that cause fluid retention. These should be avoided at most times (as the athlete may think that he or she is overweight when actually only retaining water), but particularly within seventy-two hours of competition. Even though fluid-retaining foods should be limited, it is important for the athlete to realize that *water intake is essential during this period* and that no fewer than eight glasses of fluid should be consumed each day.

CARBOHYDRATE-LOADING DIET

The carbohydrate-loading diet has received considerable publicity since it was first described in 1967, and has been used by endurance athletes with varying degrees of success since then.[9] The purpose of this diet is to enable the athlete to continue competing at a particular level of activity for an increased period of time, so the event needs to be at least two hours in length before any difference is noted. It should be realized that the carbohydrate-loading diet does *not* allow an athlete to participate more intensely. If a marathon runner usually runs at a six-minute-per-mile pace, but becomes exhausted

TABLE 24.4   Foods That Should Be Restricted Before a Weigh-in

Salt	Monosodium glutamate
All heavily salted foods	Pretzels
Breads and rolls with salt topping	Potato chips and french fries
Popcorn	Crackers
Salty and smoked fish and meats	Salted nuts
Bologna	Bacon
Frankfurters	Corned beef
Ham	Sausage
Salt pork	Kosher meats
Anchovies	Sardines
Salted cottage cheese	Herring
Peanut butter	All cheeses
Bouillon cubes	Canned soups
Soy sauce	Worchestershire sauce
Relish	Sauerkraut
Olives	Ketchup
Celery, onion, and garlic salt	Pickles
Some cocoa mixes	Horseradish

after twenty miles, a carbohydrate-loading diet *may* enable him or her to continue through twenty-six miles at a six-minute-per-mile pace; however, it probably will not allow a five-minute-per-mile pace for 26 miles.

The aim of this diet is to increase the muscle glycogen levels of the exercising muscles, so there is more glycogen available to supply energy for a longer period of time. Originally it was thought that in order to accomplish this muscle loading the muscles needed to be depleted of as much of their glycogen as possible a week before the scheduled event. This was achieved by an exhausting workout, after which very little training was done over the next six days. A high-protein, high-fat, low-carbohydrate diet was consumed for three days, followed by a high-carbohydrate, low-fat, low-protein diet for the final three days.

In its unmodified form, a carbohydrate-loading diet can be very taxing to the system and difficult to accomplish; it certainly does not suit everyone. Most athletes have modified this diet because of difficulties in following it and the side effects that have occurred. These modifications include elimination of the high-protein, high-fat, low-carbohydrate period and substitution of a continuing high-carbohydrate (80% and more) diet for at least a week prior to the event. The idea of glycogen depletion is also viewed with mixed feelings, as an exhausting run a week before may not be well tolerated. It is important not to overload with carbohydrates on the day of the event and to consume quantities of fluid.[10,11]

Those not utilizing the carbohydrate-loading diet before an endurance event should nevertheless begin their dietary preparation at least forty-eight hours before competition. The day before should consist of a light workout only, to allow the muscles to retain their stores of glycogen. Large amounts of protein, particularly meat, should be avoided, as a high-protein intake can add to the metabolic load. Also, the higher amino acid content of meat may cause some sedation (possibly related to the sedative effect of tryptophan). In addition, 20 mg of sodium nitrate in a quarter of a pound of meat can inactivate almost 6% of the hemoglobin of an average-sized adult. Complex carbohydrates are recommended.

Sugar Before and During Competition

Studies have shown that sugar, or any simple carbohydrate, taken before an event can lead to sudden reduction in the blood glucose level because of an outpouring of insulin. Therefore, the practice of consuming a simple carbohydrate such as glucose before participation should be avoided.

During continued activity, the production of insulin may decrease, allowing the athlete to consume simple carbohydrates relatively safely. Care should be taken to use only low concentrations of glucose or similar substances and to remember that high concentrations of glucose in fluid replacement solutions can decrease the rapidity of absorption.[12,13]

With endurance events of over two or three hours' duration, the body's supply of glycogen may become exhausted and there may be value in taking sugar in some form at that time. This is still a controversial subject and further research is necessary for clarification.

CONCLUSION

At the present time, scientific knowledge suggests that the nutritional needs of the athlete are no different from those of the nonathlete. It cannot be denied that individuals vary in their choice of, and response to, food. The athlete should be given sound advice but should be left to choose the foods that he or she desires, as long as these do not conflict with proven dietary principles.

It is interesting to speculate on whether future nutritional programs will explode the established truths of today. One must keep an open mind and allow time, experimentation, and adequate research to provide the answers. For the present, it appears that for athletes to reach their maximum potential, they cannot compensate for an inadequate nutritional program by excellent physical conditioning, nor should they expect superior nutrition to compensate for inadequate training.

REFERENCES

1. Tipton CM: Physiologic problems associated with the "making of weight." *Am J Sports Med* 8:449–450, 1980.
2. Houston ME, Marrin DA, Green HJ, et al: The effect of rapid weight loss on physiological functions in wrestlers. *Phys Sportsmed* 9:73–78, November 1981.
3. Hursh LM: Food and water restriction in the wrestler. *JAMA* 241:915–916, 1979.
4. Bosco JS, Terjung RL: Effects of progressive hypohydration on maximal isometric muscular strength. *J Sports Med Phys Fitness* 8:81–86, 1968.
5. Zambroski EJ, Foster DT, Gross PM, et al: Iowa wrestling study: weight loss and urinary profiles of collegiate wrestlers. *Med Sci Sports* 8:106–108, 1976.
6. Herbert WG, Ribisl PM: Effects of dehydration upon physical work capacity of wrestlers under competitive conditions. *Res Q* 43:416–422, 1972.
7. Ribisl PM: Rapid weight reduction in wrestling. *J Sports Med* 3:55–57, 1975.
8. Tipton CM, Tcheng TK: Iowa wrestling study: weight loss in high school students. *JAMA* 214:1269–1274, 1970.
9. Bergström J, Hermansen L, Hultman E, et al: Diet, muscle glycogen and physical performance. *Acta Physiol Scand* 71:140–150, 1967.
10. Costill DL, Miller JM: Nutrition for endurance sport: carbohydrate and fluid balance. *Inter J Sports Med* 1:2–14, 1980.
11. Moore M: Carbohydrate loading: Eating through the wall. *Phys Sportsmed* 9:97–103, October 1981.
12. Costill DL, Saltin B: Factors limiting gastric emptying during rest and exercise. *J Appl Physiol* 37:679–683, 1974.
13. Coyle EF, Costill DL, Fink WJ, et al: Gastric emptying rates for selected athletic drinks. *Res Q* 49:119–124, 1978.

RECOMMENDED READINGS

American College of Sports Medicine. Position stand on weight loss in wrestlers. *Sports Med Bull* 11:1–2, 1976.

Costill DL, Miller JM: Nutrition for endurance sport: Carbohydrate and fluid balance. *Inter J Sports Med* 1:2–14, 1980.

Foster C, Costill DL, Fink WJ: Effects of pre-exercise feedings on endurance performance. *Med Sci Sports* 11:1–5, 1979.

Landwer GE, Johnson GO, Hammer RW: Weight control for high school wrestlers. *J Sports Med* 3:88–94, 1975.

Ribisl PM: When wrestlers shed pounds quickly. *Phys Sportsmed* 2:30–35, July 1974.

Ryan AJ: Moderator Round Table on weight reduction in wrestling. *Phys Sportsmed* 9:78–96, September 1981.

Smith NJ: *Food for Sport*. Palo Alto CA, Bull Publishing Company, 1976.

Tcheng TK, Tipton CM: Iowa wrestling study: Anthropometric measurements and the prediction of a "minimal" body weight for high school wrestlers. *Med Sci Sports* 5:1–10, 1973.

Vincint LM: *Competing with the Sylph*. New York, Andrews and McMeel, 1979.

Williams MH: *Nutritional Aspects of Human Physical and Athletic Performance*. Springfield Ill., Charles C Thomas, 1976.

Williams RJ: *Physicians' Handbook of Nutritional Science*. Springfield Ill., Charles C Thomas, 1978.

CHAPTER 25

Thermal Injuries

HEAT INJURIES

Heat injury is preventable—yet cases of heat exhaustion and death from heat stroke continue to occur. Between 1961 and 1972, football in the United States produced at least sixty deaths from heat stroke.[1] Education and constant vigilance have subsequently greatly reduced this figure, but cases still occur.

Football is particularly likely to be associated with heat problems, for a number of reasons. The protective gear effectively reduces the ability of a large portion of the body to dissipate heat, while the added weight actually increases the amount of heat produced. In addition, football is often played during the spring and the late summer when both temperature and humidity may be dangerously high. Football players are usually highly motivated and tend to overextend themselves, particularly if encouraged to do so by their coaches. Not to be forgotten is the myth that dies hard, which states that "water deprivation makes the players tough!" Rather, water deprivation causes the players to fatigue more easily, be less effective and, most importantly, be more susceptible to heat injury.

Other sports are by no means exempt from the dangers of heat injury, particularly long-distance running, which has become increasingly popular with thousands of recreational athletes (see Chapter 21).

Physiology

When an athlete exercises, the body temperature rises. The harder the athlete exercises, the bigger the athlete, and the more subcutaneous fat present, the more heat is produced.[2]

The hypothalamus is the thermoregulatory center and controls the body's reaction to heat. This heat is dissipated by means of

1. cooling of the skin through sweat evaporation (this is the most important mechanism)
2. the lungs
3. conduction, convection, and radiation

The body is designed to work within a very narrow range of temperature fluctuation. It is constantly striving to keep the core temperature as close to 37°C (98.6°F) as possible.* It does this by producing sweat, which, when it evaporates, causes the skin to cool. Subcutaneous blood vessels dilate and blood is channeled to the skin and is cooled.

However, problems can develop if

1. sweat cannot easily evaporate, for example, if the humidity is high
2. the body is actually being heated by the environment, for example, with temperatures above 37.2°C (99°F)
3. water loss from sweat and respiration is not replaced and dehydration occurs

A combination of all three in an exercising athlete can prove rapidly fatal.

Marathoners have been observed to lose more than 5 liters of fluid during a single race (or 1.5 liters to 2.5 liters of fluid each hour), and football players who do not replace their fluid losses may lose 7 kg to 10 kg (15 lb to 20 lb) during the course of a double-

*There is a "normal" increase in temperature with exercise of up to 2.5°C (4.5°F).

day practice session. Unfortunately the thirst stimulus producing the desire to replace lost fluid is totally inadequate for the body's needs. Athletes may get thirsty only when they are already in danger, and then they usually drink far less than is required. Heat production ranges from 1,000 to 1,500 Kcal per hour or more, and radiant heat can add another 150 Kcal per hour.

Prevention

Heat injuries should not happen. They are preventable.

1. *Acclimatization.* Several physiological changes occur during the process of heat acclimatization. These include the earlier onset of sweating and increased skin blood flow, which allows the temperature regulating mechanism to come into play at a lower body temperature. Those unacclimatized will therefore reach a higher temperature before beginning to sweat adequately (Figure 25.1). The electrolyte content of sweat seems to vary, but is usually hypo-osmolar. With prolonged sweating there may be losses of 5% to 10% of the extracellular fluid sodium and chloride, and 1% to 2% of body potassium (this sodium chloride loss is less when the athlete is acclimatized).

Heat acclimatization takes at least seven days, but can take many weeks. It occurs only if the athlete works out in the heat.

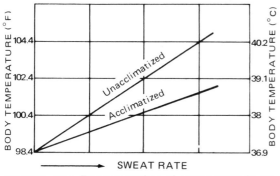

FIGURE 25.1 Representation of sweat rates in acclimatized and unacclimatized athletes

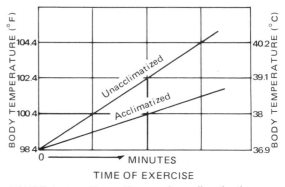

FIGURE 25.2 The effects of acclimatization on body temperature during exercise

These workouts should be carefully planned and supervised. They should be short, perhaps repeated twice a day, and then gradually increased in length and intensity, all the time ensuring adequate periods of rest and a copious supply of fluid. Clothing should be light in weight and color.

2. *Environmental conditions.* Monitoring of atmospheric conditions is vital, so the coach can judge the amount of work that can safely be handled during a particular workout session. Guesswork should be eliminated. It is necessary to know not only the temperature, but also the humidity and the *relative humidity*. Cases of severe heat injury have occurred at moderate temperatures but high humidity. It is therefore vitally important that the relative humidity be established so that a true picture of the situation can be obtained. A sophisticated apparatus for obtaining these readings is the *wet bulb globe temperature* (WBGT), but perhaps a more easily obtained and practical apparatus is the *sling psychrometer*, which measures the dry and the wet bulb temperatures and uses a scale to obtain the relative humidity (Figure 25.3).

3. *Clothing.* Football uniforms cover much of the available sweat-producing skin of the body. Those involved with the organization of practice sessions and workouts should see to it that modifications are made when the weather is hot and humid. Shorts and white

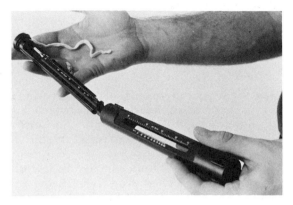

FIGURE 25.3 A sling psychrometer The trainer should use an apparatus such as this regularly before and during any practice where there is concern that the temperature and/or humidity may be above the minimally acceptable limits.

t-shirts should be worn, frequent water breaks allowed, and practices scheduled for early morning and late evening and cancelled when necessary. Net jerseys are very useful, as they allow an increased amount of skin surface to be ventilated and so aid in sweat evaporation and cooling. Any kind of sweatsuit used for the purpose of losing weight by sweating should be banned. These are highly dangerous and the weight lost, being water only, is temporary.

4. *Identifying susceptible athletes.* The physiology of each athlete varies, and so does each athlete's ability to adapt to and handle heat stress. Big athletes with large muscle mass seem particularly at risk. So are those with a thick layer of subcutaneous fat. Any athlete with a previous history of heat injury should take special precautions and should be carefully observed for early signs of a heat problem.

Athletes should be weighed before and after each practice session, in order to pick out those who might be inadequately replacing their fluid loss. A loss of up to 3% of body weight (3 kg [6 lb] in a 100 kg [200 lb] athlete) is easily corrected with normal fluid replacement. Those who have lost 3% to 5% of body weight (3 kg to 5 kg [6 lb to 10

TABLE 25.1 Planning and Conducting Practice Sessions Using a Wet Bulb Temperature Guide

Wet Bulb Temperature	Precautions
Over 24°C (76°F +)	Postpone practice until cooler, or conduct limited practice in light clothing
21.6°C to 23.9°C (71° to 75°F)	Rest periods every 30 minutes—cold water as needed
18.9°C to 21.1°C (66° to 70°F)	Cold water every 20 to 30 minutes, observe carefully
16.1°C to 18.4°C (61° to 65°F)	Observe carefully, water break, no other restrictions
15.6°C (60°F) or below	Normal practice, no restrictions, fluids
Whenever relative humidity is above 95%, irrespective of the temperature, precautions should be taken and the practice routine modified.	

Adapted from E. R. Buskirk, *Sports Medicine*, ed. A. Ryan and F. Allman (New York: Academic Press, 1974), p. 211.

lb] in a 100 kg [200 lb] athlete) are in danger of inadequately replacing their water losses unless fluids are forced. They should have almost regained their normal weight before the next practice session. Those who have lost over 5% of body weight (more than 5 kg [10 lb] in a 100 kg [200 lb] athlete) are in danger of developing major heat problems and need to be educated, as they have probably not been consuming adequate volumes of fluid. These athletes should be carefully observed on a daily basis to ensure that

1. no practice is undertaken until they have regained and maintained their weight

2. gradual underhydration over several days and eventual predisposition to severe heat problems does not occur

It should be noted that older athletes, as well as some women, have a low tolerance to heat stress, because they begin sweating at a higher temperature and it may take them longer to return their body temperatures to normal.

5. *Fluid replacement.* The single most important item in preventing heat injury is *water*. Small amounts of electrolytes may be added (*sugar in any form will delay absorption and is not necessary in athletes exercising less than two or three hours*), but it is the consumption of adequate quantities of water that has helped to radically reduce the incidence of serious heat-related injuries over the past few years.[3,4]

Athletes are easily educated in this area. They should be given a definite regimen to follow, with the understanding that bigger and heavier athletes need more water, as do athletes who are physiologically more susceptible to heat-induced problems. A suggested fluid intake scheme for preventing heat injuries follows.

1. Two hours before practice—1 liter (34 oz)
2. Fifteen minutes before practice—400 milliliters to 500 milliliters (13 oz to 17 oz)
3. Every 15 to 30 minutes during practice—400 milliliters to 500 milliliters (13 oz to 17 oz)
4. After practice—5 to 6 large glasses of fluid

The fluid should be cold water (this has been shown to be more rapidly absorbed than warm water), the exception being during early acclimatization in very hot weather, when part of the replacement fluid may contain up to ten milli-equivalents of sodium and five milli-equivalents of potassium.

As mentioned, sugar should *not* be included in the fluids because it

1. delays gastric emptying and water absorption

2. causes a sense of fullness and sometimes nausea, which decreases the athlete's ability or desire to consume more fluids and so may actually precipitate dehydration
3. causes an outpouring of insulin, which results in a secondary hypoglycemic condition a while later (this may not apply to the continuously exercising athlete)

6. *Diet.* The diet should contain much fresh salad and a variety of fruit. This helps replace many of the electrolytes that have been lost. During the acclimatization period, it may be useful to lightly salt the food, but this should not be continued once the adaptation period is over (see section on hypertension, p. 492).

It is the responsibility of those concerned with the health of the athlete to educate the coaches and the athletes in the prevention and dangers of heat injury, and to ensure that adequate steps are taken to minimize the possibility of such an injury.

HEAT-INJURY SYNDROMES

Heat-injury syndromes include:

1. Heat cramps
2. Heat fatigue
3. Heat exhaustion
4. Heat stroke
5. Mixed heat-injury syndromes

Heat Cramps

The exact etiology and pathomechanics of heat cramps remain obscure. Numerous electrolytes have been indicted, including sodium, potassium, and magnesium. Empirically it has been observed that the incidence of cramps is less when fluid intake is adequate and the diet is adjusted to include bananas, oranges, fresh salads, and a sprinkling of table salt over the food. Always ensure that the athlete does not get behind in fluid replacement. Very few athletes have ever drunk too much water!

Heat Fatigue (Heat Vasomotor Asthenia)

Heat fatigue applies to the unacclimatized athlete who becomes rapidly fatigued and weak when exposed to unusually high temperature or humidity. Recovery after exertion is also slower than normal, and allowance should be made for this to occur. Heat fatigue is a common condition that usually stops short of the more serious problems, often because the athlete is aware of what is happening and tapers off the intensity and/or the length of the exercise. Treatment is with adequate fluid replacement, keeping ahead of predicted fluid losses; adjustment of the diet to include many fresh salads and fruit; and adequate rest.

Heat Exhaustion

This is caused by excessive water loss that has been inadequately replaced.

SYMPTOMS: A throbbing headache, nausea, hair erection on the chest and upper arms, chills, unsteadiness, and fatigue. The athlete may become dizzy and lightheaded when he or she stops exercising, or may suddenly collapse (this is due to the hypovolemia causing a sudden drop in blood pressure, which is usually maintained during exercise in spite of the lack of circulating volume).

Rectal temperatures should be below 41°C (105.8°F); anything above this should be diagnosed as heat stroke. Usually temperatures range from 39°C to 40.5°C (102.2 to 104.9°F). The pulse may be rapid, but more importantly, there is a small pulse pressure (the range between the systolic and the diastolic pressure is small) and the blood pressure may fall rapidly when the athlete stands (orthostatic hypotension). The skin is usually cool and pale from vasoconstriction. Sweating is active (if it is not, consider the athlete to have heat stroke).

These athletes should be treated with intravenous fluids, electrolytes, and glucose, because hypoglycemia is often present. Though cooling is not a primary requirement, these athletes should be kept in a cool place, and iced towels may be applied.

Urine output and its appearance should be noted for at least twenty-four hours, as complications include delayed rhabdomyolysis with myoglobinuria, and renal damage. If no urine is passed within six to twelve hours, consider the athlete to have acute renal failure and refer immediately.

Heat Stroke

Heat stroke implies failure of the body's heat-controlling mechanism and constitutes a dire emergency. Chances of a fatal outcome are significant.

Heat stroke in athletes is usually the result of heat production from exercise, plus the failure of heat-loss mechanisms. Dehydration is an important factor, but heat stroke can occur in the absence of gross dehydration. The first symptoms may be unusual behavior in the form of incoherent speech, disorientation, and acute confusion or aggressiveness, followed rapidly by unconsciousness. The rectal temperature must be taken to help exclude other causes of unusual behavior or sudden unconsciousness, such as heat exhaustion or hypoglycemia. If the temperature is 41°C (105.8°F) or above, the athlete should immediately be assumed to have heat stroke and treatment with ice should be started. Other signs include the absence of sweating (though occasionally sweating persists),[5] peripheral vasodilation with flushed warm skin, and a rapid, bounding pulse. The blood pressure shows a low diastolic reading and a wide pulse pressure.

The reduction of the athlete's core temperature as rapidly as possible to 38°C to 39°C (100°F to 102°F) is vital.[6] Take the athlete out of the sun, remove most of his or her clothes, and apply wet cold towels to the trunk, abdomen, and extremities. Then place ice in liberal quantities onto the towels. Fanning to stimulate air flow is also useful. Care should be taken to protect and maintain the airway.

As soon as practical, the athlete should be transferred to an emergency room that is adequately prepared to deal with this problem. Enough ice should be loaded into the ambulance to cover the journey. The emergency room should be warned in advance of what to expect. If possible, an intravenous fluid solution should be started, but this is secondary to reducing the temperature.

If the athlete survives, there are a number of potential problems that only manifest after twenty-four hours. These include acute renal failure, acute hepatic failure, rhabdomyolysis that causes blood coagulation defects, cerebral edema, and myocardial infarction.[7]

Mixed Heat-Injury Syndromes

An athlete may present with symptoms and signs associated with both heat exhaustion and heat stroke. He or she needs to be rapidly cooled and requires fluid replacement.

TABLE 25.2   Symptoms and Signs of Heat Injury

	Heat Fatigue	Heat Exhaustion	Heat Stroke
Symptoms	Hot, fatigue	Fatigue, nausea	Disorientation, headache, incoherent speech
Mental status	Clear	Usually conscious, may faint (perhaps from orthostatic hypotension)	Confused or unconscious
Rectal temperature	38–39.5°C (100.4–103°F)	40°C + (104°F)	41°C + (105.8°F)
Skin	Flushed	Pale	Flushed
Sweat	+ +	+ +	May not be sweating (but may sweat with heat stroke)
Blood pressure		Narrow pulse pressure; may drop suddenly on standing	Low diastolic pressure with wide pulse pressure
Treatment	Oral fluids, allow to cool down	Give intravenous fluids, electrolytes and glucose, cool with ice	Cool with ice, give intravenous fluids, transfer to emergency room

Adapted from Peter G. Hanson, "Heat Injury in Runners," *Physician and Sportsmedicine* 7:6:93, June 1979.

COLD INJURIES

Cold injuries may present with peripheral problems, such as frostbite, where a finger or toe is affected, or a central problem, where there is a reduction in the body's core temperature, which can be a serious or even fatal condition. Shivering is the initial response to cold, but if the body's core temperature falls below 34°C (93°F), shivering may cease and death from hypothermia may rapidly ensue.

Cold injuries are most likely to occur when there is a combination of *cold plus high winds*. Cold by itself is not nearly as dangerous. For instance, −1°C (30°F) is not particularly cold, but if the wind is blowing at 35 miles per hour, the chill factor is such that it will reduce the actual temperature to −20.5°C (−5°F).(See Table 25.3 on page 484.) The effects of both cold and high wind are intensified if the athlete is also *wet and exhausted*. In addition, an athlete who has previously suffered from frostbite is more likely to be injured by the cold.

PREVENTION: The athlete should be educated in the dangers of the chill factor of the wind in the causation of frostbite and hypothermia. He or she should be taught how to dress for cold weather and told that multiple layers of clothing help trap air and are more effective in insulating the body then one thick layer. Because about 30% of the body's heat is lost from the surface area of the head, special attention should be paid to its insulation. Other areas that need to be covered are those farthest from the deep organs and large muscle groups, especially the nose, ears, cheeks, fingers, and toes, with the last two at particular risk of developing frostbite if shoes or gloves are too tight, and especially if they are wet. Therefore, a spare pair of dry socks and mittens should be available if the possibility of cold and rain is present.

Organizers of long-distance races should be aware of the slow runner (or the cross-country skier) at the back of the pack who may still be on the course after some of the aid stations have closed. This athlete will probably be exhausted and thus highly susceptible to cold injury.

TREATMENT: If an athlete is seen with *early signs of frostbite* (mild blanching of the skin), the part may be warmed by simply blowing through cupped hands onto the skin or by placing the extremity in the armpit and using body heat for warming. The part should never by rubbed with hands or with snow, as a permanent injury can result.

If the frostbite is deep, the part needs rewarming and should not be further exposed to the cold.[8] The warming consists of placing the part in a water bath controlled to between 40°C to 42°C (104°F to 108°F), and the rewarming should be continued until the normal color has returned to the whole area. The container should be large enough to allow movement of the part without contact with the sides. Dry heat is not advisable, and even brief exposure to high temperatures can result in serious damage.

Should the core temperature fall below 35°C (95°F), uncontrollable shivering, clumsiness, and loss of coordination and judgment will be followed by the inability to shiver, unconsciousness, and eventually death. Treatment of the hypothermic patient requires special facilities and is best performed in an intensive care unit. Immediate transfer to the nearest hospital should therefore be undertaken.

REFERENCES

1. Murphy RJ: Heat illness. *J Sports Med* 1:26–29, 1973.
2. Wyndham CH, Strydom NB: The danger of an inadequate water intake during marathon running. *S Afr Med J* 43:893–896, 1969.
3. Foster C, Costill DL, Fink WJ: Gastric emptying characteristics of glucose and glucose polymer solutions. *Res Q Exerc Sport* 51:299–305, 1980.
4. Murphy RJ, Matthews DK: Water is the key to heat problems. *Medical Opinion*, July 1976, p 39.
5. Hanson PG: Heat injury in runners. *Phys Sportsmed* 7:91–96, June 1979.

TABLE 25.3 Wind Chill Chart

TEMPERATURE (FAHRENHEIT)

Equivalent Chill Temperature

WIND (MPH)	40°	35°	30°	25°	20°	15°	10°	5°	0°	−5°	−10°	−15°	−20°	−25°	−30°	−35°	−40°	−45°	−50°	−55°	−60°
Calm	40°	35°	30°	25°	20°	15°	10°	5°	0°	−5°	−10°	−15°	−20°	−25°	−30°	−35°	−40°	−45°	−50°	−55°	−60°
5	35°	30°	25°	20°	15°	10°	5°	0°	−5°	−10°	−15°	−20°	−25°	−30°	−35°	−40°	−45°	−50°	−55°	−65°	−70°
10	30°	20°	15°	10°	5°	0°	−10°	−15°	−20°	−25°	−35°	−40°	−45°	−50°	−60°	−65°	−70°	−75°	−80°	−90°	−95°
15	25°	15°	10°	0°	−5°	−10°	−20°	−25°	−30°	−40°	−45°	−50°	−60°	−65°	−70°	−80°	−85°	−90°	−100°	−105°	−110°
20	20°	10°	5°	0°	−10°	−15°	−25°	−30°	−35°	−45°	−50°	−60°	−65°	−75°	−80°	−85°	−95°	−100°	−110°	−115°	−120°
25	15°	10°	0°	−5°	−15°	−20°	−30°	−35°	−45°	−50°	−60°	−65°	−75°	−80°	−90°	−95°	−105°	−110°	−120°	−125°	−135°
30	10°	5°	0°	−10°	−20°	−25°	−30°	−40°	−50°	−55°	−65°	−70°	−80°	−85°	−95°	−100°	−105°	−115°	−120°	−130°	−140°
35	10°	5°	−5°	−10°	−20°	−25°	−35°	−40°	−50°	−60°	−65°	−75°	−80°	−90°	−100°	−105°	−115°	−120°	−130°	−135°	−145°
40*	10°	0°	−5°	−15°	−20°	−30°	−35°	−45°	−55°	−60°	−70°	−75°	−85°	−95°	−100°	−110°	−115°	−125°	−130°	−140°	−150°

Little danger

Increasing danger
(Flesh may freeze
within one minute)

Great danger
(Flesh may freeze
within 30 seconds)

*Winds above 40 mph have little additional effect.

6. Wyndham CH: Heatstroke and hyperthermia in marathon runners. *Ann NY Acad Sci* 301:128–138, 1977.

7. Costrini AM, Pitt HA, Gustafson AB, et al: Cardiovascular and metabolic manifestations of heat stroke and severe heat exhaustion. *Am J Med* 66:296–302, 1979.

8. Mills Jr, WJ: Out in the cold. *Emergency Med* 8:134–147, 1976.

RECOMMENDED READINGS

American College of Sports Medicine position statement on prevention of heat injuries during distance running. *Med Sci Sports* 7:VII–IX, 1975.

Christensen CL, Ruhling RO: Thermoregulatory responses during a marathon—a case of a woman runner. *Br J Sports Med* 14:131–132, 1980.

Costill DL: *A Scientific Approach to Distance Running.* Los Altos, Tafnews, 1979.

Costill DL, Coté R, Miller E, et al: Water and electrolyte replacement during repeated days of work in the heat. *Aviat Space Environ Med* 46:795–800, 1975.

Costill DL, Sparks KE: Rapid fluid replacement following thermal dehydration. *J Appl Physiol* 34:299–303, 1973.

Maron MB, Wagner JA, Horvath SM: Thermoregulatory responses during competitive marathon running, *J Appl Physiol* 42:909–914, 1977.

Pugh LG, Corbett JL, Johnson RH: Rectal temperatures, weight losses and sweat rates in marathon running. *J Appl Physiol* 23:347–352, 1967.

CHAPTER 26

Illnesses, Skin Conditions, and Medications

THE MEDICAL EXAMINATION AND THE TRAINER

The trainer is often faced with a barrage of complaints, ranging in seriousness from pre-event hypochondriasis to acute emergency, and finds himself or herself in a position similar to that of a triage physician. However, the trainer is not a physician and must not be tempted to practice medicine.

The trainer's responsibility is clear: to evaluate the athlete's problem and refer as appropriate. To adequately assess a complaint, the trainer needs to:

1. evaluate the history the athlete presents. In order to do this the trainer needs to be informed of the common medical possibilities

2. undertake a screening examination to rule out serious conditions and be able to decide on the correct timing of the referral

3. have the necessary academic background to communicate with the physician on each referral

By constantly striving to adequately evaluate each problem, the trainer will advance and expand professionally and become increasingly satisfied with his or her role in the health care of the athlete.

Following is an outline of the medical screening examination of the upper respiratory tract, the chest, and the abdomen.

Examination of an Athlete with Symptoms Related to the Upper Respiratory Tract

The examination of symptoms related to the upper respiratory tract includes taking the temperature and the resting pulse. The throat should be examined for redness, the tonsils for possible exudate, and the neck for tender cervical lymph nodes. Examination of the ears should include the canal and the tympanic membrane. The trainer should become familiar with the appearance of a normal tympanic membrane, so that he or she can recognize when it is inflamed, bulging, or opaque.

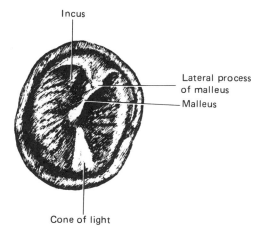

FIGURE 26.1 The tympanic membrane, as seen through an otoscope

Examination of the Chest

The trainer should always consult a physician if the athlete presents with severe chest pain. In evaluating a chest complaint, two important conditions need to be kept in mind:

1. *Pneumothorax.* Pneumothorax presents with sudden pain in the chest and shortness of breath. It may occur spontaneously or it may follow closed chest trauma such as a fracture of the ribs. A penetrating injury (such as a stab from a sharp object) can puncture the lung and cause bleeding in addition to the pneumothorax (*hemopneumothorax*).

Signs include poor air entry to one part of the lung. This is detected by asking the athlete to breathe in deeply and comparing the quality and intensity of the breath sounds in corresponding areas on both the left and the right sides of the chest. If one lung is collapsed, the breath sounds will be decreased or absent on the affected side.

2. *Asthma.* Characteristics of asthma are wheezing and difficulty in breathing. These occur when the bronchi become narrowed by spasm or by mucus secretions. Clinical detection is by the presence of wheezing heard throughout the chest on both inspiration and expiration.

Examination of an Athlete with Abdominal Pain

The examiner should be very gentle when evaluating an abdominal complaint. The examination should start with palpating away from the area of discomfort. General palpation reveals if the abdomen is soft and where the tenderness is located. The examiner should carefully feel for possible tenderness or enlargement of the liver or spleen, and for any abnormal masses. This is best done with the abdomen relaxed and the athlete inhaling deeply and rhythmically.

Signs:

1. Localized tenderness.

2. Guarding—contraction of the abdominal musculature when a tender area is palpated.

3. Rigidity—involuntary contraction of the abdominal muscles which precludes the examiner from palpating through the muscles. Rigidity is usually due to a serious underlying pathological condition.

4. Rebound tenderness—this test for abdominal peritoneal irritation should be performed very gently. The tender area should be palpated and the hand withdrawn; if positive for rebound tenderness, withdrawal of the hand causes more pain than did the downward pressure. To be certain this maneuver does not cause excessive discomfort, the abdomen should first be gently percussed. The percussion will produce a very mild form of rebound, and, if positive, the regular rebound test need not be performed. If rebound tenderness is present, the patient should immediately be referred for surgical consultation (Figure 26.2).

5. The athlete should also be asked to "blow out" or protrude the abdomen. If unable to do so because of pain, it may again signify a serious problem.

There are many causes of abdominal pain, but the trainer should be familiar with the presenting symptoms and signs of the more common serious conditions. With *appendicitis*, the athlete usually presents with nausea, vomiting, and abdominal pain. There is tenderness either in the central abdominal area or, classically, over the area midway between the umbilicus and the anterior superior iliac spine on the right side (McBurney's point). A *pelvic infection* in the female athlete may present with tenderness in both iliac fossae. An athlete with *gastric discomfort* or a *gastric ulcer* will complain of epigastric pain and discomfort, particularly related to certain foods, and the epigastrium may be tender (Figure 26.3).

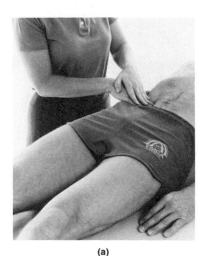

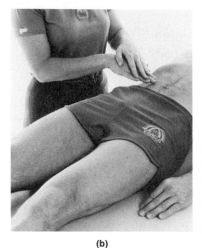

(a)   (b)

FIGURE 26.2 The rebound test for peritoneal irritation (a) Downward pressure is applied to the tender area   (b) If releasing the pressure causes an increase in the pain, peritoneal irritation should be suspected.

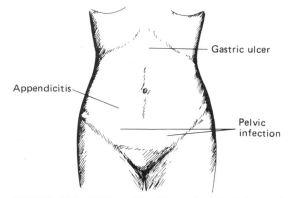

FIGURE 26.3 Differential diagnosis of abdominal pain—areas of tenderness to palpation

Evaluation of the tender abdomen is far from easy, even for experienced physicians. Always refer the athlete if there is any doubt about the significance of the symptoms or signs.

ILLNESSES AS THEY AFFECT THE COMPETING ATHLETE

Respiratory Infections

The common cold. The common cold is due to one of the viruses that affect the upper respiratory tract and is a self-limiting condition.

PREVENTION: There is no indication at this time that any medication or vitamin prevents the common cold. It has been said that large quantities of vitamin C may do so, but the evidence is still equivocal and is considered doubtful.

There is no doubt, however, that one of the precipitating factors in the onset of a cold in the competing athlete is overfatigue. The development of an upper respiratory infection may indicate that the athlete is being overtrained and should be given a few days to recover before resuming workouts.

Colds seem to occur more frequently in families or athletes living together. It would therefore be reasonable to partially isolate an affected athlete from the rest of the team.

SCREENING EXAMINATION: Screening should include taking the temperature, counting the resting pulse, examining the pharynx, and inspecting the tympanic membranes. The cervical area should be palpated for enlarged lymph nodes. If the athlete is engaged in contact sports, the abdomen should be examined to exclude the presence of an enlarged spleen or liver.

LABORATORY INVESTIGATIONS: Ordinarily no laboratory tests are required. Should a sore throat be present, however, a throat culture (streptococcal screening examination) should be started. If one suspects that the condition is due to infectious mononucleosis, a complete blood count (CBC) and a "mono spot" test should be ordered.

TREATMENT: Decongestants that do not cause drowsiness may be used. Most antihistamines cause some degree of drowsiness and are therefore not indicated for the competing athlete. Nasal sprays and nose drops have the disadvantage of causing rebound swelling of the nasal mucous membrane if used for more than a few days and may, therefore, make the problem of nasal stuffiness worse than before treatment was started. These should not be used routinely. Throat lozenges and gargles, as well as aspirin, are useful for a sore throat and fever.

Antibiotics will not affect the virus. However, bacteria frequently invade areas infected by viruses, especially after seventy-two hours. If this occurs, antibiotics are indicated to deal with that particular bacterium.

GUIDELINES FOR PARTICIPATION WITH A VIRAL INFECTION: Probably the most important criterion is whether the athlete feels motivated to compete. If the athlete feels too ill, he or she should not be coerced into participation. Many simple viral infections can be worsened by competition, and the athlete should therefore be advised to consider withdrawing if he or she feels ill. On the other hand, if the athlete wants to participate in spite of the infection, the following guidelines as to whether or not he or she should compete may be used:

1. Fever below approximately 102°F (39°C)
2. Resting pulse below 100 beats per minute
3. No complicating features such as infectious mononucleosis

If these guidelines are met, then it is probably permissible for the athlete to participate. It should be remembered, however, that these are rough guidelines only. No definite figures can be given, and each case should be judged individually.

Sore throat. A sore throat is commonly due to

1. viral infection which is part of an upper respiratory infection
2. streptococcal infection
3. infectious mononucleosis

Sometimes two of these three may coexist. For instance, it is common to find a streptococcal infection in a patient with infectious mononucleosis. It should be emphasized that the symptoms of a sore throat, whether due to a streptococcal infection or to a virus, are the same. As mentioned before, antibiotics do not influence the course of a viral infection, and a viral sore throat can indeed be very painful and distressing to the athlete.

INVESTIGATIONS: It is advisable to obtain a throat culture (streptococcal screening examination) as well as a complete blood count and mono spot test.

TREATMENT: Treatment is with the appropriate antibiotic if a streptococcal infection is present. This is usually penicillin unless the athlete is sensitive to it (drug allergy histories should always be obtained), in which case erythromycin should be used. Gargles and throat lozenges may be used as needed, as well as aspirin for fever and pain.

Canker sores. Canker sores are little ulcers that appear along the gum margins and on the mucous membrane of the mouth. They can be painful and cause considerable distress. Some athletes are susceptible to them and have recurrent attacks. There are two common types of canker sores, namely herpetic ulcers and aphthous ulcers. These may be identical in appearance, although in general aphthous ulcers are deeper and more irregular in shape.

There is no well-established treatment for herpetic ulcers, though they are usually self-limiting. The course of aphthous ulcers may be shortened to some extent by the use of a tetracycline solution (for instance, gargling with an aqueous solution of tetracycline three or four times a day for five days). Symptomatic measures include use of a local anesthetic topical gel and avoidance of acidic foods, such as tomatoes, which tend to increase the discomfort.

Otitis media.   Otitis media is often secondary to an upper respiratory infection in which there is swelling of the mucous membranes. This causes a partial or a complete block of the eustachian tube (the connection between the middle ear and the pharynx—see Figure 11.12). Blockage of this tube allows fluid to accumulate in the middle ear, predisposing it to infection, and also prevents equalization of pressure between the middle ear and the atmosphere.

SYMPTOMS: Pain in the middle ear, a blocked feeling in the ear, and sometimes a decrease in hearing.

SIGNS: The pharynx may be inflamed and there is usually redness and perhaps a bulging of the tympanic membrane (though it might be opaque in cases where there is an accumulation of fluid without actual infection in the middle ear).

TREATMENT: An antibiotic is required if there is an infection. In addition, decongestants and nasal spray (for a very limited time only) are used to try to shrink the mucous membranes and open the eustachian tubes.

The athlete should be shown how to perform the *Valsalva maneuver* if there is fluid in the middle ear after the acute infection is over. This maneuver is designed to open the eustachian tubes, equalize pressure, and allow drainage. The nose is held shut and the athlete attempts to blow out against a closed mouth and nose, thereby increasing the pressure in the pharynx and middle ear. At the same time the pressure is being increased, the athlete should swallow. The increase in pressure should not cause pain or discomfort. This maneuver may be performed a number of times a day.

Sinusitis.   One of the commonest reasons for a cold's continuing over a protracted period of time is sinusitis secondary to an upper respiratory infection.

During an upper respiratory infection, the mucous membranes that line the sinuses swell. There is an outpouring of fluid which is normally cleared by the tiny hairs lining the sinuses that sweep the excess fluid toward the sinus opening. If these hairs are immobilized by a secondary bacterial infection, or if so much fluid is produced that it cannot be removed, sinusitis develops.

SYMPTOMS: The main symptoms are facial pain, headache, blocked nose, and at times fever.

TREATMENT: Treatment is with an antibiotic (nasal cultures should be taken) and a decongestant or antihistamine.

Bronchitis.   Bronchitis is commonly part of a viral upper respiratory infection which becomes secondarily infected by bacteria, or on occasion it may be due to the mycoplasmal organism.

SYMPTOMS AND SIGNS: Fever, a hacking cough, and the production of phlegm (which may be purulent) are the main symptoms. The infection may precipitate the onset of asthma in those susceptible to the development of this condition.

TREATMENT: The sputum should be cultured. An antibiotic is indicated if a secondary infection exists, or if mycoplasma is a suspected organism. Erythromycin is the drug of choice unless hemophilus is cultured, in which case ampicillin should be used. A cough mixture and a decongestant-expectorant may also be indicated.

Pneumonia.   In the athlete, pneumonia is most commonly due to mycoplasma or a virus. On occasion, the classical pneumococcal pneumonia may occur. Investigations should include a chest X-ray, a sputum culture, and a white blood count (WBC). When mycoplasma is the responsible agent, X-ray changes may be more extensive than the clinical examination would lead one to suspect.

TREATMENT: The appropriate antibiotic is usually erythromycin for mycoplasma, penicillin for pneumococcal pneumonia, or sometimes ampicillin.

Systemic Viral Infections

Viral hepatitis.   Viral hepatitis does not occur frequently in athletes. However, an outbreak in a team that is living together can have devastating results, as occurred with members of the Holy Cross football team. Ninety-three percent of the team were found to be infected.[1,2]

ETIOLOGY: At this time it is thought that there are three groups of etiologic agents:

1. Hepatitis A virus
2. Hepatitis B virus
3. Hepatitis due to a nonspecific group of non-A and non-B agents.

It is known that the hepatitis A virus is usually transferred via the intestinal-oral route, while the hepatitis B virus is transmitted in a number of ways (via blood and blood products, saliva, sexual intercourse, and needle puncture) but not via the intestinal-oral route.

SYMPTOMS AND SIGNS: Initially the athlete complains of some fatigue, lethargy, and abdominal discomfort. Nausea and an aversion to food, particularly meat, may then be noted. The urine becomes progressively darker in color, approaching dark brown. A yellow tinge is seen in the conjunctiva in daylight (note that this yellow tinge may not be seen if the athlete is examined under an ordinary light bulb).

PREVENTION: If the athlete is a member of a team, particularly if the team is living together, blood should be drawn from every team member for a full laboratory examination. If the virus is not found to be type B, it is suggested that standard immune serum globulin (ISG) be given to all the team members. This has been found to prevent the illness from developing in 80% to 90% of exposed persons as long as it is given within one to two weeks of exposure. Close contacts of those with the B virus (e.g., spouses) may choose to have hyperimmune globulin. A team member who is suffering from infectious hepatitis should not share a room with another team member and should not actively participate until the symptoms and signs have returned to normal.

Infectious mononucleosis.   Infectious mononucleosis is one of the commonest, and possibly one of the most overtreated, illnesses occurring in young adults. Having said that, it is necessary to point out that serious complications can occur in the occasional case.

ETIOLOGY: Most cases of infectious mononucleosis are due to infection from the Epstein-Barr virus. The remainder of the cases are probably due to the cytomegalovirus or other viruses.

SYMPTOMS AND SIGNS: Sore throat and fatigue are the commonest symptoms. Any young athlete presenting with these symptoms should be suspected of having infectious mononucleosis, though of course these symptoms are completely nonspecific and might represent numerous viral or other diseases. Headache and mild generalized aching are also common symptoms. Fever is present in most but not all cases.

Lymph node enlargement may or may not be prominent. The pharynx is usually red and the tonsils are often enlarged, frequently developing characteristic patches of white exudate. Swelling around the eyes and pinpoint red patches on the palate are also characteristic signs.

The abdomen should be carefully palpated to assess if there is splenic or hepatic enlargement. Very gentle palpation is necessary, for should the spleen be heavily infiltrated with atypical lymphocytes, it could easily rupture. Jaundice develops in about 10% of cases.

One of the special features of infectious mononucleosis is a maculopapular rash which may develop if ampicillin is taken. This antibiotic is therefore avoided in an athlete with a sore throat, headache, or fever, unless there are specific indications for its use.

LABORATORY INVESTIGATIONS: A throat culture should always be taken initially, as at least 10% to 20% of cases are secondarily infected with streptococcus. The white blood cell count is the most commonly performed test, but the results vary depending on the stage of the disease. In the beginning, the count can be quite normal in 50% of the cases (5,000 to 10,000 cells per cubic millimeter); in 25% of the cases this figure may be less and in 25% it may be more. Atypical lymphocytes are also an important finding, as is a large increase in the total number of lymphocytes found on the differential count. An elevated sedimentation rate may also be present.

A positive heterophile antibody test (the mono spot test) is another important test and is fairly conclusive evidence of the diagnosis, but it should always be considered in conjunction with the blood count and with the clinical findings, as it may not become positive for up to three weeks in some cases. Liver function tests are often abnormal.

TREATMENT: Throat lozenges, aspirin for fever, and penicillin in cases of a positive throat culture for streptococcus are the only forms of treatment usually necessary. The use of corticosteroids is very controversial; some physicians feel that cortisone should be given in every case, but there do not appear to be valid statistics supporting this school of thought. Most feel cortisone should be used only for severe cases or for specific complications. The athlete should be hospitalized and carefully monitored when cortisone is used.

COMPLICATIONS: The most well-known complication is *splenic rupture*, and for this reason athletes are kept out of contact participation for four weeks or longer.[3] There

TABLE 26.1   Criteria for Return to Activity after Infectious Mononucleosis

1. Temperature should be normal.
2. Sore throat should be considerably improved.
3. There should be a general feeling of well-being.
4. There should be a decrease in the size of the spleen.
5. At least three to four weeks should have elapsed from onset to return to activity.

Though these guidelines are clinical, they are very useful and should be used in conjunction with the WBC and differential count, the sedimentation rate, and the liver function tests.

are also other complications. Death from infectious mononucleosis occurs every now and then, particularly from agranulocytosis and pneumonitis.

Hypertension

Hypertension implies blood pressure above "normal" limits as defined by age. Blood pressure is expressed as the systolic over the diastolic pressure (e.g., 120/70).

PREDISPOSING FACTORS: A history of high blood pressure in the family, particularly in the father or mother, increases the chances of an athlete's developing hypertension. This is even more significant if the athlete is black, as blacks have a higher rate of hypertension than the rest of the population. The reason for this is obscure at the present time.

Excessive salt intake (sodium chloride) is thought to be associated with the development of hypertension. Congenital abnormalities of the aorta (e.g., coarctation of the aorta) can produce hypertension that is subject to surgical correction, as is partial blockage of one of the renal arteries.

Raised blood pressure in an athlete is often detected during the physical examination. It is frequently difficult to decide if a particular reading is significant, and sometimes readings need to be repeated on a number of separate occasions while the athlete is resting in order to establish the base-line figures.

The following are guidelines evaluating blood pressure when the athlete is at rest.

Age	Mild Hypertension	Significant Hypertension
under 15	130/80	140/90
15–20	135/85	145/90
over 20	140/90	150/95

The athlete with mild or borderline hypertension should be given advice such as that in Table 26.2. He or she should also have the blood pressure checked in both arms and femoral pulses palpated (if the femoral pulses are absent, coarctation of the aorta should be suspected). Those with significantly increased blood pressure need to be investigated and possibly treated.

INVESTIGATIONS: Besides specific laboratory tests for individual cases, two important investigations that help clarify the significance of hypertension in a particular athlete are:

1. Follow-up tests of blood pressure at least three to four times a year.

2. Monitoring the rise in blood pressure during a treadmill-exercise stress test. If the blood pressure rises much above 200/95 in an athlete with borderline resting hypertension, it indicates an abnormal response to

TABLE 26.2   Advice to Athletes with Borderline Resting Hypertension

1. Decrease salt intake to a minimum.
2. Avoid gaining weight during the off-season.
3. Maintain a year-round aerobic cardiovascular program in addition to any other specialized training.
4. Have blood pressure examinations at regular intervals, e.g., every three to six months.
5. Avoid anabolic steroids.
6. Have a stress test to evaluate the exercise blood pressure response.

If this advice is followed, there should be no need to restrict the participation of an athlete with mild high blood pressure.

exercise. This may be more significant than the resting blood pressure.

Urine Abnormalities

The dipstix, or similar type of urinalysis "stix," is frequently used during the physical examination to pick up the presence of abnormal quantities of protein, glucose, or blood in the urine. If any of these are present in abnormal quantities, the athlete should be referred for further investigation.

Proteinuria.   The presence of protein in the urine can indicate

1. orthostatic (or postural) proteinuria
2. renal or urinary tract pathology
3. a false positive result, for instance, from the urine being alkaline

1. *Orthostatic proteinuria* is a condition in which there is an abnormal amount of protein in the urine without any underlying renal or urinary tract pathology. To determine if the proteinuria is due to the normal postural leakage of protein, ask the athlete to save a urine specimen that is passed before standing up in the morning (the bladder should be emptied before going to bed the night before). This should be free of protein when tested. If it is not, or if it contains casts or cells, further investigations need to be undertaken to exclude renal disease.[4,5,6,7]

2. *Renal or urinary tract pathology*: Protein, cells, and casts are usually present with renal or urinary tract pathology. Renal pathology can induce hypertension. Therefore, if protein is present in the urine, the blood pressure should be measured.

Glycosuria.   If glucose is found in the urine, a random (or fasting) blood-sugar level should be obtained and a six-hour glucose tolerance test performed to exclude the possibility of diabetes.

Hematuria.   Athletes frequently have episodes of hematuria, especially after endurance activities.[8] The exact cause of this manifestation of severe exertion is not completely understood but the condition is thought to be harmless. Some reports suggest that bladder contusions are responsible for the bleeding.[9,10] If the athlete complains of hematuria after a workout, the urine should be checked to confirm that the discoloration is actually due to blood and not myoglobinuria (discussed next). The blood pressure should also be taken.

The urine should then be checked daily before workouts. If the hematuria persists more than a day or two, further investigations may be indicated. The urine should also be examined to ensure that no casts, especially red blood cell casts (an indication of renal disease), are present.

Hematuria following exertion needs to be differentiated from acute trauma to the flank or bladder area. Hematuria resulting from such an injury needs to be immediately referred for a specialist's opinion.

A condition that can be mistaken for blood in the urine is *myoglobinuria*, which is the presence of myoglobin in large quantities in the urine. It presents with an appearance similar to blood, but the dipstix is negative. Myoglobinuria results from severe exercise by a poorly conditioned, dehydrated athlete, and as large quantities of myoglobin can lead to renal failure, its appearance in the urine indicates a potentially serious problem requiring prompt referral.[11,12]

Another condition that can cause confusion because of a macroscopic appearance suggesting hematuria is *exertional hemoglobinuria*, which is thought to be due to damaged red blood cells in the soles of the feet. The condition is considered harmless and is prevented by use of good, shock-absorbent running shoes.

Sickle-Cell Trait

Sickle-cell trait has aroused much concern in recent years, particularly since a member of a college football team collapsed during practice and subsequently died, apparently as a result of an acute sickle-cell crisis. There is still controversy as to whether the sickling was the primary cause of this athlete's death or whether it was secondary to some underlying metabolic abnormality.

The sickle-cell trait is an inherited abnormality that affects the hemoglobin content of the red blood cells (RBC). The trait is found mainly in blacks of West African descent, and in a small percentage of descendents of Mediterranean families. The abnormal hemoglobin is hemoglobin S (HbS), which makes up 30% to 40% of the hemoglobin, while the normal adult hemoglobin (HbA) makes up the other 60% to 70%. If conditions are right, such as very low oxygen tension, the abnormal hemoglobin may induce sickling of the RBC.

In a study done on professional footballers, it was noted that approximately 8% of the black athletes investigated had the trait, which is the same percentage as the natural occurrence of the trait in the general black American population. This suggests that the trait does not interfere with an athlete's ability to participate to the limits of his or her potential.

The possibility of an athlete with the trait developing a sickle-cell crisis is thought to be associated with a combination of altitude, dehydration, and overfatigue. It is therefore recommended that any such athlete be educated about the need to adequately hydrate at all times, particularly when playing at high altitudes and in hot weather. No restriction from athletic participation is recommended.[13]

Venereal Diseases

There is no doubt that venereal disease is common among athletes. Those concerned with the athlete's health should be aware of what steps to take should an athlete complain of symptoms indicative of a venereal disease. Absolute confidentiality should always be maintained, and the athlete should be aware of this confidentiality so that he or she has the confidence to discuss the matter.

The commonest venereal diseases are

1. gonorrhea
2. nonspecific urethritis
3. Trichomonas vaginitis

4. herpes progenitalis

5. syphilis

Gonorrhea. Gonorrhea is common among athletes who seem to feel a false sense of security because of the availability of penicillin. It should be realized that penicillin-resistant strains of gonococcus have resulted in difficulty in treating some cases.

Symptoms and signs include a urethral discharge, dysuria (painful urination) or both in the affected male. Some affected males may have no symptoms at all. The affected female may present with symptoms of pelvic infection or vaginal discharge, but usually will have no symptoms referable to the disease. The diagnosis is made by taking a swab from the urethra of the male or from the cervix or rectum of the female and culturing this for forty-eight hours. If the organism is sensitive to penicillin (and the patient is not), treatment should be started with either intramuscular procaine penicillin or oral ampicillin. Both of these should be supplemented beforehand with an oral dose of probenemid, which delays the urinary excretion of penicillin, increasing its effectiveness.

Nonspecific urethritis. Most of these cases are due to an infection of *Chlamydia* or *Mycoplasma*, though other organisms may be involved. The male presents with a urethral discharge and dysuria, which may be difficult to distinguish clinically from gonorrhea. A culture should therefore be performed in *every* case (in most cases the symptoms are less florid than those of gonorrhea).

Treatment is with oral tetracycline. However, if symptoms recur after this treatment, it is clinically impossible to tell a relapse from a re-infection. Both sexual partners should be treated with a three-week course of tetracycline.

Trichomonas vaginitis. A common "minor" sexually transmitted disease of the female genital tract, this seldom produces symptoms in the male. Sexual activity promotes repeated infections unless both partners are treated.

Herpes progenitalis. The herpes virus is divided into two types: type I occurs above the waist and type II occurs mainly below the waist, though there is some crossover between the two.

Herpes progenitalis is caused by the type II virus and is a sexually transmitted disease that presents with painful blisters on the genitalia. The patient is infectious during the time the lesions are present. No specific treatment is curative at the present time.

Syphilis. Though syphilis had been decreasing in frequency, it now seems to be making a comeback. There are a number of stages in the natural history of syphilis.

1. Primary syphilis presents with a lesion soon after the initial infection called a chancre. This chancre is usually found on the genitals, and is painless. Lymph node swelling of the involved region appears within one week of chancre; these nodes are painless. The chancre heals within about four weeks.

2. Secondary syphilis appears about six weeks after the chancre has healed and often presents with a rash or generalized lymph node enlargement. The secondary rash may subside within two to six weeks.

3. The patient then enters the latent phase, during which there are no clinical manifestations of syphilis on examination, but the diagnosis can be made by a positive blood test.

4. Late syphilis may present many years later with such complications as aortic aneurysm or neurological lesions.

Whenever an athlete presents with symptoms suggestive of this disease, immediate referral to the appropriate specialist is mandatory.

Allergies ("Hay Fever")

Nasal allergies to grass seed, pollens, ragweed, molds, etc., are very frequent. Where concentrations of these are high during certain times of the year, an athlete's ability to train and participate can be greatly impaired unless the condition is adequately handled. A basic rule, however, is not to make the treatment more unacceptable than the problem. It should also be remembered that asthma can develop in susceptible individuals and may require treatment.

TREATMENT:

1. *Antihistamines*—These are effective for most athletes, but they have the disadvantage of producing drowsiness and slowing reflexes, which may be incompatible with certain sports. Compromises should be sought (such as taking the antihistamines only at night) and a number of different antihistamines should be tried. However, if the medication proves unacceptable, alternative forms of therapy should be instituted.

2. *Eyedrops*—Vasoconstricting eyedrops, with or without antihistamine, are often useful. Corticosteroid eyedrops may occasionally be used for a short period, but they have serious side effects, including the possible development of glaucoma (raised intra-ocular pressure).

3. *Cromolyn sodium*—This has been used successfully in preventing asthma of allergic origin and exercise-induced asthma. It is also useful in nasal allergies when inserted into the nose. The dosage should be adjusted to the periods of greatest exposure (see exercise-induced asthma in next section).

4. *Immunotherapy*—An increasingly popular and effective treatment, this has the disadvantage of requiring desensitization injections over a long period of time.

5. *Corticosteroids*—If all else fails, and the athlete's ability to participate is greatly impaired, consideration should be given to the use of corticosteroids in one or another of the forms available.

   (a) Intra-nasal aerosol applications of corticosteroids (such as Decadron Turbinaire). These may be useful in some cases.

   (b) Intramuscular corticosteroids: While undoubtedly the mode of treatment with the highest apparent success rate, this also has the greatest potential for serious side effects and is not recommended. Once injected intramuscularly, there is no control of the blood level and no knowledge of the degree of adrenocortical suppression being produced at any given time. The length of time the corticosteroid is released from the depot in the muscle varies from individual to individual, and it is uncertain if adrenal suppression occurs or for how long it continues. By suppressing the production of immunoglobulins, it may actually exacerbate the allergy. It should not be used in an athlete who has a peptic ulcer, who is diabetic or hypertensive, or who has a positive tuberculosis (PPD) test. Should the decision be made to use an intramuscular form of cortisone, a short-acting preparation for an athlete with an initial high blood level should be chosen.

   (c) Oral cortisone: This is a viable alternative to intramuscular cortisone in some cases.

Exercise-Induced Asthma

This condition usually occurs in a known asthmatic, but it may present in some athletes only when they are exercising strenuously. The hyper-irritability of the airways is usually due to the inhalation of cold air and leads to bronchospasm during or after activity.[14] Wheezing is thus the main symptom.

In the laboratory setting, if an athlete with exercise-induced asthma is run on the treadmill for about six minutes at 70% of maximum aerobic capacity, bronchodilation occurs during the first two to four minutes. Bronchoconstriction begins three to five minutes after stopping the exercise, becoming increasingly severe and lasting up to twenty minutes in a child or teen-ager, often longer in an adult. Then it disappears.[15]

Even though wheezing usually makes a diagnosis obvious, it is important to confirm the diagnosis, as the symptoms could be interpreted as being due to lack of adequate conditioning in an athlete who is not a known asthmatic. Spirometry tests that measure the forced expiratory volume in one second (FEV_1) and the forced vital capacity (FEC) show a decrease in the FEV_1 which correlates with the symptoms.

Different sports have a different potential for stimulating the onset of an exercise-induced asthma attack, and this is thought to be related to the temperature of the air, cold air being more likely to set off an attack. Running sports produce the highest incidence in those who are susceptible, while swimmers are least likely to be affected.[16] This is probably why so many asthmatics turn to swimming, and why a number of Olympic swimmers are indeed asthmatics. The reasons why swimming is less capable of stimulating exercise-induced asthma than running are probably related to the humidity and warmth of the air in the swimming pool environment, and perhaps to lack of pollens and antigens.

TREATMENT: Some success may be obtained by teaching the athlete abdominal breathing as well as exhaling against resistance with pursed lips when exercising. If the athlete is exercising in cold weather, a cloth can be worn over the mouth to try to decrease the temperature differential of the inspired air.[17]

If the athlete is a known asthmatic, the asthma should be vigorously treated and brought under control. However, the main object in treating exercise-induced asthma is prevention. A useful drug in preventing and treating exercise-induced asthma is terbutaline sulfate (Brethīne), an aerosol sympathomimetic drug which should be taken a half hour before exercising. Cromolyn sodium (Intal) is effective in about 80% of athletes suffering from exercise-induced asthma.[18]

The action of cromolyn sodium lasts only about thirty minutes when used for this condition and it should therefore be used fairly frequently during athletic activity. Once the exercise-induced asthma has occurred, cromolyn sodium is no longer effective, and an aerosol bronchodilator should be used. Xanthines, such as theophylline, are also useful. *Note*: Cortisone and antihistamines are ineffective in preventing exercise-induced asthma, even though they are used in the treatment of asthma.

SKIN CONDITIONS

The trainer will be presented with numerous skin conditions and it is recommended that a color atlas be consulted (see Recommended Readings list at end of chapter).

Fungal Infections

The dermatophytoses are the most common fungal diseases of the skin, and they are commonly seen in athletes.

Fungal infections of the feet ("athlete's foot"). The early signs of athlete's foot (tinea pedis) are maceration, scaling, and fissuring of the toe webs, especially the fourth. This leads to desquamation of the flexor aspect of the toes and clear loculated vesicles on the instep. An important clinical feature is that the infection is asymmetrical, though both feet may be infected. A secondary bacterial infection may also be present.

DIAGNOSIS: There are other disorders of the feet that can simulate athlete's foot. It is therefore frequently necessary to obtain a microscopic examination of the skin scrapings (branching threads of mycelia crossing epithelial cells are seen in athlete's foot), and even a culture. Other conditions that should be considered include dermatitis from footwear and psoriasis, both conditions being symmetrical. A primary bacterial infection can also occur.

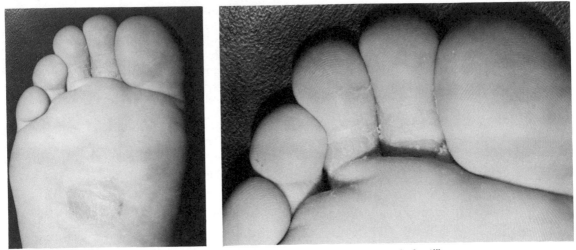

FIGURE 26.4   Tinea infection of the foot ("athlete's foot")

TREATMENT: The athlete should be instructed to carefully dry the skin between the toes and on the bottoms of the feet. Tinea pedis should be treated vigorously with an antifungal preparation such as tolnaftate (Tinactin) or clotrimazole (Lotrimin), the latter being effective against yeasts as well. These medications may be applied as creams or solutions. Occasionally oral treatment with griseofulvin is necessary.

Tinea versicolor.   Tinea versicolor is due to a mycelia, *Malassezia furfur.* It presents with brownish vesicles on white skins and as partly depigmented patches on pigmented skins. It is an innocent infection that does not seem to do harm, aside from causing skin pigment changes.

TREATMENT: Selenium sulfide (Selsun) is applied at night and washed off in the morning, and can be used three times. This usually effects a cure. Tolnaftate and clotrimazole can also be used.

"Jock itch."   Jock itch may be due to a fungal infection. Other causes include:

1. Accumulation of moisture in the groin area

2. Friction of athletic activity

3. Dermatitis caused by sensitivity to a material contained in the underwear

4. Dermatitis from sensitivity to a soap used to wash the underwear

Depending on the etiology, the problem can be treated with an antifungal, or, if the cause is not fungal, with a corticosteroid preparation.

Herpes Simplex Infection

The herpes simplex virus is divided into two types, type I occurring above the waist and type II occurring below the waist. The condition described here is usually due to the type I virus.

ETIOLOGY: Most people have been infected with herpes simplex virus before late adolescence. The virus enters nerve endings in the skin and travels through the peripheral nerves to the dorsal root ganglia, where it remains in its latent form. When the virus is re-activated, it travels down the peripheral nerve to the skin, producing the recurrent lesions which appear in about 25% of those who have been infected (but only about 7% have significant problems two or more times a year). Primary inoculation (or infection) by the herpes virus can keep occurring at different sites, from autotransmission or by contact, such as in wrestling.

In recurrent herpes, the virus travels from the dorsal root ganglia through the peripheral nerve, using an intracellular pathway that is protected from the body's immunological defense mechanisms. Recurrent herpes may be brought on by an elevation of body temperature, sunlight (ultraviolet light), or occasionally psychological conditions and tension.

INCIDENCE IN ATHLETES: Herpes simplex is a very common problem in wrestlers, occurring mainly from body-to-body contact rather than contact with the mat. For the same reasons, it is also found in rugby players, particularly in forwards. Skiers and mountain climbers, track athletes, and baseball players are likely to suffer repeated recurrent episodes when exposed to ultraviolet light.

CLINICAL COURSE:

1. *Prodromal* herpes consists of a group of symptoms such as itching, burning, or tingling in a given area before the eruption actually becomes visible. On rare occasions there may be symptoms but no lesions.

2. The *primary* infection most frequently occurs in young children, who present with ulcerated lesions in the mouth and on the tongue, as well as with cervical adenopathy, fever, and malaise. There have been reports of herpes pharyngitis in the college-age group; there are no skin signs, only a severely sore throat.

3. The *recurrent* disease first manifests with prodromal symptoms followed by a red spot (papule) which forms a blister (vesicle). After the hard vesicle breaks down, it is covered by a soft crust which later becomes hard. This process takes from five to fourteen days, depending on the size of the lesion. It is probably infectious for five days.

4. *Primary inoculation herpes* is the common type found in wrestlers. The vesicles are small and umbilicated and become pustular and crusted. They tend to form clusters of vesicles (as opposed to the recurrent disease where only one or two lesions occur), and are often mistaken for pyodermia, contact dermatitis, or herpes zoster. The diagnosis can be confirmed by isolation of the virus in tissue culture. Bacterial cultures should also be made, as there is often a secondary infection present.

The commonest areas involved in wrestlers are the cheek and the forehead, due to the lockup position which rubs the right side against the opponent's right side, but the inside of the arm may also be affected. In rugby players it is mainly the forehead and the scalp that are affected. Ultraviolet-induced recurrences in noncontact athletes occur on the face and the lips (Figure 26.5).

PREVENTION: The most important part of treating herpes simplex is prevention. Wrestlers must be removed from all contact activity as soon as they have become symptomatic (some authorities feel they should be removed as soon as the prodromal symptoms appear), and they should be kept out of contact for at least five days from the start of the eruption. Other members on the squad who were wrestling with the infected athlete should be observed daily for any signs of a

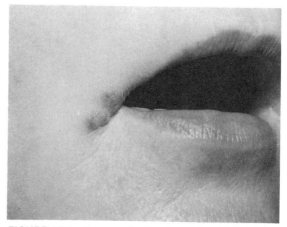

FIGURE 26.5 *Herpes simplex involving the corner of the mouth*

herpes lesion and, if this occurs, they too should be taken off all contact activities for five days.

Ultraviolet-induced herpes is prevented by application of a sunscreen to the lips, face, and other cutaneous areas that might be exposed. This sunscreen should contain para-aminobenzoic acid (PABA) and probably red veterinary petrolatum as well.

TREATMENT: An effective treatment has not been found. The athlete is advised to allow the lesion to dry and apply a "cold sore" solution or ether to encourage drying. It should be understood, however, that this will not cure the lesion or make it less infectious, but it may help hasten the course of the eruption. If the skin becomes dry when the crust develops, petroleum jelly can be used. Systemic and local antibiotics are indicated if a secondary bacterial infection is present.

Herpes Zoster

The virus that causes herpes zoster is the same as the chicken pox virus. It is thought that the condition is actually a reactivation of the chicken pox virus which has lain dormant in a sensory ganglion since the time of the primary infection.

SYMPTOMS AND SIGNS: Pain may be felt over the affected nerve root distribution, particularly the intercostal nerves, up to three days before the eruption occurs. Following the eruption, the regional lymph nodes become enlarged and tender. The rash follows a nerve root distribution—this is one of the characteristic features. The rash is initially a raised patch of erythema which becomes a cluster of umbilicated vesicles, and then may become purulent or hemorrhagic and eventually necrotic. In some cases the pain persists for a time after the rash has cleared. If the nasociliary branch or the ophthalmic branch of the temporal nerve is involved, a dangerous irritative conjunctivitis can occur in addition to scalp tenderness, headache, and enlarged lymph nodes.

TREATMENT: Treatment consists mainly of prevention of any secondary infections. In the case of nasociliary branch involvement, the athlete should be referred to an ophthalmologist. Athletes involved in direct contact, such as wrestlers, should avoid participation because they could infect those athletes who have not had chicken pox.

Impetigo

Impetigo is usually due to a staphylococcal infection. Some athletes are carriers of the bacteria, particularly in the nose, anus, and under the nails. It commonly infects blisters or damaged skin and is therefore prevalent in wrestlers. It may secondarily infect a herpes simplex or zoster area. The characteristic lesion, once seen, is easy to recognize. The skin beyond the lesion is typically normal. There may be an increase in the size of the regional lymph nodes.

PREVENTION: Carriers of staphylococci should be adequately treated with a topical antibiotic which is applied to the lesion and the nose. Oral antibiotics may be used if necessary. Wrestlers should shower before practice or participation with an antiseptic solution (Betadine or pHisoHex). Nails should be cut short and kept well cleaned. Wrestling mats should be washed daily with an antiseptic solution. All abrasions should be cleaned and treated with a topical antibiotic such as polymixin.

TREATMENT: A culture should be taken to identify the infecting organism and to determine to which antibiotic the organism is sensitive. Many staphylococci are resistant to various antibiotics, penicillins in particular.

Cellulitis

Cellulitis is generally due to a streptococcus. The initial lesion, often on the distal aspect of the limb, becomes painful and red. This may soon be followed by a red streak running up the limb. The regional lymph nodes then become swollen and painful.

TREATMENT: Antibiotics, usually penicillin or erythromycin, and a topical antibiotic are combined with rest and elevation of the limb until the infection is under control.

Urticaria

Urticaria is usually due to hypersensitivity, mainly from an allergy. It presents with itchy wheals and can develop into angioneurotic edema with respiratory and laryngeal distress.

TREATMENT: Initial treatment is with an antihistamine. If severe, adrenalin may have to be given subcutaneously or intravenously, and a corticosteroid injected intramuscularly.

Nonspecific Dermatitis

Nonspecific dermatitis is one of the most common causes of itchy skin in an athlete. The skin is dry and inflamed, particularly on the flexor aspects of the limbs. The usual cause is standing under hot showers for a long period of time or taking two or more showers a day, thus removing the natural oils from the skin and causing the itching and scaling.

TREATMENT: The treatment is to decrease the amount of soap and hot water used and to shower the minimal number of times a day possible. A moisturizing cream should be used after each shower or bath. If this does not work sufficiently, a hydrocortisone or corticosteroid preparation should be applied to the skin.

Infestations

Scabies. Scabies usually occurs as a result of close physical contact and is a very infectious condition. The scabies mite, *Sarcoptes scabiei*, burrows into the skin, usually between the fingers (60% of cases) or on the flexor aspect of the wrists, soles of the feet, or scrotum.

In a person with no previous infestation of scabies, the mite lies dormant for about one month. Dormancy is followed by development of an erythematous reaction around the burrow, and an itchy, papular, urticarial-like eruption appears, commonly on the forearms, axillae, inner thighs and buttocks, and around the ankles. Itching occurs when the athlete gets warm. The eruption is not found on the face or scalp in adults. Vesicles may appear on the hands and feet, and a secondary bacterial infection can develop.

DIAGNOSIS: Diagnosis should be made by finding the burrow on the hands, wrists, or feet (this is most easily achieved by using a magnifying glass).

TREATMENT: Gamma benzene hexachloride (Kwell) is the treatment of choice. The athlete should have a warm bath, then allow the skin to dry and cool, and apply the lotion over all body areas from the neck down. It should be left on for twelve hours, then removed by thorough washing. One application is usually all that is required. All clothing and bedding should also be thoroughly washed.

Pediculosis. Pubic lice are the most frequent form of pediculosis in the athlete, usually contracted by close sexual contact. The athlete presents with itching in the pubic area, nits are seen on the hair shafts, and secondary lymph node swelling is found. There may sometimes be a papular urticarial eruption on the trunk.

TREATMENT: The treatment for pediculosis pubis is to apply gamma benzene hexachloride (Kwell) to the hair and skin in the pubic region, the thighs, the trunk, and the axillary region. After twelve hours it is removed by thorough washing. Retreatment is usually not necessary, as long as the sexual contact is treated at the same time. All clothing or linen in contact with the affected person should be washed in hot water or else not worn or used for at least two weeks.

DRUGS AND MEDICATIONS COMMONLY USED IN ATHLETICS

The trainer should be aware of some of the details of the medications that are commonly used in an athletic environment. In particular, the anti-inflammatory medications should be carefully studied. However, the trainer is not in a position to dispense drugs unless there is a clearly written order from the physician which expressly permits him or her to do so. Under no other circumstances can the trainer dispense or advise the athlete on drug therapy.

Anti-Inflammatory Medications

Aspirin. In spite of many new preparations on the market, aspirin still has a definite place in sports medicine because of its predictable effectiveness and relatively mild side effects. It is still the basic standby because of its actions as

1. an analgesic (pain killer)

2. a mild anti-inflammatory agent

3. an antipyretic (helps to control a fever)

As an *analgesic* it is used in a dosage of two tablets (325 mg per tablet) every four to six hours. As an *anti-inflammatory* agent it has a mild but definite action if taken in a dose of two or three tablets four times a day over a period of a week or more. Aspirin can be taken before participation by athletes with overuse inflammatory lesions such as patellar tendinitis or tennis elbow. These athletes should take two or three aspirin a half hour to one hour before participation.

Some investigators feel aspirin may help stimulate regeneration of articular cartilage, particularly in those with chondromalacia of the patella, though this is still controversial.[19]

SIDE EFFECTS: The main side effects of aspirin are related to

1. the gastrointestinal tract, where gastric irritation and bleeding can be precipitated. This hazard is reduced by taking the aspirin with milk, in a buffered form (e.g., with an antacid), or in the "enteric coated" form so that it passes through the stomach into the small intestine before being released. Aspirin should not be taken with alcohol or other stomach irritants.

2. vestibular effects—tinnitus (buzzing in the ears) is a sign of aspirin intoxication, and means the dosage should be reduced.

3. hypersensitivity reactions, such as the development of bronchospasm, following ingestion.

Nonsteroidal Anti-inflammatory Agents

There are a number of nonsteroidal anti-inflammatory agents that are essentially similar in efficacy. However, a particular athlete may find one drug more effective than another and so some of these can be used in turn on a trial basis.

Ibuprofen (Motrin). Ibuprofen is a nonsteroidal anti-inflammatory agent which possesses analgesic and antipyretic properties. The usual dosage in athletes is 800 mg three times a day. It is thought to be as effective (or perhaps slightly more effective) than aspirin and is better tolerated by some people.

SIDE EFFECTS: Gastrointestinal side effects do occur, particularly nausea, and occasionally epigastric pain or diarrhea. These are relieved to some extent by combining the drug with meals, milk, or antacids. Dizziness and headache occasionally occur, as does tinnitus. On the whole, however, side effects are relatively infrequent. Other drugs include fenoprofen calcium (Nalfon), naproxen (Naprosyn), sulindac (Clinoril), and tolmetin sodium (Tolectin). *Note*: All these may produce gastrointestinal irritation and bleeding.

Phenylbutazone (Butazolidin) and oxyphenbutazone (Tandearil). Phenylbutazone and oxyphenbutazone are two drugs very similar in their structure, actions, and side effects. They are probably the most powerful nonsteroidal anti-inflammatory agents available today, but as they have the most serious side effects they should always be used with a great deal of caution. They have been on the market for many years and, though potentially hazardous drugs, they may be used if thoroughly understood.[20]

DOSAGE: A number of dosage schedules have been suggested for the athlete. For instance, phenylbutazone (Butazolidin or Butazolidin alka) can be used for seven days starting with

200 mg 4 times a day the first day (totals 800 mg)

200 mg 3 times a day the second day (totals 600 mg)

500 mg on the third and fourth days

400 mg on the fifth and sixth days

300 mg on the seventh day

The medication should always be taken at the end of a meal to avoid gastric irritation. Alternatively, 200 mg 3 times a day for 3 days and then 100 mg 3 times a day for 2 or 3 days can be used. Oxyphenbutazone (Tandearil) is most frequently used in the dosage of 200 mg 3 times a day, always taken after meals. These drugs are usually used for three to seven days at a time, but occasionally can be used for up to two weeks, certainly not longer. The three-to-seven-day course should not be administered more than two or three times during a season; the fourteen-day course only once.

SIDE EFFECTS: The most frequent side effect is related to the gastrointestinal tract, where dyspepsia, nausea, and occasionally intestinal bleeding occur. Phenylbutazone in its buffered form (Butazolidin alka) may cause less gastric irritation than without buffering; oxyphenbutazone may have a slightly lower incidence of gastrointestinal side effects but is quite likely to produce such problems if the drug is not taken at the end of the meal. Edema can occur, particularly in a woman just before her menstrual cycle.

The most significant and potentially lethal side effects relate to depression of the blood-forming tissues, resulting in agranulocytosis or aplastic anemia. These serious side effects, which have brought the phenylbutazones into ill repute, are usually but not always dose-related.

PRECAUTIONS: Phenylbutazone and oxyphenbutazone should be prescribed only after considerable thought, and the following precautions should be adhered to:

1. They should not be given to any athlete with a history of dyspepsia, peptic ulcer, or gastric bleeding.

2. The usual course of these tablets should be from three to seven days; at no time should a course of longer than two weeks be given. The number of courses given in a season should be limited.

3. The tablets should always be taken at the end of a meal with milk; they should not be taken with black coffee or alcohol or on an empty stomach.

4. If more than two courses of these anti-inflammatory agents need to be given in a season, a full blood count should be performed and the athlete should be monitored at regular intervals.

Corticosteroids

Corticosteroids are frequently used in sports medicine, but their place needs to be carefully understood. The most commonly used form is the intralesional injection. Occasionally oral or intramuscular cortisone is used, but this is exceptional. Corticosteroids are very powerful anti-inflammatory agents. However, they also have a number of serious side effects which limit their use, including

1. suppression of the adrenal glands

2. precipitation of diabetes

3. thinning of bones (osteoporosis)

4. development of glaucoma

5. mental and psychological changes.

A number of other side effects can occur if the drug is used for a longer period of time.

Intralesional corticosteroids. The injection of corticosteroids into a particular area of inflammation is very helpful in many of the injuries sustained by athletes. However, this type of administration still has potential *side effects* that are relevant to the athlete.

1. If cortisone is injected into a tendon or ligament, the structure will be weakened for at least two to six weeks.[21,22,23,24] If athletic activity is continued, the weakened tendon or ligament can undergo complete rupture, particularly if the symptoms are masked by the cortisone.[25,26,27]

2. If cortisone is injected into a joint on a number of occasions (particularly into the knee joint) intra-articular degeneration and arthritis can develop.[28,29,30]

Corticosteroid injections should thus be used with great discretion. There are a number of anatomical sites where their use is very advantageous and side effects are minimal, including:

1. Shoulder pointer (e.g., contusion of the distal clavicle and acromion process)

2. Hip pointer (e.g., contusion of the iliac crest)

3. Morton's neuroma of the foot

4. Plantar fasciitis and bursitis

5. Iliotibial tract friction syndrome

6. Tenosynovitis of the thumb extensor tendons

A number of other areas are frequently injected, but the use of cortisone in these areas is controversial.

Oral corticosteroids. These are seldom used in athletic medicine. If they are used, dosage should be limited to about five days, after which adrenal suppression may occur.

Intramuscular corticosteroids. Experiments are being conducted using intramuscular corticosteroids away from the site of injury to try to effect a more rapid decrease in inflammation following an injury. Results are uncertain at this time, though the preliminary reports are favorable.[31] The possibility of side effects still needs to be considered.

Analgesics

Acetaminophen (Tylenol). Acetaminophen is similar to aspirin in terms of analgesia but has *no* anti-inflammatory effects. It is therefore used purely as a mild pain-killer. The usual dosage is two tablets every four to six hours.

SIDE EFFECTS: With a dosage of two tablets every four to six hours there are relatively few side effects, though occasional liver and other problems have been reported.

Propoxyphene (Darvon). Propoxyphene is an analgesic with no anti-inflammatory action. It has been shown to be little more effective than aspirin and therefore probably does not need to be prescribed, particularly in view of the danger of death resulting from overdosage or when taken concurrently with alcohol.

Aspirin or acetaminophen (Tylenol) with codeine. Codeine is a narcotic analgesic that is used in combination with aspirin or acetaminophen for severe pain, for instance, after a fracture.

SIDE EFFECTS: Mainly drowsiness, nausea, and vomiting. Codeine has addictive properties.

Other Medications

Pseudoephedrine hydrochloride (e.g., Sudafed). This vasoconstrictor is useful for dealing with the symptoms of an upper respiratory infection and rhinitis. The advantage for athletes is that pseudoephedrine does not cause drowsiness, which is the main problem with most "cold medications" containing an antihistamine.

SIDE EFFECTS: Pseudoephedrine does have some side effects, however, including stimulation, which might produce hyperactivity and insomnia in sensitive athletes or if too high a dosage is taken. It should be used with caution if there is a tendency toward hypertension.

Diphenoxylate hydrochloride with atropine sulfate (Lomotil). Diphenoxylate hydrochloride is an antidiarrheal agent that contains a morphine-like derivative as its main constituent, together with atropine, and is usually effective in treating the nonspecific gastrointestinal upset that plagues many a traveling athlete. However, because of the atropine content, some athletes may have difficulty with visual focusing and mouth dryness. The usual dosage is two tablets four times a day for the adult; it should be used cautiously in children, as serious side effects can occur.

Topical antibiotics. Those using topical antibiotics should be aware of potential dangers and side effects. The most frequent side effect is hypersensitivity, which is particularly common following the administration of neomycin, though other topical antibiotics are not immune. One of the safer ones is polymyxin (Polysporin).

Antinausea agents. Severe nausea and even vomiting are frequent pre-event occurrences. Most anti-emetic drugs have side effects such as drowsiness and are therefore contra-indicated before participation. A preparation that has been found useful in such situations is Emetrol, which is an oral solution containing fructose, glucose, and orthophosphoric acid. This has a local action on the wall of the hyperactive gastrointestinal tract and reduces smooth muscle contraction. It should be taken undiluted and with no other fluid for at least 15 minutes afterwards. It helps settle the anxious athlete's stomach without side effects.

ANABOLIC STEROIDS

The widespread use of anabolic steroids by athletes was first reported in the late 1950s and the early 1960s. Since that time, they have been used by athletes in an effort to gain an advantage from the steroids' supposed strength- and bulk-producing properties.

At the present time, these drugs are banned by the International Olympic Committee and most national governing bodies, and so a highly controversial and volatile situation exists in which many athletes maintain that they cannot compete effectively against athletes from other countries who are taking the anabolic steroids unless they themselves take the drug. It is also rumored that the dosage being taken by some of the weight-athletes, such as the hammer and discus throwers and the shot putters, has continued to increase in order to keep pace with the higher standards. To enforce its ban on anabolic steroids, the International Olympic Committee has instituted highly sophisticated and expensive biochemical tests to detect steroid users.[31,32,33]

Scientific studies that have evaluated the strength-producing properties of anabolic steroids have resulted in conflicting reports. Most of the investigations published show an increase in body weight after the athlete has taken the steroids for some time, which appears to be lean body mass or fluid retention as opposed to deposition of fat. Several studies (see Table 26.3) have shown an increase in strength, particularly when the athletes have trained maximally at the same time as taking the drug and have eaten a high protein diet.[35,36,37,45]

However, these studies have been decried for their lack of adequate double-blind control and for other technical reasons.[48,49] Many well-controlled trials have failed to reveal a gain of strength (see Table 26.4) This lack of satisfactory documentation of effects that are vigorously believed by the athletes to be present may be due to these trials not having been carried out on fully

TABLE 26.3 Studies Claiming Improvement in Strength after Administration of Anabolic Steroids to Male Athletes

Steinbach[34]	1968
Johnson and O'Shea[35]	1969
O'Shea[36]	1971
Bowers and Reardon[37]	1972
Johnson et al.[38]	1972
Ariel and Saville[39]	1972
Ariel[40]	1972
Ariel[41]	1973
Ariel[42]	1973
Ward[43]	1973
Berg and Keul[44]	1974
Stamford and Moffatt[45]	1974
Win-May and Mya-Tu[46]	1975
Freed et al.[47]	1975

trained athletes at the peak of their fitness when performing intense training and ingesting a high protein diet. On the other hand, there may just be no strength-gaining effect.

In addition, since the use of anabolic steroids is against the rules of most organizations, any scientific work carried out on these athletes is unlikely to be published in the scientific literature. It is probably for these same reasons that very few harmful ef-

TABLE 26.4 Studies Showing No Improvement in Strength after Administration of Anabolic Steroids to Male Athletes

Fowler et al.[50]	1965
Weiss and Muller[51]	1968
Munson[52]	1970
O'Shea and Winkler[53]	1970
Casner et al.[54]	1971
Fahey and Brown[55]	1973
Golding et al.[56]	1974
Stromme[57]	1974
Hervey[58]	1975
Johnson et al.[59]	1975
Keul et al.[60]	1976
Hervey et al.[61]	1976
Loughton and Ruehling[62]	1977

fects have been recorded in the medical press. Many authorities have warned about the potentially harmful action of anabolic steroids, particularly since there is a close clinical relationship to testosterone and other androgenic agents, although the anabolic steroids in current use have a high anabolic activity relative to the androgenic activity, which may potentially lessen some of the side effects. However, they may stimulate precocious puberty and premature closure of the epiphyses in adolescents, cause reduced testicular function, be responsible for various liver abnormalities including liver cancer and cyst formation, and possibly precipitate diabetes.[79-63]

In the studies reported in the literature, anabolic steroids appear to have caused few, if any, lasting side effects in the male athlete. Changes in liver function, as demonstrated by a rise in the SGOT and LDH levels, and side effects such as increased blood pressure, headache, nausea, reduced sexual interest, and acne have been published. These effects seem to disappear in the male after discontinuing the drug. It should be noted, however, that female athletes do definitely develop side effects which may be long-lasting (see Chapter 23).[63]

The present-day concern is also related to the large doses reportedly used by some athletes and also to the length of time these athletes continue taking the steroids. Even with these high doses, there is *as yet* little documented evidence of long-term problems developing in male athletes. Certainly, athletes continue taking the drug even though it is barred for international competition and even though the medical profession has pointed out on numerous occasions the potential dangers to health.[48,49,63]

It appears that athletes will continue to use these medications until even more definite clinical evidence of health hazards is produced, or until there is an adoption of higher ethical standards by both the athlete and his or her coach.[49] The question is— should athletes continue to take the drug subversively, possibly in violation of the doctrine of sportsmanship (supposing that the strength gain is actually achieved), or should they be allowed to take it under medical guidance and supervision?

The trainer is caught in the middle of this controversy and may need to educate athletes as to the potential dangers and lack of adequate documentation of strength gains. The moral and ethical questions should also be openly discussed.

REFERENCES

1. Morse LJ, Bryan JA, Hurley JP, et al: The Holy Cross College football team hepatitis outbreak. *JAMA* 219:706–708, 1972.

2. Bowman JF: Infectious hepatitis in a college football player. *Am J Sports Med* 4:101–106, 1976.

3. de Shazo WF: Returning to athletic activity after infectious mononucleosis. *Phys Sportsmed* 8:71–72, December 1980.

4. Ryan AJ: Moderator Round Table on Proteinuria in the athlete. *Phys Sportsmed* 6:45–55, July 1978.

5. Bailey RR, Dann E, Gillies AH, et al: What the urine contains following athletic competition. *NZ Med J* 83:309–313, 1976.

6. Castenfors J: Renal clearance and urinary sodium and potassium excretion during supine exercise in normal subjects. *Acta Physio Scand* 70:207–214, 1967.

7. Anderson RE: The significance of proteinuria in athletes. *J Sports Med* 3:133–135, 1975.

8. Siegel AJ, Hennekens CH, Solomon HS, et al: Exercise-related hematuria: Findings in a group of marathon runners. *JAMA* 241:391–392, 1979.

9. Blacklock NJ: Bladder trauma in the long distance runner. *Am J Sports Med* 7:239–241, 1979.

10. Hoover DL, Cromie WJ: Theory and management of exercise-related hematuria. *Phys Sportsmed* 9:90–95, November 1981.

11. Schiff HB, MacSearraigh ET, Kallmeyer JC: Myoglobinuria, rhabdomyolysis and marathon running. *Quart J Med* 47:463–472, 1978.

12. Demos MA, Gitin EL: Acute Exertional Rhabdomyolysis. *Arch Intern Med* 133:233–239, 1974.

13. McCurdy PR: Moderator Round Table: Should sickle cell trait ban sports participation? *Phys Sportsmed* 4:58–65, January 1976.

14. Burton RM: Case report: Exercise induced asthma in cold weather. *Phys Sportsmed* 9:131–132, September 1981.

15. Godfrey S: Exercise-induced asthma—Clinical, physiological and therapeutic implications. *J Allergy Clin Immunol* 56:1–17, 1975.

16. Fitch KD: Exercise-induced asthma and competitive athletics. *Pediatrics* 56:942–943, 1975.

17. Brenner AM, Weiser PC, Krogh LA, et al: Effectiveness of a portable face mask in attenuating exercise-induced asthma. *JAMA* 244:2196–2198, 1980.

18. Godfrey S, König P: Suppression of exercise-induced asthma by salbutamol, theophylline, atropine, cromolyn, and placebo in a group of asthmatic children. *Pediatrics* 56:930–934, 1975.

19. Chrisman OD, Snook GA, Wilson TC: The protective effect of aspirin against degeneration of human articular cartilage. *Clin Orthop* 84:193–196, 1972.

20. Black HM, Cox JS, Straugh WR: Use of phenylbutazone in sports medicine: Understanding the risks. *Am J Sports Med* 8:270–273, 1980.

21. Kennedy JC, Baxter Willis R: The effects of local steroid injections on tendons. A biomechanical and microscopic correlative study. *Am J Sports Med* 4:11–21, 1976.

22. Unverferth LJ, Olix ML: The effect of local steroid injection on tendon. *J Sports Med* 1:31–37, 1973.

23. Kretzler Jr, HH: Tendons and cortisone. AMA, *Med Aspects Sport* 16:31–33, 1974.

24. Matthews LS, Sonstegard DA, Phelps DB: A biomechanical study of rabbit patellar tendon: Effects of steroid injection. *J Sports Med* 2:349–357, 1974.

25. Melmed EP: Spontaneous bilateral rupture of the calcaneal tendon during steroid therapy. *J Bone Joint Surg* 47B:104–105, 1965.

26. Ismail AM, Balakrishnan R, Rajakumar MK: Rupture of the patella ligament after steroid infiltration. Report of a case. *J Bone Joint Surg* 51B:503–505, 1969.

27. Lee HB: Avulsion and rupture of the tendocalcaneus after injection of hydrocortisone. *Brit Med J* 2:395, 1957.

28. Bentley G, Goodfellow JW: Disorganization of the knees following intra-articular hydrocortisone injections. *J Bone Joint Surg* 51B:498–502, 1979.

29. Salter RB, Gross A, Hall JH: Hydrocortisone arthropathy: an experimental investigation. *Can Med Ass J* 97:374–377, 1967.

30. Ishikawa K: A study of deleterious effect of intra-articular corticosteroids on knee joint. II. The factors of joint impairments. *J Japanese Orthop Assoc* 52:1761–1781, 1978.

31. Brooks RV, Firth RG, Sumner NA: Detection of anabolic steroids by radioimmunoassay. *Brit J Sports Med* 9:89–92, 1975.

32. Pop T, Dragan I, Uta I, Petou, E: A new modern method of making evident anabolic steroids in the urine of high performance sportsmen. *Med Sport (Turin)* 29:10–12, 1976.

33. Ward RJ, Shackleton CHL, Lawson AM: Gas chromatographic-mass spectrometric methods for the detection and identification of anabolic steroid drugs. *Br J Sports Med* 9:93–97, 1975.

34. Steinbach M: Über den Einfluss anaboler Wirkstoffe auf Körpergewicht Muskelkraft und Muskeltraining. *Sportarzt Sportmed.* 11:485–492, 1968.

35. Johnson LC, O'Shea JP: Anabolic steroid: effects on strength development. *Science* 164:957–959, 1969.

36. O'Shea JP: The effects of an anabolic steroid on dynamic strength levels of weight lifters. *Nutr Rep Int* 4:363–370, 1971.

37. Bowers R, Reardon J: Effects of methandrostenolone (Dianabol) on strength development and aerobic capacity. *Med Sci. Sports* 4:54, 1972.

38. Johnson LC, Fisher G, Silvester LJ, Hofheins CC: Anabolic steroid: effects on strength, body weight, O_2 uptake and spermatogenesis in mature males. *Med. Sci Sports* 4:43–45, 1972.

39. Ariel G, Saville W: Effect of anabolic steroids on reflex components. *J Appl Physiol* 32:795–797, 1972.

40. Ariel G: The effect of anabolic steroid (methandrostenolone) upon selected physiological parameters. *Athletic Training* 7:190–200, 1972.

41. Ariel G: The effect of anabolic steroid upon skeletal muscle contractile force. *J Sports Med Phys Fitness* 13:187–190, 1973.

42. Ariel G: The effect of anabolic steriod (methandrostenolone) upon the voluntary force of skeletal muscle. University of Massachusetts, 1973. Ph. D. thesis.

43. Ward P: The effect of an anabolic steroid on strength and lean body mass. *Med Sci Sports* 5:277–282, 1973.

44. Berg A, Keul J: Der Einfluss von anabolen Substanzen auf das Verhalten der freien Serumaminosäuren von Normalperson und Schwerathleten in Ruhe und bei Korperarbeit. *Oesterr Z Sportsmed* 4:11–18, 1974.

45. Stanford BA, Moffat R: Anabolic steriod: effectiveness as an ergogenic aid to experienced weight trainers. *J Sports Med Phys Fitness* 14:191–197, 1974.

46. Win-May M, Mya-Tu M: The effect of anabolic steroids on physical fitness. *J Sports Med Phys Fitness* 15:266–271, 1975.

47. Freed DLJ, Banks AJ, Longson D, Burley DM: Anabolic steriods in athletics: cross-over double blind trial on weightlifters. *Br Med J* 2:471–473, 1975.

48. Ryan AJ: "Athletics" in *Handbook of Experimental Pharmacology.* Ed. Born GVR et al. Heidelberg, Springer-Verlag, 1976.

49. Ryan AJ: Anabolic steroids are fools' gold. *Federation Proceedings* 40:12, 0038–0044, 1981.

50. Fowler WM. Jr, Gardner GW, Egstrom GH: Effect of an anabolic steriod on the physical performance of young men. *J Appl Physiol* 20:1038–1040, 1965.

51. Weiss V, Muller H: Zur Frage der Beeinflüssung des Kraftstrainings durch anabole Hormone. *Schweiz Z Sportmed* 6:79–89, 1968.

52. Munson AR: Some effects of anabolic steroids during weight training. Los Angeles, University of Southern California, 1970. Ed.D. thesis.

53. O'Shea JP, Winkler W: Biochemical and physical effects of an anabolic steroid in competitive swimmers and weight lifters. *Nutr Rep Int* 2:351–362, 1970.

54. Casner S, Early R, Carlson BR: Anabolic steroid effects on body composition in normal young men. *J Sports Med Phys Fitness* 11:98–103, 1971.

55. Fahey TD, Brown CH: The effects of an anabolic steroid on the strength, body composition and endurance of college males when accompanied by a weight training program. *Med Sci Sports* 5:272–276, 1973.

56. Golding LA, Freydinger JE, Fishel SS: Weight, size and strength—unchanged by steroids. *Physician Sportsmed* 2:39–45, 1974.

57. Stromme SB, Meen HD, Aakvaag A: Effects of an androgenic-anabolic steroid on strength development and plasma testosterone levels in normal males. *Med Sci Sports* 6:203–208, 1974.

58. Hervey GR: Are athletes wrong about anabolic steroids? *Br J Sports Med* 9:74–77, 1975.

59. Johnson LC, Roundy ES, Allsen PE, et al: Effect of anabolic steroid treatment on endurance. *Med Sci Sports* 7:287–289, 1975.

60. Keul J, Deus B, Kindermann W: Anabole Hormone: Schädigung, Leistungsfähigkeit und Stoffwechsel. *Med Klin* 71:497–503, 1976 (Engl. abstr.).

61. Hervy GR, Hutchinson I, Knibbs AV, et al: Anabolic effects of methandienone in men undergoing athletic training. *Lancet* 2:699–702, 1976.

62. Loughton SJ, Ruhling RO: Human strength and endurance responses to anabolic steroid and training. *J Sports Med Phys Fitness* 17:285–296, 1977.

63. American College of Sports Medicine: Position statement on "The Use and Abuse of Anabolic–Androgenic Steroids in Sports," 1977.

64. Bagheri SA, Boyer JL: Peliosis hepatis associated with androgenic-anabolic steroid therapy. *Ann Int Med* 81:610–618, 1974.

65. Bernstein MS, Hunter RL, Yachmin S: Hepatoma and peliosis hepatis developing in a patient with Fanconi's anemia. *N Engl J Med* 284:1135–1136, 1971.

66. Burger RA, Marcuse PM: Peliosis hepatis, report of a case. *Am J Clin Pathol* 22:569–573, 1952.

67. Falk H, Thomas LB, Popper H, Isaak KG: Hepatic angiosarcoma associated with androgenic-anabolic steroids. *Lancet.* 2:1120–1122, 1979.

68. Farrell GC, Joshua EE, Uren RF, et al: Androgen-induced hepatoma. *Lancet* 1:430–431, 1975.

69. Guy, JT, Auslander MO: Androgenic steroids and hepato-cellular carcinoma. *Lancet* 1:148, 1973.

70. Henderson JT, Richmond J, Sumering MD: Androgenic-anabolic steroid therapy and hepato-cellular carcinoma. *Lancet* 1:934, 1972.

71. Johnson FL, Feagler JR, Lerner KG, et al: Association of androgenic-anabolic steroid therapy with development of hepatocellular carcinoma. *Lancet* 2:1273–1276, 1972.

72. Kintzen W, Silny J: Peliosis hepatis after administration of fluoxymesterone. *Can Med Assoc J* 83:860–862, 1960.

73. McDonald EC, Speicher CE: Peliosis hepatis associated with administration of oxymetholone. *J Am Med Assoc* 240:243–244, 1978.

74. Meadows AT, Naiman JL, Valdes-Dapena MV: Hepatoma associated with androgen therapy for aplastic anemia. *J Pediatr* 84:109–110, 1974.

75. Nadell J, Kosek J: Peliosis hepatis. *Arch Pathol Lab Med* 101:405–410, 1977.

76. Prat J, Gray GF, Stolley PD, Coleman JW: Wilm's tumor in an adult associated with androgen abuse. *J Am Med Assoc* 237:2322–2323, 1977.

77. Recant L, Lacy P, eds: Fanconi's anemia and hepatic cirrhosis. *Clin Conf Am J Med* 39:464–475, 1965.

78. Usatin MS, Wigger HJ: Peliosis hepatis in a child. *Arch Pathol Lab Med* 100:419–421, 1976.

79. Ziegenfuss J, Carabasi R: Androgens and hepatocellular carcinoma. *Lancet* 1:262, 1973.

RECOMMENDED READINGS

Busse WW: Exercise-induced asthma. Clinical symposium. *Am J Sports Med* 9:194–196, 1981.

Lucking MT: Steroid hormones in sports, Paper presented at the International Conference on Sports Medicine, Utrecht, The Netherlands, 23–26 March 1981.

McFadden ER, Ingram RH: Exercise-induced asthma. *New Eng J Med* 301:763–769, 1980.

Maki DG, Reich RM: Infectious mononucleosis in the athlete. Diagnosis, complications, and management. *Am J Sports Med* 10:162–173, 1982.

Mitchell SC, Blount SG, Blumenthal S, et al: The pediatrician and hypertension. *Pediatrics* 56:3–5, 1975.

Prokop L: Drug abuse in international athletics. *J Sports Med* 3:85–87, 1975.

Rassner G: *Atlas of Dermatology.* Edited by Kahn G. Baltimore, Urban and Schwarzenberg, 1978.

Ryan AJ: Editorial on sickle cell trait and sports. *Phys Sportsmed* 4:76, January 1976.

Saver GC: *Manual of Skin Diseases,* 4th Ed. New York, JB Lippincott, 1980.

APPENDIX

Training Room Forms

Release of Information—for Colleges and Universities (General)

RELEASE AND AUTHORIZATION

We are required to provide the _____ Conference and the NCAA with certain information for the purpose of determining eligibility, scholarships, awards, and other honors. Under _____ student records policy, we are unable to release information such as transcripts of courses and grades, entrance examination scores, and other information which is required by the _____ and NCAA without your written consent.

I, _____, hereby authorize _____ to release the following information to the Department of Intercollegiate Athletics:

   1. All information requested by the _____ Conference.

   2. All information requested by the NCAA.

I further authorize the _____ Department of Intercollegiate Athletics to release this information to the _____ Conference and the NCAA.

I have been informed of _____ student records policy and it is my intention that this release and authorization remain in full force and effect as long as I am a student at _____, or until I terminate this release and authorization in writing, whichever event occurs earlier.

_____   _____

Student-Athlete   *Date*

_____   _____

Witness   *Date*

Release of Medical Information—NATA-suggested Form

RELEASE OF INFORMATION AUTHORIZATION

I, _____, Do—Do Not, give my consent for the team physician, athletic trainers, or other medical personnel of _____, to
(name of school)

release such information regarding my medical history, record of injury or surgery, record of serious illness, and
rehabilitation results as may be requested by the scout or representative of any professional or amateur athletic organization seeking such information.

I understand that such scout or representative of the team has made representations to the team physician,
athletic trainer or other medical personnel of _____, that the
(name of school)

purpose of this request for my medical information is to assist the organization he or she represents in making
a determination as to offering me employment.

I understand that a record will be kept of all individuals requesting such information and the date of the request. This information is normally confidential and except as provided in this Release will not be otherwise released by the parties in charge of the information. This Release remains valid until revoked by me in writing.

Signed: _____ *Dated:* _____

Reprinted by permission of the National Athletic Trainers Association.

Release of Medical Information (*continued*)—NATA-suggested Log of Transaction

	Information Discussed
_____	_____
(*Name*)	_____
_____	_____
(*Organization*)	_____
_____	_____
(*Date*)	_____
_____	_____
(*Interview or telephone*)	_____

Reprinted by permission of the National Athletic Trainers Association.

Training Room Record

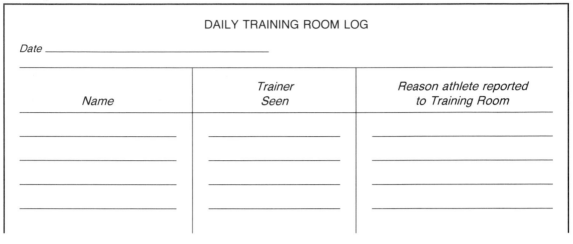

DAILY TRAINING ROOM LOG

Date _____

Name	Trainer Seen	Reason athlete reported to Training Room
_____	_____	_____
_____	_____	_____
_____	_____	_____
_____	_____	_____

Daily Injury Report to the Coach

DAILY INJURY LIST

Date _____

Name	Injury	Time Off
No practice		
Limited practice (specify)		
Minor injury—for information only		

Emergency Information (to be filled in at the start of participation by the athlete)

SPORTS MEDICINE

Name _____ Age _____

Address _____

Phone _____ SS# _____

Sport _____

List two persons to contact in case of emergency:

Name _____ Home Phone _____

Address _____ Work Phone _____

Relationship _____

Name _____ Home Phone _____

Address _____ Work Phone _____

Relationship _____

Insurance Co. _____ Policy No. _____

IMPORTANT

Are you allergic to any drugs? _____ If so, what? _____

Do you have any other allergies? (i.e. bee sting, dust) _____

Are you on any medication? _____ If so, what? _____

Do you wear contacts? _____

Other:

Signature _____ *Date* _____

Injury Record

REPORT OF INJURY

Name of athlete _____

Date _____

Time _____

Attending athletic trainer _____

Mechanism of injury _____

_____

_____

Type of injury _____

Anatomical area involved _____

Extent of injury _____

First aid administered: _____

_____

_____

Other treatment administered: _____

_____

Referral action: _____

_____

Athletic Trainer (*signature*)

Individual Cumulative Medical Record

SPORTS MEDICINE

Name: _____ SS# _____

Sport(s): _____

Tetanus toxoid: _____

Allergies: _____

Routine medication: _____

Previous injuries _____

_____

Chronic injuries: _____

Current Injury or Complaint	*Current Medication*
_____	_____
_____	_____
_____	_____
_____	_____

GLOSSARY

abduction   movement of the limb away from the midline of the body

actin   protein of the myofibril of the muscle; together with myosin is responsible for muscle contraction and relaxation

adduction   movement of the limb towards the midline of the body

anoxia   lack of oxygen

aortic stenosis   narrowing of the aortic orifice of the heart

aponeurosis   a tendinous expansion that helps to connect a number of muscles to bone

apophyseal injury   an injury involving the non-weight-bearing area of the growth plate (epiphyseal plate), to which a tendon is usually attached

arthrogram   an X-ray study in which radio-opaque material is injected into a joint

bursa   a sac-like cavity that allows a muscle or tendon to slide over bone

calorific value   the availability of calories to an individual according to his or her specific metabolic capability. It is that value which produces calories in an individual's metabolic conversion cycle.

chondromalacia   softening and destruction of articular cartilage

crepitus   a crackling sound or feeling sometimes found in fractures or tenosynovitis

cricothyroid cartilage   tissue connecting the cricoid and thyroid cartilages

ecchymosis   bleeding visible beneath the skin as a blue or purple patch

epiphyseal injury   an injury involving the growth plate (epiphyseal plate)

Frohlich type body   Frohlich syndrome is a condition in which there is a large amount of body fat together with lack of sexual development.

genu recurvatum   hyperextension of the knees

glycolytic enzyme   helps break down glycogen without oxygen

hemarthrosis   blood within a joint

hematocrit   volume (%) of erythrocytes (red blood cells) in whole blood

hemoglobin   the oxygen-carrying component of the red blood cells

isokinetic resistance   resistance varies; the speed is constant

isometric resistance   fixed resistance; no movement takes place

isotonic resistance   the resistance is constant; the speed of movement varies

Kager's triangle   a triangular space anterior to the Achilles tendon which is normally visible on X-ray as a radiolucent area

kinesiology   study of the motion of the human body

myopia   nearsightedness

myosin   protein of the myofibril of the muscle; together with actin is responsible for muscle contraction and relaxation

pinna   the external portion of the ear

podiatrist   specialist in podiatry; dealing with the study and care of the foot

pyelogram   an X-ray study in which radio-opaque dye is injected in order to outline the kidney, ureter and bladder

"Q" angle   the angle formed by a line drawn from the anterior superior iliac spine, to the mid-point of the patella and then to the tibial tubercle

retrograde amnesia   inability to recall events which occurred before a head injury

sprain   an injury to a ligament. The severity of the injury is graded by degree:

    first degree — minimal damage

    second degree — partial tearing of the ligament

    third degree — complete ligamentous disruption

strain   injury involving the muscle, tendon, or musculotendinis unit. classified into degrees of severity (*see* sprain)

subluxation   incomplete or partial dislocation of a joint

tenosynovitis   inflammation of a tendon sheath

valgus stress   a force that is applied to a joint in which the distal aspect of the limb is moved away from the midline

varus stress   a force that is applied to a joint in which the distal aspect of the limb is moved towards the midline

vascularization   the development of blood vessels within tissue

INDEX